Hepatic Radiography

Hepatic Radiography

Edited by

Michael E. Bernardino, M.D.
Professor of Radiology
Director, Abdominal Radiology
Emory University School of Medicine
Atlanta, Georgia

Peter J. Sones, Jr., M.D.
Clinical Professor of Radiology
Emory University School of Medicine
Atlanta, Georgia

MACMILLAN PUBLISHING COMPANY
NEW YORK

Collier Macmillan Canada, Inc.
TORONTO

Collier Macmillan Publishers
LONDON

Copyright © 1984, Macmillan Publishing Company, a division of Macmillan, Inc.

Printed in the United States of America

All rights reserved. No part of this book may be reproduced or transmitted in any form or by any means, electronic or mechanical, including photocopying, recording, or any information storage and retrieval system, without permission in writing from the Publisher.

Macmillan Publishing Company
866 Third Avenue, New York, New York 10022

Collier Macmillan Canada, Inc.
Collier Macmillan Publishers · London

Printing 1 2 3 4 5 6 7 8   Year: 4 5 6 7 8 9 0 1 2

Library of Congress Cataloging in Publication Data
Main entry under title:

Hepatic radiography.

  Includes bibliographies and index.
  1. Liver—Radiography. 2. Liver—Diseases—Diagnosis.
3. Diagnosis, Radioscopic. I. Bernardino, Michael E.
II. Sones, Peter J., 1937–   . [DNLM: 1. Liver—
radiography. WI 700 H5265]
RC846.H47   1984   616.3′620757   84-11295
ISBN 0-02-308650-5

Preface

The past several years have seen significant advances in diagnostic and interventional radiology. These advances have been particularly rewarding for the study of liver disease. Improved imaging and therapeutic procedures in oncology have generated changes in treatment protocols and in evaluating the results of therapy for hepatic malignancies. Our enriched understanding of the anatomic and hemodynamic aspects of the portal system has greatly benefited patients with portal hypertension. Now we are confidently more aggressive in our therapeutic approach to the variceal bleeder, and we have modified our approach to the preservation of portal flow following shunt.

All of the diagnostic modalities used to evaluate the liver are represented in this book. In its structure and organization this volume goes beyond a historical overview of imaging to present greater insight into the current state of the art, as well as possible future developments. Each chapter is designed to elucidate the advantages and weaknesses of the various diagnostic modalities. We have attempted to clarify the relationship of the various diagnostic modalities to the appropriate diagnostic approach in respect to the patient's particular clinical problem. Ideally, this book will serve as a reference source, allowing both radiologists and other clinicians to gain rapid access to diagnostic information.

The interventional approach to the liver is emphasized in recognition of its increasing impact on the practice of radiology. We firmly believe that to detect a lesion is not the only goal of the radiologist. Biopsy or drainage should be the next step in the hepatic examination. Many of the formerly undetected lesions (some are as small as half a centimeter)—now accessible to us through improved imaging techniques—are nonspecific in their appearance. A combination of the interventional approach and improved detection should give a histologic answer in the majority of cases. In consequence, the patient is better served because the cost of the procedure is significantly reduced, and increased benefits are reaped with minimal complications.

We should like to thank all the authors who have participated in this undertaking. Each was chosen for expertise in the area of his or her contribution. They have helped us to reach our goal of clarifying an optimal overall approach to radiology of the liver.

MICHAEL E. BERNARDINO
PETER J. SONES, JR.

Contributors

William A. Berkman, M.D.,
Assistant Professor of Radiology,
Department of Radiology,
Emory University School of Medicine,
Atlanta, Georgia

Michael E. Bernardino, M.D.,
Professor of Radiology and
Director of Abdominal Radiology,
Department of Radiology,
Emory University School of Medicine,
Atlanta, Georgia

David C. P. Chen, M.D.,
Assistant Professor of Radiology,
Division of Nuclear Medicine,
USC Medical Center,
Los Angeles, California

J. Luther Clements, Jr., M.D.,
Professor of Radiology,
Department of Radiology,
Emory University School of Medicine,
Atlanta, Georgia

William A. Fajman, M.D.,
Assistant Professor of Radiology,
Division of Nuclear Medicine,
Emory University School of Medicine,
Atlanta, Georgia

Michael P. Federle, M.D.,
Associate Professor of Radiology,
University of California, San Francisco
    General Hospital,
San Francisco, California

R. Kristina Gedgaudas-McClees, M.D.,
Associate Professor of Radiology,
Department of Radiology,
Emory University School of Medicine,
Atlanta, Georgia

Thomas L. Lawson, M.D.,
Professor of Radiology,
Department of Radiology,
Medical College of Wisconsin,
Milwaukee, Wisconsin

Errol Lewis, M.D.,
Assistant Professor of Radiology,
Department of Radiology,
M. D. Anderson Hospital,
Houston, Texas

Thomas W. Oliver, Jr., M.D.,
Fellow, Interventional Radiology,
Department of Radiology,
Emory University School of Medicine,
Atlanta, Georgia

Richard C. Reba, M.D.,
Professor of Radiology,
Division of Nuclear Medicine,
George Washington University
    Medical Center,
Washington, D.C.

James V. Rogers, Jr., M.D.,
Professor of Radiology,
Department of Radiology,
Emory University School of Medicine,
Atlanta, Georgia

Peter J. Sones, Jr., M.D.,
Clinical Professor of Radiology,
Department of Radiology,
Emory University School of Medicine,
Atlanta, Georgia

William E. Torres, M.D.,
Associate Professor of Radiology,
Department of Radiology,
Emory University School of Medicine,
Atlanta, Georgia

Arina van Breda, M.D.,
Attending Radiologist,
The Alexandria Hospital,
Alexandria, Virginia;
Assistant Clinical Professor of Radiology,
George Washington University Medical
    Center,
Washington, D.C.

Arthur C. Waltman, M.D.,
Professor of Radiology,
Department of Radiology,
Harvard Medical School,
Boston, Massachusetts

Contents

Preface — v

Contributors — vii

1. Plain Film Diagnosis of the Liver — 1
   James V. Rogers, Jr., William E. Torres, J. L. Clements, Jr., and R. Kristina Gedgaudas-McClees

2. Hepatic Scintigraphy — 50
   Richard C. Reba, David C. P. Chen, and William A. Fajman

3. Hepatic Sonography — 82
   William A. Berkman, Michael E. Bernardino, and Errol Lewis

4. Hepatic Computed Tomography — 109
   Michael E. Bernardino

5. Magnetic Resonance Imaging of the Liver — 146
   Thomas L. Lawson and Michael E. Bernardino

6. Radiographic Evaluation of Hepatic Trauma — 167
   Michael P. Federle

7. Hepatic Biopsies and Abscess Drainages — 197
   Michael E. Bernardino

8	Diagnostic Hepatic Angiography: Mass and Diffuse Disease *Arina van Breda and Arthur Waltman*	*214*
9	Hepatic Angiography: Portal Hypertension *Thomas W. Oliver, Jr. and Peter J. Sones, Jr.*	*243*
10	Vascular Interventional Techniques in Liver Disease *Peter J. Sones, Jr. and Thomas W. Oliver, Jr.*	*276*
	Index	*307*

Hepatic Radiography

1

Plain Film Diagnosis of the Liver

JAMES V. ROGERS, JR. • WILLIAM E. TORRES
J. L. CLEMENTS, JR. • R. KRISTINA GEDGAUDAS-McCLEES

INTRODUCTION

One of the first examinations obtained routinely in abdominal radiography is the plain radiograph of the abdomen. The liver occupies anywhere from 15 to 30 percent of the area on such examinations. Thus, it is important to pay particular attention to the region of the liver and obtain as much information as possible from these films.

The purpose of this chapter is to review the normal radiographic anatomy and pathology. Also, pathologic calcifications, gas collections, unusual collections of fat, and the systemic manifestations of hepatic disease are discussed within this chapter.

HEPATIC ANATOMY

Evaluation of the liver on abdominal plain films is usually difficult for the radiologist. Many physicians have problems in remembering gross anatomical facts pertaining to the liver—anatomic facts that have increased in importance with the advent of CT (computerized tomography) and ultrasound.

The liver, situated in the uppermost part of the right upper quadrant, is the largest solid organ in the human body, weighing between 1 and 2 kg in the adult. The liver, usually larger in the male than the female, measures approximately 10.0 to 12.5 cm in its anteroposterior dimension, 20.0 to 22.5 cm in its transverse diameter and 15.0 to 17.5 cm vertically. The largest portion fits under the right hemidiaphragm, while the smaller or thinner portion extends into the left subdiaphragmatic space. The majority of the superior aspect of the right lobe is situated below the right lung, except for a portion that is in contact with the anterior abdominal wall. The smaller left lobe lies beneath the heart and to a lesser extent below the left lung. The right and left lobes of the liver differ in size, with the right lobe approximately six times larger than the left (1–4).

The liver is divided into two lobes, right and left, each containing two segments. The main lobar fissure divides the liver into right and left lobes; this fissure is demarcated by a line drawn from the gallbladder fossa to the inferior vena cava (Figure 1–1). The right lobe is further divided into anterior and posterior segments by the right segmental fissure, while the left lobe is separated by the left segmental fissure into medial and lateral segments. The caudal portion of this last division, the falciform ligament, is easily seen on gross examination of the liver. It is the classic, but incorrect, idea of the dividing line between the right and left hepatic lobes. The quadrate lobe is a portion of the medial segment of the left lobe. The smaller caudate lobe is the posterior portion of the liver, which lies between the fissure of the ligamentum venosum and the fossa of the inferior vena cava (2,4–6) (Figure 1–2).

The liver has two surfaces, a diaphragmatic, or superior surface and a visceral, or inferior surface. The superior surface is seen as a smooth, convex structure conforming to the shape of the diaphragm, whereas the inferior surface is slightly concave, with ridges and indentations corresponding to adjacent organs; the right lobe comprises the major portion of the inferior surface. Grooves are present on the inferior surface of the liver for the underlying organs. Beginning on the right, grooves are present for the hepatic flexure of the colon, the right kidney, the adrenal gland, the first portion of the duodenum, the gallbladder, and to the left, the stomach (2,3) (Figure 1–3).

Considerable amounts of fat may be present adjacent to the liver, often interposing itself between the liver and adjacent organs. The more peripheral portions of the right lobe are adjacent to properitoneal fat, whereas the majority of the inferior aspect of the liver is in contact with retroperitoneal fat, especially around the right kidney. This relationship between the liver and surrounding fat is important and helpful in identifying liver borders (2,7).

On plain abdominal films, the liver is often defined by contiguous fat or by gas in adjacent bowel. The right lobe can be outlined laterally and often inferiorly by fat, except in asthenic individuals. Superiorly, the surface of the right lobe of the liver cannot be defined because of its confluence with the diaphragm and lack of fat, nor can the left lobe, which lies beneath the heart. Inferiorly, the border of the left lobe is at times

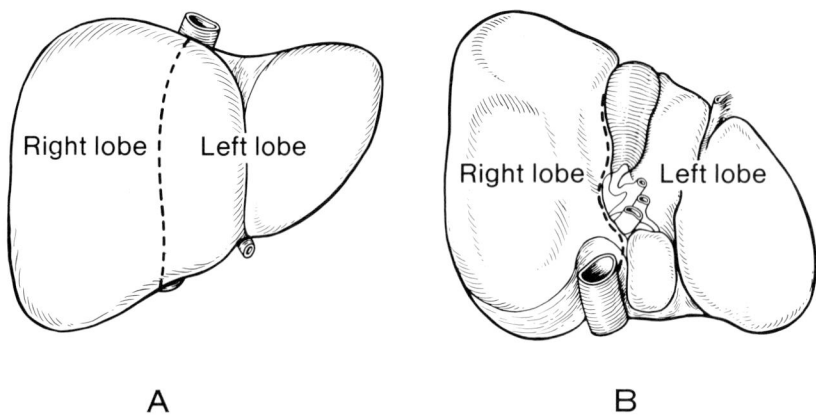

Figure 1–1. Anterior (*A*) and posterior (*B*) views of liver depicting division of right and left lobes by the main lobar fissure extending from the inferior vena cava to the gallbladder fossa.

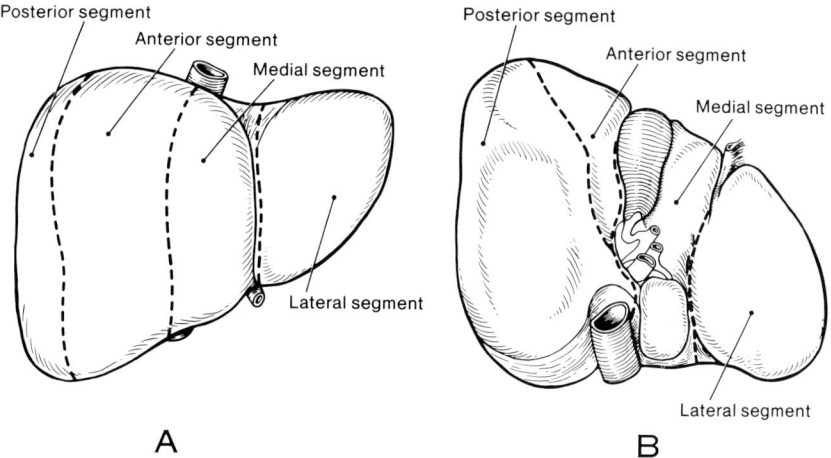

Figure 1-2. Anterior (*A*) and posterior (*B*) views of segmental anatomy of the liver showing anterior and posterior segments of the right lobe, and medial and lateral segments of the left lobe.

demarcated by the stomach air. The hepatic borders adjacent to or outlined by bowel are often a rough guide to liver size (2,7).

There is marked variation in the size and shape of the liver. McAfee *et al.* (8) divided normal variations in liver shape in the frontal projection into twelve patterns; the triangular configuration of the liver constituted about two thirds of normal livers without disease. It is not possible, however, to separate normal from abnormal livers on the basis of configuration alone. Because of its great regenerative ability, the shape of the liver can change following disease or vascular alterations (9).

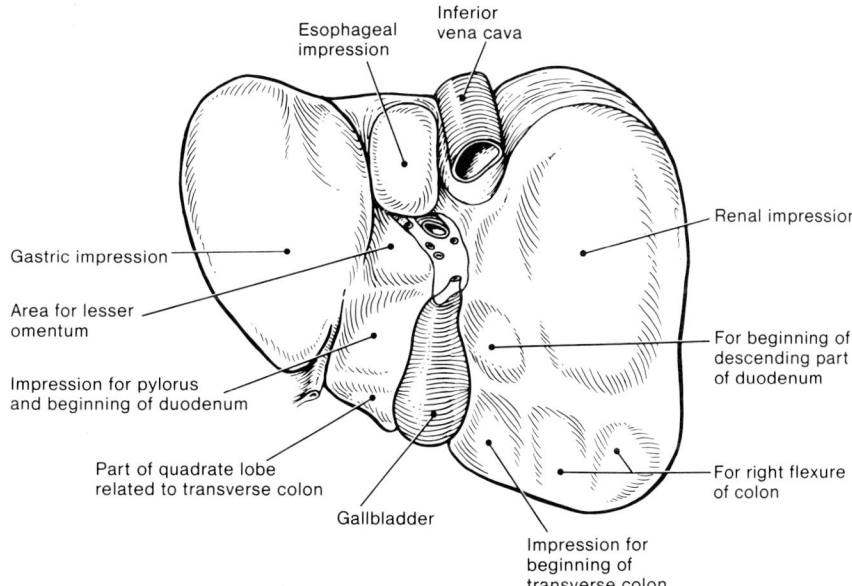

Figure 1-3. Various grooves on the inferior portion of the liver for the underlying organs.

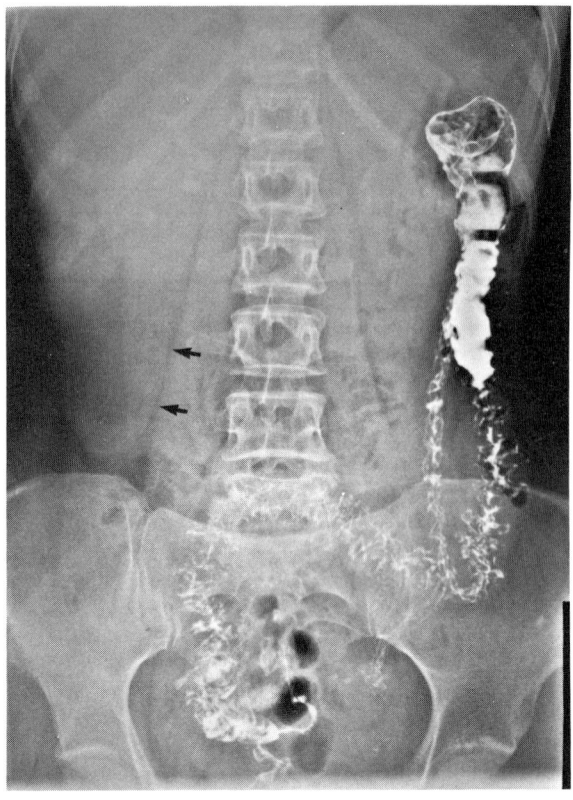 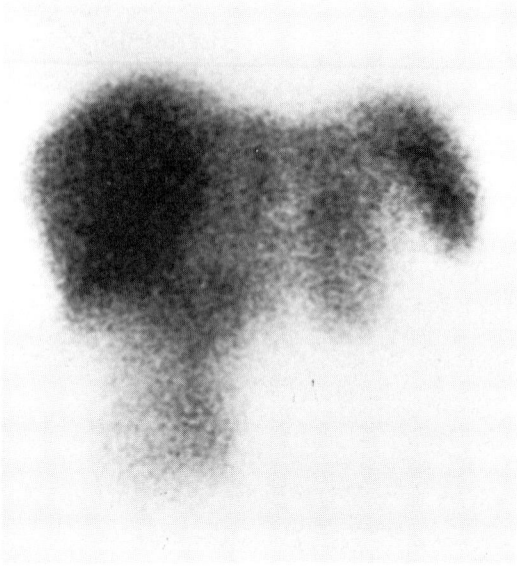

Figure 1-4. Riedel's lobe. *A.* Plain film of abdomen (arrows). *B.* Anterior view, radionuclide liver scan.

A variety of asymptomatic hepatic abnormalities of form or position can be produced. The clinical significance of these abnormalities lies in a differentiation from disease processes. With atrophy or aplasia of the left lobe, a rare occurrence, compensatory hypertrophy of the right lobe occurs. Complete absence of the left lobe is not an uncommon phenomenon. This allows the stomach and duodenum to rotate upward and to the right and can simulate a small liver, as seen in some patients with cirrhosis. Riedel's lobe is a tonguelike protrusion from the right lower lobe; in the past it was thought to be associated with intraabdominal disease (Figure 1-4). Other hepatic anomalies include the appendicular lobe, which displaces the stomach downward and to the left, and localized anomalous enlargements of normal lobes, which cause varying degrees of displacement of adjacent organs (1,2,4).

Since the borders of the liver are often difficult to visualize on radiographic examinations, organs adjacent to the liver play an important role in evaluating the liver for changes in size or contour. A complex relationship exists between the liver and some of the intraperitoneal and extraperitoneal organs. For changes in liver size to be seen on plain films, one must depend on displacement of adjacent organs and tissues, but these changes can be seen only if a difference in density is present between the liver and the adjacent structure. Even though the liver is an intraperitoneal organ, it can still displace retroperitoneal organs. The structures adjacent to the liver that can be recognized radiographically and that can be displaced by an enlarged liver are the gallbladder, kidney, stomach, duodenum, colon, diaphragm, and occasionally, the esophagus. Changes in liver size must be significant enough to produce displacement of the adjacent organs to be recognized on conventional radiographs (2,10).

The dome of the diaphragm, and therefore the upper margin of the liver in the supine position, is at the level of the ninth posterior rib at moderate inspiration. Gross degrees of hepatomegaly cause diaphragmatic elevation and restrict motion of the diaphragm. Conversely, a decrease in size of the liver does not cause depression of the diaphragm (4,10).

Hepatomegaly causes gastric displacement downward, posteriorly, and to the left (Figure 1–5). The left lobe of the liver, the most anterior structure in the left upper quadrant, will displace the stomach backward when there is a localized mass or hepatomegaly. Conversely, a shrunken liver can cause displacement of the stomach in the opposite direction; this is felt to be secondary to the "pull" on the stomach by the hepatogastric ligament or by a "vacuum mechanism." This kind of displacement without

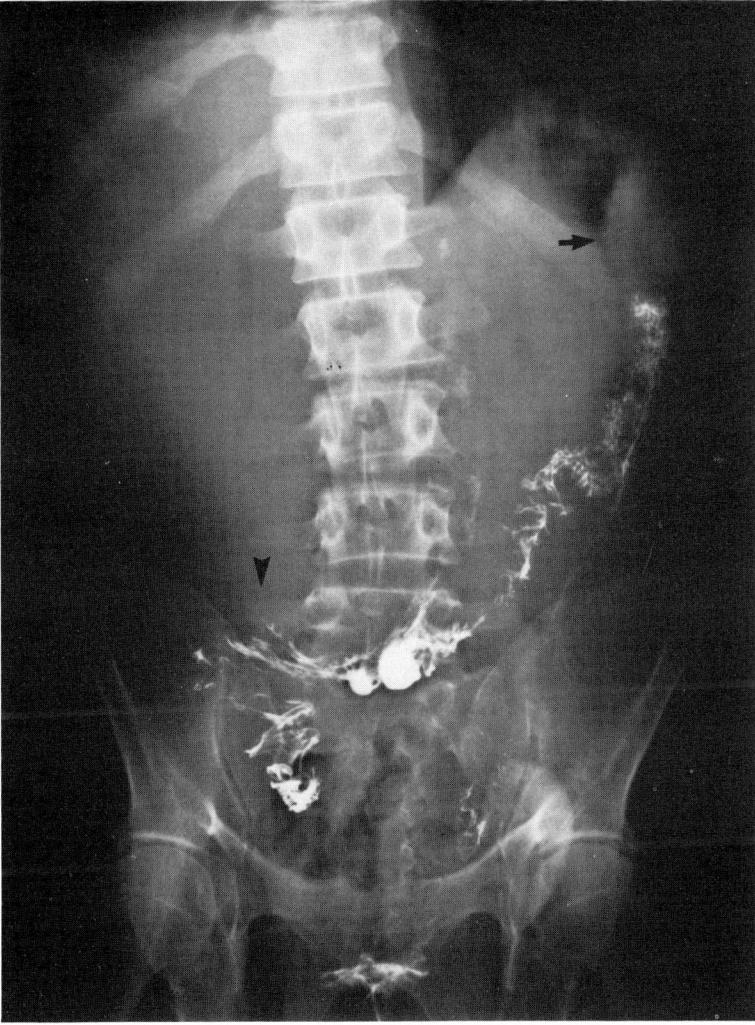

Figure 1–5. Elevation of hemidiaphragm, displacement of stomach to the left (arrow), and depression of colon by enlarged liver (arrowhead).

other known pathology, such as eventration of the right diaphragm, should raise the possibility of a cirrhotic liver (10–12).

Generalized enlargement of the liver causes the duodenum to be displaced downward and to the left. Since the spine is situated behind the duodenum, the duodenum is compressed instead of displaced backward. A more localized enlargement of the liver will cause the duodenum to be indented or displaced in the direction of growth (10,13).

Generalized hepatic enlargement displaces the transverse colon and the hepatic flexure downward and posteriorly (Figure 1–5). The displacement ends abruptly in the left upper quadrant where the colon is no longer related to the liver. Upward displacement of the colon, as well as other abdominal organs related to the liver, is noted when there is loss of hepatic volume, as seen in severe cases of cirrhosis. Chilaiditi's syndrome is an uncommon entity in which the right part of the transverse colon lies high in the abdomen above the shadow of the liver (10,14).

The gallbladder is closely related to the visceral surface of the right lobe of the liver. Hepatic enlargement will cause the gallbladder to be displaced downward and medially (10).

Hepatic masses cause the right kidney to be displaced in any direction except anteriorly or laterally, with downward displacement being the most common. There is usually concomitant rotation of the kidney with this downward displacement. This displacement should be distinguished from that caused by an enlarged suprarenal gland. The right kidney, instead of being displaced by the liver, can be compressed by a mass in the liver and, therefore, give a wider appearance on the anterior-posterior (AP) view. A decrease in the size of the liver may cause upward displacement of the kidney (10,14).

CALCIFICATIONS IN THE LIVER

Although more than forty causes of hepatic calcification have been reported (4), intrahepatic calcification is extremely unusual, other than the calcified granulomas from a previous tuberculous or histoplasmosis infection, or the calcification associated with an echinococcus infestation. Fewer than three hundred instances of radiographically demonstrable hepatic calcifications due to other etiologies are recorded in the world literature. These must be distinguished from other calcifications in the liver area by radiographs in the appropriate projection. Occasionally fluoroscopy, conventional tomography, or computed tomography may be necessary for localization. In some cases, contrast studies such as cholecysto-cholangiography, pyelography, upper gastrointestinal series, or colon studies may be helpful. The most common calcifications overlying the hepatic area are in costal cartilages, or extrahepatic gallstones. Infrequently calcification in the lung base, pancreas, kidneys, skin, subcutaneous tissue, subphrenic space, retroperitoneal area, adrenals, porta hepatis lymph nodes, or blood vessels may be confusing.

Since calcifications within the liver always indicate an abnormality, in certain cases additional imaging procedures may be necessary to outline the extent of the liver involvement. These include ultrasound, CT scanning, and radionuclide scanning. In many cases, the pattern of the calcification may be pathognomonic of the underlying pathology and the activity of the disease. In selected cases, however, invasive procedures such as splenoportography, hepatic angiography, percutaneous transhepatic cholangiography, ERCP, percutaneous biopsy, or even laparotomy may be indicated for more definitive diagnosis and treatment planning.

Infectious and Granulomatous Calcification

Tuberculosis and histoplasmosis (15-18) account for most of the calcified liver granulomas, and their patterns are so similar radiographically that differentiation usually cannot be made without appropriate laboratory or skin tests. Tuberculous granulomas are more prevalent worldwide. However, in endemic areas of histoplasmosis, granulomas on this basis are much more common. Both are nearly always inactive or quiescent, few in number (occasionally solitary), have discrete margins, and may be rounded or oval. They are commonly amorphous or laminated calcium deposits, usually 1 to 3 mm in diameter and rarely exceeding 5 mm. Accompanying calcifications in the spleen and/or calcified pulmonary parenchymal granulomas or nodes are almost certain confirmatory signs of the proper diagnosis (Figures 1-6,1-7). Larger solid or "popcorn"-type calcifications may be seen rarely (16) (Figure 1-8).

Hepatic nodules from 0.5 to 2.0 mm in size were found by Zipser *et al.* (19) in 80 to 100 percent of autopsied patients with disseminated miliary tuberculosis and in 50 to 80 percent of patients with nondisseminated tuberculosis. In this series, only one case with macronodular involvement was encountered and none showed calcification. Astley *et al.* reported a case with innumerable small calcified granulomas that were possibly tuberculous (20). Active tuberculosis with macronodular calcified hepatic involvement is reported only rarely (21).

Schwarz *et al.*, in an autopsy series, found 1 to 3 mm laminated calcifications in the spleen characteristic of histoplasmosis (22). Tuberculous calcification tended to be more irregularly rounded.

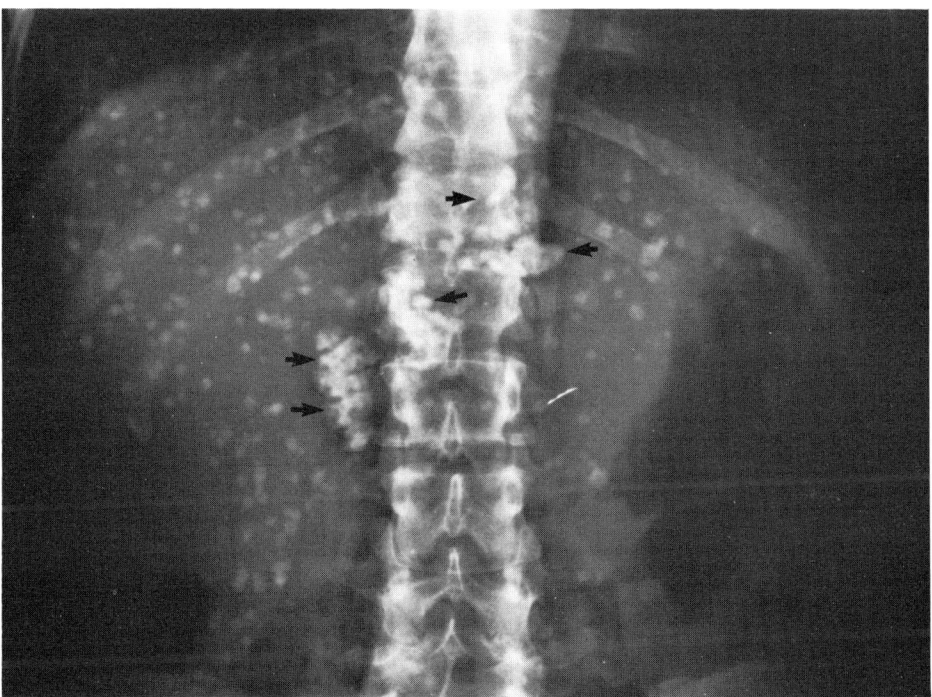

Figure 1-6. Numerous small calcified granulomas of liver, spleen, and celiac and paraaortic lymph nodes (arrows). Asymptomatic.

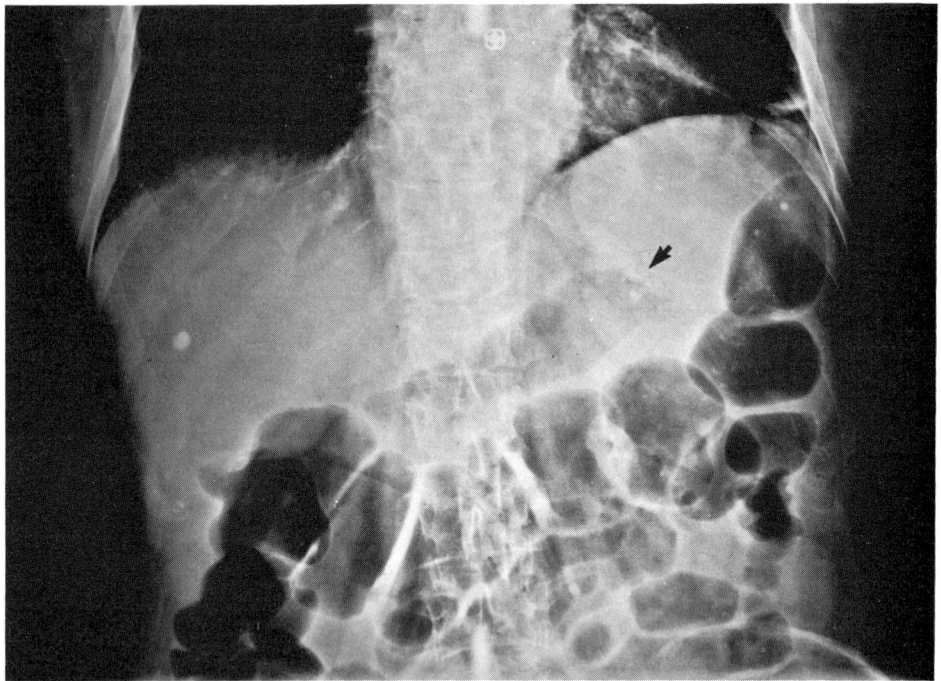

Figure 1-7. Solitary calcified granuloma of liver with small calcified splenic granulomas. AP radiograph. Calcification is also noted in the splenic artery (arrow).

Hepatic calcification on the basis of syphilitic gumma has been reported rarely. These occur apparently in a small percentage of the patients with hepar lobatum (syphilitic cirrhosis). Symmers et al. reported 19 gummas in 102 cases of hepar lobatum (23). None contained calcification. The reported cases exhibited large, well-defined, localized areas of mottled calcification (24,25).

Calcified brucella granulomas have only rarely been reported in the liver and/or spleen (26-28). Several discrete granulomas may be present, with the individual lesion measuring about 1 cm in diameter with a range of 2 to 23 mm. These granulomas tend to be sharply circumscribed with a solid dense center and a thin peripheral rim of calcification that may be rounded or serpiginous, giving a halo effect. These may be connected by radiating, "pseudopodlike," thin, calcified, sometimes branching strands, giving a snowflake appearance. *Brucella suis* is the usual offender in such granulomas rather than *brucella melitensis,* or *brucella abortus.*

Chronic granulamotous disease of childhood, although uncommon, is complicated frequently by chronic liver abscesses, sometimes with calcification (16,21,29,30). In this and other related neutrophil dysfunction syndromes, there is impairment of the ability of peripheral blood neutrophils and monocytes to kill opsonized, ingested bacteria. Chronic and recurrent pneumonia is an almost constant complication. Other foci of chronic or recurrent infections are clues to this disorder in affected children, especially inflamed cervical nodes, sometimes with calcification. The hepatic calcifications may be small, scattered clusters of speckled calcifications or rounded, macronodular, irregular calcifications. Calcified splenic granulomas are sometimes seen.

Hydatid disease from the larval stage of *Echinococcus granulosus* is by far the most common cause of rim calcifications in a liver cyst (4,15,16,21,31). Although worldwide

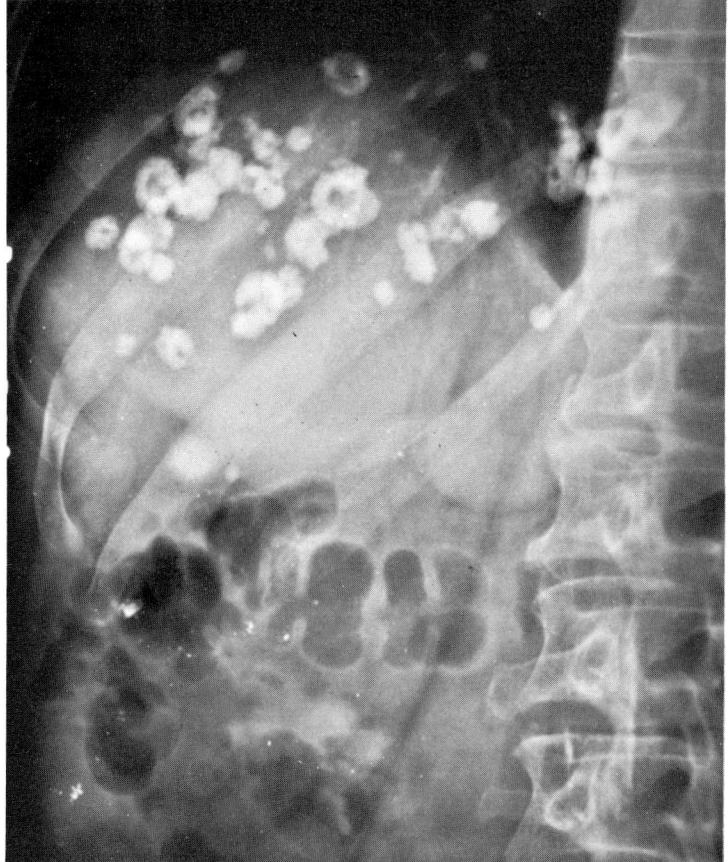

Figure 1-8. Multiple large calcified liver granulomas, an incidental finding. (Courtesy of James V. Rogers, III, M.D., Seattle, Washington.)

in distribution, these are especially prevalent in parts of South America, Asia, southern Europe, Australia, and New Zealand (31). These hepatic cysts are unilocular, usually single, but multiple in 30 percent of cases, and vary from 3 cm to over 40 cm in diameter (32). Fifty-five to 65 percent of hydatid cysts are located in the liver. They may also be found in the lungs, kidneys, bones, or occasionally in virtually any other organ or tissue. The cyst is usually present 5 to 10 years or more before calcification develops in the pericyst. At first, it is semilunar in distribution (Figure 1-9) but eventually becomes circumferential and fissured (Figure 1-10). This is virtually pathagnomonic of an inactive cyst. More than 10 percent of the cysts exhibit radiographically demonstrable calcification (32-34), and calcification of the internally located daughter cysts that are sometimes present is virtually pathognomonic of hydatid disease. Occasionally, focal areas of amorphous calcification may be present within the cyst on the basis of necrotic tissue, purulent material, or hemorrhage.

Other rim calcifications, although rare, may occur in the wall of a pyogenic abscess (18), amebic abscess (16,35,36), or congenital or acquired nonparasitic cyst (37,38) and have an appearance indistinguishable from a hydatid cyst. A calcified gallbladder wall or neoplastic rim calcification may rarely be mistaken for a hydatid cyst.

The larval stage of *Echinococcus multilocularis* is much less common in humans, but it is a much more malignant infestation than *Echinococcus granulosus*. The daughter cysts form external to the parent cyst with progressive involvement of the liver. In

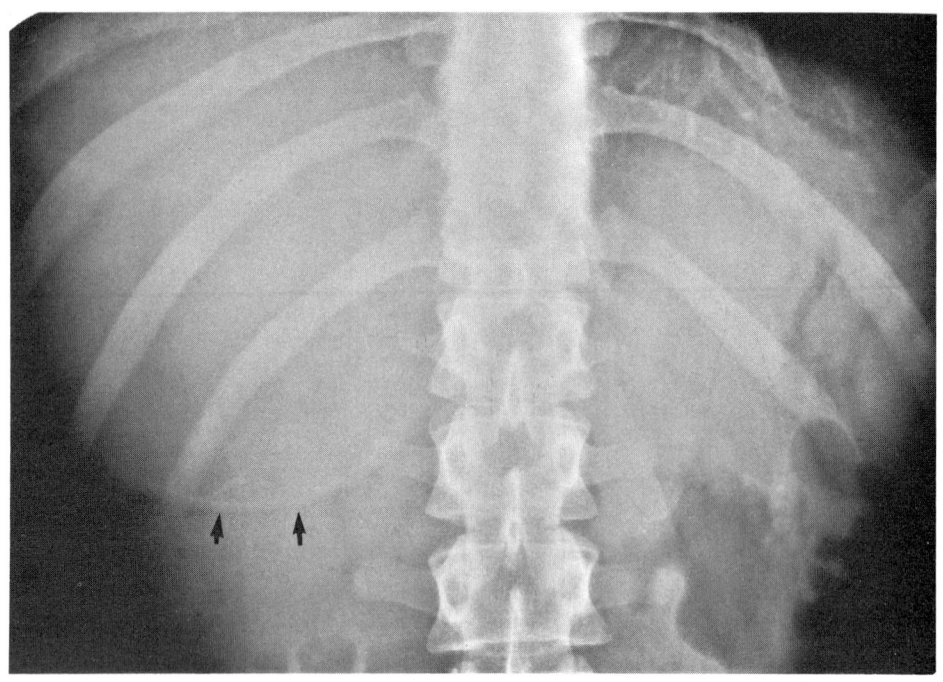

Figure 1-9. Partial "rim" calcification (arrows) in an *Echinococcus granulosus* liver cyst in a Japanese student.

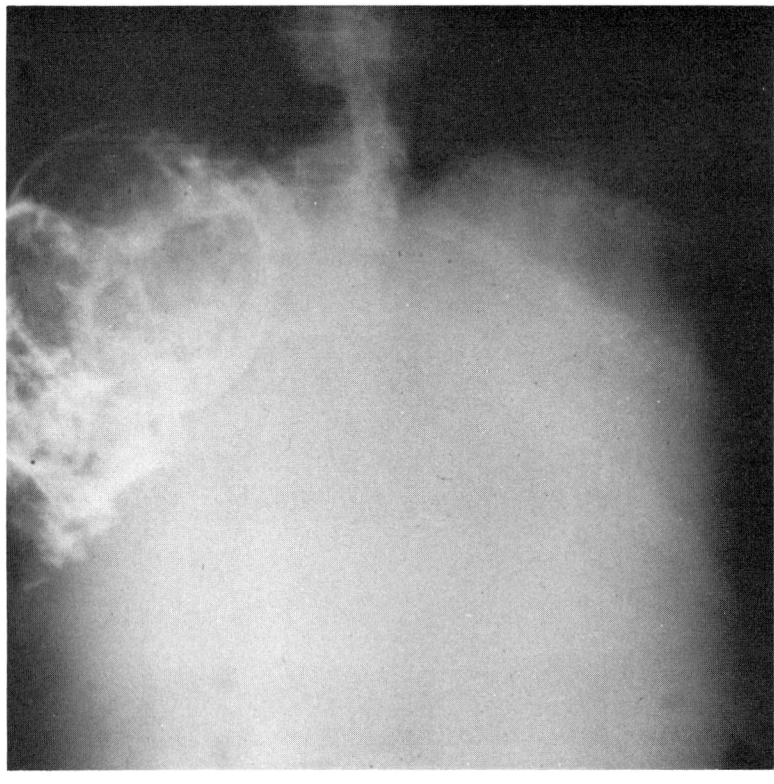

Figure 1-10. Complete circumferential calcification in an *Echinococcus granulosus* liver cyst; this extensive calcification indicates inactivity.

over 50 percent of cases, there are associated extensive areas of amorphous calcification in the liver, with interspersed small 2- to 4-mm ringlike, or rim, calcifications characteristic of the disease (39,40).

On rare occasions, other parasitic infestations may cause hepatic calcification. There has been a case report of the liver fluke *Fasciola gigantica,* commonly found in Africa, apparently gaining access to the liver parenchma and producing a fairly large area of necrosis with an irregular 7-cm, somewhat lobulated, amorphous area of calcification in which *Fasciola gigantica* eggs were identified pathologically (41). The nymphs of *Armillifer armillatus,* a tongue worm, may infest humans and produce multiple "C" or comma-shaped calcifications 4 to 7 mm in diameter in the liver, peritoneal cavity, or other abdominal organs. The adult parasite is found principally in the upper respiratory tract of snakes, usually pythons from West Africa, and human infestation (porencephalosis) results from accidental ingestion of their saliva or excreta (4,42,43). The guinea worm, *Dracunculus medinensis,* has been reported calcified in the liver (16,44) (Figure 1-11). *Paragonimus westermani* is a rare cause of liver calcification. Cysticer-

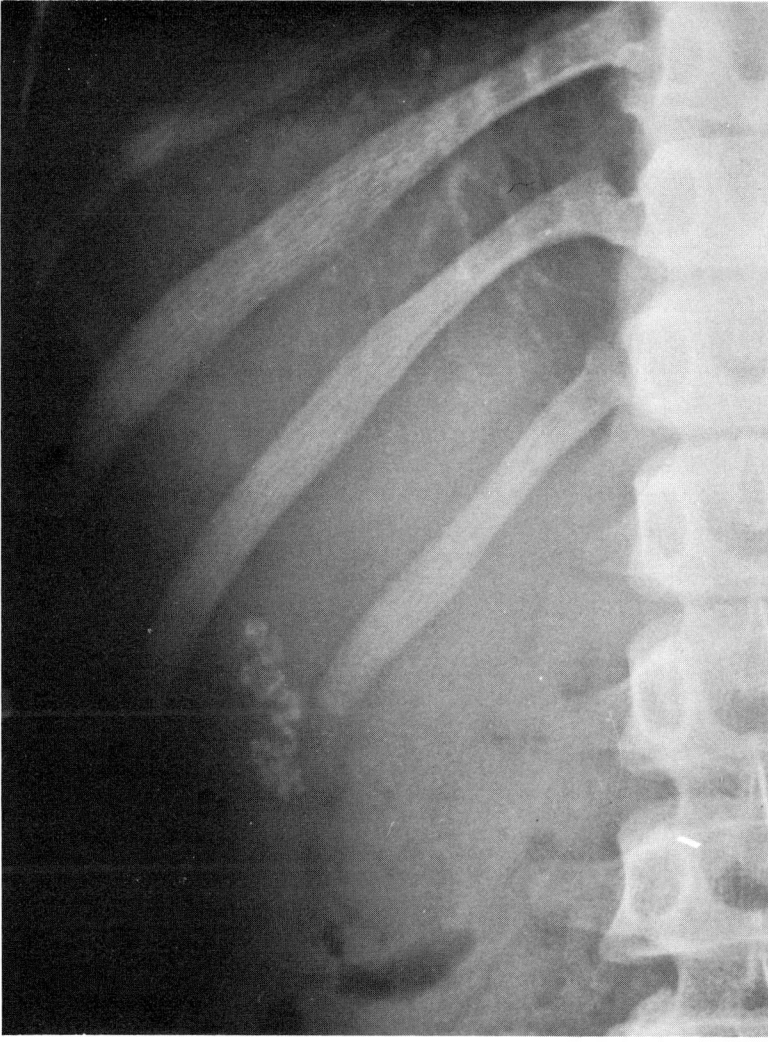

Figure 1-11. Calcified parasite in the liver. Several similar cases have been seen at Grady Hospital, Atlanta, Ga. Since *Dracunculus medinensis* is not endemic to the area and no histologic proof has been obtained, these have been nicknamed facetiously "Dracunculus gradyensis."

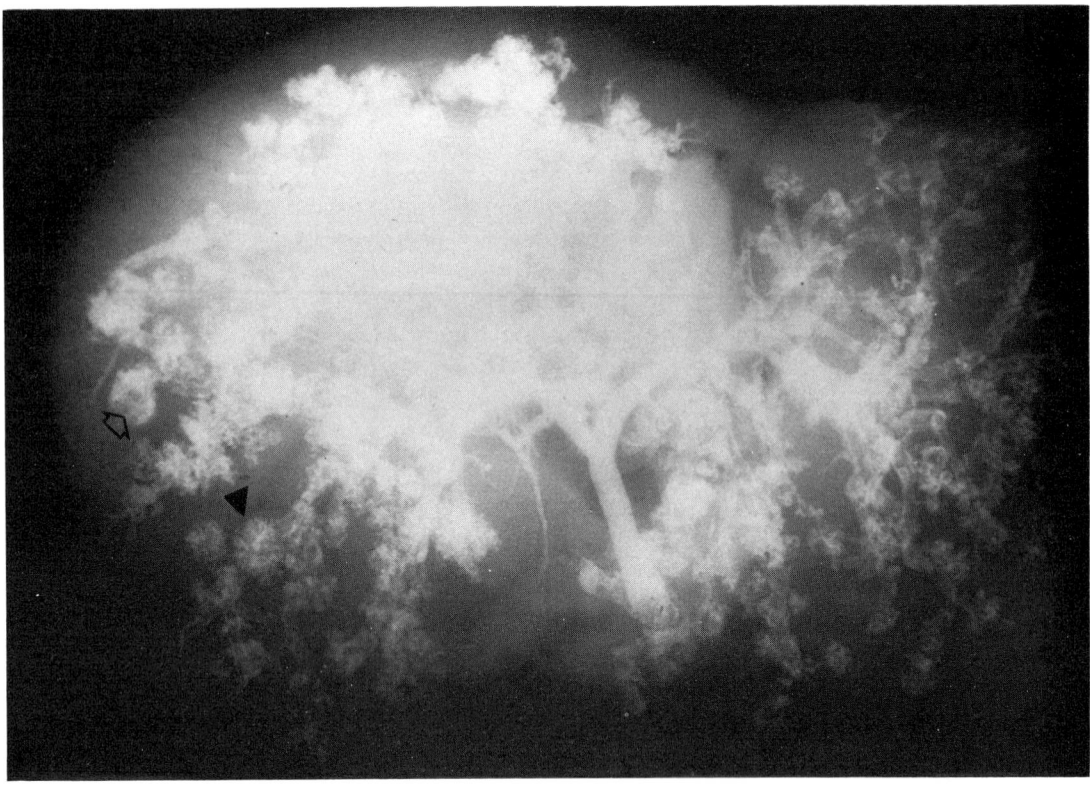

Figure 1-12. Clonorchiasis: a surgical liver specimen with contrast injected into the biliary tree demonstrates the characteristic calculi (black arrowhead) and bile thrombi (open arrowhead) formed as denuded epithelium and clonorchis ova conglomerate in the ducts, creating stasis, bacterial infection, strictures, or tumors.

cosis, the larval stage of *Taenia solium,* as well as trichinosis, the larval stage of *Taenia saginata,* have been suggested as rare causes of liver calcification. Their characteristic appearance in the muscles and other areas of the body should aid in radiographic identification. A single case has been reported of generalized hepatic calcification in advanced *Schistosomiasis Japonica* (45). Nodular liver calcifications have been reported secondary to transplacental infection from toxoplasmosis as well as herpes simplex (46). Gallstones, or rarely, common duct calcifications may result from infestation by the liver fluke, *Chlonorcis sinensis* (47) (Figure 1-12), or the roundworm, *Ascaris lumbicoides.*

Coccidiomycosis and sarcoid have been mentioned as rare causes of liver calcification (16). Cytomegalovirus has also been suggested. One suspects that in time all pathogens affecting the liver will be implicated.

Neoplastic Calcification

Tumors from *primary carcinoma of the liver in adults* rarely contain calcification. In a review of the literature, Hall *et al.* found only 30 reported cases (48). Mixed malignant tumors containing hepatic and cholangiomatous cells, as well as mesenchymal elements, were the most common. In addition to amorphous areas of dystrophic calcification, areas of metaplastic bone formation may sometimes be present. Two such cases of mixed malignant tumor have been reported (49). One had hypertrophic pulmonary osteoarthropathy and multiple spider angiomata of the skin.

Although hepatocellular carcinoma is three times as frequent as cholangiocarcinoma, calcification is reported much more frequently in duct cell carcinoma (18,25,48,50–52) (Figure 1–13). The cholangiocarcinomas exhibited multiple irregular, amorphous, flaky, granular, nodular, or cystic calcifications in a large area. Haddow *et al.* reported one case of hepatocellular carcinoma with a large solid area of calcification with spiculated margins (25). Seventy percent of hepatocellular carcinomas are associated with cirrhosis, compared to 30 percent of cholangiocarcinomas. Clustered, granular calcifications have been observed in at least three hemangioendotheliomas of the liver (53,54). The association of this tumor with thorium deposition in the liver several years following intravascular thorium dioxide injection has been well-substantiated in over 50 patients (53,55,56) (Figure 1–14).

Tumors from primary carcinoma of the liver in children occur infrequently. In a survey over a ten-year period of children with liver tumors who had surgery, 375 cases were found, 252 with malignant tumors and 123 with benign tumors (57). Of the malignant tumors, 129 were hepatoblastomas and 98 were hepatocellular carcinomas. Seven other less common malignant tumors accounted for the other 25 cases. Ishak *et al.* reviewed cases registered at the Armed Forces Institute of Pathology and found 3 cases with mottled amorphous calcification in the 35 hepatoblastomas of mixed epithelial and mesenchymal origin and no calcifications in 12 hepatocellular carcinomas (58). Others

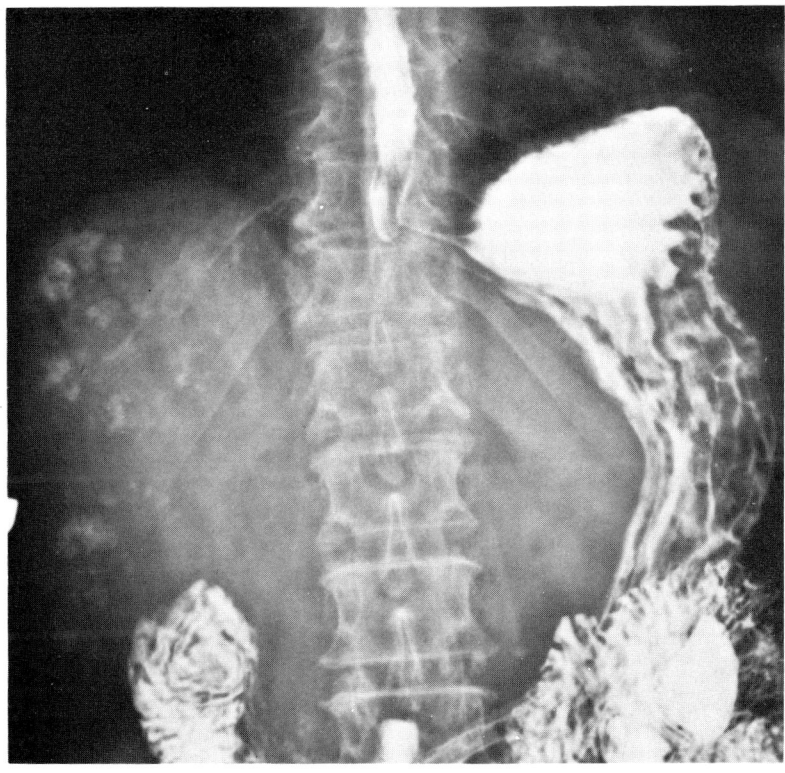

Figure 1-13. This 70-year-old female with autopsy-proven cholangiocarcinoma was reported previously by Schroder (52) without illustrations.

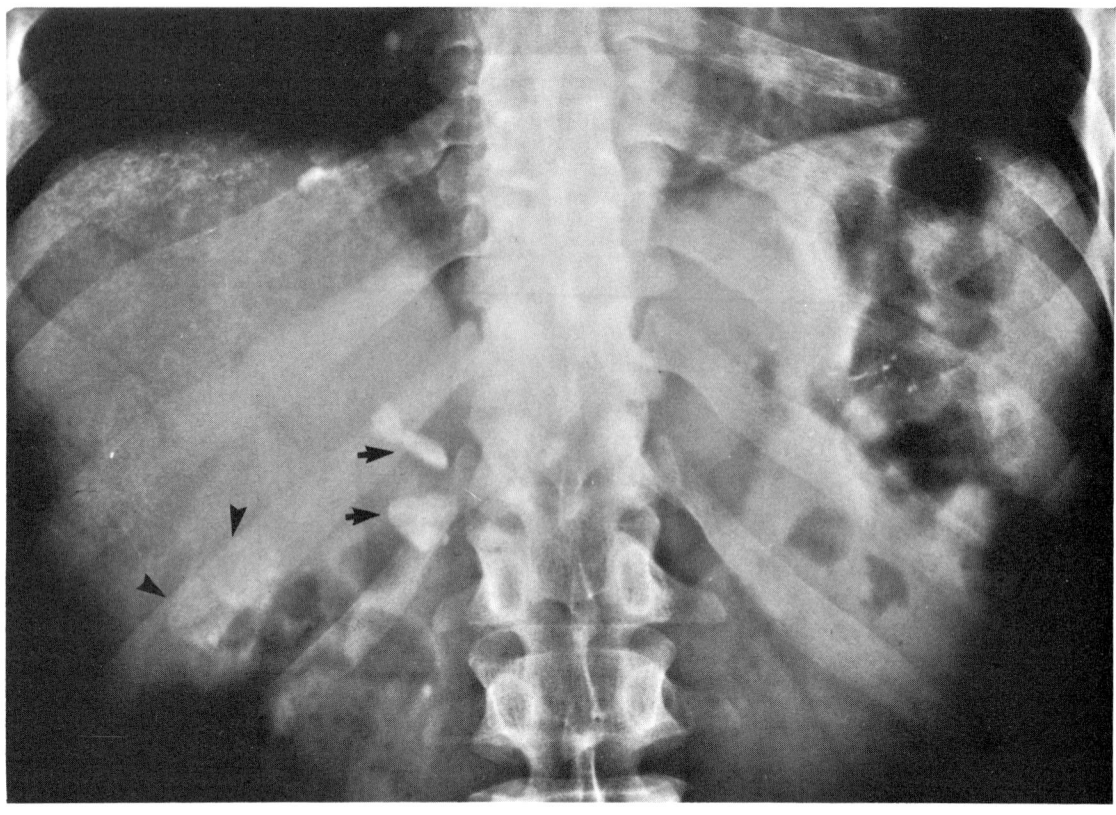

Figure 1-14. This patient had a carotid arteriogram using 35 ml. of Thorotrast 17 years earlier. Lacy, somewhat granular opacity of the liver with granular opacity of the spleen and densely opaque peripancreatic nodes (arrows) characteristic of the presence of thorium in the reticuloendothelial system for years. Earlier, there is a more diffuse density of the liver and spleen without the lymph node opacification. Incidental gallstones (arrowheads).

have reported calcifications in 3 of 11 cases with hepatoblastomas (59). Sorsdahl and Gay reported 2 cases of hepatomas with calcification (Figure 1-15) (60).

Benign hepatic neoplasms rarely contain calcifications. Cavernous hemangioma is the most common primary hepatic tumor, but it rarely exhibits calcification. In those cases that do, however, the pattern may be characteristic with a central amorphous calcification and calcific strands radiating peripherally in something of a "spoke-wheel" pattern, as may be seen in hemangiomas of other body parts (61,62). In infantile hemangioendothelioma and cavernous hemangioma of infancy, clustered granular calcifications have been reported (Figure 1-16) (63,64). Phleboliths have not been reported in hemangiomas of the liver. Arcuate calcification has been mentioned in hamartoma of the liver.

Metastatic hepatic neoplasms are many times more common than primary malignancies. This accounts largely for the more frequent occurrence of calcification in metastatic tumors. The usual calcification occurring with hepatic neoplasms, primary or metastatic, is dystrophic in nature, on a degenerative basis, and associated with tissue necrosis, ischemia, or hemorrhage. The calcifications may be granular, nodular, irregular, extensive, but rarely "rimlike." These are usually associated with an obvious mass or enlarged liver. Mucous-producing adenocarcinoma of the colon is the most common

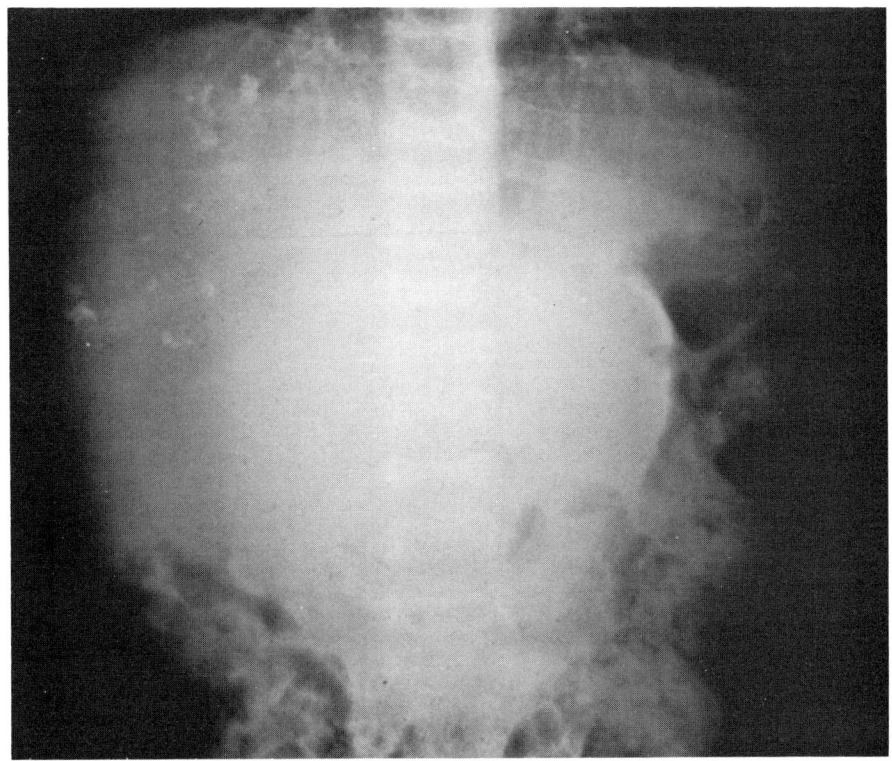

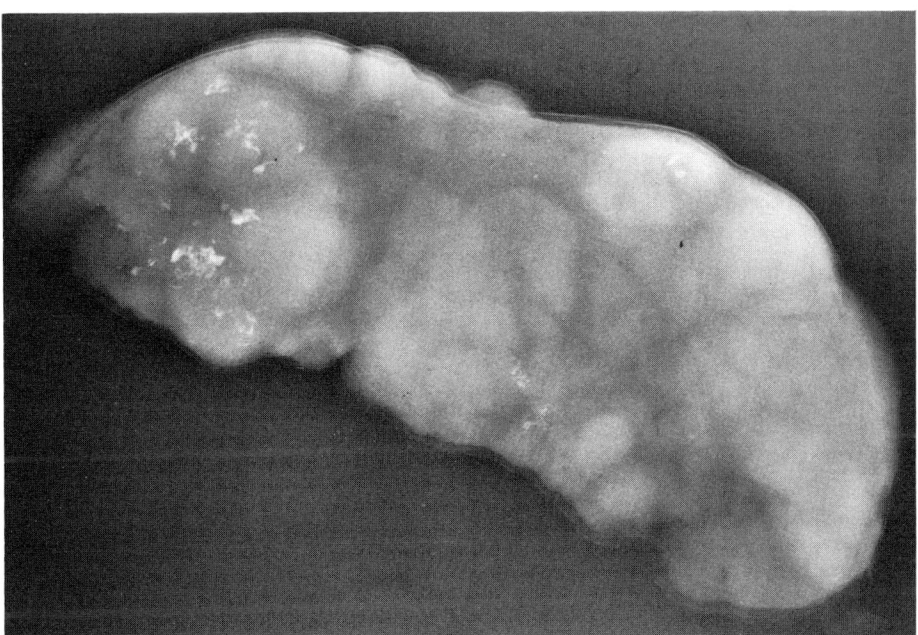

Figure 1-15. *A.* One-year-old male with pathologic diagnosis of hepatoma, embryonic type (Sorsdahl and Gay, 1967) (60). Note multiple foci of gross amorphous calcification in a large mass of the right lobe of the liver. *B.* Radiograph of gross specimen after right lobectomy.

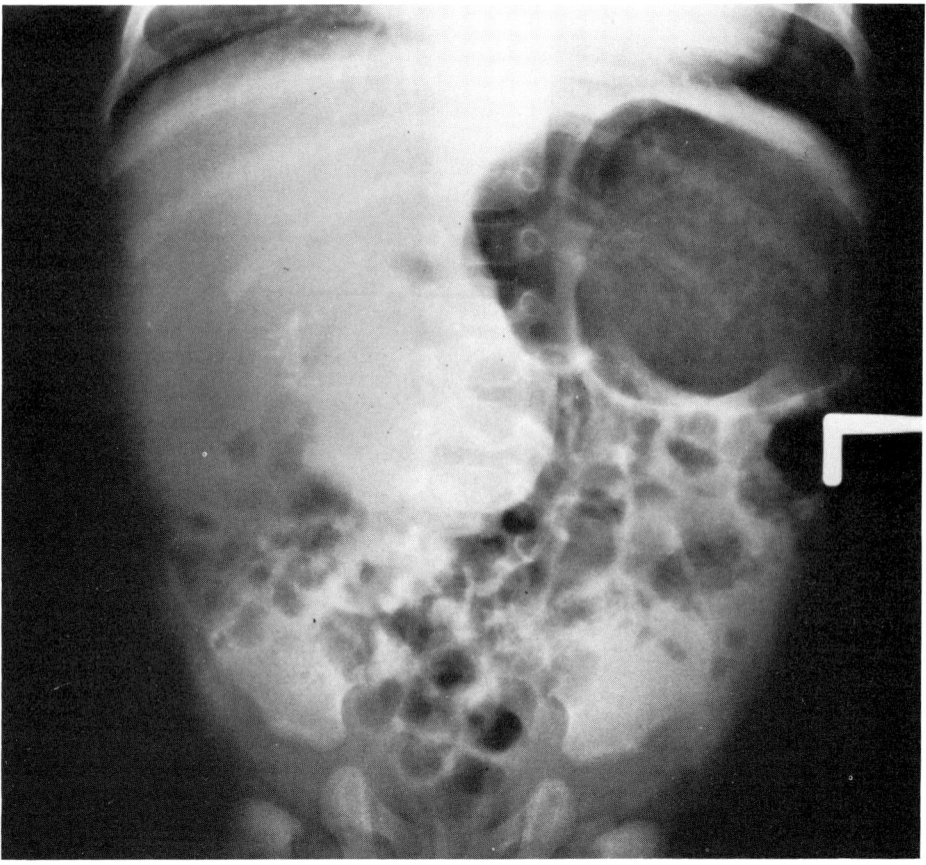

Figure 1-16. Three-month-old male infant with mass containing clustered, focal calcifications in the enlarged right lobe of the liver. Pathological diagnosis: infantile hemangioendothelioma.

metastatic neoplasm with calcification. These metastases usually have a characteristic appearance consisting of extensive, multiple, diffuse, fine granular, or "poppy seed" calcifications, most of which are located in mucin pools (Figure 1-17). It has been suggested (65) that the mucin may act as an ion exchange resin for calcium deposition in these cases. The individual calcifications average 2 to 4 mm in diameter and are variable in density. Although this pattern of calcification can occur from mucin-producing tumors from other sites in the gastrointestinal tract, ovary, or breast, the colon is by far the most common site of origin (52,66–70). Calcifications in abdominal metastases occur most commonly on the basis of cystadenocarcinoma of the ovary (71). But these do not cause calcified liver metastases as frequently as the colon, although many of the peritoneal metastases may overlay the liver. The metastases from cystadenocarcinoma of the ovary may be dystrophic (72). In some cases, however, diffuse, fine, punctate, psammomatous calcifications varying from 5 to 100 μ in diameter may produce a cloudlike density in the metastatic area. These calcifications are not dystrophic, and are located in actively growing tissue. Several cases have been reported (16,25,73) with calcifications in liver metastases from breast carcinoma. There is an ever-increasing list

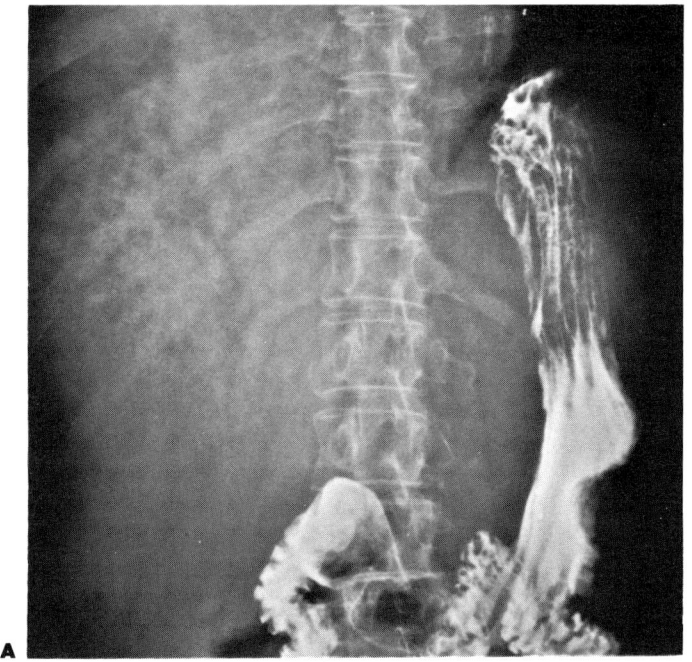

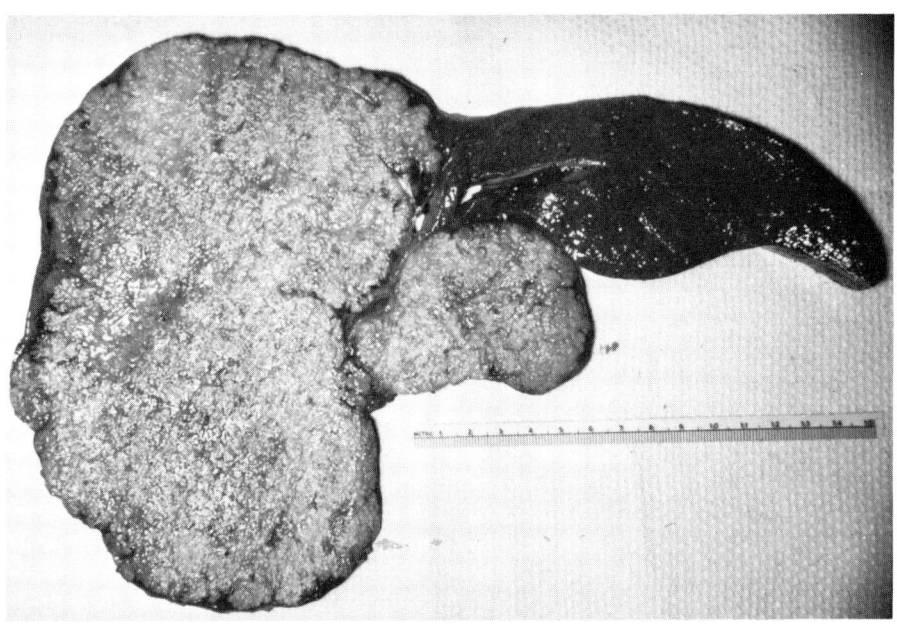

Figure 1–17. *A.* Case 2 of Schroder (52). Carcinoma of the rectum with autopsy-proven liver metastases with diffuse granular "poppyseed" pattern on AP radiograph. *B.* Photograph of pathology specimen showing diffuse involvement of the right lobe of the liver.

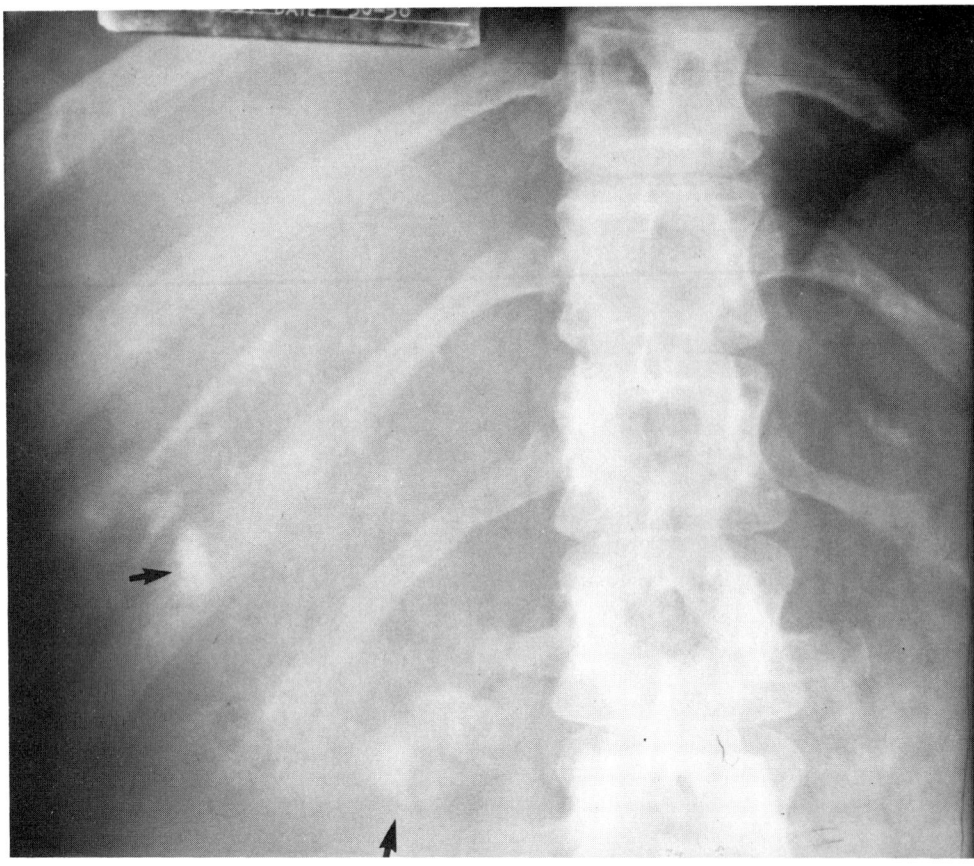

Figure 1-18. Case 3 of Schroder (52). Biopsy-proven chondromyxocarcinoma of salivary gland. Sixty-one-year-old female (arrows).

of primary neoplasms that are rarely associated with calcification in liver metastases (4,15,16,17,21). These include malignant melanoma, neuroblastoma, mesothelioma, rhabdomyosarcoma, embryonal testicular tumors, retroperitoneal mesenchymoma, osteosarcoma, leiomyosarcoma, carcinoid, myeloma, Hodgkin's disease, and salivary gland carcinoma (18,21,52,74-77) (Figure 1-18). Dystrophic calcification is likely to occur in some neoplasms following radiation therapy or chemotherapy (78).

Vascular Calcifications

Hepatic artery aneurysms are quite rare (79). These are more common in the extrahepatic portion of the artery and only a small percentage have calcification in the arterial wall. Appropriate contrast studies would be required for accurate diagnosis. Arteriosclerotic calcification of the hepatic artery is extremely unusual.

Calcified thrombi in the portal vein or inferior vena cava have been reported occasionally. The portal venous thrombi usually occur in adults with a characteristic location and vascular pattern (25) (Figures 1-19 and 1-20). Calcified thrombi in the splenic or

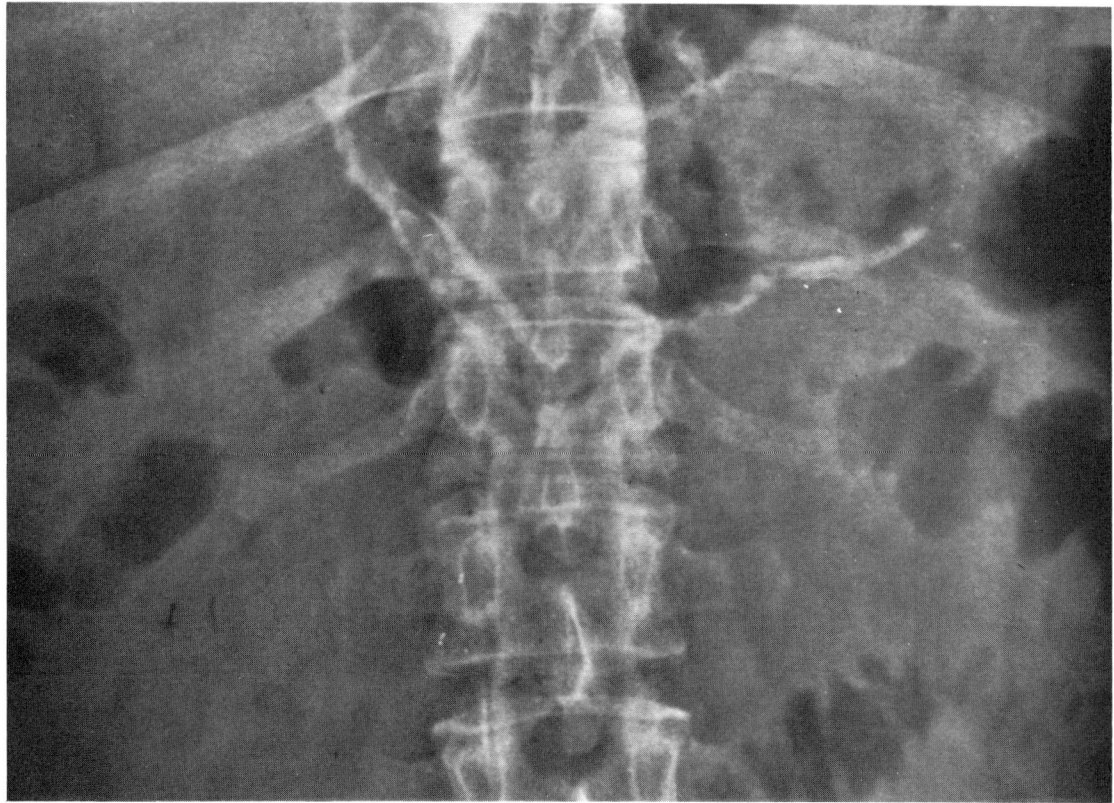

Figure 1-19. Typical appearance of calcified thrombus in portal and splenic veins.

superior mesenteric veins may also be found. These are frequently not completely obstructive and can be readily evaluated by splenoportography. In infants, a "bullet-shaped" calcific density to the right of the twelfth dorsal interspace or first lumbar vertebra is characteristic of a thrombus in the intrahepatic portion of the inferior vena cava (80,81). If symptomatic, thrombectomy is required.

Miscellaneous Causes of Hepatic Calcification

Simple nonparasitic cysts, either congenital or acquired, are quite rare, usually single, but sometimes multiple, and infrequently have spherical "rim" calcification (37,38) (Figure 1-21). The necessity for differentiation from hydatid disease has already been mentioned. About one third of the cases with polycystic disease have both kidney and liver involvement, and there has been one case report of "rim" calcification in the hepatic cysts (82).

Calcified primary intrahepatic calculi are quite rare (83,84) and cholangiography may be necessary to establish an accurate diagnosis. Most primary intrahepatic calculi are associated with Caroli's disease (21,84). However, these are usually radiolucent. Secondary intraphepatic calculi from stones in the extrahepatic biliary tree or occa-

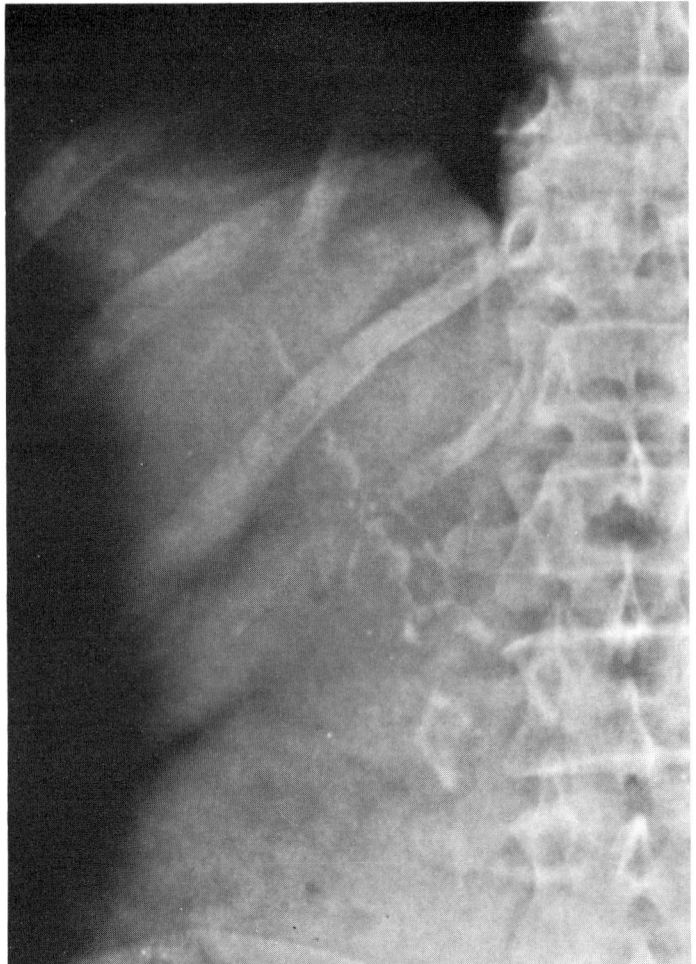

Figure 1-20. *A.* Calcification of portal vein thrombus. *B.* Splenoportogram showing partial patency of the portal vein.

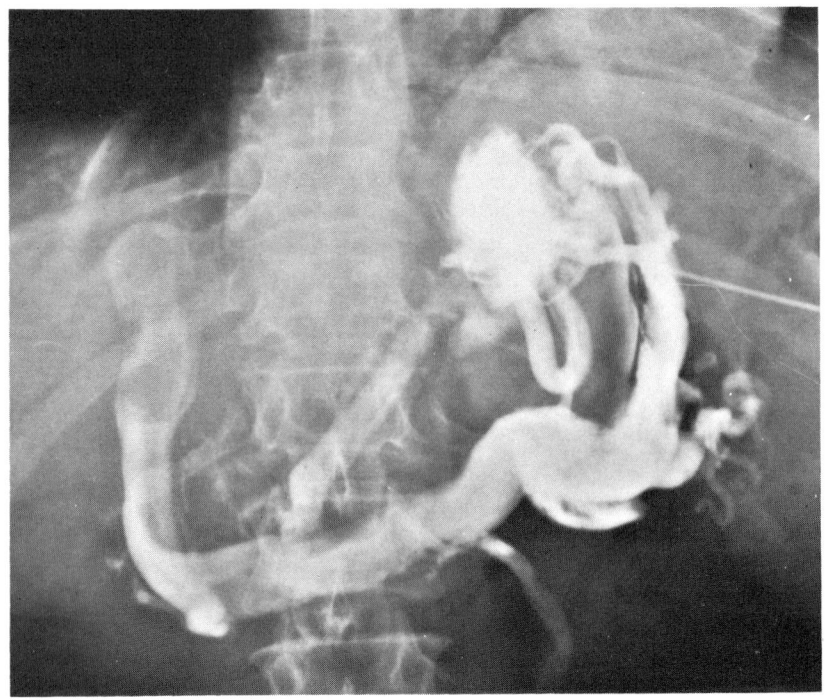

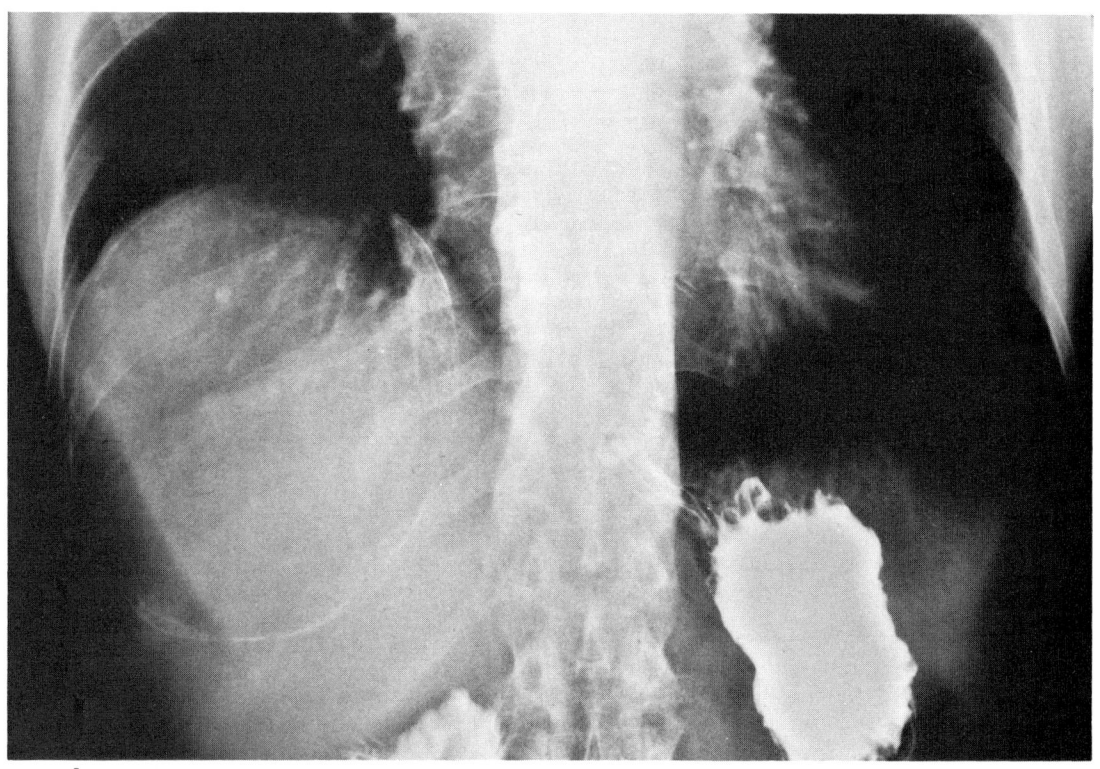

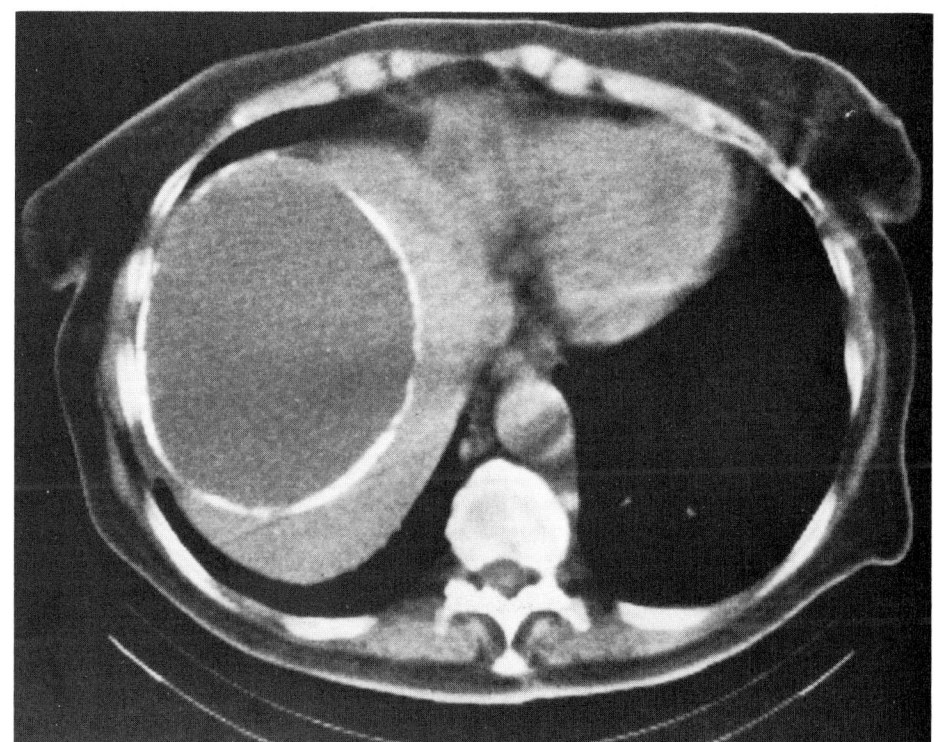

Figure 1-21. *A*. AP radiograph showing surgically proven nonparasitic liver cyst with "rim" calcification in a 68-year-old white female. *B*. Computed tomographic demonstration of the cyst.

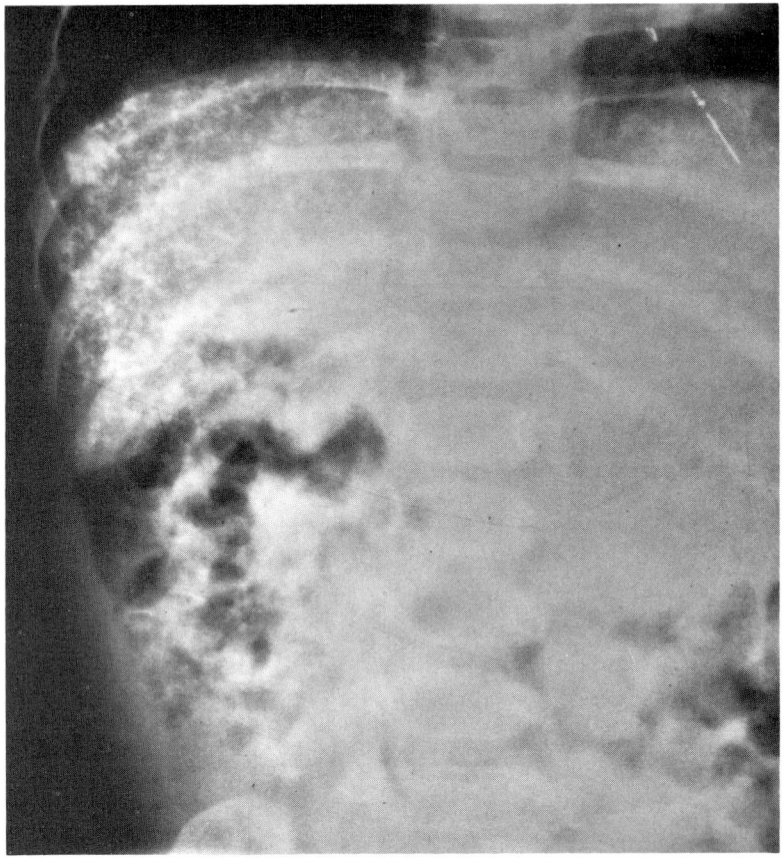

Figure 1-22. Eighteen-month-old male with diffuse liver calcification following omphalitis and *Escherichia coli* sepsis in early infancy. There was no liver calcification observed radiographically at 10 months of age. Liver biopsy at 18 months revealed diffuse granulomatous changes.

sionally from noncalculous obstruction are much more common, but are also rarely calcified.

Capsular calcification has been mentioned as a rare occurrence in alcoholic cirrhosis, pyogenic infection, meconium peritonitis, lipoid granulomatosis following peritoneal instillation of mineral oil, pseudomyxoma peritoneii, and after trauma (16).

Other miscellaneous causes of liver calcification include calcifications associated with umbilical vein catheterization or injection of hypertonic solution in neonates (85). These may be calcified thrombi at the catheter site in an intrahepatic branch of the portal vein, or focal calcifications adjacent to the catheter tip apparently on the basis of focal hepatic necrosis. Focal or extensive calcification following transplacental infection with toxoplasmosis or herpes simplex has already been mentioned (46).

Cholesterol ester storage disease has been implicated in focal calcification of the liver and spleen (86). Omphalitis in the newborn has been followed by massive liver calcification (Figure 1-22). Posteclampsia, regenerating nodules in cirrhosis or following massive liver necrosis, and hematoma have all been mentioned as rare causes of hepatic calcification.

HEPATIC/PERIHEPATIC RADIOLUCENCIES

Fat

On the plain film of the abdomen, fat lucencies may be appreciated in the right upper quadrant in contrast to the water density of the liver. The most common fat lucency that can be appreciated in the hepatic area is the retroperitoneal, or properitoneal, fat line. The amount of fat in the extraperitoneal area varies with the nutritional status of the patient. This extraperitoneal fat allows identification of the lateral and posterior-inferior margins of the right lobe of the liver (7). The lateral margin of the liver is defined by the extraperitoneal fat in the flank area, which is contiguous with the posterior pararenal space. When ascitic fluid accumulates between the lateral margin of the liver and extraperitoneal fat, separation of the liver margin from the fat can be appreciated. It has been shown that ascitic fluid has a different attenuation coefficient than normal liver tissue (87).

The right posterior-inferior margin of the liver is identified by the retroperitoneal fat in the anterior pararenal space. It has been pointed out that there is often a discrepancy in the radiographic and the clinical evaluations of liver size, since the anterior margin of the liver is palpated on physical examination but not visualized on the abdominal radiograph. The posterior margin is visualized on radiographs by contrast between the water density of the liver and the fat in the anterior pararenal space. The overall liver size cannot be accurately evaluated on plain films of the abdomen (7).

Loss of the detail of the interface between the posterior-inferior margin of the liver and the fat in the anterior pararenal space can occur as a result of the accumulation of ascitic fluid within the peritoneal space. With the patient in supine position, free intraperitoneal fluid has a tendency to accumulate in the right subhepatic space at the interface between the upper pole of the kidney and the liver margin (Morison's pouch) (7).

The extraperitoneal fat extends from the posterior pararenal space onto the inferior surface of the right hemidiaphragm and the parietal peritoneum. The lucency of this fat line is usually obscured by the air-filled right lung base. However, when there is a thick layer of extraperitoneal fat in this area and a right pleural effusion, air-space, or interstitial infiltrate in the right lung base, this lucent fat stripe can be appreciated on plain films. On occasion it may be so prominent as to suggest the presence of free intraperitoneal air. The presence of intraperitoneal air can be excluded by films in different positions, such as erect or decubitus views (7).

It has been pointed out that retroperitoneal hemorrhage, such as that occurring with ruptured abdominal aneurysm, can cause radiolucent shadows as a result of the dissection of blood into the planes of the retroperitoneal fat (88). When this occurs in the right upper quadrant, it may suggest emphysema in the liver or the perihepatic space (Figure 1–23).

Physiological accumulation of fat can occur in the periportal, pericholecystic, and falciform ligament areas (7,89,90). The radiolucencies produced by the fat in these areas are seldom of sufficient lucency to suggest the possibility that they represent gas shadows. If there is suspicion that these lucencies may represent gas, films in various projections, such as erect and decubitus views, would be of value in excluding the possibility of intrahepatic or perihepatic gas.

Fat infiltration of the liver can result from a number of pathological conditions. This infiltration is readily appreciated on computed tomography by the decreased attenuation of the photon beam, but it cannot be appreciated on plain films of the abdomen in the adult. Appreciation of fatty infiltration by increased lucency in the liver area has

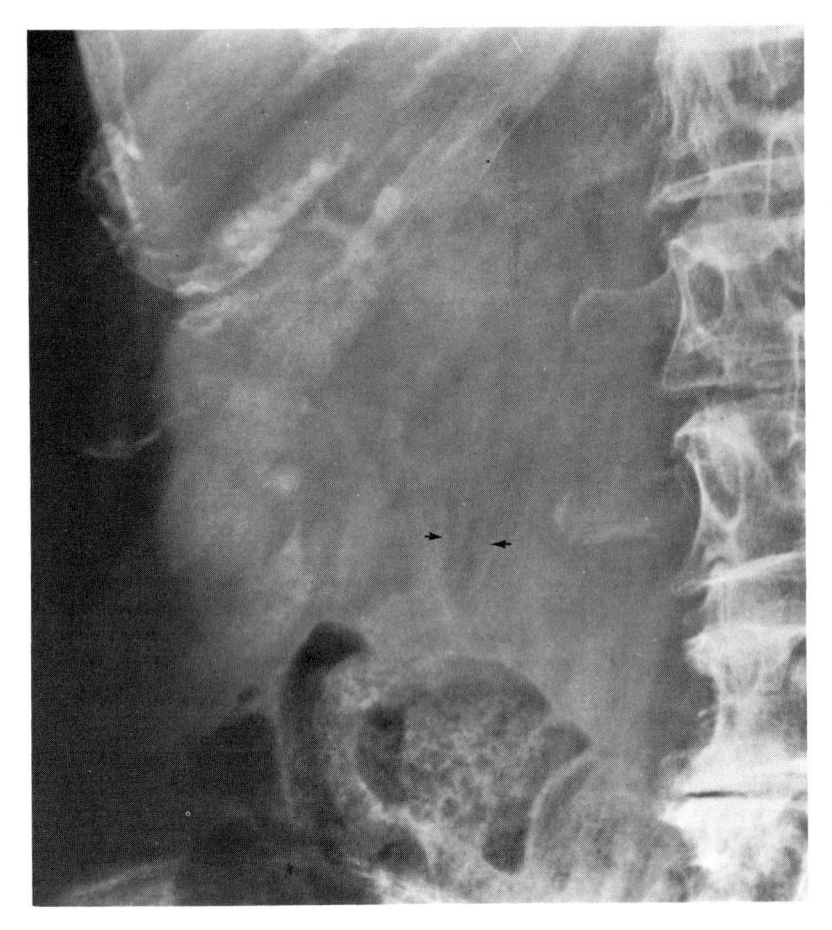

Figure 1-23. Retroperitoneal hemorrhage secondary to ruptured abdominal aortic aneurysm. The blood dissecting into the retroperitoneal fat in the right upper quadrant demonstrates linear lucent areas (arrows) of fat outlined by retroperitoneal blood simulating gas in the liver or subhepatic area.

been described in the pediatric patient, particularly those undergoing pyelography with large doses of contrast material resulting in "total body opacification" (91).

Gas/Air

Air/gas within the gallbladder is readily appreciated on the plain radiograph of the abdomen. The presence of radiolucent gas shadows in the gallbladder area should always be considered an abnormal finding. This gas can occur as a result of a number of etiologies. These include infection with a gas-producing organism, internal biliary fistula as a result of calculi, peptic ulcer disease, or neoplasm. Gas can also occur as a result of prior surgical procedures that anastomose the gallbladder or bile duct to the intestinal tract.

Emphysematous cholecystitis is the result of infection of the gallbladder by a gas-forming organism (7,92). Radiographically, gas within the gallbladder has a fairly characteristic appearance, assuming the pear-shaped configuration of the gallbladder in the right upper quadrant (Figure 1-24). On erect films, air-fluid levels may be identified within the lumen of the gallbladder. In addition, gas is frequently present outlining the wall of the gallbladder (pneumatosis) (Figure 1-24). Gas shadows within the wall of the gallbladder are usually a thin lucent line along the margins of the gallblad-

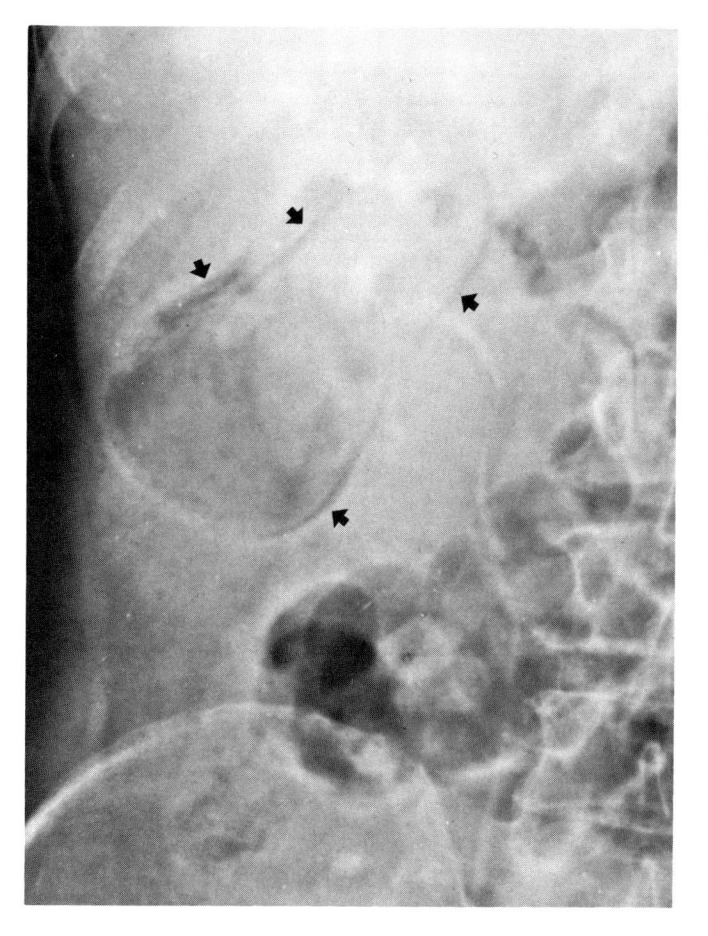

Figure 1-24. Emphysematous cholecystitis demonstrating gas within the lumen of the gallbladder as well as linear accumulation of gas within the wall of the gallbladder (arrows).

der. The most common infecting organisms are clostridial or colon bacteria (92). This condition has been reported to be more common in men than women and may be associated with diabetes mellitus (92).

The presence of the pneumatosis of the gallbladder wall suggests necrosis secondary to gangrenous cholecystitis. This condition is considered to be more of a surgical emergency than acute cholecystitis without gas within the gallbladder lumen or wall. Mortality and morbidity in this condition is considered to be greater than in the more common form of acute cholecystitis (7). Associated gas within the bile duct system indicates that there is no associated obstruction to the cystic duct (Figure 1-25).

Internal biliary fistula with a fistulous communication between the gallbladder and some segment of the gastrointestinal tract is the most common cause for the detection of gas within the gallbladder on plain films of the abdomen. Internal biliary fistula can result from biliary calculus disease, peptic ulcer disease, neoplasm, or the results of a previous surgical procedure (92-95).

Fistula secondary to calculi account for 90 percent of cholecystoenteric fistulae (94). The most frequent site of biliary fistula is gallbladder to duodenum (92,94). Biliary enteric fistula occur as a result of long-standing calculus gallbladder disease. A gallstone may temporarily obstruct the cystic duct, with pressure erosion of the calculus into an

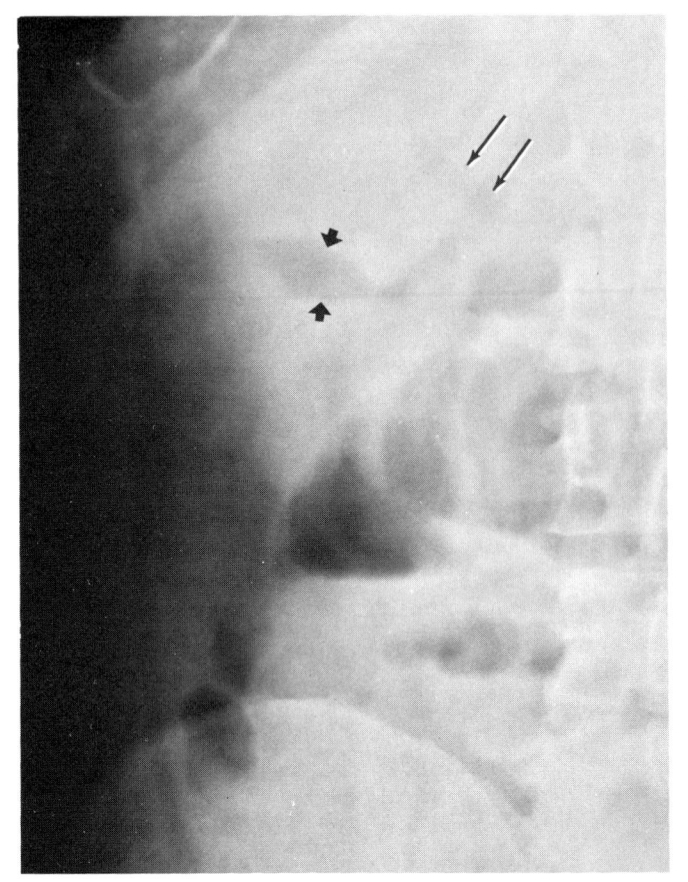

Figure 1-25. Plain erect film of the right abdomen in a patient with gallstone ileus. Gas is demonstrated within the gallbladder (large arrows). Also gas is present outlining the common hepatic bile duct (small arrows), indicating the cystic duct to be patent.

adjacent viscus, most commonly the duodenum. The next most commonly involved viscus is the colon. Erosion of a stone into the stomach is the least common event (94). Fistula to the colon with extrusion of a gallstone into the colon usually produces no obstruction unless a preexisting stenotic lesion is in the distal colon. With extrusion into the duodenum or stomach, the gallstones, if they are small, will pass readily through the intestinal tract with no evidence of obstruction (92). When larger stones are extruded into the duodenum or stomach, they may impact and obstruct at the level of the duodenum or ligament of Treitz. However, they obstruct most commonly in the distal ileum.

When small bowel obstruction occurs secondary to extrusion of a gallstone into the intestinal tract, a clinical and radiological syndrome occurs referred to as gallstone ileus or gallstone obturation (92,94-97). The radiologist plays a major role in the diagnosis of this condition. Early diagnosis is important since there is increased morbidity with delay in diagnosis or failure to diagnose this condition preoperatively.

In the radiologic diagnosis, there is a classic triad of findings: (1) air in the gallbladder and/or bile ducts, (2) obstructive small bowel pattern, and (3) opaque gallstone visualized outside the gallbladder area or disappearance or change in the position of a previously demonstrated gallstone in the right upper quadrant (94,97). Frequently all three features of this triad are not encountered radiologically (Figure 1-25). The most constant feature is the presence of ileus. A frequent pitfall in the diagnosis of gallstones ileus is the inability to discern air within the biliary tree (95). A characteristic finding has been described of air-fluid level within the duodenum on the erect film, due to duodenal ileus, and a second adjacent air-fluid level in the right upper quadrant representing the gallbladder (94). The gallstone producing the ileus may not be sufficiently opaque for detection on a plain film of the abdomen. With a high index of suspicion, barium studies are of value in proving the diagnosis. The cholecystoduodenal fistula could be filled by this method (Figure 1–26) and on occasion gallstones can be identified on subsequent films after adminstration of barium by mouth. The barium enema examination with reflux of the terminal ileum has demonstrated on occasion the obstructing gallstone in the distal ileum (Figure 1–27).

Peptic ulcer disease of the duodenum is a less common cause of internal biliary fistulae than is biliary calculus disease. Six percent of fistulae are attributable to peptic

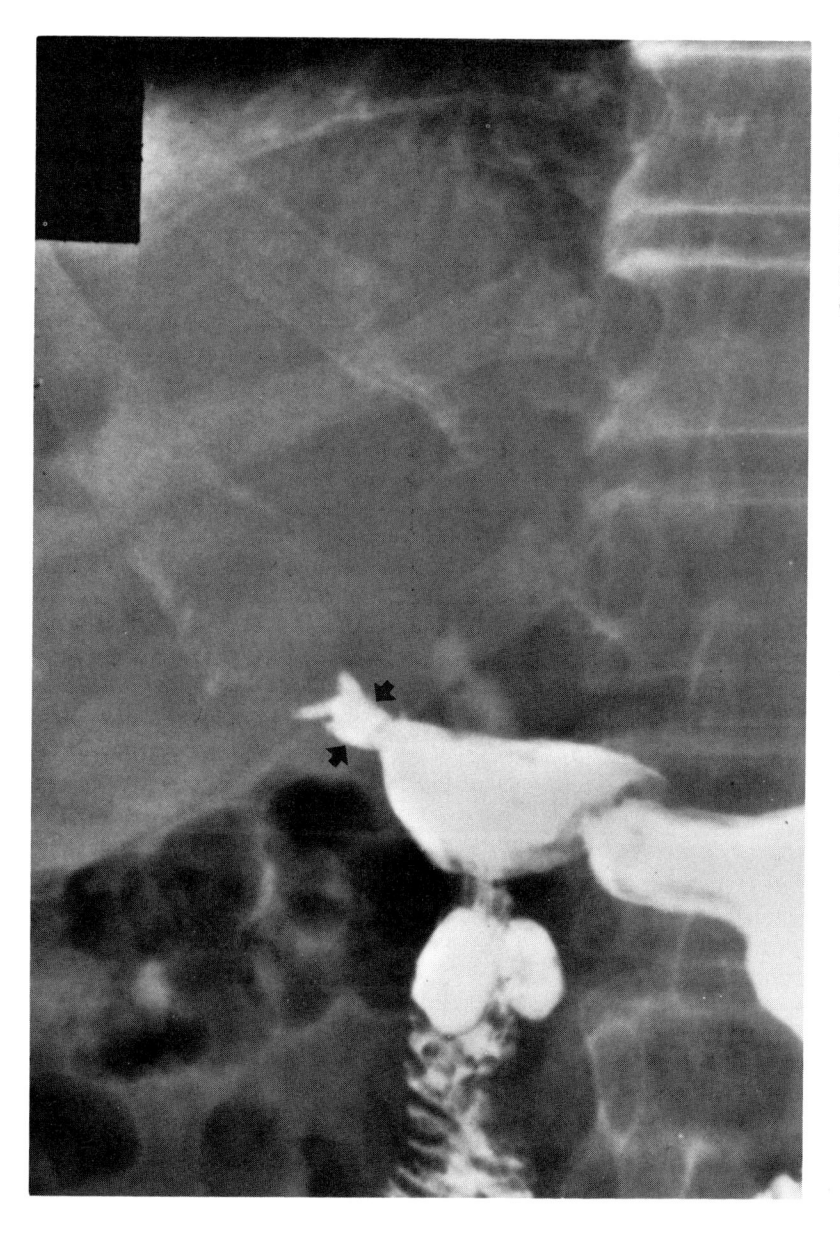

Figure 1–26. Barium contrast study demonstrating the cholecystoduodenal fistula in a patient with gallstone ileus. A small segment of the neck of the gallbladder is filled (arrows).

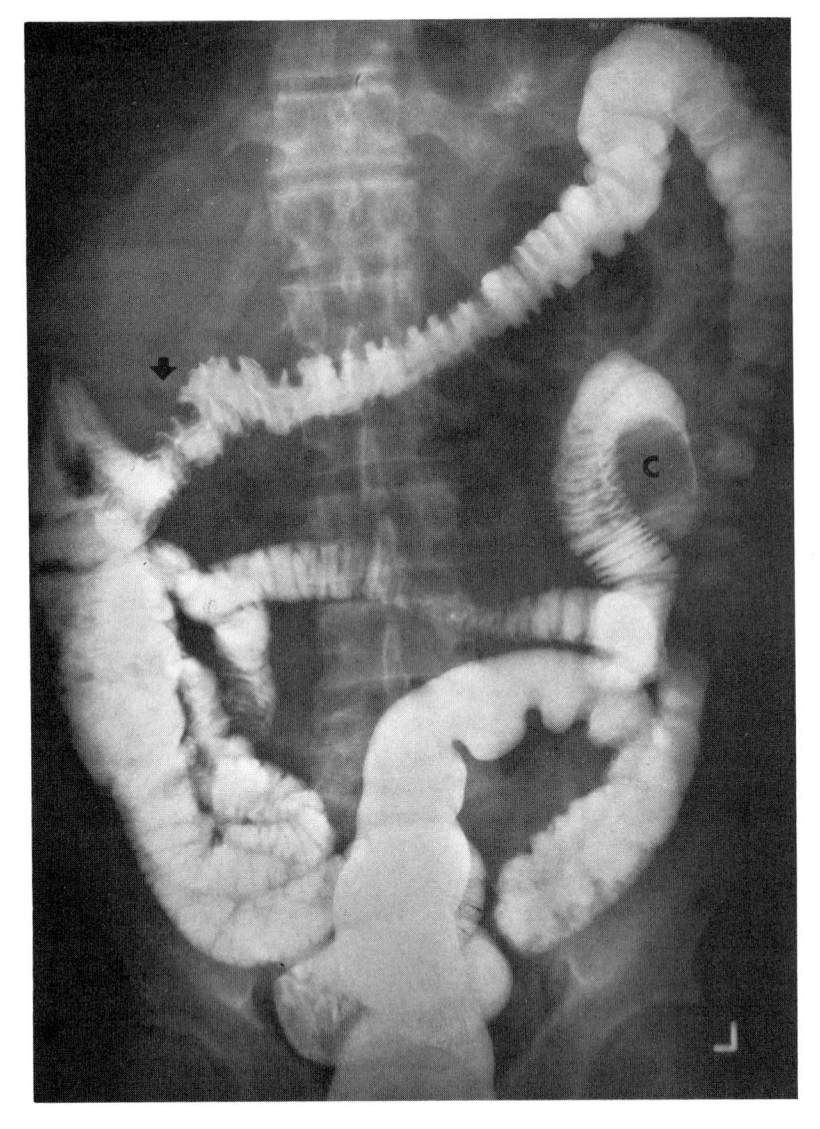

Figure 1-27. Barium enema examination performed on a patient with gallstone ileus. A long segment of the distal ileum was refluxed with demonstration of the obstructing nonopaque gallbladder calculus (C). A small amount of gas is demonstrated within the gallbladder (arrow).

ulcer perforation and 4 percent are attributable to a malignant process or the results of trauma.

Intestinal gas in the right upper quadrant may simulate air within the gallbladder. A distended duodenal bulb due to duodenal ileus could simulate gas within the gallbladder because of the anatomical proximity of these two structures. Contrast material by mouth would readily rule out the possibility of gas within the gallbladder.

Gas within the bile duct system is most commonly caused by communication with the gastrointestinal tract in the postoperative patient following sphincterotomy or choledochoenterostomy (7). More rare causes of gas within the bile duct system include incompetence of the sphincter of Vater secondary to a patulous sphincter in the elderly, pancreatitis, recent passage of calculi, and juxtaampullary neoplasm or inflammation secondary to peptic ulcer disease.

Gas in the bile duct system secondary to gas-forming organisms is rare. However, this has been described with pyogenic cholangitis (98) and may also occur when there is communication between the bile duct system and a liver abscess. Calculus disease rarely causes choledochointestinal fistulae.

Gas in the portal venous system is identified radiographically in the liver area as a branching radiolucent linear pattern extending to the periphery of the liver area (Figure 1-28). This portal vein gas is differentiated from gas within the bile ducts by its peripheral location. Gas in the bile duct system accumulates in the larger central ducts. This phenomenon has been attributed to the direction of flow of portal vein blood to the periphery, carrying gas bubbles with it; the flow of bile tends to localize gas in the more central ductal system (99,100).

Radiographic detection of gas in the portal venous system is an abnormal finding, usually secondary to a necrotic bowel and/or bacteremia. The mortality rate is extremely high in this group of patients (99-101). In the adult, gas in the portal venous

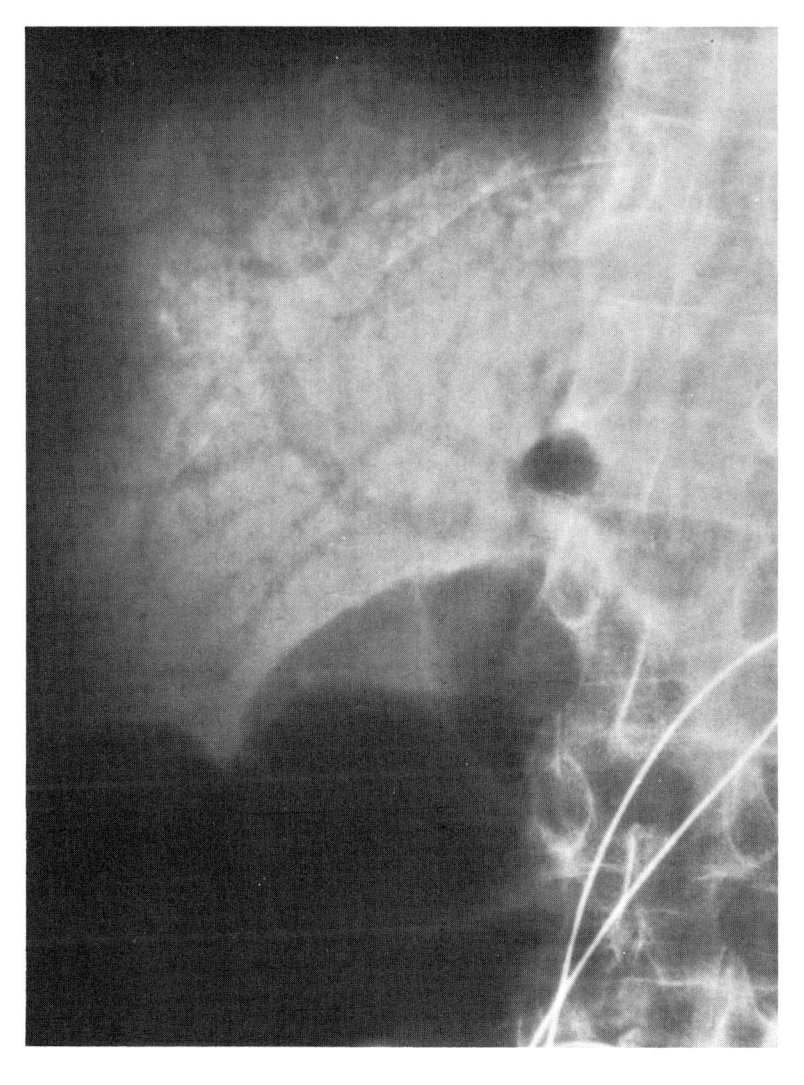

Figure 1-28. Portal venous gas in an adult with necrotizing colitis secondary to leukemia with chemotherapy. Extensive air is demonstrated throughout the portal venous system.

system is most commonly the result of ischemic bowel disease. In the infant, it is most commonly associated with necrotizing enterocolitis of the newborn (7). Less common, but also life-threatening, conditions that result in gas in the portal venous system include generalized sepsis, mechanical obstruction with bowel wall necrosis, diabetic coma, and pelvic and intraabdominal abscesses (7,101,102). Gas in the portal venous system is rarely associated with more benign etiologic conditions such as gastric and duodenal distention, gastric and duodenal peptic ulcer disease, hydrogen peroxide enemas, jugular and umbilical vein catheterization, and—following air-contrast barium enema examination of the colon in patients with inflammatory bowel disease—both ulcerative colitis and Crohn's disease (103). Thus gas in the portal venous system is not always a grave prognostic sign. The significance of this finding should be considered in the light of the patient's clinical condition.

The mechanism of gas accumulation in the portal venous system is not fully understood. Possible causes include passage of intraluminal gas from the distended bowel lumen through compromised mucosa into the mesenteric venous system, with embolization to the intrahepatic portal radicals, or actual invasion of the bowel wall and veins by gas-forming bacteria (99–102).

Intestinal pneumatosis, or air within the bowel wall, occurs when the integrity of the bowel wall has been compromised by ischemia, necrotizing enterocolitis, or caustic burns of the gastrointestinal tract. The linear accumulation of gas bubbles in association with gas in the portal venous system may be seen to suggest the etiology of the portal venous gas. However, gas may be present within the bowel wall and not be identified because of the associated gaseous distention of the bowel lumen.

Gas within the liver parenchyma is caused most commonly by gas formation within a liver abscess and gas gangrene of the liver. Radiologically, gas within a liver abscess can present as a single loculated air-fluid level or multiple loculated air-fluid levels, or multiple small air bubbles without air-fluid levels (92,104–107). The latter is seen most often with gas gangrene (clostridial infection) of the liver (106,107). Occasionally gas may be seen in the liver following penetrating wounds of this organ (7). Liver abscesses result most commonly from portal venous drainage system infection, biliary tract obstruction and infection, and generalized sepsis (7,104). Less common causes of liver abscess include trauma, tumor, or adjacent infection. The majority of liver abscesses do not contain gas (7). Amebic liver abscesses do not contain gas unless secondary bacterial infection (Figure 1–29) (92) or air is introduced into the abscess at the time of drainage. The radiologic differential diagnosis of a gas-containing abscess within the liver includes most commonly subphrenic abscess. Other entities include emphysematous cholecystitis, renal and perinephric abscesses, subhepatic abscess, and interposition of the right colon between the liver and the anterior abdominal wall (Chilaiditi's syndrome) (108,109). In the plain film evaluation of abnormal gas lucencies in the right upper quadrant, films in upright and in both decubitus positions are a necessity, as are well-penetrated films of the thoracoabdominal region, including the lower portions of both pleural spaces. Contrast examinations of the upper gastrointestinal tract and colon may be necessary on occasion to confirm the extraluminal nature of gas shadows in the right upper quadrant.

The differential diagnosis between right subphrenic abscess and liver abscess is difficult. Generally with liver abscess there is more tissue between the abscess cavity and the diaphragmatic margin than with subphrenic abscess. The lack of pleural reaction or effusion in the right pleural space and no limitation of motion of the right hemidiaphragm indicate liver abscess over right subphrenic abscess (104).

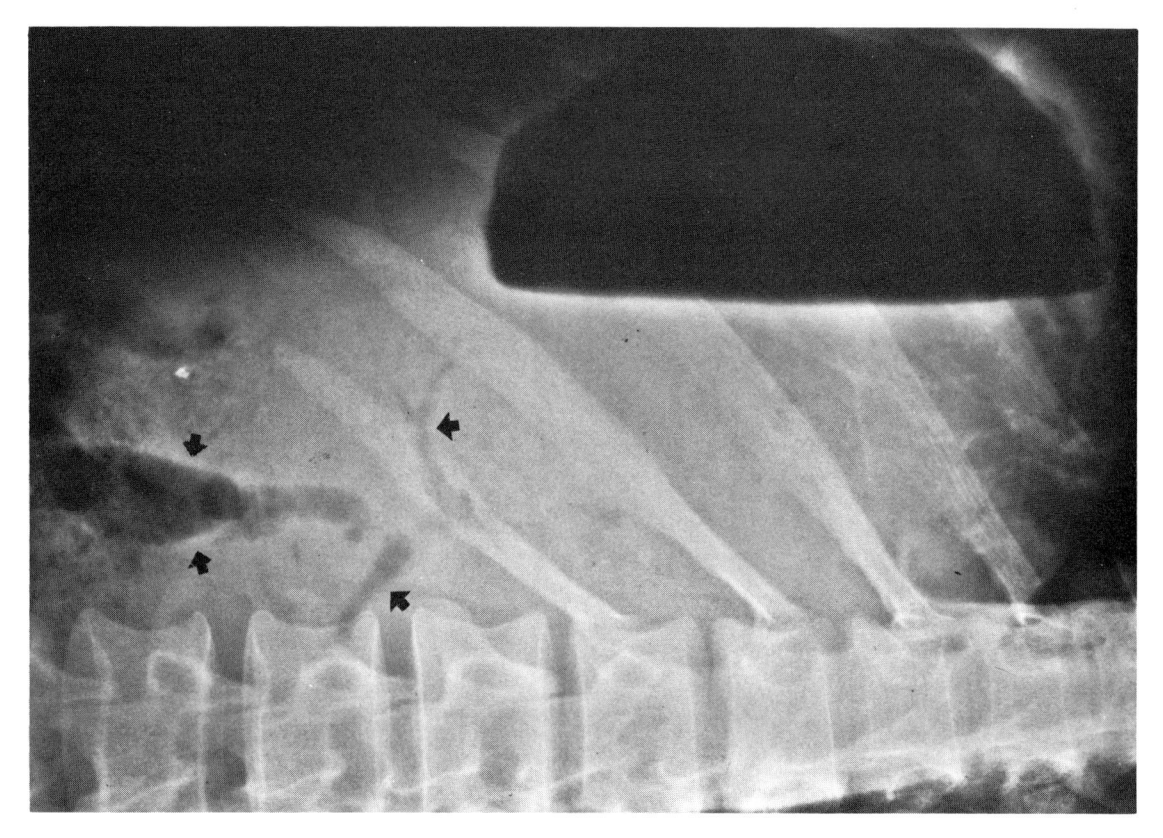

Figure 1-29. A secondarily infected amebic abscess. The left lateral decubitus film demonstrates the large smoothly outlined cavity with an air-fluid level. In addition, gas is identified within the bile duct and gallbladder (arrows), indicating that the abscess communicates with the ductal system.

In the evaluation of suspected right upper quadrant inflammatory process, other modalities of abdominal imaging are more efficient than plain films in the detection and localization of loculated inflammatory process. These include nuclear liver scanning, ultrasound, and computed tomography of the abdomen (104,110). Of these modalities, computed tomographic examination of the abdomen is considered the most accurate and efficient (110).

Perihepatic gas can result from perihepatic abscess (Figures 1-30,1-31,1-32), pneumoperitoneum, and interposition of the right colon between the liver and anterior abdominal wall. Perihepatic abscesses occur most commonly following abdominal surgery, secondary to anastomotic leaks. They are less commonly the result of gastric and duodenal peptic ulcer disease, biliary tract disease, pelvic inflammatory disease, and appendicitis (7).

Whalen (111) has classified the potential spaces of localization of perihepatic abscesses by the divisions created by the ligamentous attachments of the liver. The right subphrenic space is divided from the right subhepatic space by the coronary ligament, which attaches to the liver posteriorly. The inferior leaf of the coronary ligament parallels the right eleventh rib, delineating the superior extent of the right subhepatic

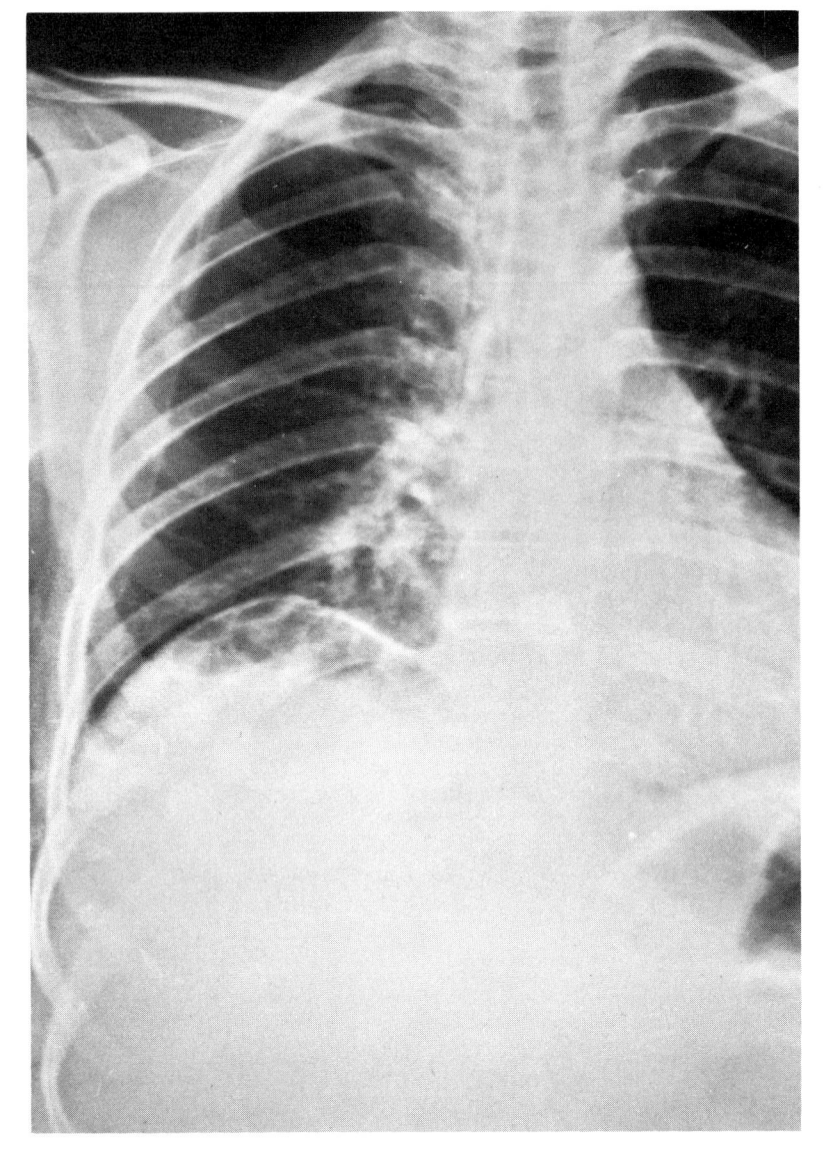

Figure 1-30. Chest film demonstrating right subphrenic abscess secondary to pelvic abscess. There is minimal reaction in the base of the right lung.

space. On the left, the coronary ligament separates the anterior and posterior left subphrenic spaces. The falciform ligament separates right and left anterior subphrenic spaces. The gastrohepatic ligament divides the left subhepatic space into anterior and posterior (lesser sac) compartments.

As discussed earlier, the differentiation of right subphrenic abscess from liver abscess can be difficult on plain films, and more definitive information can be obtained by computerized tomography, ultrasound, and nuclear liver scanning (110). A right subhepatic abscess is usually confined below the eleventh right rib by the inferior leaf of the coronary ligament. Secondary intrathoracic changes are usually absent. On the left, contrast media in the stomach helps differentiate a left lobe abscess from left subphrenic abscess. An enlarged left lobe of the liver displaces the stomach posteriorly,

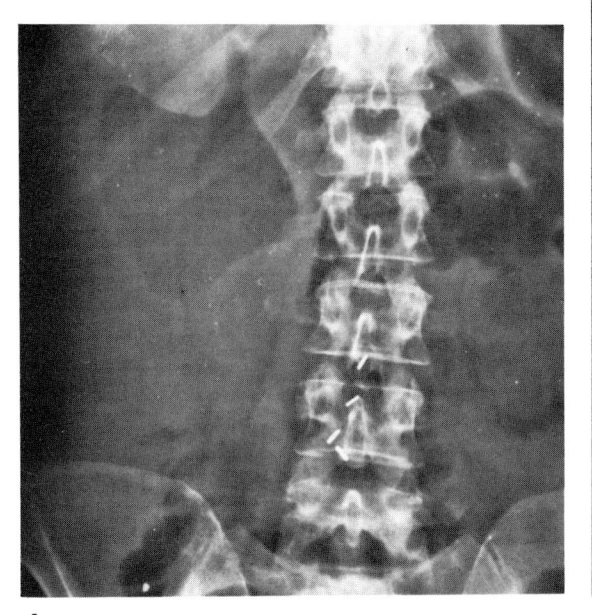

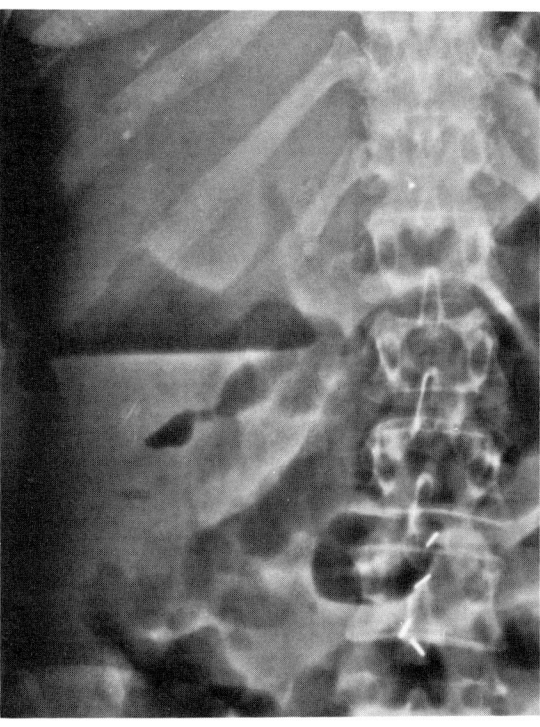

Figure 1-31. Recumbent (*A*) and erect (*B*) films of the right abdomen in a patient with a right subhepatic abscess secondary to pelvic abscess. On the erect film, the loculated gas does not extend above the level of the eleventh rib.

whereas a left subphrenic abscess displaces the stomach inferiorly. An abscess in the posterior subhepatic space (lesser omental sac) usually displaces the stomach superiorly and anteriorly.

Pneumoperitoneum occurs most commonly as a result of perforated gastric or duodenal peptic ulceration, perforated colonic diverticulum, and traumatic rupture of an abdominal viscus (112). Localized air in the right upper quadrant is the most frequent plain film finding with the patient in recumbent position. Menuck and Siemers (112) described the two most common patterns as: (1) a linear lucency along the posterior-inferior liver margin, and (2) a triangular lucency lying over the superior portion of the right kidney. Both of these areas are in the region of the posterior extent of the right subhepatic space (Morison's pouch). Other recumbent plain film findings of free air include visualization of the outer wall of intestinal loops, a rounded lucency in the anterior abdomen, and visualization of the falciform ligament (Figure 1-33) (112,113). Erect films of the chest, erect and lateral decubitus films of the abdomen, and the supine lateral film of the abdomen utilizing a horizontal x-ray beam are much more efficient in the diagnosis of pneumoperitoneum and the differentiation from perihepatic abscess.

Interposition of the colon between the liver and anterior abdominal wall (Chilaiditi's syndrome) may on occasion simulate free perihepatic air (108,109). Usually, colonic haustra can be identified by an outline of intraluminal air, indicating the intraluminal location of the gas. Contrast examination of the colon without preparation can readily

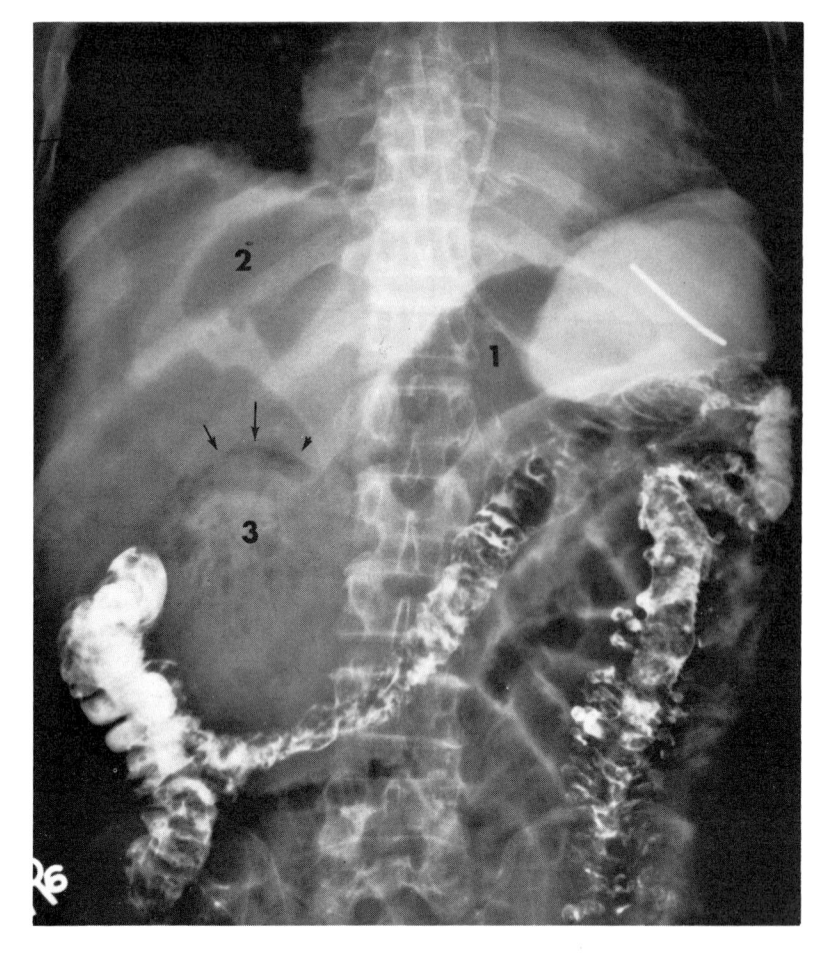

Figure 1–32. Multiple periphepatic abscesses secondary to perforated gastric carcinoma. Abscess in the left posterior compartment (lesser sac) (1). Right subphrenic abscess (2). Right subhepatic abscess (3). The curved linear gas shadow indicated by the arrows represents gas trapped in the posterior extent of the right subhepatic space (Morison's pouch). Barium is present in the colon from prior barium enema and water-soluble contrast material is present in the fundus of the stomach.

confirm the presence of the interposed colon and rule out both pneumoperitoneum and subphrenic or hepatic abscess.

HEPATIC ABNORMALITIES WITH ACCOMPANYING SYSTEMIC MANIFESTATIONS OF HEPATIC DISEASE

Cirrhosis

Cirrhosis is defined as extensive hepatic fibrosis with nodule formation, the result of hepatocyte necrosis (4). Causes of cirrhosis include alcoholism, hepatitis, prolonged cholestasis, cardiac failure, hemochromatosis, Wilson's disease, hepatic venous obstruction, malnutrition, congenital syphilis, and a variety of drugs and toxins. Cirrhosis can be diffuse (as seen in patients with alcoholism), for example, micronodular cirrhosis; focal, for example, macronodular cirrhosis; or mixed (114). Despite the type of injury, the liver's response is identical: fatty degeneration, formation of fibrous septa, and nodular regeneration (115). The eventual outcome is portal hypertension and liver failure.

The clinical signs of cirrhosis include jaundice, ascites, fever, encephalopathy, and fine tremors of the upper extremities. Laboratory data reflect liver failure with elevation

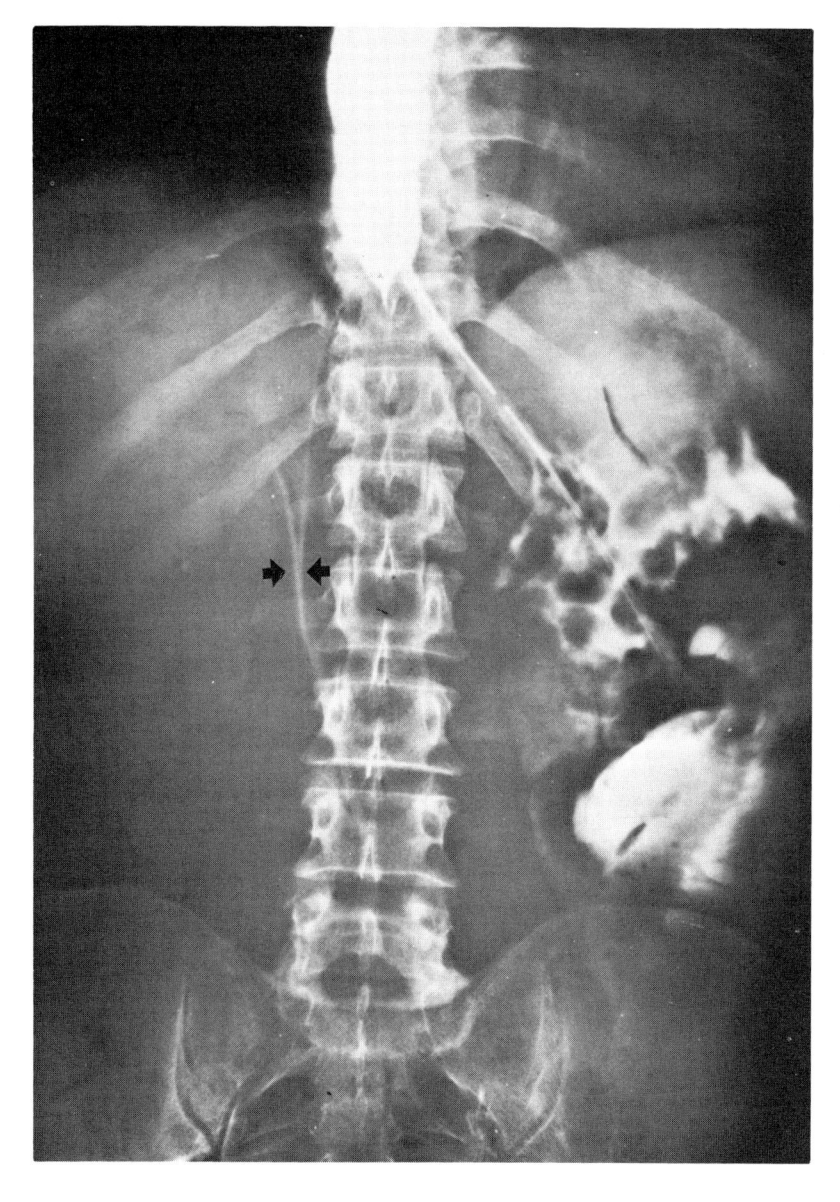

Figure 1-33. Massive pneumoperitoneum as a result of perforation of the stomach secondary to gastric volvulus. Water-soluble contrast material partially outlines the stomach. The recumbent film demonstrates diffuse lucency throughout the entire abdomen. The linear density indicated by the arrows represents the falciform ligament outlined by the free air in the peritoneal cavity.

of bilirubin and transaminase levels, decrease in serum albumin, and prothrombin deficiency. Complications of cholelithiasis, pancreatitis, peptic ulcer disease, and eventually hepatoma can also occur.

The radiographic plain film manifestations of cirrhosis include findings in the abdomen, lungs, and bones. The plain film of the abdomen can reflect hepatosplenomegaly, ascites, gallstones (Figure 1-34), and calcifications of the pancreas in chronic pancreatitis.

Occasionally, a contracted cirrhotic liver can appear to be denser than usual, especially when ascites is present surrounding it. It is uncertain whether this is due to the increased fibrosis or to the relative increase in density as the result of contrast with adjacent retroperitoneal fat. (10).

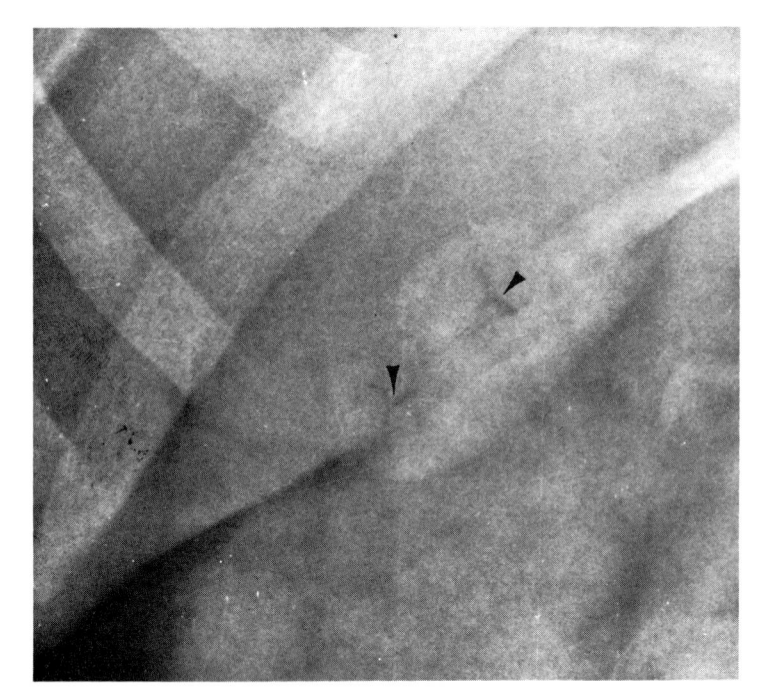

Figure 1-34. Noncalcified gallstones (arrows) demonstrating "Mercedes Benz" sign of gas within gallstone fissures (black arrowheads).

Figure 1-35. Twenty-five-year-old male cirrhotic with hepatic osteoarthropathy. Note the dense periostial new bone along the medial and lateral aspects of the distal femur (arrowhead).

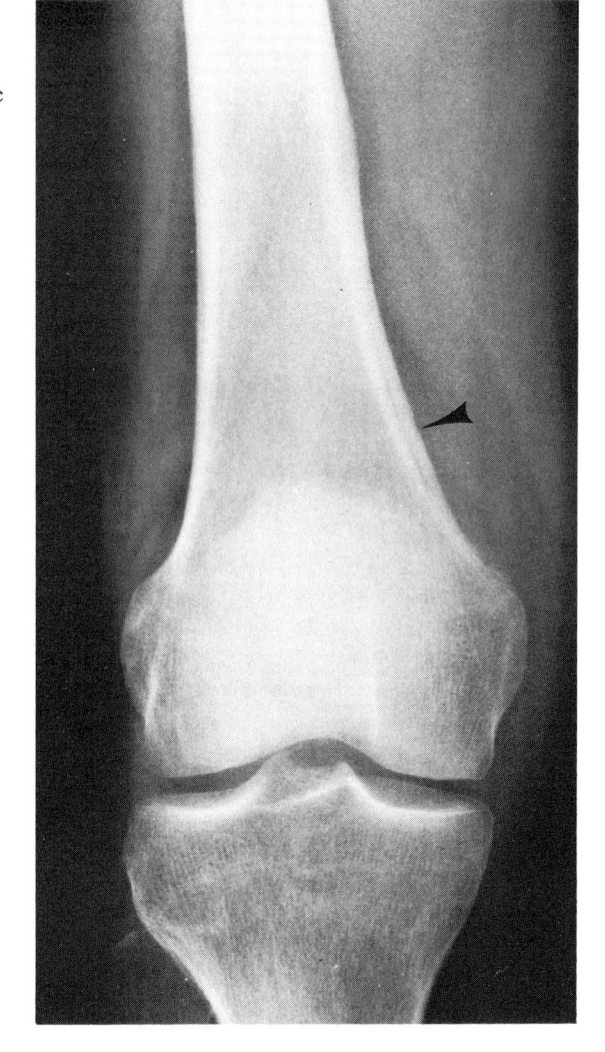

Reports of visibly fatty livers have also been published (116,117). These have been primarily in children whose cirrhosis was secondary to fibrocystic disease with diffuse fatty metamorphosis, although children with malnutrition, viral hepatitis, kwashiorkor, Cushing's syndrome, Type I glycogen storage disease, familial hyperlipidemia, fructose intolerance, and liver toxins have also been described (91,118,119).

Long bone abnormalities have been well-described. Chronic biliary cirrhosis and post hepatic cirrhosis (as well as other chronic diseases, such as benign biliary strictures, bile duct carcinoma, and chronic active hepatitis) have been associated with a dense hypertrophic osteoarthropathy of the long bones (Figure 1–35) (120–124). Symmetric involvement of the distal tibia and fibula is seen in 95 percent of cases, with distal femoral, metatarsal, and phalangeal changes noted less commonly (Figure 1–36). The

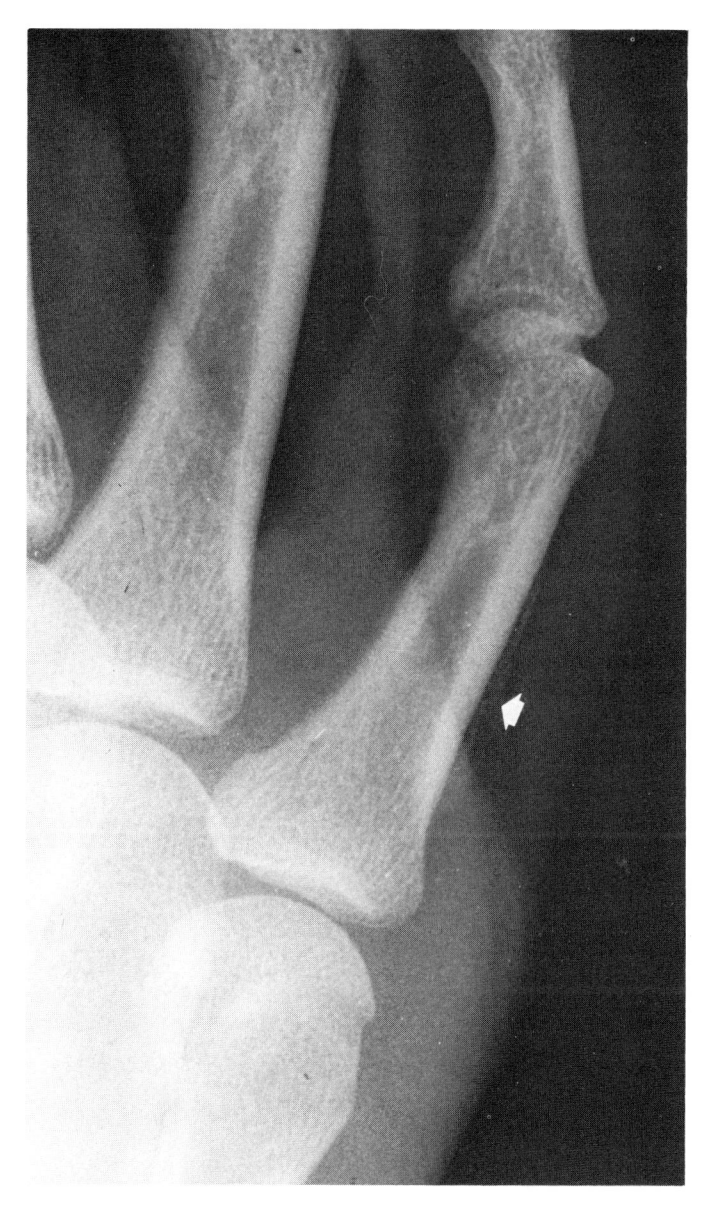

Figure 1–36. Same patient as in Figure 1–35 with hepatic osteoarthropathy demonstrated as more subtle periostial new bone in the proximal fifth phalanx (arrowhead).

periostial reaction begins distally and spreads proximally (125). Ninety percent of these patients are jaundiced; 95 percent have clubbing. The bone changes are generally asymptomatic, however. The extent of bone change does not correlate with the degree of liver disease.

Aseptic necrosis, especially in the femoral heads, has been described in patients with liver disease (Figure 1-37). Presumably, showers of emboli from the fatty liver are implicated (126). This same etiology has been presumed to cause infarcts in the metaphyses of infants.

Patients with cirrhosis and portal hypertension commonly develop portal-systemic collateral veins. These have been described on chest x-rays as lobulated posterior mediastinal masses when distal esophageal varices are present (127). Enlargement of the azygos vein to diameters of 20 mm or greater has also been noted (128). Pulmonary edema can also occur in patients with liver failure, probably of neurogenic origin, possibly also, in part, due to altered vascular permeability (129–131), creating an adult respiratory distress syndrome (ARDS) pattern.

Arteriovenous shunting is present (132) due to small intraacinar vessels (133), creating tiny pulmonary nodules on the chest x-ray. These nodules represent the dilated vessels (134,135). Right-to-left shunting has also been reported in these patients during lung perfusion scans (136,137).

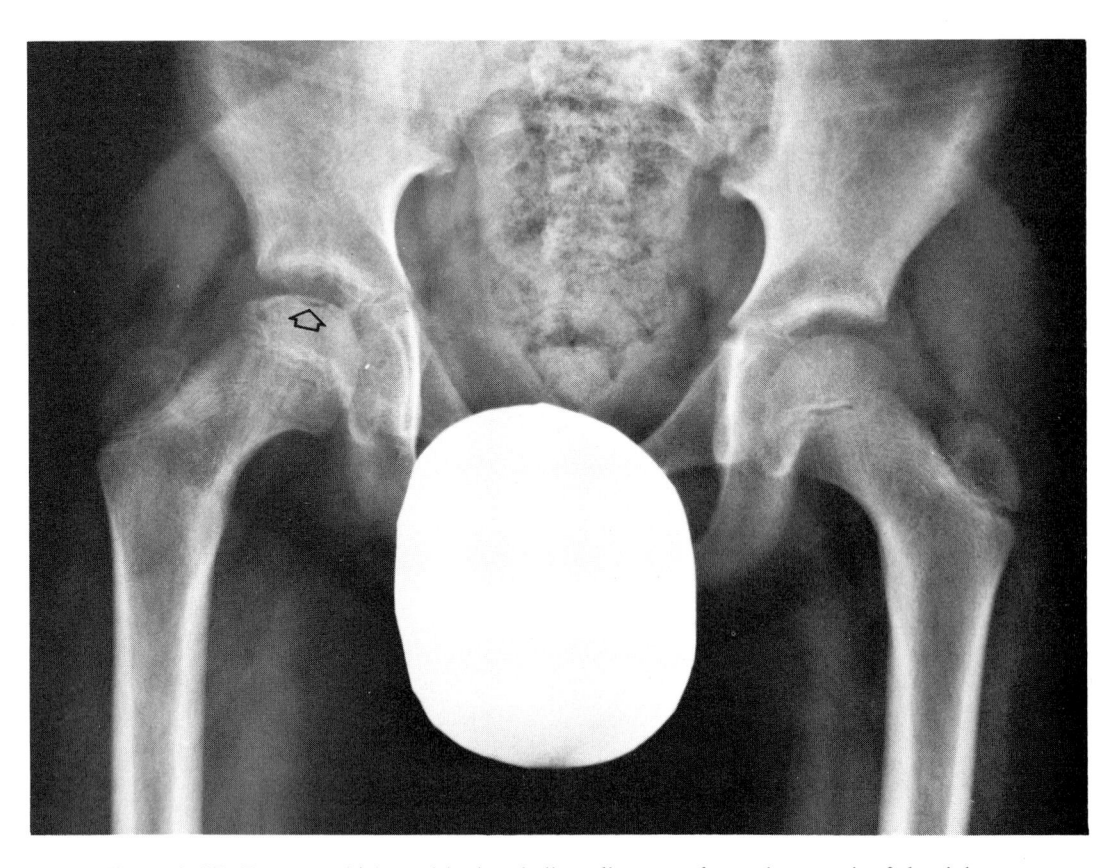

Figure 1-37. Ten-year-old boy with chronic liver disease and aseptic necrosis of the right femoral head (arrowhead).

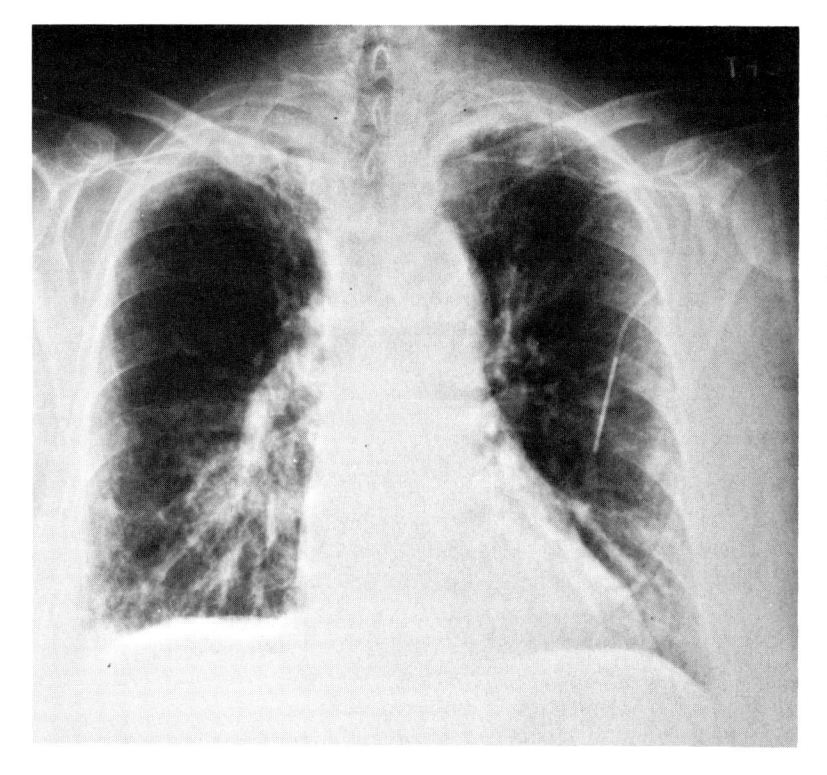

Figure 1-38. Fifty-five-year-old man with subacute viral hepatitis demonstrating bibasilar interstitial infiltrates (lymphocyte interstitial pneumonia).

In the precirrhotic stage of viral hepatitis, bibasilar interstitial infiltrates can occur, so-called lymphocytic interstitial pneumonia (LIP) (138) (Figure 1-38). Similar changes have also been reported histologically in the liver (139).

Anemia

Sickle cell disease results from the effect of a genetically transmitted abnormal hemoglobin in which the red blood cells assume a sickle shape when exposed to low levels of oxygen.

In such cases the marrow becomes hyperactive, creating widened medullary cavities and generalized osteoporosis (140). Vertebrae have a "fish-mouth," or biconcave, appearance secondary to focal ischemic changes in the centers of the end-plates. Cortical and medullary infarcts have also been noted (141).

Infants exhibit dactylitis clinically with widening of bones, lytic changes, and periostitis secondary to osteomyelitis. Children demonstrate delayed maturation and osteonecrosis of the humeral and femoral heads secondary to localized infarctions leading to osteoarthritis in later life.

Thalassemia is a hereditary defect in the synthesis of hemoglobin that causes destruction of erythrocytes (142). This condition is divided into thalassemia major (more severe cases), and thalassemia minor. The liver is enlarged markedly as is the spleen, especially in thalassemia major. Bones show widened medullary spaces and the long and tubular bones show thinned cortices. The skull has widened diploe, creating the classic "hair-on-end" appearance.

Table 1-1. Classification of Glycogen Storage Diseases by Enzymatic Defect

Type	Disease	Organs Affected
I	von Gierke's	Liver, kidneys, small bowel
II	Pompe's	Heart, central nervous system, muscle, general, leukocytes
III	Cori's (Forbes')	Liver, heart, muscle, leukocytes
IV	Anderson's (amylopectinosis)	Liver, general
V	McArdle's	Skeleton, muscles
VI	Her's	Liver, leukocytes

Glycogen Storage Disease

These diseases are autosomal recessive disorders of carbohydrate metabolism. Six inborn errors of metabolism cause defects in enzymes responsible for glycogen storage in many organs, creating an excess of normal or abnormal glycogen. The types of glycogen storage disease are classified by the enzymatic defect and are listed in Table 1-1 (143).

In all but Types II and V, 95 percent have marked hepatomegaly, often occupying a large portion of the abdomen and pelvis. The hepatocytes of these patients show marked infiltration with abnormal glycogen, as well as fatty metamorphosis. Cirrhosis can occur in Types III and VI (144). Hepatic cell adenomas have been reported (145–147), which can undergo malignant transformation (147).

Children with glycogen storage disease are growth retarded, reflecting the changes of hypoglycemia on bone physiology. A generalized osteoporosis is present with widening of the diaphyses and ribs, kyphoscoliosis, multiple fractures (Types I, III, and IV), spiculation of the growth plates and metaphyses (Types I, II, III, IV, and VI) (143,144) and gout (Types I and III).

Gaucher's Disease

This disease is a familial metabolic defect in which abnormal deposits of cerebrosides are identified within the reticuloendothelial system. A definite Jewish predilection is present.

Two forms occur. The infantile form is fatal, with survival not past 18 months. The chronic or progressive form is variable in intensity and in the degree of involvement of various organs (liver, spleen, bones). Eighty percent of cases have marked hepatomegaly (14). The bones are packed with Gaucher's cells, causing widening of the medullary cavities and pressure atrophy of the cortices. This creates an Erlenmeyer flask deformity. Irregular areas of rarefaction are also present as the result of mass effect of the abnormal cells on the trabeculae (Figure 1-39) (148–150).

Wilson's Disease

This disease is an autosomal recessive disorder in which abnormal amounts of copper are absorbed from the gastrointestinal tract and deposited in various other organs. It is rarely apparent clinically before the age of 6 years, usually presenting when the

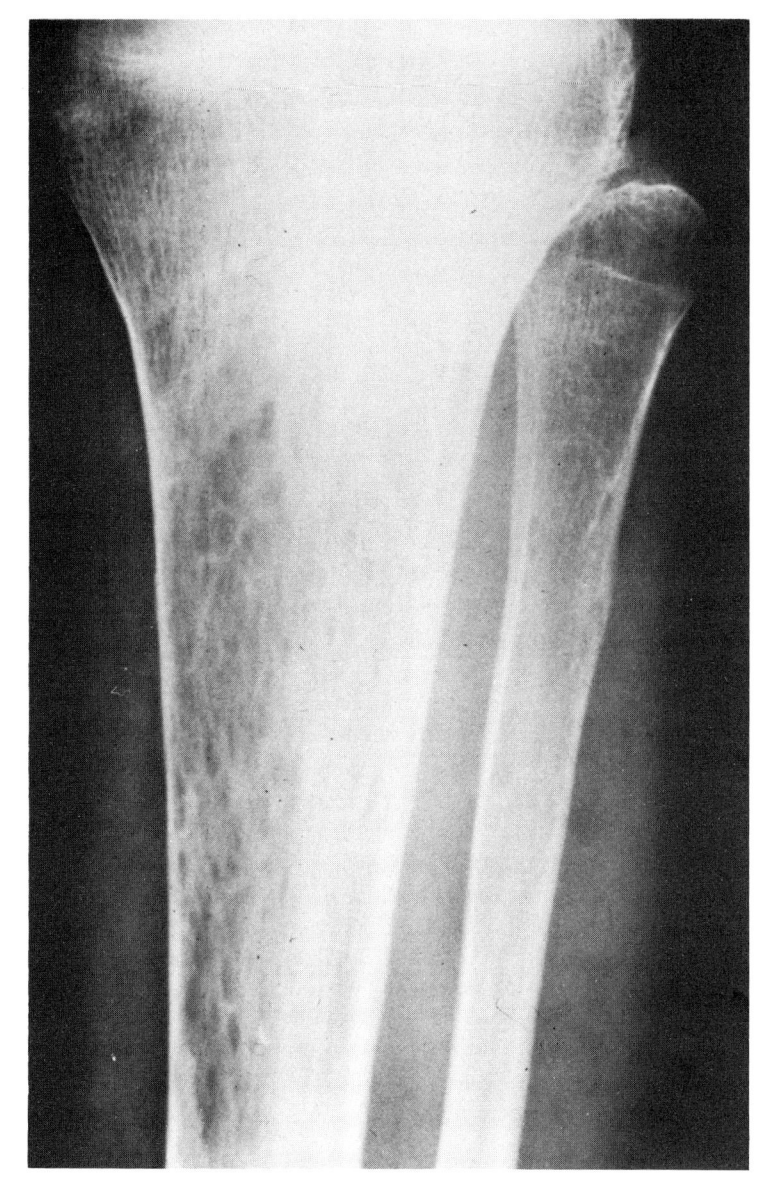

Figure 1-39. Twenty-four-year-old male with Gaucher's disease. There is a marked honeycomb pattern in the medullary cavity of the proximal tibia, reflecting the coarsened and widely spaced trabeculae.

patient is 12 to 20 years of age. When present in the liver and brain, hepatolenticular degeneration exists (151). Wilson's disease is often associated with psychiatric and neurological symptoms, arthropathies, and renal tubular acidosis.

The liver is usually involved and cirrhosis is commonly present (152–154). When it occurs, it can be present months to years before it is clinically apparent. It is seldom the dominant clinical feature (152). Eighty-five percent of cases have minor bone changes, such as osteomalacia, pseudofractures, microlocular and multilocular cysts at sites of tendon and ligamentous insertion, bone fragmentation, and anterior vertebral body compression deformities (153). Cartilaginous degeneration secondary to premature degenerative changes is seen in young patients. Chondrocalcinosis (Figure 1–40) is not uncommon (140,152).

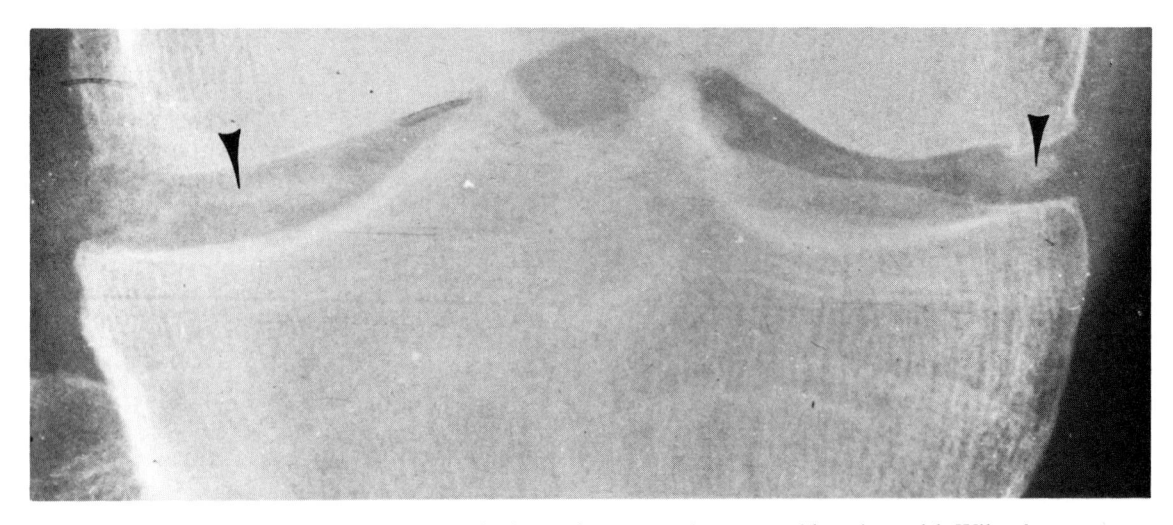

Figure 1-40. Chondrocalcinosis in the knee of a twenty-three-year-old patient with Wilson's disease (arrowheads).

Cholangitis

Pericholangitis is an inflammatory cholestatic process localized to the periductal regions of the liver. It can eventually result in chronic active hepatitis, postnecrotic cirrhosis, or biliary cirrhosis (151). It is manifested clinically by jaundice, fever, chills, pain, leukocytosis, and hepatosplenomegaly. Rarely, pericholangitis has been diagnosed subsequent to the diagnosis of ulcerative colitis.

Sclerosing cholangitis is a rare inflammatory disease affecting the submucosal and subserosal layers of the common bile duct and, occasionally, intrahepatic ducts (155). The end result is fibrosis and a thickening of the wall, with marked narrowing creating biliary cirrhosis and portal hypertension. It most commonly affects males in the fourth to fifth decades. It has been associated with other inflammatory or immunological disorders, such as Riedel's struma, retroperitoneal and mediastinal fibrosis, ulcerative colitis, porphyria, disseminated vasculitis, and immune deficiency diseases (151). The diagnosis can only be made radiographically by opacification of the bile ducts.

Cystic Diseases

Cystic disease of the liver is rare and often associated with cysts of other organs, especially the kidneys (156). Liver cysts, per se, are usually asymptomatic unless they rupture or bleed. Larger cysts can create pressure effects on other structures and may create symptoms in this manner.

These cysts are difficult to diagnose but have three presentations on plain films of the abdomen: (1) their outer rims may form a thin ring of calcium; (2) they may displace adjacent structures, such as the stomach, gallbladder and right diaphragm; or (3) they may be radiolucent, best demonstrated with tomography or after intravenous pyelogram (IVP) (157) (Figure 1-41).

Polycystic renal disease can be divided into two major categories: infantile and adult types. Both are genetically, clinically, and morphologically unrelated. The infantile type

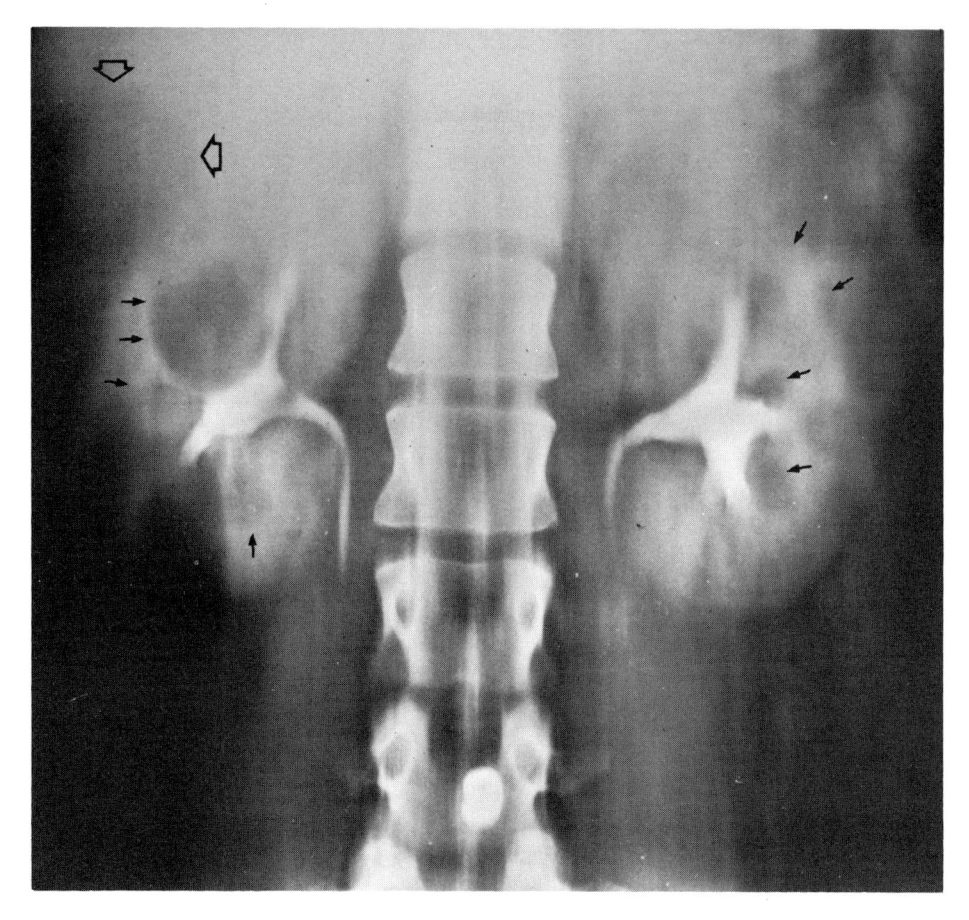

Figure 1-41. Twenty-year-old woman with hepatic cystic disease. This tomographic study during an IVP demonstrates a large lucent defect in the inferior margin of the right lobe of the liver representing a solitary liver cyst (open arrowheads). There are multiple renal cysts bilaterally (arrows).

is autosomal recessive. Four subtypes are present: perinatal, neonatal, infantile, and juvenile (158). These types generally relate to the age and degree of onset of diffuse cystic changes in the collecting tubules. In the juvenile form, liver disease predominates with portal fibrosis encasing the ducts. Hepatomegaly and portal hypertension are present.

The adult type is inherited by an autosomal dominant trait, clincially detected in the 40- to 50-year-old population, although it can be seen in infancy (159). The renal cysts involve not only the collecting tubules, but also the nephrons. Fifty percent of patients with cystic livers have polycystic renal disease. Only 20 to 30 percent with polycystic disease will have hepatic cysts. Liver cysts are felt to be developmental defects of the bile ducts. No cirrhosis or portal hypertension is present in the adult form. Ten percent of cases have pancreatic cysts; 10 percent have berry aneurysms.

Zellweger's disease is a rare condition of biliary dysgenesis, cirrhosis, and fibrosis, also associated with renal cysts (160).

REFERENCES

1. Bockus HL (ed): Gastroenterology. Philadelphia: Saunders, 1965.
2. Gelfand DW: Anatomy of the liver. Radiol Clin North Am 1980;18(2):187–194.
3. Goss GM (ed): Gray's Anatomy of the Human Body. Philadelphia: Lea & Feibiger, 1973, pp 1244–1250.
4. McNulty JG. Radiology of the Liver. Philadelphia: Saunders, 1977.
5. Kane RA: Sonographic anatomy of the liver. Seminars in Ultrasound 1981;7(3):190–197.
6. Marks WM, Filly RA, Callen PW: Ultrasonic anatomy of the liver: A review of new applications. J. Clin Ultrasound 1979;7:137–146.
7. Mindelzun R, McCort J: Hepatic and perihepatic radiolucencies. Radiol Clin North Am 1980;18:221–238.
8. McAfee JG, Ause RG, and Wagner HN: Diagnostic value of scintillation scanning of the liver. Arch Intern Med 1965;116:95.
9. Okuda K, Ilo M: Radiologic Aspects of the Liver and Biliary Tree. Igaku Shoin Pub., distributed by Year Book Med. Pub., Chicago, 1976.
10. Kattan KR: The effect of changes in liver volume on the adjacent viscera. Radiol Clin North Am 1980;18:195–207.
11. Friedman E, Lewi Z: Gastric displacement in atrophic liver cirrhosis. Radiology 1962;79:644–646.
12. Meyers HI, Jacobson G: Displacement of stomach and duodenum by anomalous lobes of the liver. AJR 1958;79:789.
13. Kattan KR, Moskowitz M: Position of the duodenal bulb and liver size. AJR 1973;119:78–83.
14. Whalen JP: Radiology of the Abdomen: Anatomic Basis. Philadelphia: Lea & Febiger, 1976.
15. Baker SR, Elkin M: Plain Film Approach to Abdominal Calcifications. Saunders Monographs in Clinical Radiology, vol. 21. Philadelphia: Saunders, 1983.
16. Darlak JJ, Moskowitz M, Kattan KR: Calcifications in the liver. Radiol Clin North Am 1981;18:209–219.
17. Gelfand DW: The liver: Plain film diagnosis. Semin Roentgenol 1975;10:177–185.
18. Karras BG, Cannon AH, Zanon B Jr.: Hepatic calcifications. Acta Radiol 1962;57:458–468.
19. Zipser RD, Rau JE, Ricketts RR, Bevans LC. Tuberculous pseudotumors of the liver. Am J Med 1976;61:946–951.
20. Astley R, Harrison N: Miliary calcification of the liver: Report of a case. Br J Radiol 1949;22:723–724.
21. Clemett AR: Radiology of the liver and bile ducts. In Margulis AR, Burhenne HJ (eds): Alimentary Tract Radiology vol. 2:1371–1433, 3rd ed. St. Louis: Mosby, 1983.
22. Schwartz J, Silverman FN, Adriano M, et al.: The relation of splenic calcification to histoplasmosis. N Eng J Med 1955;252:887–891.
23. Symmers D, Spain DM: Hepar lobatum. Arch Pathol Lab Med 1946;66:64–68.
24. Alergant CD: Gumma of the liver with calcification; Case report. AMA Arch Intern Med 1956;98:340–343.
25. Haddow RA, Kemp-Harper RA: Calcifications in the liver and portal system. Clin Radiol 1967;18:225–236.
26. McGarity WC, Serafin D: Brucellosis: Indication for splenectomy. Am J Surg 1968;115:355–363.
27. Spink WW: Suppuration and calcification of the liver and spleen due to long standing infection with Brucella Suis. N Eng J Med 1957;257:209–210.
28. Yow EM, Brennan JC, Nathan MH, Israel L: Calcified granulomata of the spleen in long standing Brucella infection. Ann Intern Med 1961;55:307–313.
29. Caldicott WJH, Baehner RL. Chronic granulomatous disease of childhood. AJR 1968;103:133–139.

30. Gold RH, Douglas SD, Preger L, et al.: Roentgenographic features of the neutrophil dysfunction syndromes. Radiology 1969;92:1045–1054.
31. Bonakdarpour A: Echinococcus disease: Report of 112 cases from Iran and a review of 611 cases from the United States. AJR 1967;99:660–667.
32. Gonzalez LR, Marcos J, Illanas M, et al.: Radiologic aspects of hepatic echinoccosis. Radiology 1979;130:21–27.
33. Hadidi A: Sonography of hepatic echinococcal cysts. Gastrointest Radiol 1982;7:349–354.
34. McAfee JG, Donner MW: Differential diagnosis of calcifications encountered in abdominal radiographs. Am J Med Sci 1962;243:609–650.
35. Landay MJ, Hartona S, Hirsh G, et al.: Hepatic and thoracic amebiasis. AJR 1980;135:449–454.
36. Reeder MM: Tropical diseases of the liver and bile ducts. Semin Roentgenol 1975;10:229–243.
37. Caplan LH, Simon M: Nonparasitic cysts of the liver. AJR 1966;96:421–428.
38. Coutsoftides T, Hermann RE: Nonparasitic cysts of the liver. Surg Gynecol Obstet 1974;138:906–910.
39. Heilbrun N, Klein AJ: Massive calcification of the liver: Case report with a discussion of its etiology on the basis of alveolar hydatid disease. AJR 1946;55:189–192.
40. Thompson WM, Chisholm DP, Tank R: Plain film roengenographic findings in alveolar hydatid disease: *Echinococcus Multilocularis.* AJR 1972;116:345–358.
41. Grange D, Drumeaux D, Couzineau P, et al.: Hepatic calcification due to fasciola gigantica. Arch Surg 1974;108:113–115.
42. Chartres JC: Radiological manifestations of parasitism by the tongue worms, flat worms, and the round worms more commonly seen in the tropics. Br J Radiol 1965;38:503–511.
43. Samuel E: Roentgenology of parasitic calcification. AJR 1950;63:512–522.
44. Khajani A: Guinea worm calcification: A report of 83 cases. Clin Radiol 1968;19:433–435.
45. Okuda K, Jinnouchi S, Arakawa M, et al.: Generalized calcification of the liver in advanced schistosomiasis japonica: A case report. Acta Hepatogastroenterol 1975;22:98–102.
46. Shackelford GD, Kirks DR: Neonatal hepatic calcification secondary to transplacental infection. Radiology 1977;122:753–757.
47. Ameres JP, Levine MP, DeBlasi HP: Acalculous clonorchiasis obstructing the common bile duct: A case report and review of the literature. Am Surg 1976;42:170.
48. Hall M, Winkelman EI, Hawk WA, Hermann RE: Calcifications in the liver, an unusual feature of ductal cell hepatic carcinoma: Report of a case. Cleve Clin Q 1970;37:93–105.
49. Ludwig J, Grier MW, Hoffman HN, McGill DB: Calcified mixed malignant tumors of the liver. Arch Pathol Lab Med 1975;99:162–169.
50. Allen RW, Holt AH: Calcification in primary liver carcinoma. AJR 1967;99:150–152.
51. Meyers A: Calcification in cholangiocarcinoma. Br J Radiol 1968;41:65–66.
52. Schroder JS: Calcifications in the liver. J Med Assoc Ga 1959;48:398–401.
53. Curry JL, Johnson WG, Feinberg DH, Updegrove JH: Thorium induced hepatic hemangioendothelioma. AJR 1975;125:671–677.
54. Davis GM: Hemangioendothelioma of the liver with unusual roentgenologic findings: Report of a case. Gastroenterology 1961;40:253–258.
55. Janower ML, Miettinen OS, Flynn ML: Effects of long term thorotrast exposure. Radiology 1972;103:13–20.
56. MacMahon HE, Murphy AS, Bates MI: Endothelial cell sarcoma of the liver following thorotrast injections. Am J Pathol 1947;23:585–611.
57. Exelby PR, Filler RM, Grosfeld JL: Liver tumors in children in the particular reference to hepatoblastoma and hepatocellular carcinoma: American Academy of Pediatrics surgical section survey 1974. J Pediatr Surg 1975;10:329–337.
58. Ishak KG, Glunz PR: Hepatoblastoma and hepatocarcinoma in infancy and childhood: Report of 47 cases. Cancer 1967;20:396–422.

59. Margulis AR, Nice CM, Rigler LG: The roentgen findings in primary hepatoma in infants and children. Radiology 1956;66:809–817.
60. Sorsdahl OA, Gay BB: Roentgenologic features of a primary carcinoma of the liver in infants and children. AJR 1967;100:117–127.
61. Aspray M: Calcified hemangiomas of the liver. AJR 1945;53:446–452.
62. Plachte A: Calcified cancerous hemangioma of the liver: Review of the literature and report of 13 cases. Radiology 1962;79:783–788.
63. Stanley P, Gates GF, Ross LE, Miller SW: Hepatic covernous hemangiomas and hemangioendotheliomas in infancy. AJR 1977;129:317–321.
64. Selke AC, Cornell SH: Infantile hepatic hemangioendothelioma. AJR 1969;106:200–203.
65. Ghahremani GG, Meyers MA, Port RB: Calcified primary tumors of the gastrointestinal tract. Gastrointest Radiol 1978;2:331–339.
66. Appleby A, Hacking PM: Calcification in hepatic metastases. Br J Radiol 1958;31:449–450.
67. Green PA, Stephens DH: Hepatic calcification in cancer of the large bowel. Am J Gastroenterol 1971;55:466–470.
68. Khilnani MT: Calcified liver metastasis from carcinoma of the colon. Am J Dig Dis 1961;6:229–232.
69. Miele AJ, Edmonds HW: Calcified liver metastases: A specific roentgen diagnostic sign. Radiology 1963;80:779–785.
70. Wells J: Calcified liver metastases. N Eng J Med 1956;255:639–640.
71. Fred HL, Eiband JM, Collins LC: Calcifications in intra-abdominal and retroperitoneal metastases. AJR 1964;91:138–148.
72. Nathanson L: Calcified metastatic deposits in the peritoneal cavity, liver and right lung field from papillary cystadenocarcinoma of the ovary. AJR 1950;64:467–469.
73. Shonfeld EM, Guarino AV, Bessolo RJ: Calcified hepatic metastases from carcinoma of the breast: Case report and review of the literature. Radiology 1973;106:303–304.
74. Ross P: Calcification in liver metastases from neuroblastoma. Radiology 1965;85:1074–1079.
75. Zimmer, FE: Islet-cell carcinoma treated with alloxan: Associated with calcified hepatic metastases and thyroid myopathy. Ann Intern Med 1964;61:543–549.
76. Persaud V, Bateson EM, Bankay CD: Pleural mesothelioma associated with massive hepatic calcification and unusual metastases. Cancer 1970;26:920–928.
77. Oh KS: Mottled areas of intra-abdominal calcification. JAMA 1969;208:521–523.
78. Dolan A: Tumor calcification following therapy. AJR 1963;89:166–174.
79. Jarvis L, Hodes PJ: Aneurysm of the hepatic artery demonstrated roentgenographically. AJR 1954;72:1037–1040.
80. Silverman NR, Borns PF, Goldstein AH, et al.: Thrombus calcification in the inferior vena cava: A specific roentgenologic entity. AJR 1969;106:97–102.
81. Singleton EB, Rosenberg HS: Intraluminal calcification of inferior vena cava. AJR 1961;86:556–560.
82. Kutcher R, Schneider M, Gordon DH: Calcification in polycystic disease. Radiology 1977;122:77–80.
83. Galambos A: Intrahepatic lithiasis with multiple locations. Am J Dig Dis 1954;21:95–96.
84. Pridgen JE Jr., Aust JB, McInnis WD: Primary intrahepatic gallstones. Arch Surg 1977;112:1037–1043.
85. Ablow RC, Effman EL: Hepatic calcifications associated with umbilical vein catheterization in the new born infant. AJR 1972;114:380–385.
86. Carter AR, France NE, Lewis BW, Shaw DG: Cholesterol storage disease: Radiological features. Pediatr Radiol 1974;2:135–136.
87. Love L, Demos TC, Reynes CJ, et al.: Visualization of the lateral edge of the liver in ascites. Radiology 1977;122:619–622.

88. Nichols GB, Schilling PJ: Pseudo-retroperitoneal gas in rupture of aneurysm of abdominal aorta. Am J Roentgenol 1975;125:134–137.
89. Govoni AF, Meyers MA: Pseudopneumobilia. Radiology 1976;118:526.
90. Haswell DM, Berne AS, Schneider B: Plain film recognition of the ligamentum teres hepatis. Radiology 1975;114:263–267.
91. Melhem RE: The radiolucent liver. Pediatr Radiol 1976;4:153–156.
92. McSherry CK, Stubenbord WT, Glenn F: The significance of air in the biliary system and liver. Surg Gynecol Obstet 1969;128:49–61.
93. Scott MG, Pygott F, Murphy L: The significance of gas or barium in the biliary tract. Br J Radiol 1954;27:253–265.
94. Bergner LH: Internal biliary fistulas. Am J Gastroenterol 1965;43:11–22.
95. Balthazar EJ, Schechter LS: Air in gallbladder: A frequent finding in gallstone ileus. Am J Roentgenol 1978;131:219–222.
96. Balthazar EJ, Schechter LS: Gallstone ileus: The importance of contrast examinations in the roentgenographic diagnosis. AJR 1975;125:374–379.
97. Figiel LS, Figiel SJ, Wietersen FK, Dranginis EJ: Gallstone obturation: Clinical and roentgenographic considerations. AJR 1955;74:22–37.
98. Wastie ML, Cunningham GE: Roentgenologic findings in recurrent pyogenic cholangitis. AJR 1973;119:71–76.
99. Susman N, Senturia HR: Gas embolization of the portal venous system. AJR 1960;83:847–850.
100. Wiot JF, Felson B: Gas in the portal venous system. AJR 1961;86:920–929.
101. Tedesco FJ, Stanley RJ: Hepatic portal vein gas without bowel infarction or necrosis. Gastroenterology 1975;69:240–243.
102. Traverso LW: Is hepatic portal venous gas an indication for exploratory laparotomy? Arch Surg 1981;116:936–938.
103. Sadhu VK, Brennan RD, Madan V: Portal vein gas following air-contrast barium enema in granulomatous colitis: Report of a case. Gastrointest Radiol 1979;4:163–164.
104. Foster SC, Schneider B, Seaman WB: Gas-containing pyogenic intrahepatic abscesses. Radiology 1970;94:613–618.
105. Harley HRS: Peri- and intrahepatic abscess. Proc R Soc Med 1969;63:319–322.
106. Elson MW: Antemortem radiographic demonstration of gas gangrene of the liver. Radiology 1960;74:57–60.
107. Beetlestone CA, Bohrer SP: Right upper quadrant gas shadows. JAMA 1976;236:1397–1398.
108. In Edwards DAW, Shanks SC, Kerley P (eds): The Diaphragm. A Text Book of X-ray Diagnosis, Vol 4, Alimentary Tract. Philadelphia: Saunders, 1970, p. 268.
109. Behlke FM: Hepatodiaphragmatic interposition in children. AJR 1964;91:669–673.
110. Lundstedt C, Hederstrom E, Holmin T, et al.: Radiological diagnosis in proven intraabdominal abscess formation: A comparison between plain films of the abdomen, ultrasonography and computerized tomography. Gastrointest Radiol 1983;8:261–266.
111. Whalen JP, Bierny JP: Classification of perihepatic abscesses. Radiology 1969;92:1427–1437.
112. Menuck L, Siemers PT: Pneumoperitoneum: Importance of right upper quadrant features. AJR 1976;127:753–756.
113. Miller RE: Perforated viscus in infants: A new roentgen sign. Radiology 1960;74:65–67.
114. Sherlock S: Diseases of the Liver and Biliary System, 5th ed. London: Blackwell, 1975.
115. Baggenstoss AH, Stauffer MH: Post-hepatic and alcoholic cirrhosis: Clinical-pathologic study of 43 cases of each. Gastroenterology 1952;22:157–164.
116. Griscom NT, Capitanio MA, Wagoner ML, et al.: The visibly fatty liver. Radiology 1975;117:385–389.
117. Steinbach HL, Crane JT, Bruyn HB: The roentgen demonstration of the liver with fatty metamorphosis: Report of a case due to congenital fibrocystic disease. Radiology 1954;62:858–860.

118. Fletcher K: Observations on the origin of liver fat in infantile malnutrition. Am J Clin Nutr 1966;19:170–174.
119. Swischuk LE: A new and unusual roentgenographic finding of fatty liver in infants. Am J Roentgenol 1974;122(1):159–164.
120. Epstein O, Ajdukiewicz AB, Dick R, et al.: Hypertrophic hepatic osteoarthropathy: Clinical, roentgenologic, biochemical hormonal, and cardiorespiratory studies, and review of the literature. Am J Med 1979;67:88.
121. Buchanan DJ, Mitchell DM: Hypertrophic osteoarthropathy in portal cirrhosis. Ann Intern Med 1967;66:130.
122. Caffey J, Silverman FN: Pediatric X-ray Diagnosis, 7th ed. Chicago: Year Book Med. Pub., 1978.
123. Guenter CA, Hammersten JF: Hypertrophic osteoarthropathy in cirrhosis of the liver. Am Rev Respir Dis 1970;101:590.
124. Han SY, Collins LC: Hypertrophic osteoarthropathy in cirrhosis of the liver. Radiology 1968;91:795.
125. Pais MJ: Disease states affecting both liver and bone. Radiol Clin North Am 1980;18:253–267.
126. Jones JP Jr, Jameson RM, Engleman EP: Alcoholism, fat embolism and avascular necrosis. J Bone Joint Surg 1968;50A:1065.
127. Moult PJA, Waite DW, Dick R: Posterior mediastinal venous masses in patients with portal hypertension. Gut 1975;16:57.
128. Doyle FH, Read AE, Evans KT: The mediastinum in portal hypertension. Clin Radiol 1961;12:114.
129. Trewby PN, Warren R, Contini S, et al.: Incidence and pathophysiology of pulmonary edema in fulminant hepatic failure. Gastroenterology 1978;74:859.
130. Bynum LJ: Hepatic failure and respiratory distress. Gastroenterology 1978;74:995.
131. Sandweiss D, Thomson B: The adult respiratory distress syndrome: the predisposing role of liver disease. Ariz Med 1973;30:264.
132. Bashour FA, Miller WR, Chapman CB: Pulmonary venoarterial shunting in hepatic cirrhosis: Including a case of cirsoid aneurysm of the thoracic wall. Am Heart J 1961;62:350.
133. Berthelot P, Walker JG, Sherlock S, et al.: Arterial changes in the lungs in cirrhosis of the liver—lung spider nevi. New Eng J Med 1966;274:291.
134. Stanly NN, Woodgate DJ: Mottled chest radiograph and gas transfer defect in chronic liver disease. Thorax 1972;27:315.
135. Williams A, Trewby P, Williams R, et al.: Structural alterations to the pulmonary circulation in fulminant hepatic failure. Thorax 1979;34:447.
136. Stanley NN, Ackrill P, Wood J: Lung perfusion scanning in hepatic cirrhosis. Br Med J 1972;4:639.
137. Wolfe JD, Tashkin DP, Holly EE, et al.: Hypoxemia of cirrhosis: Detection of abnormal small pulmonary vascular channels by a quantitative radionuclide method. Am J Med 1977;63:746.
138. Swett HA, Greenspan RH: Thoracic manifestations of liver disease. Radiol Clin North Am 1980;18:269–279.
139. Sabesin S, Levinson M: Acute and chronic hepatitis: multisystemic involvement related to immunologic disease. Adv Intern Med 1977;22:421.
140. Murray RO, Jacobson HG: The radiology of skeletal disorders, 2nd ed. New York: Churchill Livingstone, 1977.
141. Moseley JE: Skeletal changes in the anemias. Semin Roentgenol 1974;9:169.
142. Nathan DG: Thalassemia. New Engl J Med 1972;286:586.
143. Miller JH, Stanley P, Gates F: Radiography of glycogen storage diseases. Am J Roentgenol 1979;132:379.
144. Preger L, Saunders GW, Gold RH, et al.: Roentgenographic skeletal changes in the glycogen storage diseases. Am J Roentgenol 1969;107:840.

145. Howell RR, Stevenson RE, Ben-Menachem Y, et al.: Hepatic adenoma with type 1 glycogen storage disease. JAMA 1976;236:1481–1484.
146. Miller JH, Gates GF, Landing BH, et al.: Scintigraphic abnormalities in glycogen storage disease. J Nucl Med 1978;19:354–358.
147. Landing BH: Tumors of the liver in childhood. In K Okuda, RL Peter (eds), Hepatocellular Carcinoma. New York: Wiley, 1976, pp 205–226.
148. Martel W, Sitterley BH: Roentgenologic manifestations of osteonecrosis. Am J Roentgenol 1969;106:509.
149. Rourke JA, Heslin DJ: Gaucher's disease. Am J Roentgenol 1965;94:621.
150. Strickland B: Skeletal manifestations of Gaucher's disease with some unusual findings. Br J Radiol 1958;31:246.
151. Rabinowitz JG: Abnormalities of the liver and other organs. Radiol Clin North Am 1980;18:281–295.
152. Finby N, Bern AG: Roentgenographic abnormalities of the skeletal system in Wilson's disease (hepatolenticular degeneration). Am J Roentgenol 1958;79:603.
153. Mindelzun R, Elkin M, Scheinberg IH, et al.: Skeletal changes in Wilson's disease. Radiology 1970;94:127.
154. Rosenoer VM, Michell RC: Skeletal changes in Wilson's disease (hepatolenticular degeneration). Br J Radiol 1959;32:805.
155. Tinkler L: Primary sclerosing cholangitis. Postgrad Med J 1971;47:666.
156. Brun B, Palbol J: Polycystic disease of the liver. Acta Radiol (Diagn) 1977;18:241.
157. Mitty HA, Shapira H: Total body opacification in the adult. Am J Roentgenol 1972;115:630.
158. Blyth H, Ockenden B: Polycystic disease of the kidney and liver presenting in childhood. J Med Genet 1971;8:257.
159. Ross DG, Travers H: Infantile presentation of adult type polycystic kidney disease in a large kidney. J Pediatr 1975;187:760.
160. Poznanski AK, Nosanchuk JS, Baublis J, et al.: Cerebrohepatorenal syndrome (Zellweger's syndrome). Am J Roentgenol 1970;109:313.

2
Hepatic Scintigraphy

RICHARD C. REBA • DAVID C. P. CHEN
WILLIAM A. FAJMAN

INTRODUCTION

Radionuclide imaging of the liver has been available for more than 25 years. The instruments and pharmaceuticals have undergone great change and have been refined so that satisfactory resolution and target-specific radiotracers are now available. Currently, radionuclide hepatic scanning is a valuable technique for investigating the morphology and function of the liver. The method is relatively simple, safe, noninvasive, and widely available throughout the world.

In this chapter, the radiopharmaceuticals most commonly used for liver scanning, i.e., radiocolloid and iminodiacetic acid derivatives, will be described. We will discuss the use of hepatic scintiscanning in the differential diagnosis of malignant and benign focal liver disease, for the evaluation of diffuse hepatic disease, for the differential diagnosis of acute and chronic cholecystitis, and for the evaluation of jaundice. Finally, comparison of radionuclide imaging to other imaging techniques, such as computed tomography and gray scale ultrasound, is also included where pertinent.

Radionuclide hepatic imaging is based on the ability of the liver to extract and concentrate a radiolabeled compound that has been injected into the blood stream. Following the injection, the rate of hepatic uptake, the spatial distribution within the liver, and the rate of hepatic clearance of the radiolabeled compound gamma-ray emission is accomplished with an external scintillation detector. The mass of the injected radiolabeled compound is many times less than that which produces a pharmacologic action, that is, there is no interference with the normal hepatic metabolic processes. Images can be displayed on x-ray or Polaroid film (analog display), or by use of a digital computer and a cathode ray (digital display).

RADIOPHARMACEUTICALS

Two physiologic mechanisms are employed to achieve hepatic accumulation of injected radiolabel: the phagocytic function of the Kupffer cells and the ability of the parenchymal polygonal cells to extract certain classes of compounds.

Phagocytic Function

The group of radiopharmaceuticals that rely on the phagocytic function of the fixed reticuloendothelial cells includes a number of colloids which have been labeled with either I-131, Au-198, In-113m or Tc-99m. Tc-99m sulfur colloid is the most commonly used radiotracer because of its desirable nuclear properties and general availability. Indium-113m colloid remains an acceptable alternative liver scanning agent, particularly in the regions of the world where receipt of the Mo generator is unreliable. However, the photon energy of In-113m (393 Kev) is burdensome to collimate, and the probability of interaction of the 393 Kev gamma ray with the ½-inch-thick NaI crystal of the camera is only about 15 percent.

The reported average size of the colloid particles that have been used is variable. The best estimates are that the average TC-99m sulfur colloid is 100 to 400 nm, and In-113m Fe(OH)^3 colloid varies from 3,000 to 4,000 nm (1). The colloid particles are trapped by the reticuloendothelial cells and, for all practical purposes, remain permanently within the cell. The size and number of the particles are important since the precise diameter of a colloid appears to be related to its distribution within the reticuloendothelial system (2). In general, the smaller the particle, the more likely it is to be deposited in the bone marrow phagocytes (3). Since a change in particle distribution is used in many interpretation schemes, one should be aware of the preparation method and the expected normal *in vivo* distribution of the radiocolloid employed.

The critical organ for radiation is the liver, and the absorbed dose from Tc-99m sulfur colloid is approximately 0.2 to 0.4 rads per mCi. The standard preparation of Tc-99m sulfur colloid is relatively simple and may be completed within 15 minutes. The vial in which the pertechnate, thiosulfate, and hydrochloric acid reaction occurs is in a water bath (95 ± 5C, 10 ± 2 minutes), which will produce the preferred particle size. However, the longer the vial is in the water bath, apparently the larger the particles will be. Normally, about 85 to 90 percent of injected colloid is rapidly extracted by the liver, 5 to 10 percent extracted by the spleen, and 2 to 3 percent by the bone marrow. The half-time of clearance from the plasma is approximately 2½ to 3 minutes. Since the lung also contains fixed phagocytes, diffuse pulmonary activity may also be seen when the particle size distribution has been altered or in certain disease states (4–6).

Hepatic Parenchymal Agents

The following have been shown to be extracted by the hepatic parenchymal cells and subsequently excreted into the biliary system: rose bengal, an iodinated flourescein dye; iodinated contrast materials, such as iodiapamide and ioglycamic acid; thiol complexes; amine complexes; amino acid Schiff base complexes, such as pyridoxylidene glutamate; and iminodiacetic acid complexes (IDA). Because of their rapid plasma clearance, hepatic transit time, and hepatic clearance, the Tc-99m-labeled IDA analogs have the greatest hepatobiliary specificity and are the most frequently used hepatobiliary compounds.

The structural characteristics necessary for hepatobiliary accumulation and excretion have been studied by Firnau (7). The most important characteristics for hepatobiliary specificity are a molecular weight range between 300 and 1,000 daltons, possession of a strong polar group, at least a two-ring system in different planes, and a firm binding to albumin. Tc-99m-labeled IDA derivatives possess these features.

Normally, after intravenous administration, 85 to 95 percent of the Tc-99m IDA drugs are extracted by the liver by an active transport process. Minor differences in the physical and chemical nature of the specific derivative, particularly with regard to the polar characteristics, will determine the degree of renal excretion, but as a class, 5 to 15 percent of the administered dose is excreted by the kidneys. Usually, intrahepatic distribution of Tc-sulfur colloid matches that of Tc-IDA during the early (5 to 10 minutes) parenchymal phase; however, dichotomy in regional patterns has been described. For example, sulfur colloid "cold" defects that were "hot" or normal following Tc-IDA have been seen in patients with cirrhosis, hepatocarcinoma, hepatic ademona, focal nodular hyperplasia, and biloma (8).

Bilirubin will compete with the IDA drug for the hepatocyte carrier transport sites. However, even with serum total bilirubin concentrations of 20 to 30 mg/dl, diisopropyl-IDA achieves adequate hepatic extraction and biliary excretion suitable for clinical interpretation. Therefore, it is possible to evaluate patients with suspected acute cholecystitis and, early in their course, differentiate medical from surgical jaundice in patients with moderately severe hyperbilirubinemia.

Experimental Radiopharmaceuticals

Receptor-Binding. Eckelman *et al.* have identified a new class of radiopharmaceuticals and have discussed their potential for elucidating disease mechanisms (9). Krohn *et al.* have reported preliminary work describing the use of a new radiopharmaceutical, Tc-99m neogalactoalbumin (Tc-NGA), designed to measure specific liver functions (10). These investigators have demonstrated that the Tc-NGA binds to specific receptors on hepatic parenchymal cells (hepatic-binding protein, or HBP) and have proposed a mathematical model that can be used to quantitate hepatic blood flow, the affinity constant and concentration of the HBP receptor, and the rate of lysosome catabolism of the receptor-binding HBP radiopharmaceutical. The use of this compound and the proposed mathematical model has been demonstrated in animals under basal conditions. Investigators who believe changes in receptors are fundamental to the basic understanding of disease processes are optimistic that this type of *in vivo* study can be extended to humans in order to monitor changes in receptors as a function of specific disease states.

Metabolic Substitutes. Analogs of glucose and mannose labeled with 18-F have been proposed as metabolic substrates suitable for quantifying malignant tumor metabolism and tumor response to chemotherapy in the liver. The eventual role of this example of *in vivo* biochemistry is uncertain. The subject has been reviewed by Welch (11).

FOCAL LIVER DISEASE

The radiocolloid liver scan is a sensitive technique for the detection of an intrahepatic mass (12–14). A multiple view radiocolloid scan of the liver can locate an intrahepatic mass, but the study does not provide information regarding the precise nature of an abnormality. A major disadvantage of radionuclide liver scanning is its limited ability in detecting a "cold" lesion in a "hot" background. The current planar imaging technology does not allow the detection of lesions smaller than 1 to 2 cm in diameter. Anatomic location of an abnormality may also influence its detectability by radionuclide liver scanning. For example, in order to be detected, a mass that occurs in the center of the right lobe must be larger than one located at the margin of the thin left lobe. Therefore, anatomic location and instrument resolution are the primary determinants of the false-negative results of liver scanning for detection of focal defects. As in the interpretation of all imaging techniques, knowledge of regional anatomy (Figure 2–1) and an appreciation of anatomic variants are generally the major factors influencing the false-

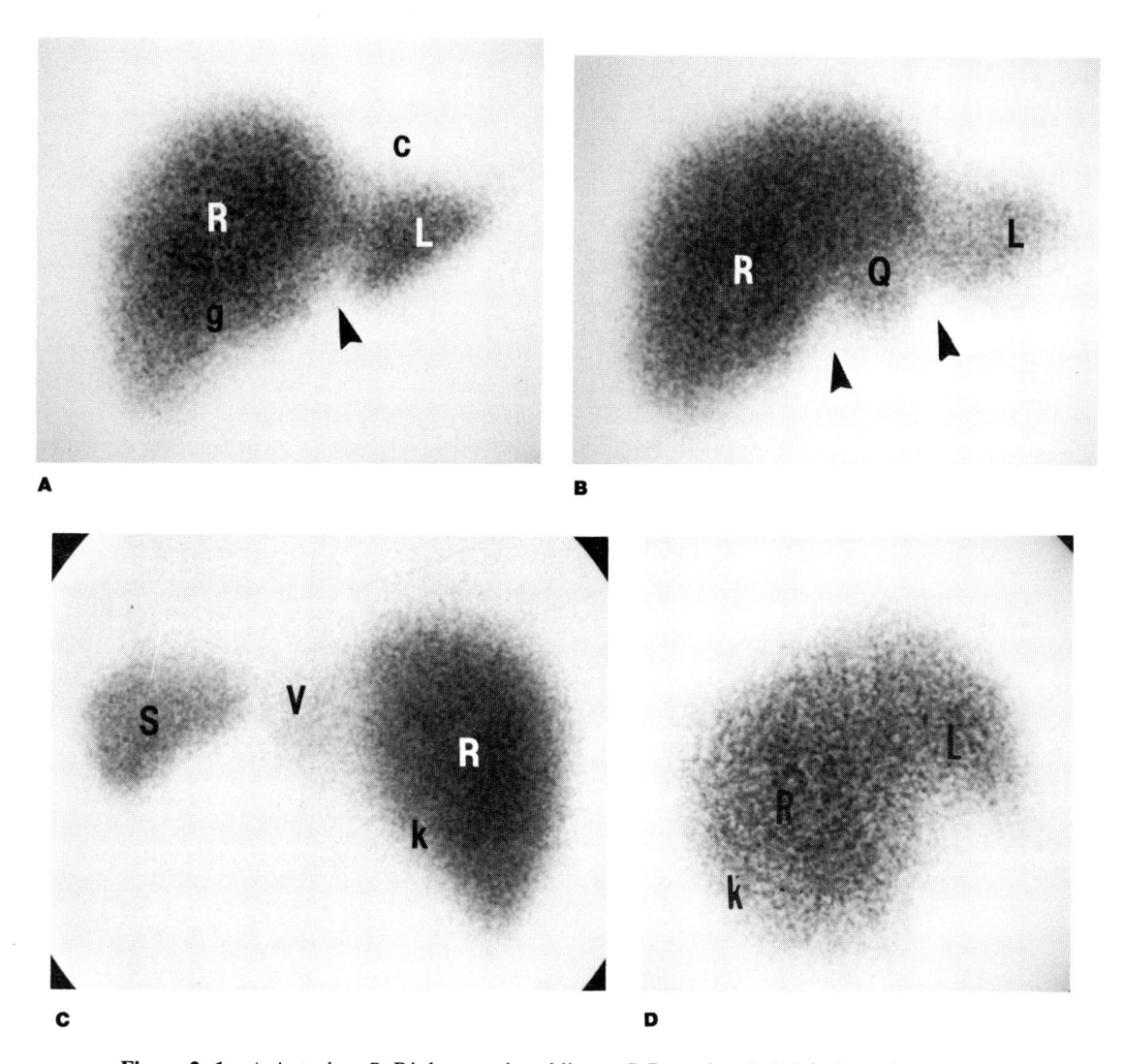

Figure 2–1. *A.* Anterior. *B.* Right anterior oblique. *C.* Posterior. *D.* Right lateral. Arrows represent the interlobar fissures; R = right lobe; L = left lobe; Q = quadrate lobe; C = cardiac impression; g = gallbladder fossa; K = renal impression; V = vertebral attenuation; and S = spleen.

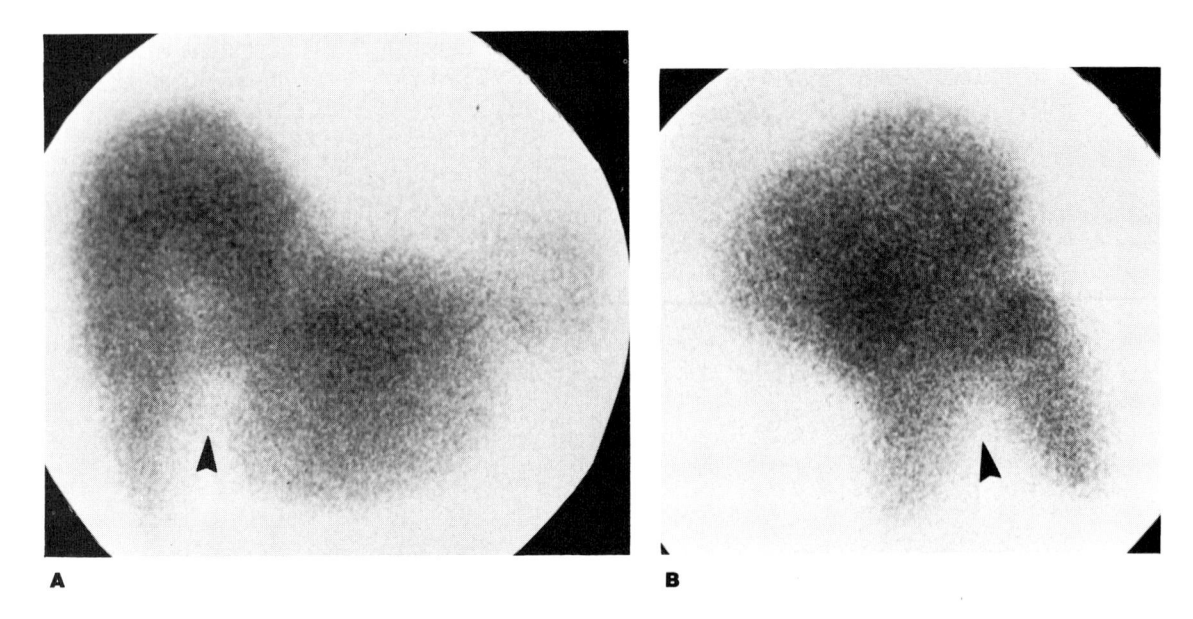

Figure 2-2. Anterior (*A*) and right lateral (*B*) views showing a prominent gallbladder fossa (arrow). This is enhanced by hypertrophy of the left lobe. This configuration of the dome is observed commonly in eventration of the diaphragm.

positive rate (15,16). However, in addition to the presence of an anatomic variant such as a thin left lobe or a prominent intrahepatic gallbladder fossa (Figure 2-2), a false-positive interpretation may result from fibrosis secondary to cirrhosis, a benign tumor or cyst, or any number of associated conditions, including extrinsic compression (Figures 2–3 and 2–4).

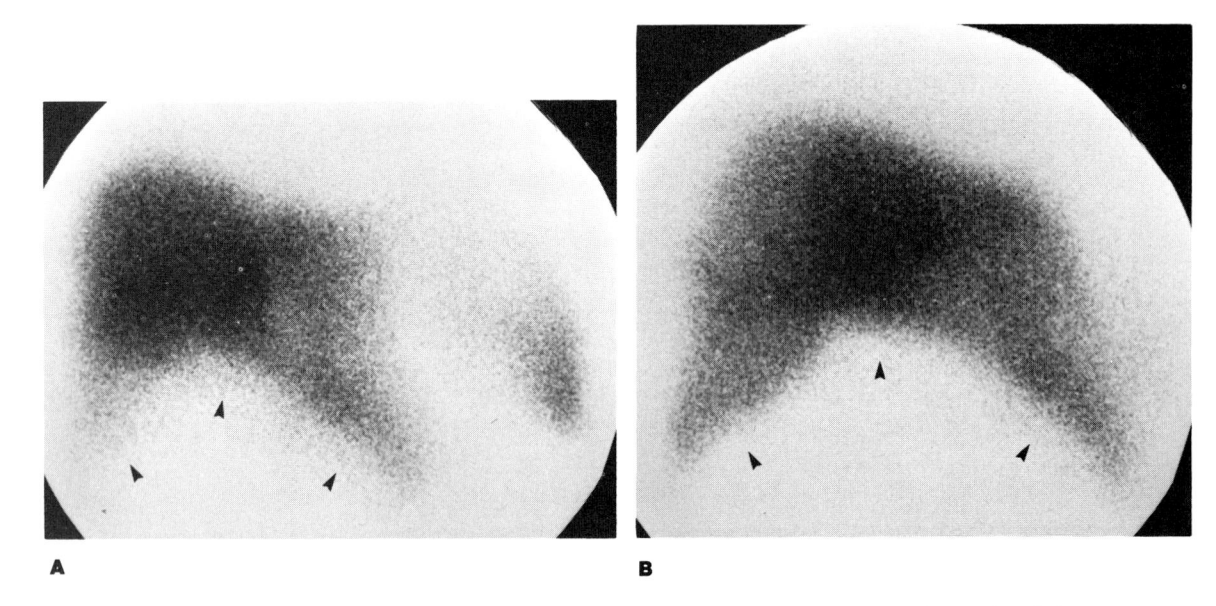

Figure 2-3. Anterior (*A*) and right anterior oblique (*B*) views show marked deformity of the liver edge, suggesting a mass (arrows). In actuality, this was loculated ascitic fluid.

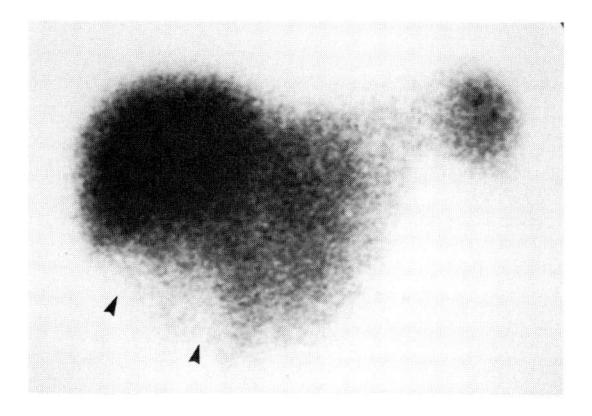

Figure 2-4. Anterior view of the liver shows irregularity of the inferior right lobe (arrows), which could easily be mistaken for an intrahepatic mass. A large polycystic kidney compressing the liver was the actual cause.

Metastatic Hepatic Malignancy

The most widely used indication for performing a liver scan is for the detection of metastatic hepatic malignancy. The liver is a common site for metastatic deposits of malignant tumors from the stomach, colon, pancreas, and skin (melanoma), as well as advanced cancer of the breast, lung, and prostate. Primary cancers of the ovary, kidney, and uterus metastasize less frequently to the liver. In children, Wilm's tumor and neuroblastoma often metastasize to the liver.

The sensitivity and specificity of radiocolloid liver scan for the detection of metastatic disease is variable. Reliability of a scan depends on many features, such as the pathology of the tumor (accuracy is higher when the primary is of gastrointestinal origin rather than a nongastrointestinal malignancy), the stage of the disease, variations in interpretation criteria, instrumentation used, and even in the type of colloid preparation (17,18). The results of different studies reporting the sensitivity and specificity of the liver scan in patients with metastatic liver disease indicate that overall sensitivity is about 85 percent, with a range of 80 to 95 percent, depending on the interpretation criteria used, the pathology, and the stage of the tumor. Specificity is about 85 percent with a range of 70 to 95 percent, depending on the same features and the incidence and frequency distribution of other diseases in the population from which the patient is being examined. False-negative results are more frequent when the liver is normal in size and when metastatic deposits are smaller than 2 cm or lie deep in the liver mass. The sensitivity for the detection of liver metastasis may be as low as 50 percent in patients with a normal-size liver (19). However, it has also been cautioned that in patients with a history of malignancy, a normal-size liver, and normal biochemical liver function tests, liver scanning will reveal the presence of metastases in 10 to 15 percent (20).

Specific image patterns are characteristic of specific primary tumors. For example, several large, or occasionally solitary, lesions with a discrete margin are typical of metastases from a primary gastrointestinal tract malignancy (Figure 2-5). Multiple small lesions with an ill-defined border are more common from metastasis of a lung, breast, or melanoma primary (Figures 2-6, 2-7).

Metastatic liver disease appears occasionally on the liver scan as a nonspecific diffuse and patchy distribution that is similar to that seen in patients with any diffuse parenchymal disease, such as cirrhosis. Thus, differentiating between metastatic liver disease and cirrhosis, as well as other diffuse parenchymal diseases of the liver, becomes difficult (Figure 2-8). Broadening the criteria for liver scan positivity by including sub-

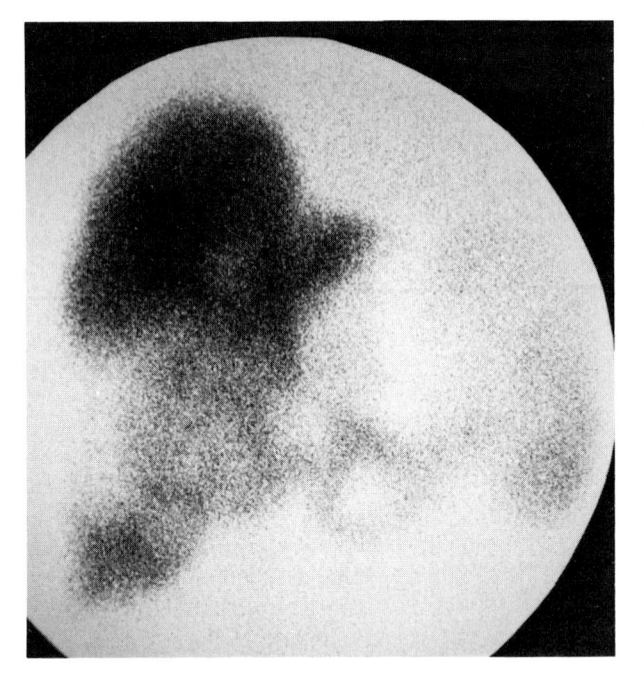

Figure 2-5. Anterior view of the liver, with multiple large defects in a patient with metastatic adenocarcinoma of the colon.

jective nonhomogeneous colloid distribution and hepatomegaly in patients with a history of breast cancer will increase the sensitivity dramatically, but at the expected cost of increasing the false-positive rate (17). Adoption of this strategy to patients with colorectal cancer does not improve sensitivity. Visible bone marrow concentration of colloid is useful to differentiate cirrhosis from metastatic disease (21). While there are exceptions, in general, a focal hepatic defect seen with prominent bone marrow and spleen activity is more likely to be the result of severe diffuse hepatic parenchymal disease than of metastatic liver disease.

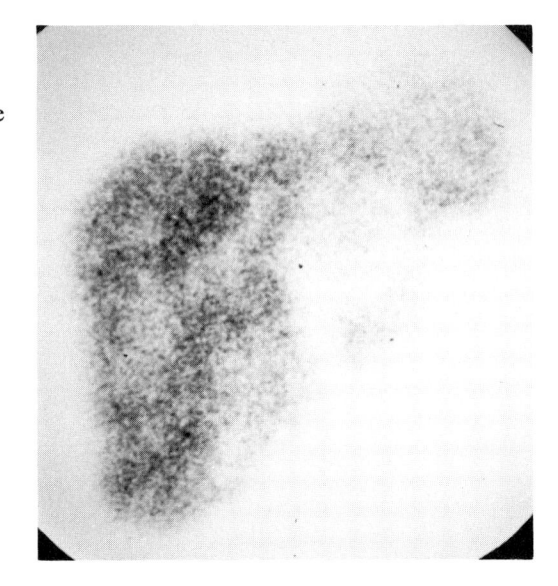

Figure 2-6. Anterior view of the liver showing diffuse small focal lesions in a patient with breast carcinoma metastases.

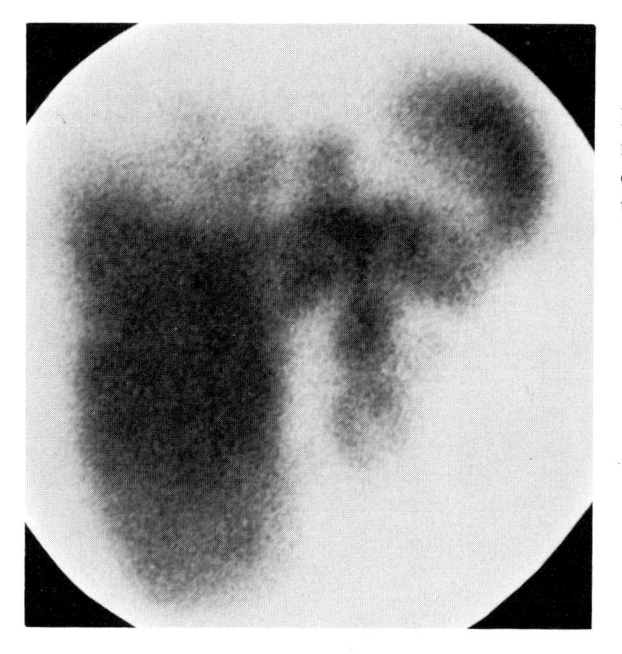

Figure 2-7. Anterior view of the liver shows multiple small defects in a patient with breast carcinoma. Smaller defects are more easily seen in the thin left lobe.

Most reports evaluating the sensitivity and specificity of liver scans for metastatic disease have correlated the results to percutaneous liver biopsy, peritoneoscopy, laporotomy, or autopsy. Random percutaneous biopsy has a false-negative rate of approximately 50 percent (22,23). Likewise, limitations of peritoneoscopy result in a reported false-negative rate of 36 percent (24). Even direct inspection and palpation during surgical laporotomy may fail to detect metastatic disease in 10 percent of patients (25). In the largest reported experience correlating liver scans with short interval (28 days) post-mortem findings, the false-positive rate was 10 percent and the false-negative rate, 17 percent (26). This study again emphasized that the factor that most limited scan accuracy was the inability to detect consistently lesions smaller than 2 cm.

Sensitivity, specificity, and predictive value are expressions that are now used widely to define test utility and to compare the relative efficacy of different testing techniques. As discussed by Reba and Kleinman (27), the false-negative rate and the a priori probability of disease prevalence have a profound effect on test outcome and influence the positive predictive value of the test much more than sensitivity. For example, if a liver scan (sensitivity = 71 percent; specificity = 95 percent) is performed on a patient from a general practice in which a reasonable estimate of the prevalence of hepatic malignancy is 1 percent, an abnormal liver scan will result in a positive probability of only 12.5 percent that the patient has hepatic metastases. However, if a liver scan is performed from an oncology clinic, or from a hospital inpatient population in which a reasonable estimate of the prevalence of malignancy might be as high as 25 percent, a positive liver scan will result in an 85 percent probability that the patient has hepatic metastases. In the first case, when the positive probability of hepatic metastasis increased from 1 percent to 13 percent, the practitioner probably would not recommend liver biopsy or peritoneoscopy to confirm the diagnosis. However, in the second instance, when the probability is increased from 25 percent to 83 percent, the recommendation for further testing is on much firmer ground. With regard to the effects of the false-positive rate, if diagnostic criteria for a test are selected that result in a false-positive rate of 10 percent, when used in a patient from a population with a disease prevalence

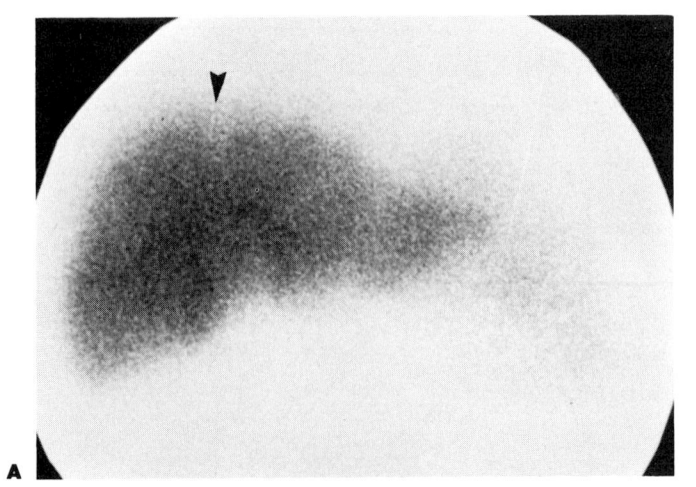

Figure 2-8. *A.* Right anterior oblique view of the liver is mildly inhomogeneous, with a single area suggesting a focal defect (arrow). *B.* The CT scan showed multiple metastases in this patient with carcinoma of the lung.

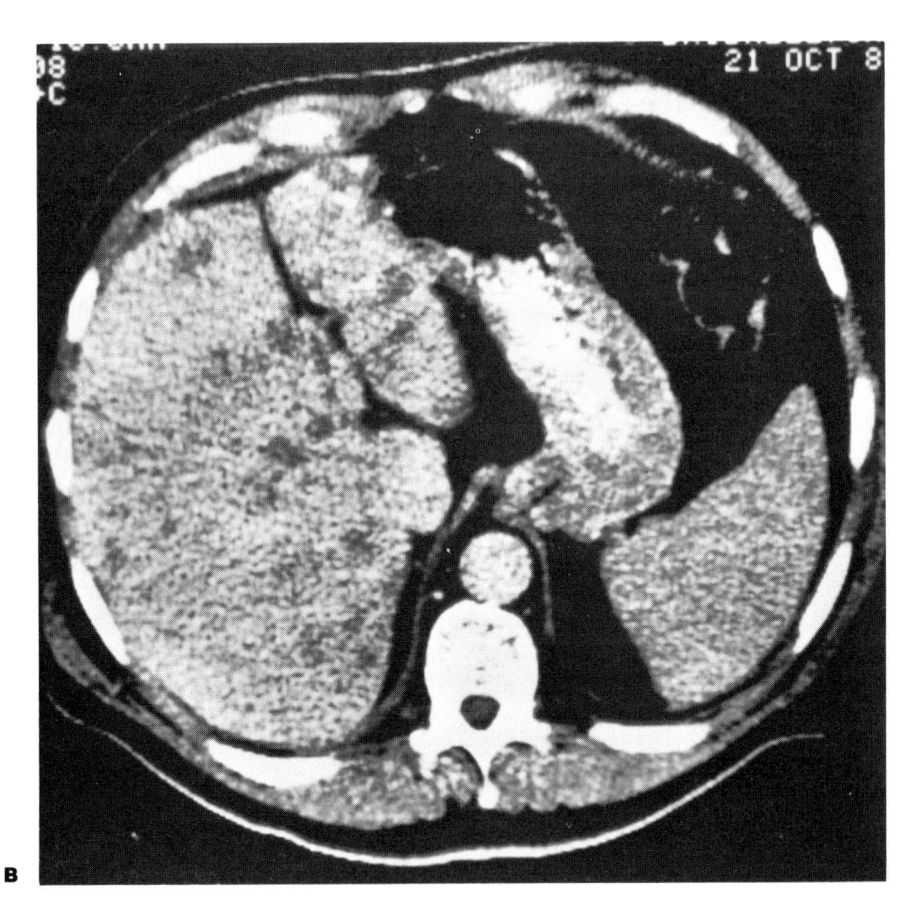

of 10 percent, increasing test sensitivity from 90 percent to 99 percent only increases the positive predictive value of the test from 50 percent to 52 percent. However, in this test with a sensitivity of 90 percent in the same population with a disease prevalence of 10 percent, decreasing the false-positive rate from 10 percent to 4 percent will increase the predictive value of a positive test from 50 percent to 72 percent.

The strategy of serial testing has been employed by incorporating carcinoembryonic antigen (CEA) titers, where an abnormal CEA titer is required before considering an abnormal liver scan to be positive for malignancy. Sugerbaker *et al.* have reported in one series of patients with breast cancer that the false-positive rate of liver scanning is decreased from 14 percent to 0 percent (28). Similar results have been described in a large number of patients with colorectal cancer (29).

The major considerations in choosing which test to apply first are that the cost and discomfort involved should be less for the initial test since it is applied to the larger population. With the implementation of the Diagnostic Related Groups (DRGs), it will be prudent to adopt some type of multiple discriminant analysis of the proper diagnostic algorithm for each defined patient population and suspected disease stage to result in the most effective and cost-beneficial operational scheme to be used for each (average) patient.

In summary, the sensitivity of liver radiocolloid scanning for detection of hepatic metastases is approximately 80 ± 10 percent. Most false-positive results are due to unappreciated anatomical variants in the gallbladder fossa, the renal fossa, a thin biconcave left lobe, or prominent attentuation from the hepatic vein, ribs, or structures within the porta hepatis; the false-negative rate is primarily a reflection of the limitations in resolution. In addition to detecting metastases in patients with malignancy, the liver scan is useful to monitor the progress of disease, to monitor changes during treatment, and specifically is useful to assess adequacy of hepatic artery catheter placement for isolated liver perfusion (vide infra).

Special Forms of Hepatic Scintiscanning for Malignancy

Metastatic Carcinoma Detected with Radiolabeled Antibody. Although the concept that tumor antibodies could be used to detect sites of metastases was proposed first in 1953 (30), it was not until the work of Goldenberg and co-workers (31) that the real potential of the technique could be appreciated. These investigators used I-131-labeled, purified, high-affinity goat antibody to carcinoembryonic antigen and reported an approximate 85 percent sensitivity for the detection of metastases from a number of different tumor types. Circulating antigen did not interfere with the test results. The technique requires subtraction of a sulfur colloid liver scan and a blood-pool scan from the antibody scan. This subtraction technique and the slow blood clearance, which results in scans being performed after 48 hours or more, are believed to be minor inconveniences. In recent as yet unpublished work from this same group, radioimmunodetection scans were significantly more sensitive for the detection of hepatic metastases (97 percent) than were radionuclide colloid scans (85 percent), ultrasound (80 percent) or x-ray computed tomography (80 percent) in a selected group of approximately 30 patients. NMR comparison was made in a smaller group of patients, and the sensitivity was similar to the traditional imaging techniques, that is, the results were less favorable than the radioimmunodetection method. The original methods of using polyclonal antibody have been extended to investigate monoclonal antibody, Fab fragments and second antibody injection in efforts to simplify the imaging techniques (32–34). The radiolabeled antibody imaging techniques have great promise for improved diagnosis and treatment of solid tumors.

Hepatic Arterial Perfusion Scanning. The exclusive hepatic arterial blood supply of liver tumors has allowed the use of the regional arterial perfusion therapy of hepatic neoplasms. Using hepatic arterial infusion delivery of chemotherapeutic drugs or radioactive-labeled microspheres results in a higher concentration of therapeutic agent delivered to the tumor while minimizing systemic exposure to these toxic agents. Injection of Tc-99m macroaggregated serum albumin permits evaluation of arterial catheter placement by assessing the perfusion patterns (35,36).

Primary Hepatic Malignancy

One of the most explicit indications for a radionuclide liver scan is in patients suspected of having a hepatocellular carcinoma. Hepatocellular carcinoma comprises about 80 percent of primary hepatic malignancies. Currently, 85 to 90 percent of patients with hepatocellular carcinoma are inoperable because of the extent of the primary tumor or because of disseminated disease. Early diagnosis of focal hepatocellular carcinoma may result in useful surgical intervention.

Hepatocellular carcinoma is usually visualized as a large solitary focal defect on radionuclide scan (Figure 2–9). Since hepatomas can originate as multifocal tumors,

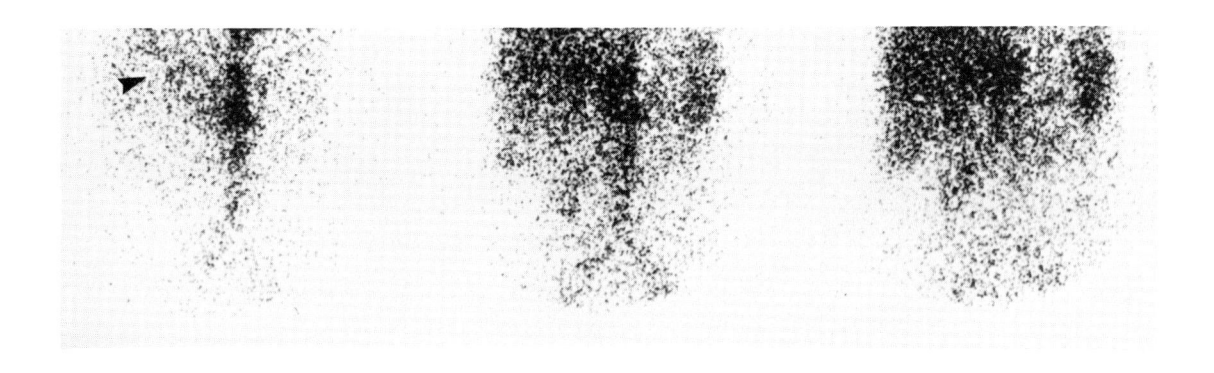

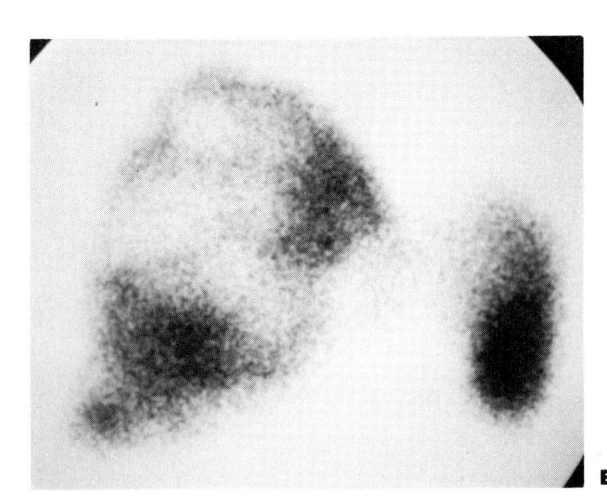

Figure 2-9. *A.* Radionuclide angiogram shows prominent early arterial flow (arrow). *B.* The anterior image shows a large focal lobulated defect. Although not always observed and nonspecific, these findings can be seen in hepatocellular carcinoma, as in this case.

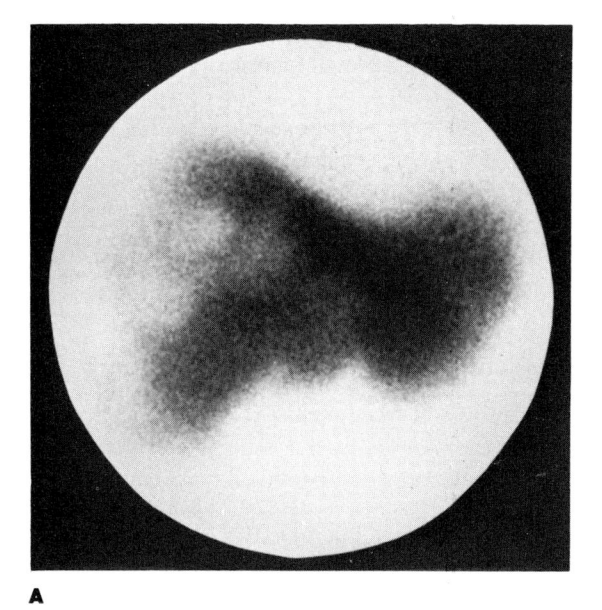

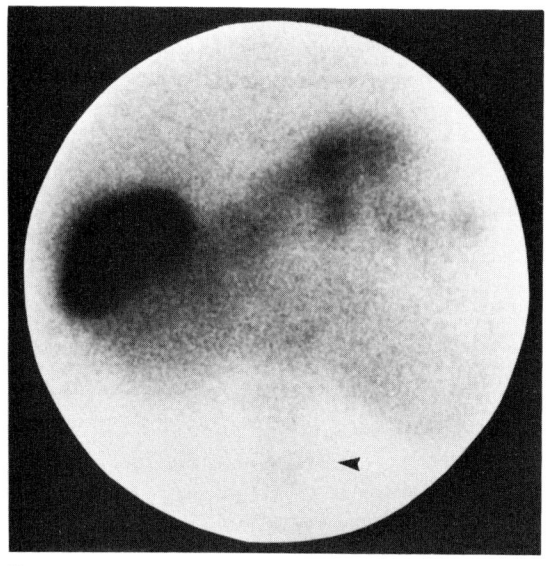

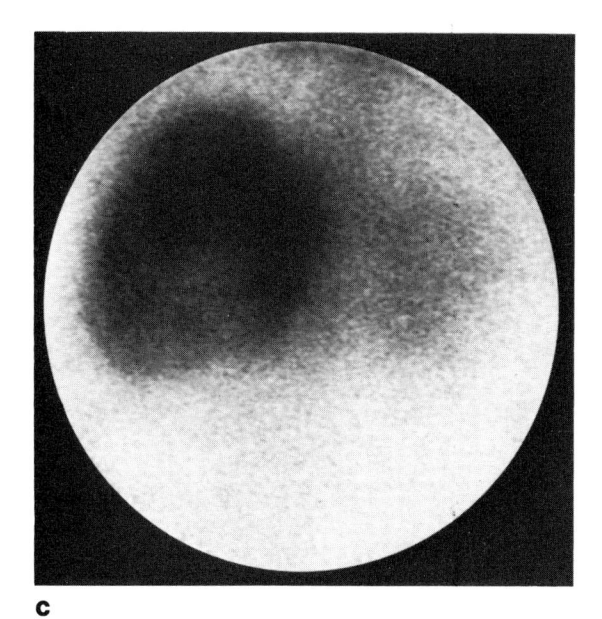

Figure 2-10. *A.* The anterior ^{99m}Tc sulfur colloid image demonstrates a large lobulated mass. *B.* The posterior view demonstrated increased splenic activity and bone marrow activity (arrow), consistent with underlying parenchymal liver disease. *C.* The anterior ^{67}Ga citrate image shows intense activity. In the appropriate clinical setting, this is consistent with hepatocellular carcinoma, as in this case.

multiple focal defects do occur, as reported in 21 percent of a limited number of patients (37). Although none of these patients has a normal scan pattern, a nonhomogeneous pattern is not unexpected because of the frequent association with cirrhosis. Active accumulation of gallium-67 by hepatocellular carcinoma is reported widely and is the basis for radionuclide detection of this tumor (38–39). More than 90 percent of primary hepatocellular carcinomas show significant gallium concentration (Figure 2–10), while less than 50 percent of hepatic metastasis show significant gallium-67 concentration. There is not universal agreement on the mechanism for the gallium uptake and concentration by hepatocellular carcinoma cells. Larsen *et al.* postulate a multistep process by which gallium, when bound to its transport protein transferrin, binds to transferrin receptor on the cell surface. This metal-protein complex is then transported to the cell interior and delivered to the lysosome, where the metal is released and binds to acceptor molecules within the cell cytoplasm (40).

Gallium imaging is performed 48 or more hours following intravenous injection of 3 to 5 mCi Ga-67 citrate. Bowel preparation for these patients is similar to that used prior to a barium enema since the major route of excretion of the gallium is via the gastrointestinal tract. Normally, gallium concentration is seen in the liver, spleen, and bone marrow, and if images are obtained within 24 hours of administration, gallium may also be seen in the kidneys and urinary bladder.

Focal Nodular Hyperplasia and Hepatoadenoma

Although a rare condition, focal nodular hyperplasia is more common than hepatoadenoma, occurs more often in women, and is not associated with a history of oral contraceptives (41,42). Patients are usually asymptomatic, and an abdominal mass can be palpated. The tumor is typically hypervascular with tortuous irregularly granular vessels demonstrated during contrast angiography (43). Focal nodular hyperplasia tends to be unencapsulated, usually presents as multiple nodules, and histologically is composed of an abundance of Kupffer cells. Thus, radiocolloid distribution is usually normal (Figure 2–11), or perhaps a mild focal nonhomogeneous appearance is present unless the lesion is large or hemorrhage has occurred, in which case a focal decrease in radiocolloid localization will be seen. Rarely, the appearance will be that of a relative increased activity, that is a "hot spot" (44).

Hepatoadenoma was quite rare before the widespread use of oral contraceptives. It occurs almost exlcusively in women of childbearing age and is nearly always associated with the use of oral contraceptive drugs (41). Significant increased risk is related to the prolonged use of contraceptives, age greater than 30 years, and the use of high-potency hormones (45). Patients present with vague abdominal discomfort and a palpable abdominal mass, but the onset may be abrupt if hemorrhage occurs. Such patients represent an abdominal emergency. Liver function tests are typically normal. This tumor

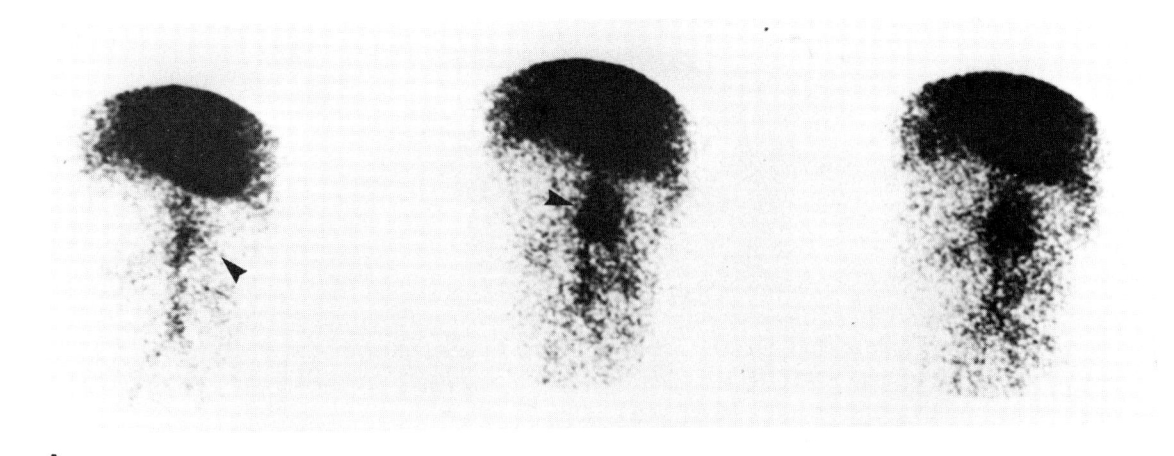

A

Figure 2–11. *A.* The radionuclide angiogram shows prominent focal increased flow to a focus in the left lobe (arrows).

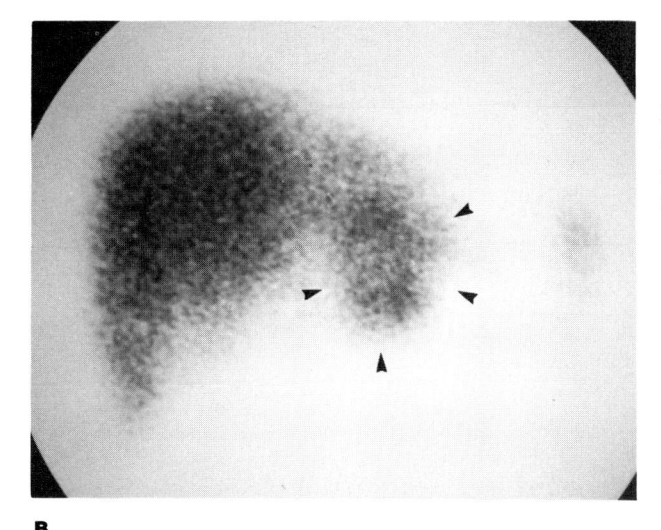

Figure 2-11. *B.* The anterior view shows colloid to be present in the mass (arrows), a finding consistent with the diagnosis of focal nodular hyperplasia.

is usually solitary and varies widely in size, although the majority are 8 to 15 cm in diameter. They are more common in the right lobe, frequently are in a subcapsular position, project from the surface, and may occasionally be pedunculated. The tumor is usually encapsulated and relatively soft so that the appearance is similar to normal liver parenchyma and may be considered benign. However, malignant adenomatous change has also been described (46). Microscopically, the tumor is composed of sheets or cords of normal or slightly atypical homogeneous hepatocytes with only a few biliary ducts, no portal tracts or central veins, and no Kupffer cells (41). Since this tumor contains no Kupffer cells, the radiocolloid scan appearance is one of a solitary focal intrahepatic mass (Figure 2-12). Belfar *et al.* (47) reported a case of hepatoadenoma with a focal defect on sulfur colloid scan that accumulated Tc-99m methyl iminodiacetic acid (HIDA) but did not excrete the radioactivity. It is believed that these findings were due to uniform hepatocytes present in the hepatoadenoma, but absence of bile ducts.

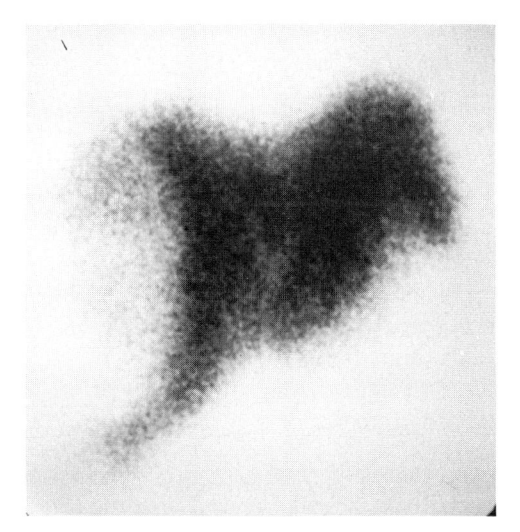

Figure 2-12. Anterior view of the liver shows an area of decreased activity in the right lobe in this patient taking birth control pills. This proved to be an adenoma with hemorrhage.

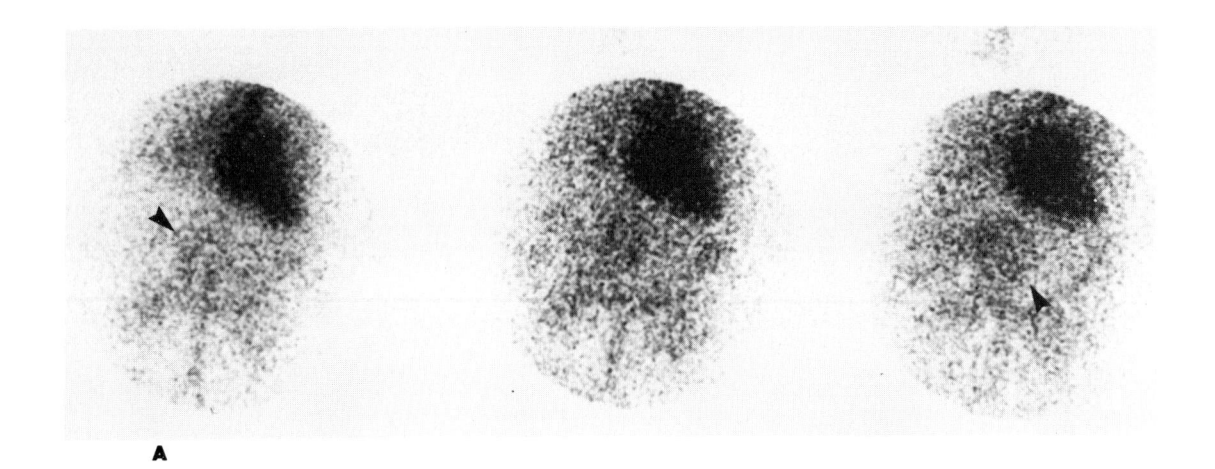

Figure 2-13. *A.* The radionuclide angiogram shows nonspecific increased flow to the left lobe (arrows).

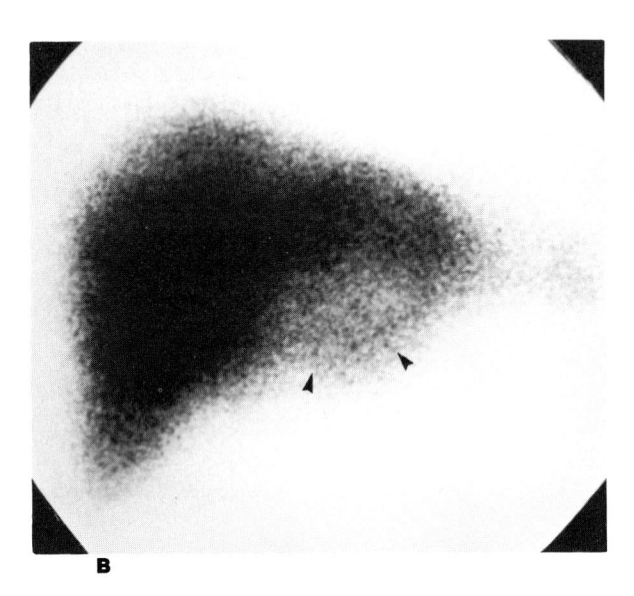

Figure 2-13. *B.* The anterior view shows that this area does not concentrate sulfur colloid. A hemangioma was diagnosed subsequently.

Hemangioma

Hemangioma is the most common benign tumor, but constitutes only a small fraction (less than 5 percent) of all liver neoplasms (48). The tumor is of mesodermal origin and may be capillary or cavernous. Capillary hemangiomas have a reddish-purple appearance; they may be disseminated throughout the organ or may be present as a single hemangioma less than 2.5 cm in diameter. Cavernous hemangioma usually consist of relatively small (1 to 2 cm diameter), solitary, dark red compressible vascular spaces lined with endothelium and filled with blood.

The appearance of hemangiomas on Tc-99m sulfur colloid scan is nonspecific, that is, a single large lesion or multiple focal defects. Recent studies have demonstrated that the intravascular blood pool of a hemangioma can be visualized after Tc-99m-labeled red blood cell injection, on the so-called delayed blood pool images (49–51). The scan appearance is unpredictable on radionuclide angiography and has little differential diagnostic value (Figure 2–13). In contrast to the sulfur colloid abnormality, the lesion has much higher activity than the liver in the 1 to 2 hour delayed blood-pool images. Furthermore, this finding is specific, as only hemangioma will produce increased (delayed) blood-pool activity. Engel *et al.* (51) reported no false-positive results and only one false-negative study (scan demonstrated isoactive blood-pool image) in 9 patients with one or more hemangiomas and in 12 patients with either primary or metastatic disease, cyst, or cirrhotic nodule. The Tc-99m red blood cell (RBC) scan should be performed as the procedure of choice in separating hemangioma from other hepatic lesions. It is recommended that the Tc-99m RBC blood-pool scan be the initial procedure and that contrast computed tomography or angiography be reserved for those patients who demonstrate an isoactive blood pool.

Hepatic Abscess

Pyogenic infection is the primary etiology of an hepatic abscess in patients from industrialized nations, while on a worldwide basis, *Entamoeba histolytica* is the most frequent cause of a hepatic abscess. Early diagnosis of a hepatic abscess is crucial to avoid moribund complications such as generalized sepsis. An abscess of the liver or spleen may be detected with a high degree of sensitivity using radiocolloid scan (14,52,53). The appearance of an abscess on scanning is as one or more focal defects. The size and shape of the abscess, as well as the extent of hepatic involvement, can be readily displayed from multiple projection views of the organ. This information provides excellent guidance for successful drainage. Recently, the preferred treatment for many pyogenic and amebic abscesses has become conservative, and open surgical drainage is less frequently used. The radionuclide scan can be used to document response to therapy and progress toward resolution of liver abscesses, as many patients have been described that have been treated successfully by antibiotics alone or antibiotics combined with percutaneous drainage.

Gallium and indium-111 oxine-labeled autologous leukocytes have been used to localize intraabdominal abscess with good results (54–58). The precise mechanism for Ga-67 accumulation in the abscess is unknown, but is believed to be due to increased capillary and cell permeability in the abscess region (Figure 2–14). Thus, bound or unbound Ga-67 will diffuse into the abscess and bind to lactoferrin, which is present in high concentration (57, 58).

Although the scan patterns of pyogenic abscess by radiocolloid and Ga-67 are similar to that found in hepatocellular carcinoma, clinical findings, such as abdominal pain, liver tenderness or hepatic friction rub, pyrexia, and nocturnal sweating can usually distinguish the two disorders. The specificity of diagnosis can be increased by needle aspiration guided by the scan or by ultrasound. Although gallium does not concentrate within an amebic abscess, frequently one can appreciate relative circumferential gallium concentration about the periphery. This pattern is believed to be secondary to the cellular inflammatory reaction known to occur along the border of an amebic abscess.

There are good data to suggest that the leukocyte scan is useful primarily in patients with an infection of short duration. Sfakianakis *et al.* performed a prospective study to compare the utility of gallium-67 and indium-111 leukocyte scanning in 32 patients with moderate to high clinical suspicion of having a focal infection (59). Their results suggest that In-111 leukocyte scanning is a reliable technique to detect focal sepsis in patients who were septic less than 2 weeks, but in those with more prolonged infections,

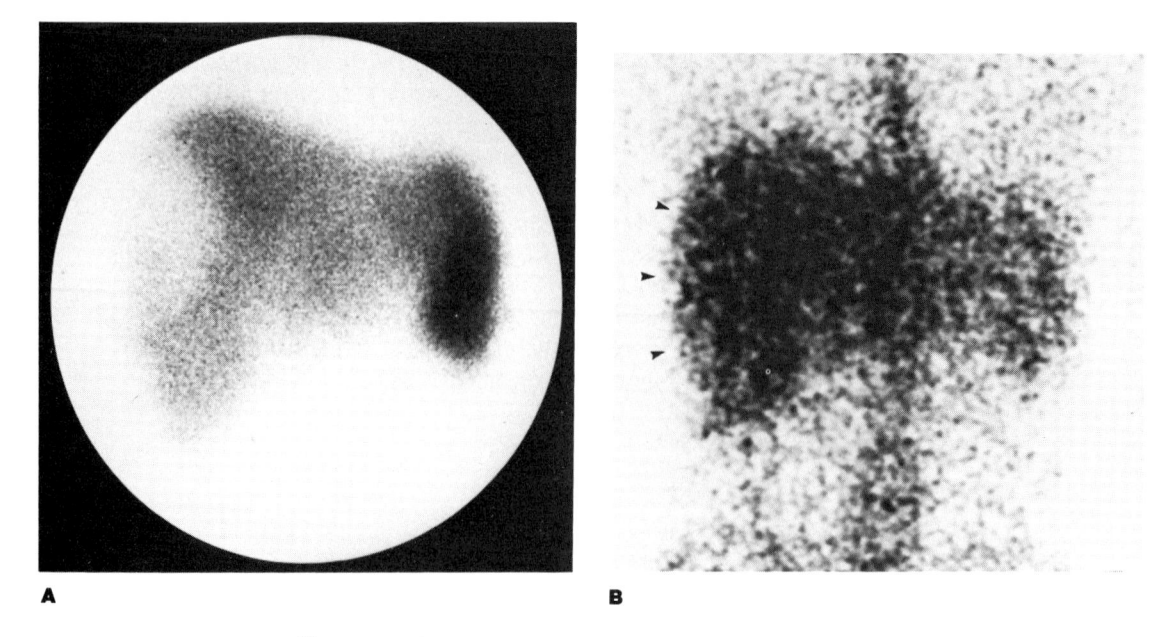

Figure 2–14. *A.* ^{99m}Tc colloid image shows a large defect in the right lobe in this patient with a suspected abscess. *B.* The ^{67}Ga citrate scan shows activity in the same area, but not greater than the surrounding liver. By virtue of the positive liver scan defect, this becomes a positive ^{67}Ga citrate image. Not all pyogenic abscesses concentrate ^{67}Ga citrate prominently. This study emphasizes the need for a liver scan prior to ^{67}Ga citrate imaging.

the WBC scan loses much of its sensitivity and may be falsely negative. In such an instance, if the In-WBC scan is negative, a gallium scan should be considered.

Indium-111-labeled leukocytes (WBC) have been used to diagnose hepatic abscess and to differentiate hepatic abscess from tumor (56,60). At present, the In-111 WBC technique has not received New Drug Application approval from the FDA, but its promise is believed to be great (61).

Cyst

Gray scale ultrasonography is the procedure of choice if a hepatic cyst is suspected. Simple hepatic cysts are often demonstrated during routine ultrasonography of the abdomen performed for other reasons. The cysts are usually too small to be detected by radiocolloid scanning techniques. A large cyst may produce hepatomegaly and, in some instances, displace the liver from its normal position. Radiocolloid scan appearance of a cyst is a nonspecific discrete focal decrease in activity that cannot be distinguished from other solid masses (Figure 2–15).

FOCAL INCREASED UPTAKE IN RADIOCOLLOID SCAN

A focal increased uptake on a radiocolloid scan, the liver scan "hot spot," is seen often in patients with obstruction of the superior or inferior vena cava and has also been described in the presence of thrombosis of the hepatic veins (Budd-Chiari syndrome), hepatic tumors, cirrhosis, and focal nodular hyperplasia (5).

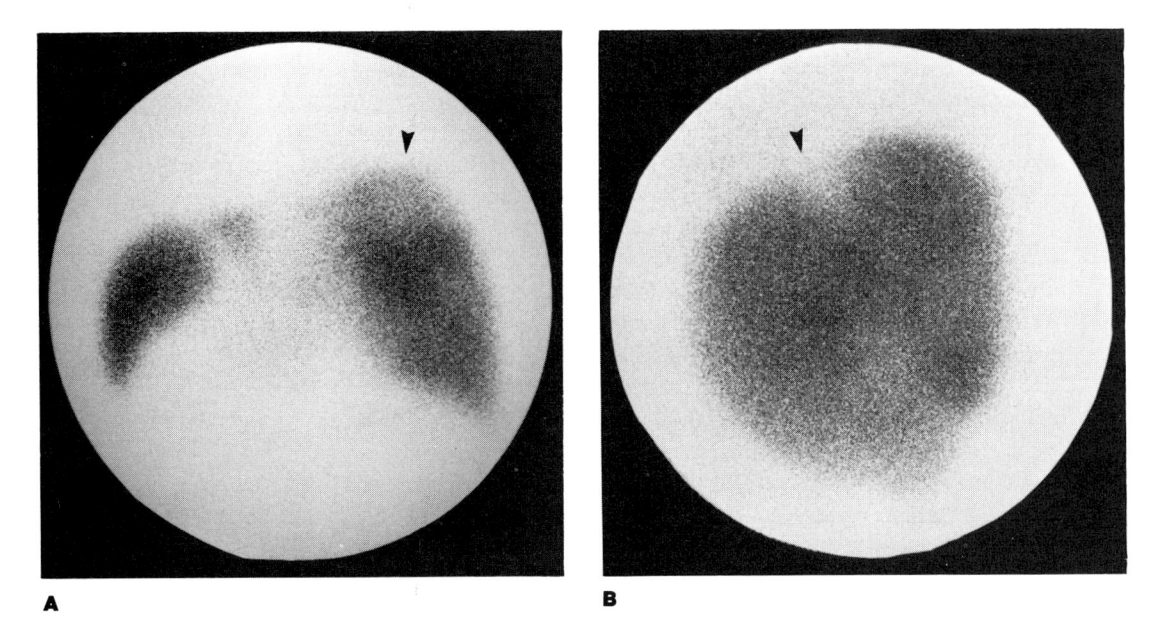

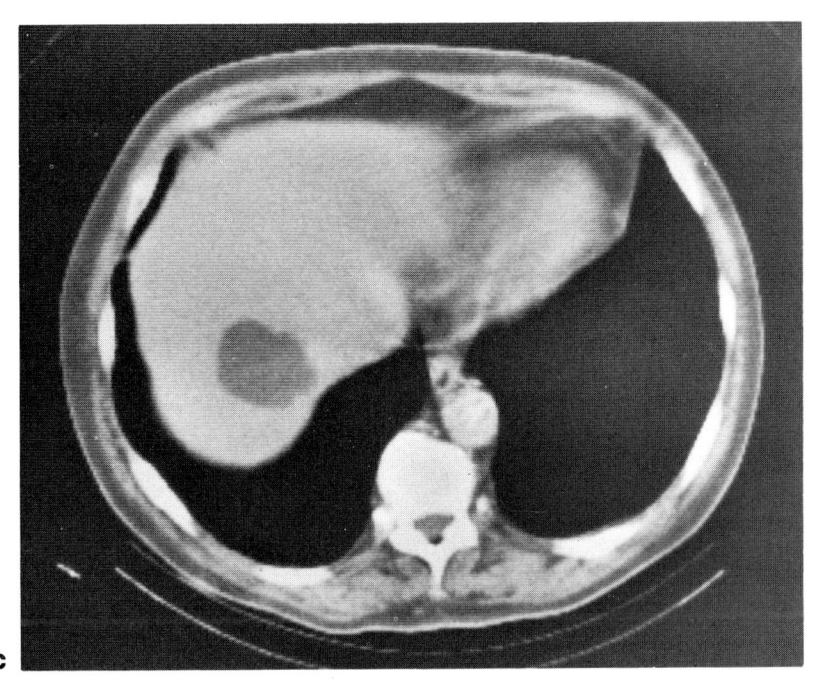

Figure 2-15. Posterior (*A*) and right lateral (*B*) views show a single focal defect (arrows). Clinically, the suspicion of metastases was low and further workup was done. *C.* CT scan showed the lesion to be a liver cyst.

Superior venal caval (SVC) obstruction produces venous distention and edema in the head and upper extremities, and often, dilated venous collaterals are seen over the upper portion of the thorax and abdomen. The most common cause of this condition is malignancy by either direct extension into the vessel or metastatic lymph nodes. SVC obstruction is also seen in patients with an intrathoracic aneurysm, lymphoma, or inflammatory lymph node enlargement. Because restricted venous return results in reduced cardiac output and venous hypertension produces cerebral edema, obstruction of the SVC may produce cardiovascular collapse. Therefore, the appearance of SVC obstruction is a medical emergency that demands immediate diagnosis and therapy. The diagnosis may be accomplished simply and rapidly by radionuclide venography and liver scanning. The factors that influence the characteristics of the "hot spot" are the site and extent of the obstruction and the individual variation in the anatomy of the collateral venous channels (62). Although the liver flow or "perfusion" study is not particularly useful, the vascular pattern can document the collateral circulation that results in the uneven delivery of colloid in patients with SVC obstruction. This finding would be in contrast to what would be seen in patients with Budd-Chiari syndrome or focal nodular hyperplasia in which the "hot spot" is secondary to intrahepatic disease and not vena cava obstruction.

Significant vena cava obstruction will produce a specific focal increased uptake in the central portion of the liver on radiocolloid scan (Figure 2–16). This occurs because the collateral channels divert the colloid via the umbilical vein into small segments of the liver (62).

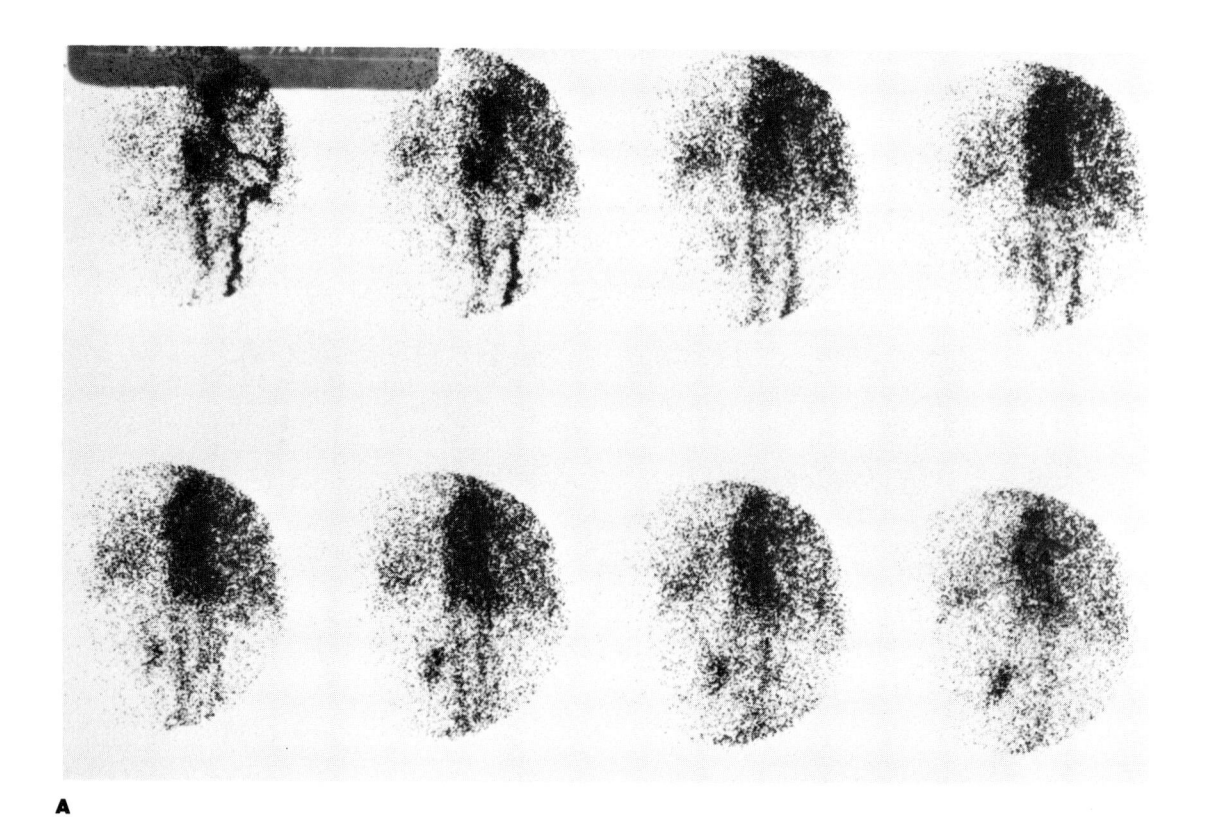

Figure 2–16. *A.* Radionuclide angiogram shows serpiginous vessels crossing the abdomen.

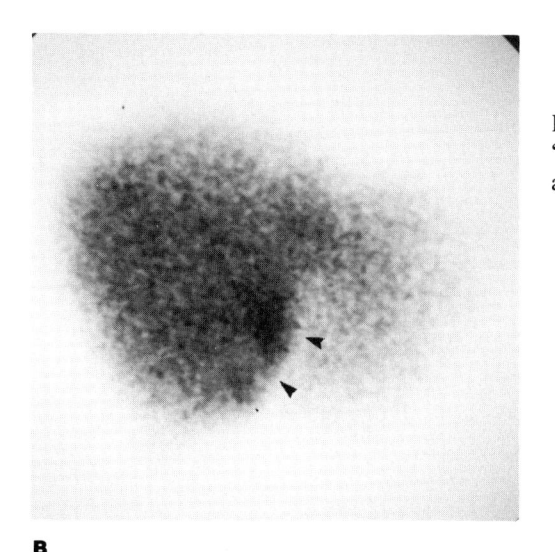

Figure 2-16. *B.* The anterior view shows the semilunar "hot" spot in the region of the ligamentum teres, a finding almost pathognomonic of superior vena cava occlusion.

In patients with Budd-Chiari syndrome (occlusion of hepatic veins), the liver is diffusely enlarged, tender, and severe intractable ascites is present. Symptoms may appear rapidly and lead to death from liver failure within a week, or a more indolent course may last several years. Radiocolloid liver scan of a patient with hepatic vein thrombosis will show an increased uptake of radioactivity located centrally in the anterior view and posteriorly in the right lateral view (63) (Figure 2-17). This localization occurs in the caudate lobe, a region that has independent venous drainage directly into the inferior vena cava without passing through the hepatic vein. The appearance is variable, and in some patients only nonhomogeneous liver uptake is noted. This pattern is difficult to distinguish from that produced by diffuse hepatic parenchymal disease.

EVALUATION OF HEPATIC FUNCTION: DIFFUSE HEPATIC DISEASE
Radiocolloid Scanning

Current biochemical tests of liver function play an important role in the assessment of hepatic cellular integrity. Bromsulphalein retention has been used widely as a sensitive indicator of hepatic cell dysfunction, but normal plasma retention is not specific for any particular category of hepatic disturbance. Indeed, most biochemical tests of liver function are nonspecific. Various serum enzyme activities are sensitive indicators of liver cell damage and quite useful in the evaluation of acute liver disease. However, such tests are not helpful for the assessment of functional hepatic reserve during the late stages of liver diseases such as cirrhosis.

Liver scanning is relatively insensitive to changes in parenchymal function and should not be obtained as another test of liver function. The scan may be of some value in patients with moderate to severe dysfunction, particularly to record objectively changes in liver and spleen size, the extent of scar formation, repair, and extrahepatic shunting. Although the Kupffer cells and the hepatic polygonal cells have different embryological origins and different functions, it is generally agreed that most pathologic processes affect both cell populations relatively equally. Thus, quantification of the rate and the degree of colloid uptake probably represents integrity of hepatocyte function and, therefore, global hepatic function. As an aside, it should be appreciated that data

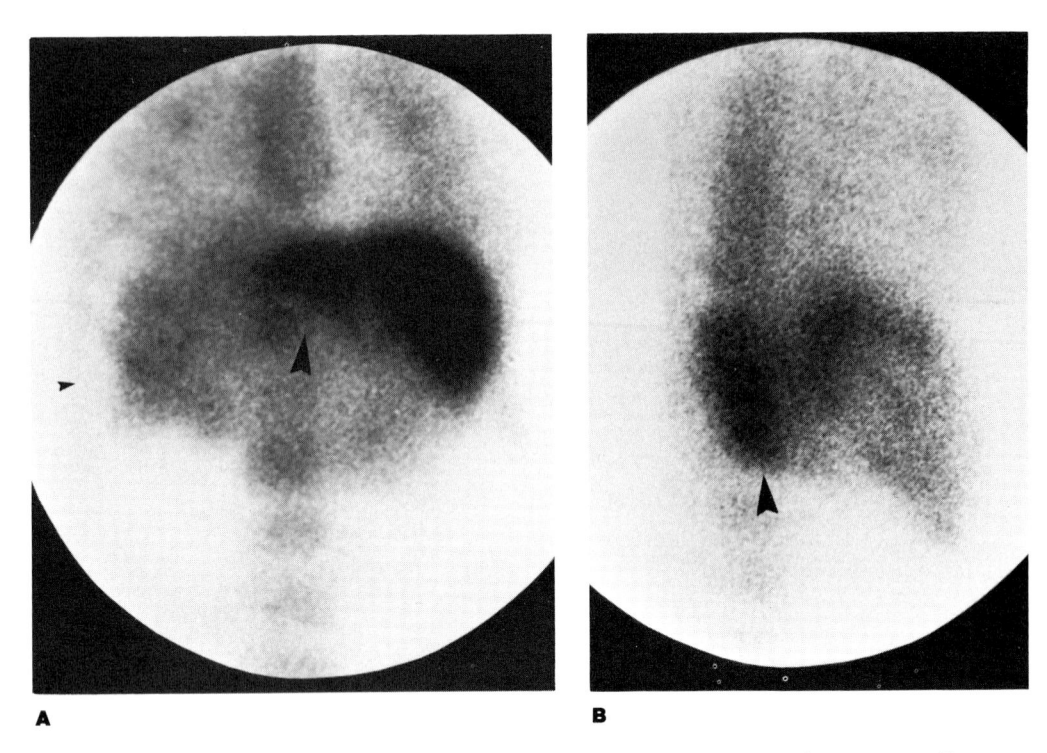

Figure 2-17. Anterior (*A*) and right lateral (*B*) views of the liver show inhomogeneous liver activity, prominent bone marrow and spleen activity, and evidence of ascites manifested by separation of liver and rib activity (small arrows). Focal increased activity is noted in the caudate lobe (large arrows). The caudate lobe has direct communication with the vena cava and may, therefore, be prominent in cases of hepatic vein occlusion.

derived from early measurements of change in liver activity following injection of colloid (Kupffer cell) or IDA-type compound (polygonal cell) must be "corrected" for liver blood flow before absolute cell function can be estimated.

The liver contains about 85 percent to 90 percent of the fixed reticuloendothelial system. The normal liver receives approximately 25 percent of its blood from the hepatic artery and 75 percent from the portal vein. Colloid uptake in the liver is dependent on liver *blood flow* and on the *extraction efficiency* of the Kupffer cells. As function of the parenchymal cells deteriorates, such as in cirrhosis, the hepatic artery flow may account for a greater proportion of the total blood supply to the liver. Most hepatic neoplasms derive their blood supply predominantly from the hepatic artery.

The scan appearance of the liver in patients with cirrhosis depends on the stage and severity of the infammatory process. Early in the cirrhotic process, mild hepatomegaly due to fat infiltration and mild redistribution of colloid to the spleen and bone marrow are noted. As a cirrhotic process progresses, atrophy of the right lobe with compensatory hypertrophy of the left lobe frequently develops. A marked reversal of the usual right-to-left hepatic lobe distribution of radiocolloid resulting in disproportionate prominence of the left lobe is the most sensitive liver scan finding in patients with cirrhosis (64). During the terminal stages of the disease, scans show a smaller liver that contains much less colloid with correspondingly intense activity in the bone marrow and spleen (Figure 2-18). Splenomegaly is often noted; however, the size of the spleen is variable. Sple-

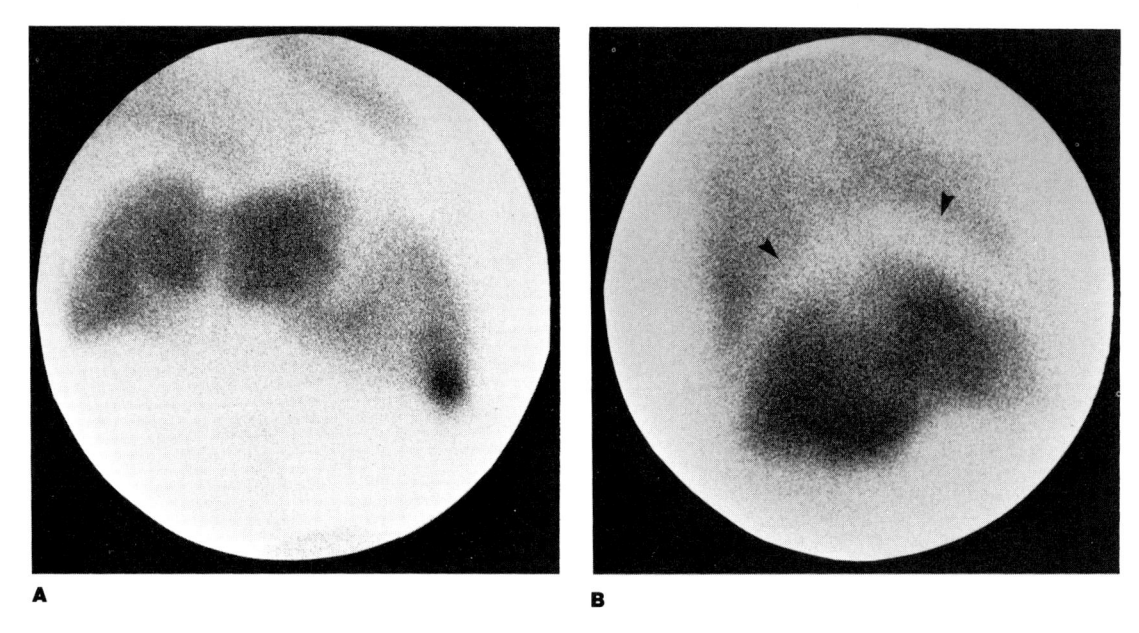

Figure 2-18. Anterior (*A*) and right lateral (*B*) views show a small inhomogeneous liver. Bone marrow and lung activity is prominent, and a "halo" of ascitic fluid is visible between the liver and lung activity (arrows). These findings are typical of advanced cirrhosis.

nomegaly and the relative increased concentration of colloid seen in the spleen when compared with the liver (normal spleen/liver ratio is 0.8 to 1.2) are related to changes in portal pressure and/or changes in portal blood flow that are sequelae of the disease. Following portal decompression, the spleen may not return to normal size.

The distribution of radiocolloid in the cirrhotic liver is usually nonhomogeneous, and with regeneration and formation of fibrous tissue, there may be areas of relative decreased and relative increased tracer concentration (Figure 2-19). The mechanism for these changes is related to the overall reduction of Kupffer cells per volume of tissue, as well as the result of inflammation, fibrosis, necrosis, or by regenerating parenchymal cells. Intrahepatic shunting may also produce a focal decrease in activity (65).

The mechanism of increased bone marrow and splenic activity seen in scans of patients with chronic liver disease has been discussed. Although the redistribution of colloid on the scan induced by changes in portal pressure can not be separated precisely from those produced by changes in portal blood flow, such as shunting, portal hypertension is believed to be primarily responsible for the characteristic redistribution of colloid in these patients. The intensity of bone marrow or splenic uptake of colloid and the measured wedge hepatic vein pressure in these patients are directly related (66,67). However, the abnormal scan pattern seen in chronic liver disease remains fixed and does not reverse when portal hypertension is relieved by surgical decompression (68, 69). Another factor involved in this long-term redistribution pattern appears to be intrahepatic shunting. This shunting results in portal blood bypassing the hepatic sinusoids and thus becomes more available for the nonhepatic reticuloendothelial cells. In the normal situation, hepatic extraction efficiency of the liver for colloid is about 95 percent (68,70). Theoretically, a reduction in the number of hepatic reticuloendothelial cells would result in similar scan findings, but there is no evidence to support this hypothesis (71).

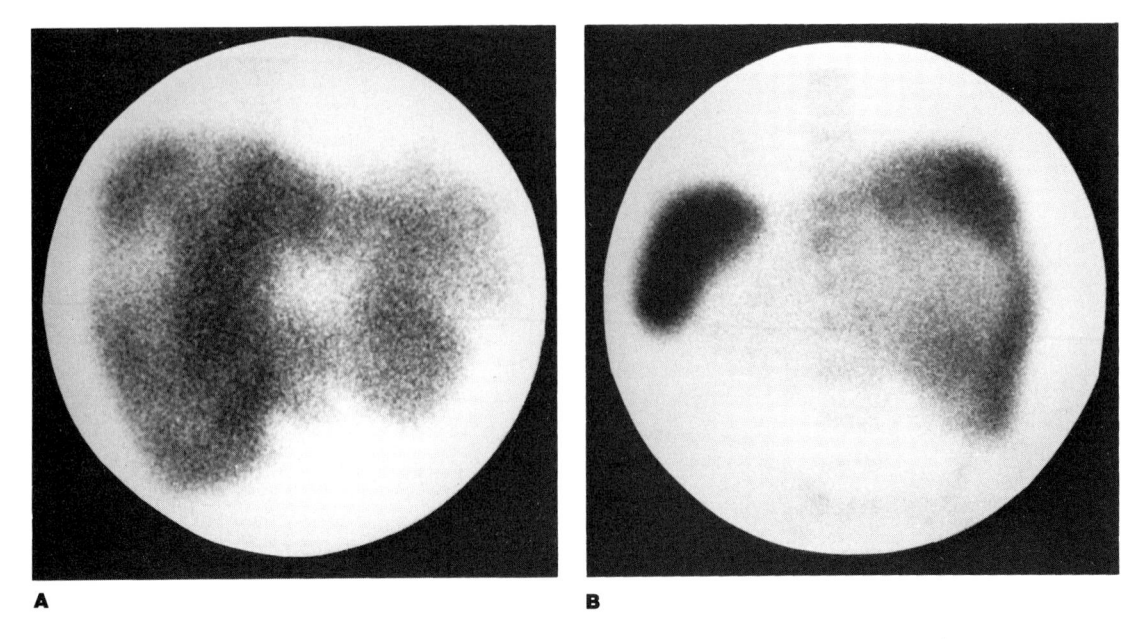

Figure 2-19. Anterior (*A*) and posterior (*B*) views of the liver show multiple irregular defects in the liver. Increased splenic activity and prominent bone marrow activity are present. These areas were diagnosed as pseudomasses in a patient with alcoholic liver disease. The helpful diagnostic feature is the abnormal colloid distribution, which is uncommon in metastatic disease.

Increases in spleen and bone marrow concentration are most often seen in patients who have cirrhosis, but anemia from any cause, including iron deficiency, and proliferative bone marrow disease may produce a similar pattern (72). The mechanism is complex and, in addition to extrahepatic shunting, includes interstitial edema with resulting venous drainage impairment, such as seen in patients with acute severe hepatitis, passive chronic congestion, hepatic vein obstruction, recent general anesthesia, and replacement of liver tissue, for example, fibrosis, extensive metastases, chronic granulomatous disease, fat, and glycogen.

An absolute increase in splenic concentration of colloid without apparent decrease in liver activity is seen in patients with myeloproliferative diseases, in association with rheumatoid arthritis, particularly Felty's syndrome, and in those patients in whom the RES has been stimulated, such as during septicemia or by the administration of various drugs. Extrahepatic shift of colloid has been described as one of the transient findings associated with cancer chemotherapy (73). Detailed reviews of drug-induced change in the biological distribution of radiopharmaceuticals have appeared (74,75).

Hepatobiliary Scanning

The large hepatic polygonal cells, the hepatocytes, comprise 80 to 90 percent of the hepatic parenchymal mass and are metabolically active cells. These cells are responsible for the extraction and excretion of a large number of chemicals, pigmented materials, drugs, and products of metabolism into the biliary system. An early application of nuclear medicine suggested that the use of a radiolabeled substance extracted by the hepatocytes and excreted into the biliary system might be useful to evaluate hepatocyte integrity and, therefore, represent a measure of total hepatic function. In 1955, Taplin *et al.* introduced I-131-labeled rose bengal (76). This dye is selectively excreted by hepatic cells exclusive of Kupffer cell function. Moreover, once excreted into the intestinal tract, rose bengal is not reabsorbed. Thus, the known pharmacokinetics of the dye appear to share many desired characteristics of a suitable liver function test. Early studies indicated that the hepatic uptake and excretion curves following intravenous administration of I-131-labeled rose bengal were useful to evaluate liver function. However, because of the poor physical characteristics of the I-131 nuclide, the technique was never widely adapted.

There was a great resurgence of interest in hepatobiliary imaging following the introduction of Tc-99m-labeled iminodiacetic acid (IDA) derivatives. A variety of IDA analogues are available, but currently the most popular is diisopropyliminodiacetic acid (DISIDA). Following injection, this class of drugs is rapidly extracted by the hepatocytes and excreted into the bile. Since this is a study of dynamics rather than morphology alone, images are usually obtained at frequent intervals initially and then as needed. The normal study shows rapid uptake by the liver with visualization of the bile ducts, gallbladder, and bowel by 1 hour (Figure 2-20).

Cholelithiasis and its complications are the most common cause of abdominal surgery (77). This diagnosis of cholecystitis is a frequent consideration in patients with acute right upper quadrant pain. Acute cholecystitis is most often associated with cystic duct obstruction by stones (77). Hepatobiliary imaging allows evaluation for cystic duct obstruction with a high degree of accuracy. Gallbladder visualization by 1 hour virtually excludes the diagnosis (78,79). Failure to visualize the gallbladder by 1 hour with normal biliary to bowel transit is a sensitive finding in acute cholecystitis. Although chronic cholecystitis may mimic these findings at 1 hour, an image at 4 hours will usually dif-

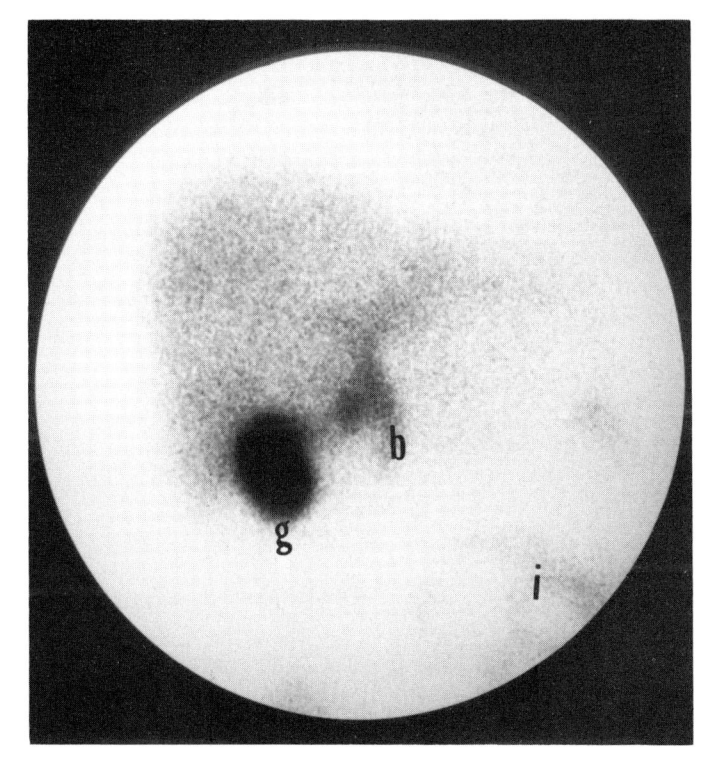

Figure 2-20. Normal 30-minute anterior ^{99m}Tc-DISIDA image showing: g = gallbladder; b = common bile duct; i = intestinal activity.

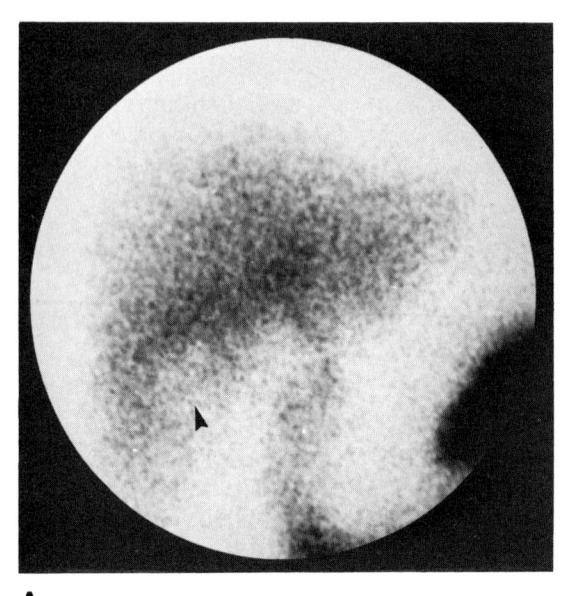

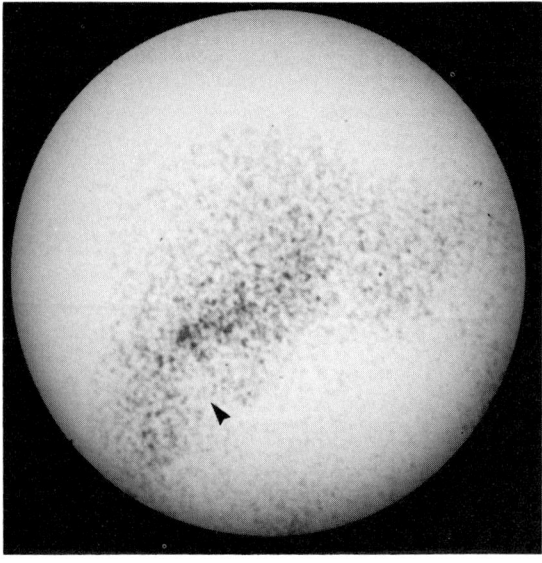

Figure 2-21. Anterior images at 60 minutes (*A*) and 4 hours (*B*) from a ^{99m}Tc-DISIDA study with gallbladder fossa devoid of activity (arrows), consistent with acute cholecystitis found at surgery.

ferentiate the two (Figure 2-21). In chronic cholecystitis, the gallbladder typically will visualize at 4 hours (78,79). the accuracy of hepatobiliary imaging in diagnosing acute cholecystitis has been reported to be greater than 95 percent by several authors (78-81).

Although acute acalculous cholecystitis was thought to be a potential problem for hepatobiliary imaging, this has not proven to be the case, and hepatobiliary imaging may be the procedure of choice when this entity is suspected (82).

False-positive results may occur secondary to a nonfasting state (83), in alcoholics, and in patients receiving total parenteral nutrition (84).

The use of hepatobiliary imaging in cholestasis has been shown to be useful, but is dependent upon the bilirubin level. Biliary obstruction is characterized by good clearance of the agent with no visualization of the bile ducts or bowel (Figure 2-22). Hepatocellular disease shows poor hepatic concentration and delayed visualization or nonvisualization of the ducts and bowel (Figure 2-23). Pauwels and co-workers were able to differentiate obstruction from hepatocellular disease with an accuracy of 90 percent (85). At high bilirubin levels (>20 mg/dl), the accuracy decreased markedly. The study appears most useful in diagnosing obstruction rather than excluding it. In acute obstruction, the findings may occur prior to enzymatic or sonographic abnormality (86). Partial obstruction is demonstrated by delayed filling of the bowel (78, 85), but this finding must be interpreted with caution when meperidine or morphine have been administered (87).

In the pediatric age group, biliary atresia is a devastating disease. Distinguishing this entity from neonatal hepatitis is paramount. Portoenterostomy shows promising results if performed before 4 months of age (88), and even better prognosis when performed before 10 weeks of age (88, 89). Quantitation of fecal excretion has been helpful in the differential diagnosis (90). Atresia demonstrates less than 5 percent excretion

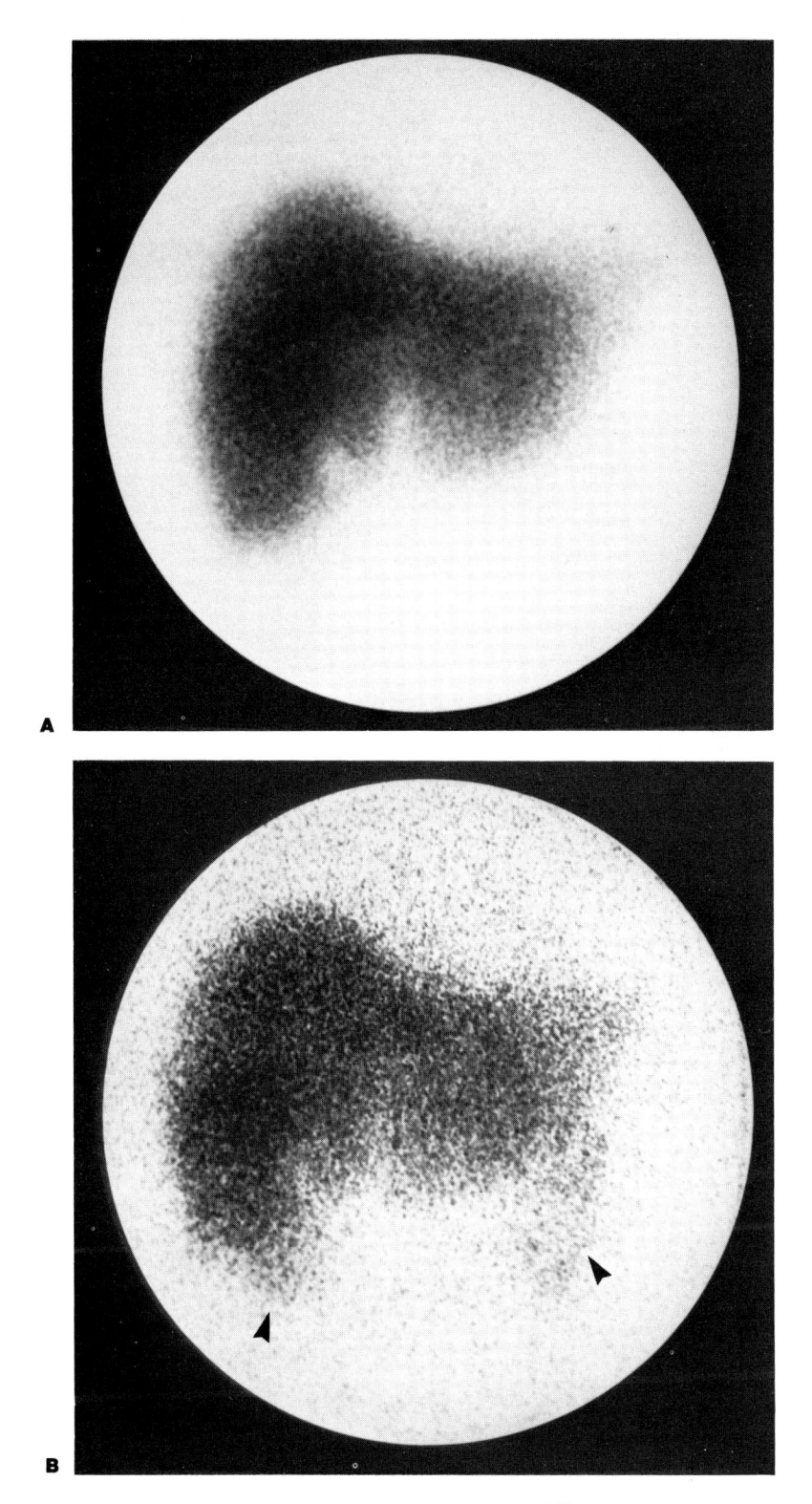

Figure 2-22. Images at 4 hours (*A*) and 24 hours (*B*) from a ^{99m}Tc-DISIDA show no excretion into the intestine, but good hepatic uptake. At 24 hours, the kidneys are visualized, since they represent the secondary route of excretion (arrows). A stone had completely obstructed the patient's common bile duct.

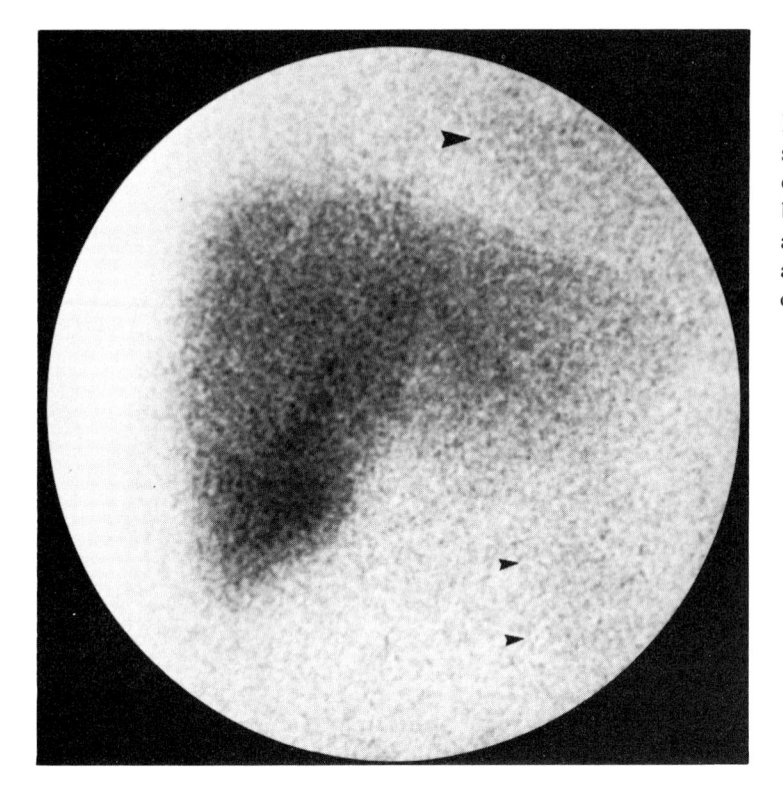

Figure 2–23. Four-hour view of study in a patient with hepatocellular disease showing persistent cardiac blood-pool activity (arrow), but faint activity in the intestine (small arrows), consistent with no obstruction.

Figure 2–24. A 4-hour ^{99m}Tc-DISIDA image demonstrating good hepatic uptake, but no evidence of excretion into the bowel. Obvious bladder activity is present. Findings are consistent with biliary atresia.

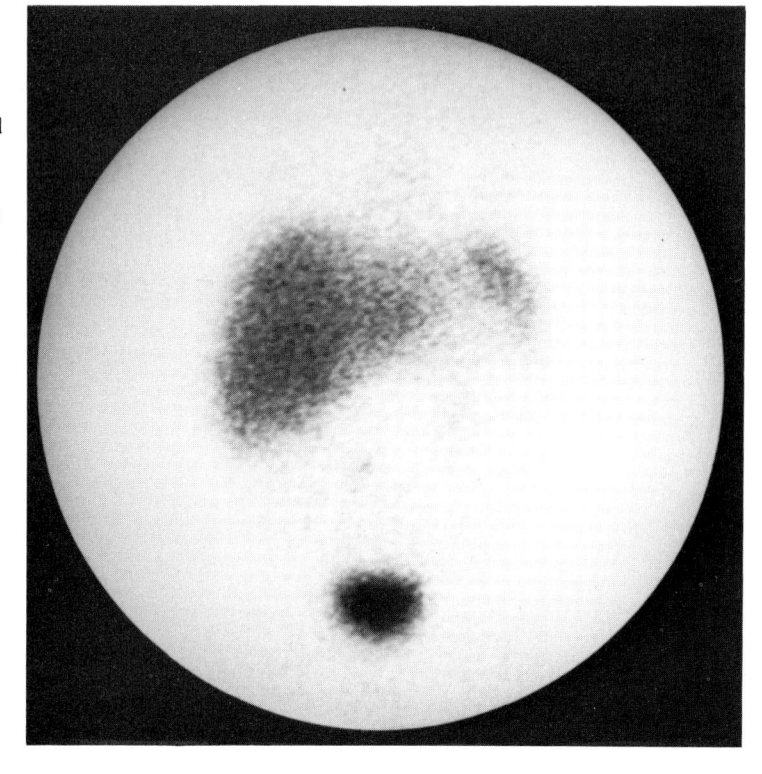

after 72 hours, and values greater than 10 percent are associated with neonatal hepatitis. Obviously, it is difficult to get accurate results unless samples are collected without urine contamination. Imaging has been utilized with some success using ^{131}I-rose bengal (91). The false-positive rate is approximately 20 percent, however, in which case needless surgery would be performed. The use of the ^{99m}Tc-hepatobiliary agents has resulted in variable success rates. Collier and co-workers (92) compared ^{131}I-rose bengal with ^{99m}Tc-BIDA and found the 6-hour half-life of ^{99m}technetium to be a limiting factor. The ^{99m}technetium agent failed in three of five patients with neonatal hepatitis. Others have reported greater success with accuracies in the 90 percent range (93,94). Oral phenobarbital may be helpful in improving the results (94). A pattern of good extraction by the liver and no excretion is most often associated with atresia (Figure 2–24), whereas poor extraction and no excretion are more likely to be associated with neonatal hepatitis. These findings are obviously most helpful earlier in the course of biliary atresia, before parenchymal damage ensues. The use of other isotope labels such as Ru-97 is under investigation (95), because the longer half-life (2.9 days) should allow more prolonged imaging than 24 hours.

Other uses of the hepatobiliary agents include evaluation for bile leaks (96) and patency of surgical anastomoses (86). Obviously, the use of the ^{99m}Tc agents allows evaluation of areas or lesions detected with ^{99m}Tc sulfur colloid that are suspected to be in communication with the biliary tract (97). The superior resolution of these agents also allows detection of focal disease that may have gone unsuspected (98) (Figure 2–25).

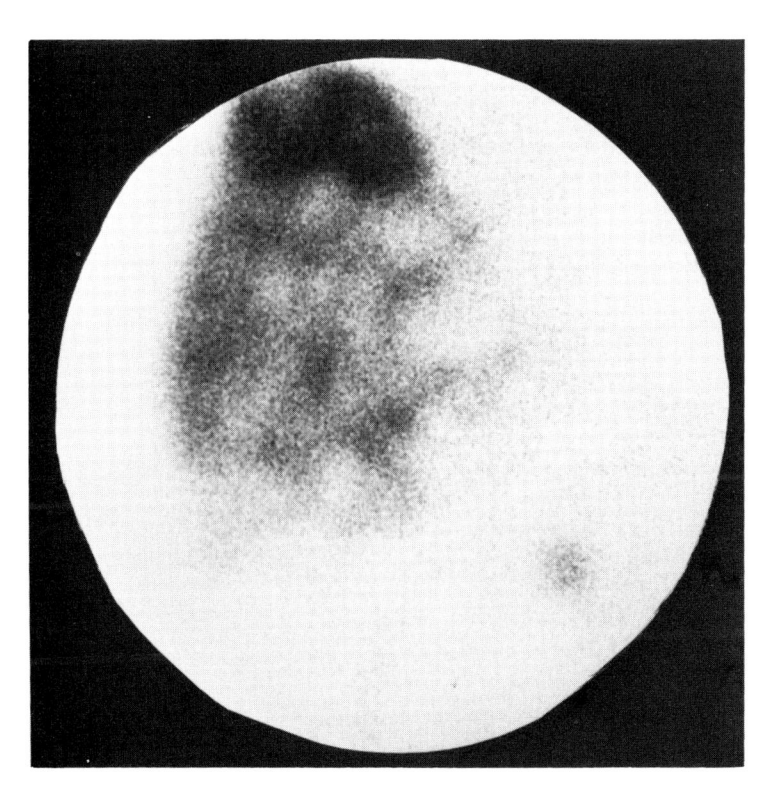

Figure 2–25. Early parenchymal ^{99m}Tc-DISIDA image showing multiple focal defects that proved to be metastatic lesions.

REFERENCES

1. Warbick A, Ege GN, Henkelman RM, et al.: An evaluation of radiocolloid sizing techniques. J Nucl Med 1977;18:827–834.
2. Atkins HL, Hauser W, Richards P: Factors affecting distribution of technetium-sulfur colloid. J Reticuloendothel Soc 1970;8:176–184.
3. Saba TM: Physiology and physiopathology of the reticuloendothelial system. Arch Intern Med 1970;126:1031–1050.
4. Hinkle GH, Leonard JC, Krous HF, Alexander JB: Absence of hepatic uptake of Tc-99m sulfur colloid in an infant with Coxsakie B_2 viral infection. Clin Nucl Med 1983;8:246–248.
5. Stadalnik RC: Gamut. "Hot spots"—liver imaging. Semin Nucl Med 1979;9:220–221.
6. Sy WM, Malach M: Editorial. Lung uptake on 99m technetium liver scan. Chest 1975;68:613–614.
7. Firnau G: Why do Tc-99m chelates work for cholescintigraphy? Eur J Nucl Med 1976;1:137–139.
8. Lamki L: A dichotomy in hepatic uptake of 99m-Tc-IDA and 99mTc-colloid. Semin Nucl Med 1982;12:92–94.
9. Eckelman WC, Reba RC, Gibson RE, et al.: Receptor-binding radiotracers: A Class of potential radiopharmaceuticals. J Nucl Med 1979;20:350–357.
10. Krohn KA, Vera DR, Stadalnik RC: A complimentary radiopharmaceutical and mathematical model for quantitating hepatic-binding protein receptors. In WC Eckelman (ed), Receptor-Binding Radiotracers, vol. 2. Boca Raton, Fla.: CRC Press, 1982, pp. 41–59.
11. Welch MJ: New radiopharmaceuticals for studying liver function. J Nucl Med 1982;23:1138–1139.
12. Holder LE, Saenger EL: The use of nuclear medicine in evaluating liver disease. Semin Roentgenol 1975;10:215–222.
13. Oster ZH, Larson SM, Strauss HW, Wagner HN: Analysis of liver scanning in a general hospital. J Nucl Med 1975;16:450–453.
14. Drum DE: Current status of radiocolloid hepatic scintiphotography for space-occupying disease. Semin Nucl Med 1982;12:64–74.
15. McAfee JG, Ause RG, Wagner HN Jr: Diagnostic value of scintillation scanning of the liver. Arch Intern Med 1965;116:95–110.
16. Shi W-J, Reba RC, DeLand FH: Causes of focal hepatic portal defect on 99m-Tc-sulfur colloid scintigraphy. Semin Nucl Med 1983;13:171–173.
17. Drum DE: Optimizing the clinical value of hepatic scintiphotography. Semin Nucl Med 1978;8:346–357.
18. Drum DE, Beard JO: Liver scintigraphic features associated with alcoholism. J Nucl Med 1978;19:154–160.
19. Poulose KP, Reba RC, Cameron JC, Wagner HN Jr: The value and limitations of liver scanning for the detection of hepatic metastases in patients with cancer. J Indian Med Assoc 1973;61:199–205.
20. Hatfield PM: Role of liver scanning in the diagnosis of hepatic metastases. Med Clin North Am 1975;59:247–276.
21. Simon TR, Neuman AL, Gorelick FS, et al.: Scintigraphic diagnosis of cirrhosis: A receiver operator characteristic analysis of the common interpretative criteria. Radiology 1981;138:723–726.
22. Conn HO: Rational use of liver biopsy in the diagnosis of hepatic cancer. Gastroenterology 1972;63:142–146.
23. Dixon AG, Burns WA: Liver biopsies in patients with malignancy: a postmortem study. Lab Invest 1973;28:405 (abstract).
24. Bleiberg H, Rozencweig M. Longeval E, et al.: Peritoneoscopy as a diagnostic supplement to liver function tests and liver scans in patients with carcinoma. Surg Gynecol Obstet 1977;145:821–825.

25. Ozarda A, Pickren J: The topographic distribution of liver metastasis. Its relation to surgical and isotope diagnosis. J Nucl Med 1962;3:149–152.
26. Ostfeld DA, Meyer JE: Liver scanning in cancer patients with short-interval autopsy correlation. Radiology 1981;138:671–673.
27. Reba RC, Kleinman JC: The sensitivity, specificity, and predictive value of diagnostic tests. In BA Rhodes (ed), Quality Control in Nuclear Medicine. St. Louis; Mosby, 1977, pp. 53–64.
28. Sugarbaker PH, Beard JO, Drum DE: Detection of hepatic metastases from cancer of the breast. Am J Surg 1977;133:531–535.
29. Szymendera JJ, Wilczynska JE, Nowacki MP, et al.: Serial CEA assays and liver scintigraphy for the detection of hepatic metastases from colorectal carcinoma. Dis Colon Rectum 1982;25:191–197.
30. Pressman D: Radiolabelled antibodies. Ann NY Acad Sci 1957;69:644–650.
31. Goldenberg DM, DeLand F, Kim E, et al.: Use of radiolabeled antibodies to carcino embryonic antigen for the detection and localization of diverse concerns by photoscanning. N Engl J Med 1978;298:1384–1388.
32. Goodwin DA, Meares CF, Diamanti CI, et al.: Use of specific antibody for rapid clearance of circulating blood background from radiolabeled tumor imaging proteins. J Nucl Med 1983;24:P31 (abstract).
33. Moldofsky PJ, Powe J, Mulbern CB Jr, et al.: Metastatic colon carcinoma detected with radiolabeled F(ab')$_2$ monoclonal antibody fragments. Radiology 1983;149:549–555.
34. Powe J, Pak KY, Paik CH, et al.: Labeling monoclonal antibodies and F(ab')$_2$ fragments with (^{111}In) indium using cyclic DTPA anhydride and their in vivo behavior in mice bearing human tumor xenografts. Cancer Drug Delivery 1984, in press.
35. Bledin AG, Kim EE, Haynie TP: Technetium Tc-99m-macroaggregated albumin angiography and perfusion. JAMA 1983;250:941–943.
36. Ziessman HA, Thrall JH, Gyves JW, et al.: Quantitative hepatic arterial perfusion scintigraphy and starch microspheres in cancer chemotherapy. J Nucl Med 1983;24:871–875.
37. Poulose KP, Reba RC, Deland FH, Wagner HN Jr: Role of liver scanning in the preoperative evaluation of patients with cancer. Br Med J 1968;4:585–587.
38. James O, Wood EJ, Sherlock S: 67-gallium scanning in the diagnosis of liver disease. Gut 1974;15:404–410.
39. Waxman AD, Richmond R, Juttner H, et al.: Correlation of contrast angiography and histologic pattern with gallium uptake in primary liver-cell carcinoma: noncorrelation with alpha-feto protein. J Nucl Med 1980;21:324–327.
40. Larsen SM, Racey JS, Allen DR, et al.: Common pathway for tumor cell uptake of gallium-67 and iron-59 via a transferrin receptor. J Natl Cancer Instit 1980;64:41–53.
41. Kew MC: Tumors of the liver. In D Zakim and TD Boyer (eds), Hepatology. Philadelphia: Saunders, 1983, pp. 1048–1083.
42. Vera J, Murphy GP, Aronoff BL, Baker HW: Primary liver tumors and oral contraceptives. JAMA 1977;238:2154–2158.
43. Casarella WJ, Knowles DM, Wolff M, Johnson PM: Focal nodular hyperplasia and liver-cell adenoma: radiologic and pathologic differentiation. Am J Roentgenol 1978;131:393–402.
44. Piers DA, Houtoff JH, Krom RAF, et al.: Hot spot liver scan in focal nodular hyperplasia. Am J Roentgenol 1980;135:1289.
45. Rooks JB, Ory HW, Ishak KG, et al.: Epidemiology of hepatocellular adenoma: the role of oral contraceptive use. JAMA 1979;242:644–648.
46. Halling TS, Wood WG: Oral contraceptives and cancer of the liver: a review with two additional cases. Am J Gastroenterol 1982;77:504–508.
47. Belfar AJ, Grijm R, van der Schoot JB: Hepatic adenoma: Imaging with different radionuclides. Clin Nucl Med 1979;4:375–378.
48. Ishak KG, Rabin L: Benign tumors of the liver. Med Clin North Am 1975;59:995–1013.

49. Front D, Royal HD, Israel O, et al.: Scintigraphy of hepatic hemangiomas: the value of Tc-99-labeled red blood cells. J Nucl Med 1981;22:684–687.
50. Hall FM, Hurwitz EFI, Royal HD: Radionuclide and CT diagnosis: cavernous hemangioma of liver (letter to the editor). Am J Roentgenol 1980;135:424–425.
51. Engel MA, Marks DS, Sandler MA, Shetty P: Differentation of focal intrahepatic lesions with 99m-Tc-red blood cell imaging. Radiology 1983;146:777–782.
52. Schraibman IG: Non-parasitic liver abscess. Br J Surg 1974;61:709–712.
53. Ranson JHC, Madayag MA, Localio SA, Spencer FC: New diagnostic and therapeutic techniques in the management of pyogenic liver abscesses. Ann Surg 1975;181:508–518.
54. Lavender JP, Lowe J, Barker JR, et al.: Gallium 57-citrate scanning in neoplastic and inflammatory lesions. Br J Radiol 1971;44:361–366.
55. Segal AW, Thakur ML, Arnot RN, Lavender JP: Indium-111-labelled leucocytes for localization of abscesses. Lancet 1976;2:1056–1058.
56. Fawcett HD, Lantieri RL, Frankel A, McDougall IR: Differentiating hepatic abscess from tumor: combined 111-In white blood cell and 99m-Tc liver scans. Am J Roentgenol 1980;135:53–56.
57. Tsan MF: Studies on gallium accumulation in inflammatory lesions: III. Role of polymorphonuclear leukocytes and bacteria. J Nucl Med 1978;19:492–495.
58. Hoffer PB, Huberty J, Kayama-Bushi H: The association of Ga-67 and lactoferrin. J Nucl Med 1977;18:713–717.
59. Sfakianakis GN, Al-Sheikh W, Heal A, et al.: Comparisons of scintigraphy with In-111 leukocytes and Ga-67 in the diagnosis of occult sepsis. J Nucl Med 1982;23:618–626.
60. Rovekamp MH, van Royen EA, Reinders Folmer SCC, van der Schoot JB: Diagnosis of upper-abdominal infections by In-111 labeled leukocytes with Tc-99m colloid subtraction technique. J Nucl Med 1983;24:212–216.
61. Reba RC, Chandeysson PC: The clinical usefulness of indium-111 labeled leukocytes for the detection of infection. In ML Thakur, MD Ezekowitz, and MR Hardeman (eds), Radiolabeled Cellular Blood Elements, The Hague: Martinus Nijhoff, 1984.
62. Shafer RB, Wolff JM: Vascular dynamics of the "hot spot" liver scan (editorial). Clin Nucl Med 1980;5:523–524.
63. Tavill A, Wood E, Kreel L, et al.: Liver physiology and disease. Gastroenterology 1975;68:509–518.
64. Shreiner DP, Barlai-Kovach M: Diagnosis of alcoholic cirrhosis with the right-to-left hepatic lobe ratio. J Nucl Med 1981;22:116–120.
65. Waxman AD: Scintigraphic evaluation of diffuse hepatic disease. Semin Nucl Med 1982;12:75–88.
66. Fernadez JP, O'Rourke RA, Cooper JN, et al.: The extra-hepatic uptake of 198Au as an index of portal hypertension. Am J Digestive Dis 1970;15:883–893.
67. Gourgoutis GD, Das G, Lindsay N: Splenic uptake of 99m technetium sulfur colloid as an index of portalhypertension. Am J Gastroenterol 1972;57:435–442.
68. Horisawa M, Goldstein G, Waxman AD, Reynolds T: The abnormal hepatic scan of chronic liver disease. Its relationship to hepatic hemodynamics and colloid extraction. Gastroenterology 1976;71:210–213.
69. Davis G, Alazraki N, Taketa R, Halpern SE: Parameters of liver spleen scans as an indication of portal hypertension. Am J Gastroenterol 1976;65:31–36.
70. Hoefs H, Sakimura I, Reynolds T: Direct measurement of intrahepatic shunting by the portal vein injection of microspheres. Gastroenterology 1978;75:968 (abstract).
71. Shaldon S, Chiandussi L, Guevara L, Caesar J: The estimation of hepatic blood flow and intrahepatic shunted blood flow by colloidal heat-denatured human serum albumin labeled with I-131. J Clin Invest 1961;40:1346–1354.
72. Bekerman C, Gottschalk A: Diagnostic significance of the relative uptake of liver compared with spleen in 99m-Tc-sulfur colloid scintiphotography. J Nucl Med 1971;12:237–240.
73. Kaplan WD, Drum DE, Tokich JJ: The effect of cancer chemotherapeutic agents on the liver-spleen scan. J Nucl Med 1980;21:84–87.

74. Hladik WB III, Nigg KK, Rhodes BA: Drug-induced changes in the biological distribution of radiopharmaceuticals. Semin Nucl Med 1982;12:184–218.
75. Lentle BC, Scott JR, Nouijaim AA: Iatrongenic alterations in radionuclide biodistribution. Semin Nucl Med 1979;9:131–143.
76. Taplin GV, Meredith OM, Kade H: The radioactive (131-I-tagged) rose bengal uptake-excretion test for liver function using external gamma-ray scintillation counting techniques. J Lab Clin Med 1955;45:665–678.
77. Schein CJ: Acute Cholecystitis. New York: Harper & Row, 1972.
78. Weissmann HS, Badia J, Sugarman LA, et al.: Spectrum of cholescintigraphic patterns in acute cholecystitis. Radiology 1981;138:167–175.
79. Zeman RK, Burrell MI, Cahow CE, Caride V: Diagnostic utility of cholescintigraphy and ultrasonography in acute cholecystitis. Am J Surg 1981;141:446–451.
80. Szlabick RE, Catto JA, Fink-Benett D, Ventura V: Hepatobiliary scanning in the diagnosis of acute cholecystitis. Arch Surg 1980;115:540–544.
81. Suarez CA, Block F, Bernstein D, et al.: The role of HIDA/PIPIDA scanning in diagnosing cystic duct obstruction. Ann Surg 1980;191:391–396.
82. Weissman HS, Berkowitz D, Fox MS, et al.: The role of technitium-99m Iminodiacetic Acid (IDA) cholescintigraphy in acute acalculous cholecystitis. Radiology 1983;146:177–180.
83. Klingensmith WC, Spitzer VM, Fritzberg AR, Kuni CC: The normal fasting and postprandial diisopropyl-IDA Tc 99m Hepatobiliary study. Radiology 1981;141:771–776.
84. Shuman WP, Gibbs P, Rudd TG, Mack LA: PIPIDA scintigraphy for cholecystitis: false positives in alcholism and total parenteral nutrition AJR 1982;138:1–5.
85. Pauwels S, Piret L, Schoutens A, et al.: Tc-99m-Diethyl-IDA imaging: clinical evaluation in jaundiced patients. J Nucl Med 1980;21:1022–1028.
86. Weissman HS, Sugarman LA, Freeman LM: The clinical role of Technitium-99m Iminodiacetic Acid cholescintigraphy. In LM Freeman and HS Weissman (eds), New York: Raven Press, 1981, pp. 35–89.
87. Taylor A, Kipper MS, Witztum K, et al.: Abnormal ^{99m}Tc-PIPIDA scans mistaken for common duct obstruction. Radiology 1982;144:373–375.
88. Kasai M, Watanabe I, Oli R: Followup studies of long-term survivors after hepatic portoenterostomy for "noncorrectable" biliary atresia. J Pediatr Surg 1975;10:173–182.
89. Altman RP: The portoenterostomy procedure for biliary atresia: a five year experience. Ann Surg 1978;188:351–358.
90. Ghadimi H, Suss-Korstak A: Evaluation of the radioactive rose-bengal test for the differential diagnosis of obstructive jaundice in infants. N Engl J Med 1961;265:351–358.
91. Silverberg M, Rosenthall L, Freeman LM: Rose bengal excretion studies as an aid in differential diagrams of neonatal jaundice. Pediatrics 1973;67:140–145.
92. Collier BD, Treves S, Davis MA, et al.: Simultaneous ^{99m}Tc-P-Butyl-IDA and ^{131}I-rose bengal scintigraphy in neonatal jaundice. Radiology 1980;134:719–722.
93. Gerhold JP, Klingensmith WC, Kuni CC, et al.: Diagnosis of biliary atresia with radionuclide hepatobiliary imaging. Radiology 1983;146:499–504.
94. Majd M, Reba RC, Altman RP: Hepatobiliary scintigraphy with Tc-99m-PIPIDA in the evaluation of neonatal jaundice. Pediatrics 1981;67:140–145.
95. Schachner ER, Gil MC, Atkins HL, et al.: Ruthenium-97 hepatobiliary agents for delayed studies of the biliary tract I: Ru-97 PIPIDA: Concise communication. J Nucl Med 1981;22:352–357.
96. Weissman HS, Chun KJ, Frank MS, et al.: Demonstration of traumatic bile leakage with cholescintigraphy and ultrasonography. Am J Roentgenol 1979;133:893–847.
97. Bhaskara KR, Bheram P, Lieberman LM: Evaluation of focal defects on Technetium-99m sulfur colloid scans with new hepatobiliary agents. Radiology 1980;136:497–499.
98. Weissman HS, Sugarman LA, Frank MS, Freeman LM: Serendipity in Technetium-99m Dimethyl Iminodiacetic Acid cholescintigraphy. Radiology 1980;135:449–454.

3

Hepatic Sonography

WILLIAM A. BERKMAN • MICHAEL E. BERNARDINO • ERROL LEWIS

INTRODUCTION

During the 1970s, technological advances in both ultrasound and computed tomography (CT) have improved and dominated noninvasive imaging of the liver. Prior to the advent of ultrasound and CT, radionuclide liver scintigraphy was the primary noninvasive modality. Unlike radionuclide imaging, CT and ultrasound provide more definitive anatomic and pathologic information. They provide this information quickly with better resolution and evaluate not only the liver but other areas of the abdomen. The additional information gained in "staging" the abdomen is a distinct advantage over radionuclide scanning. These two modalities are complementary and, when considered together, provide solutions to many diagnostic dilemmas.

This chapter will review proper sonographic scanning technique, discuss normal anatomy, and characterize focal and diffuse liver disease. Sonographic accuracy, sensitivity, and the capabilities of hepatic sonography will be examined. Also, present and possible future developments that could redefine the proper role and indications for hepatic sonography will be discussed.

TECHNIQUE

The key to a successful and complete hepatic sonographic evaluation is a meticulous study with active physician participation. Whether using a static-B scanner or a real-time unit, a consistent and logical approach using multiple views and patient positions is necessary. Besides multiple views and positions, proper attention to technical factors, such as choice of transducers, is necessary.

Transducers

When using static imaging, an ideal transducer should have a focal zone of between 7 and 11 cm with a penetration depth of at least 17 cm (1). The echo pattern throughout the liver should be homogeneous, yielding both a near and far field of equal echogenicity. In an average-size patient, a 3.5 MHz medium or long focus transducer would be used to survey most of the liver. Over thin areas such as the lateral segment of the left lobe, a 5.0 MHz transducer could be used. In large patients, a 2.25 MHz transducer may be required to penetrate the entire depth of the liver. Proper adjustment of the time-gain compensation curve is necessary to insure a uniform demonstration of the hepatic parenchyma.

A complete static examination of the liver is performed at 1-cm intervals in longitudinal, transverse, and oblique planes, with adjustment of transducer frequencies for deep or superficial areas of the liver. A subcostal technique is utilized to scan the anterior liver. Compound scanning is used for depicting the transverse representation of the entire hepatic anatomy, but may introduce pseudolesions due to misregistration (2). Other pseudolesions can be caused by improper scanning techniques or by failure to identify anatomic variations. Generally, the most useful information for evaluation of the liver is obtained from longitudinal scans, since artifacts secondary to ribs and respiration can be avoided. However, the static-B scanning technique has multiple disadvantages: the examination requires considerable operator expertise and time, and the anterior portion, dome, and lateral portions of the liver are difficult to scan completely. Areas such as the lateral segment of the left lobe, as well as the central vascular anatomy, may be better visualized with transverse views.

A standardized protocol (3) encompassing the entire liver and performed by residents, physicians and/or technologists in 15 minutes will decrease the number of false negative diagnoses due to either incomplete hepatic examination or false positive diagnoses due to the production of pseudolesions. This protocol relies on an aggressive real-time approach to the liver. The initial drawbacks of real-time scanning (lower resolution transducers and a smaller field of view) are not a problem at present. More recently, real-time sector transducers with a wide field of view and excellent resolution have become available. These developments allow the physician to play a more active role in evaluating the liver similar to a fluoroscopic examination of the gastrointestinal tract.

The approach that we advocate consists of an initial complete abdominal survey examination with a wide-angle real-time transducer. While examining the liver, specific identification of the hepatic veins, portal veins, IVC, common bile duct, and their branches is accomplished and identification of any parenchymal focal or diffuse abnormalities is noted. Following this brief real-time examination, specific static images of the liver in appropriate scanning planes are performed in order to obtain an overall picture of the liver and abdomen. With the use of small-size transducers without the articulating scanning arm, intercostal and subcostal scanning is facilitated, and subsequently areas previously unable to be scanned are now examined. The freedom of real-time scanners also enables patients to be more easily positioned for lateral decubitus scanning. Frequently, this position salvages studies that would have been incomplete with static-B scanners because of inadequate visualization of the liver.

Despite the introduction of digital ultrasound machines, the actual sensitivity has not improved and ultrasound remains less sensitive than CT. Data manipulation with either pre-data or post-data processing has added to one's confidence in identifying a lesion, but does not increase its sensitivity (4). Also, present digital ultrasound units are limited by our lack of knowledge about the interaction of tissue with the sound beam, by the small size of the computer memories, and by the lack of adequate software.

Sonographic Anatomy of the Liver

The normal hepatic parenchyma has a homogeneous echo intensity that is greater than the renal cortex and less than or equal to the pancreas. The parenchyma is interrupted by branching tubular structures representing portal and hepatic veins. Portal veins are encased in a collagen sheath, which accounts for the hyperreflectivity of the vessel walls. While more echogenic walls usually distinguish portal veins from hepatic veins, this distinction fails in about 30 percent of the cases in which the hepatic veins are echogenic (Figure 3-1). This increased echogenicity is usually noted in the distal portions of long hepatic veins. A more reliable way to distinguish hepatic veins from portal veins is to follow the course of the vessel to its origin. Another feature that distinguishes the portal from hepatic vein branches is that the branching hepatic veins form apices that are directed toward the diaphragm and inferior vena cava, while the portal vein branches form apices directed toward the porta hepatis (5,6). Also, portal vein caliber increases toward the porta hepatis, while hepatic vein caliber increases toward the diaphragm and inferior vena cava.

The portal vein originates at the junction of the superior mesenteric vein and the splenic vein, just to the right of midline and anterior to the inferior vena cava. It then courses into the porta hepatis and divides into an anterior left branch and a more laterally directed right branch. The right branch then divides into an anterior and posterior division. The left portal vein originates slightly to the right of the midline and then passes anteriorly and to the left. It gives off branches to the quadrate lobe, lateral segment of the left lobe and the caudate lobe. Occasionally the left portal vein may appear as an echodense line within the left lobe and should not be confused with the posterior margin of the left lobe of the liver (7). This is generally a problem with static scanning and real-time imaging will clarify the relationship of this line to the portal vein.

The inferior vena cava and the gallbladder fossa define the major hepatic fissure, a plane that separates the liver into right and left lobes (Figure 3-1). The right lobe of the liver is then divided into an anterior and posterior portion by the right hepatic vein. The anterior and posterior branches of the right portal vein enter the corresponding segments of the right hepatic lobe. The left lobe of the liver is divided into a medial segment (traditional quadrate lobe) and a lateral segment by the left hepatic vein. The caudate lobe is functionally a separate entity since it receives blood supply from both the right and left hepatic arteries. Prior to surgical resection of primary and solitary hepatic metastatic lesions, knowledge of the functional and vascular anatomy is necessary.

The various ligaments and fissures of the liver contain fat, collagen, and vessels, making them highly echogenic relative to the hepatic parenchyma. These structures provide important anatomic landmarks and guidelines that could be confused for pathologic findings (8). In the transverse plane, the ligamentum teres, ligamentum venosum, and fissure between the quadrate and right hepatic lobes can be identified. The falciform ligament contains the ligamentum teres and the umbilical vein remnant. It appears as an echogenic focus in transverse scans (Figure 3-1). It extends from the diaphragm to the umbilicus in a sagittal plane (9). Thus, it separates the lateral segment of the left lobe from the quadrate lobe of the liver. While this ligament typically appears as a round echogenic focus in the transverse plane, longitudinal orientation of the transducer will give a more linear appearance, helping to differentiate the ligament from an ech-

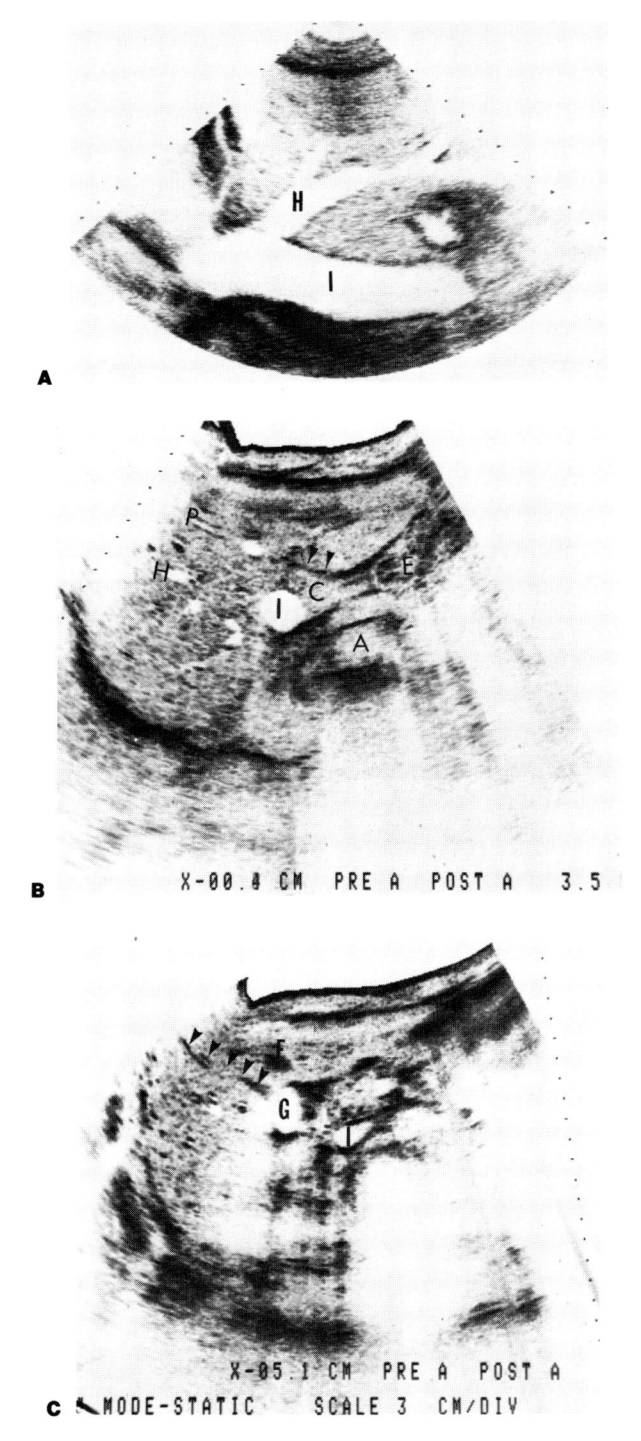

Figure 3-1. *A.* Normal anatomy. Longitudinal scan in plane of the inferior vena cava (I) shows hepatic veins (H) draining into the IVC. A normal homogeneous echo pattern of the hepatic parenchyma is present. *B.* Transverse sonogram through liver at the level of the intrahepatic portion of the interior vena cava (I). The caudate lobe (C) is separated from the lateral segment of the left lobe of the liver by the ligamentum venosum (black arrows). The homogeneous echo pattern of the liver is interrupted by portal veins (P) and hepatic vein (H) branches. The portal vein walls are highly reflective, while the hepatic vein walls are not. E = esophagus; A = aorta. *C.* Transverse scan through liver. The echogenic falciform ligament (F) separates the lateral segment of the left lobe of the liver from the quadrate lobe and should not be mistaken for an echogenic lesion. The gallbladder (G) and inferior vena cava (I) define the major hepatic fissure (black arrows) dividing the liver into right and left lobes.

ogenic lesion. The medial margin of the quadrate lobe is the falciform ligament and ligamentum teres, and the lateral margin is the gallbladder fossa. The ligamentum venosum is seen as a transversely oriented structure that defines the anterior margin of the caudate lobe and the posterior margin of the left lobe. The ligamentum venosum extends from the porta hepatis transversely and superior to the caudate lobe, dividing it from the left lobe of the liver. Posteriorly, the caudate lobe is bordered by the inferior vena cava.

FOCAL HEPATIC MASSES

Hepatocellular Carcinoma

Hepatoma formation is commonly associated with predisposing diseases such as cirrhosis, hepatitis, hemochromatosis, and syphilis. A higher incidence of hepatocellular carcinoma is seen in Chinese and African blacks. Kamin *et al.* (10) described three types of ultrasound patterns in hepatocellular carcinoma. These included densely echogenic masses, diffuse disease, and a mixture of the two. Akuda *et al.* (11) described the various vascular patterns in hepatoma: (1) discrete hypervascular mass, (2) diffuse irregular tortuous vessels, and (3) a mixture of the two patterns. Good correlation was found between the sonographic pattern and type of vascularity. The most common finding was that of hepatomegaly with diffuse distortion of the normal internal architecture. Each of these patterns is not unique to hepatocellular carcinoma. They may be noted in other forms of focal and diffuse hepatic disease (Figure 3–2).

Metastatic Disease

In evaluating metastatic disease of the liver in 93 cases, Green *et al.* (12) described five ultrasound patterns. These include:

1. Discrete hypoechoic masses, 23 percent
2. Discrete echogenic masses, 30 percent

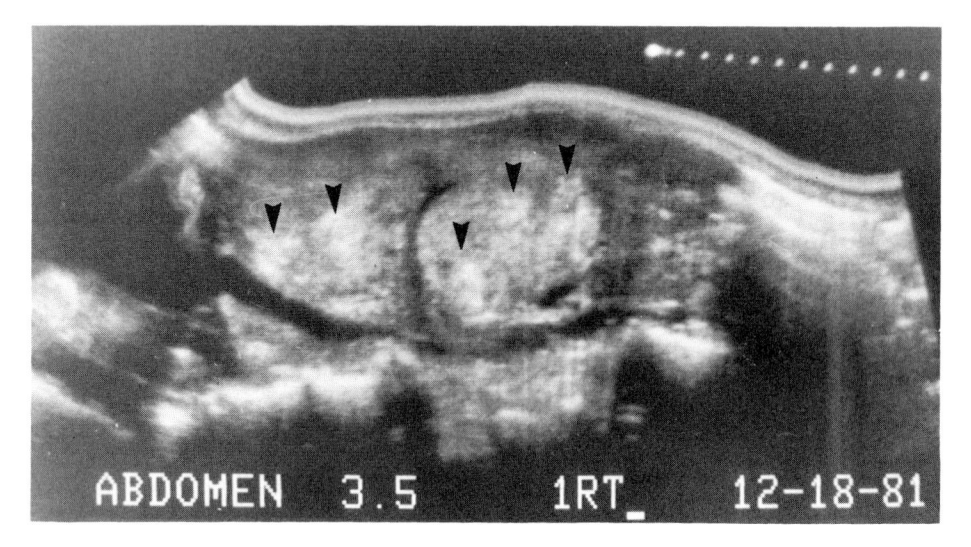

Figure 3–2. A transverse sonogram through the liver shows multiple densely echogenic lesions (black arrows) representing metastases from an islet cell tumor. This appearance would be difficult to differentiate from multifocal hepatoma.

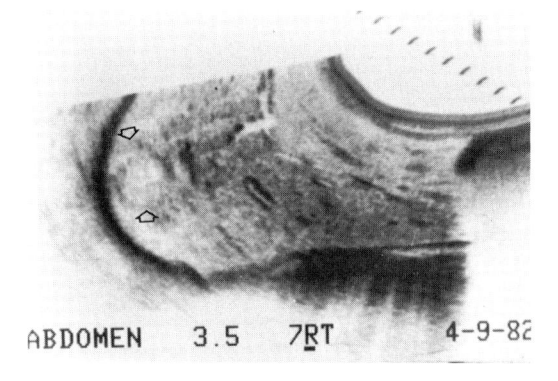

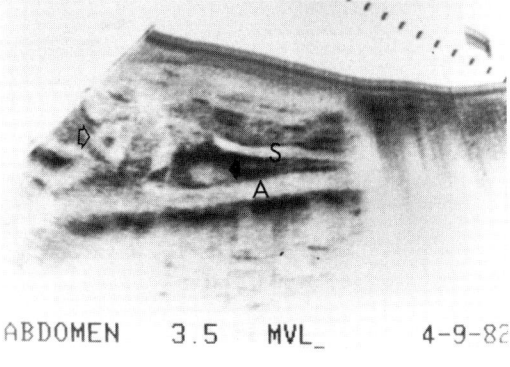

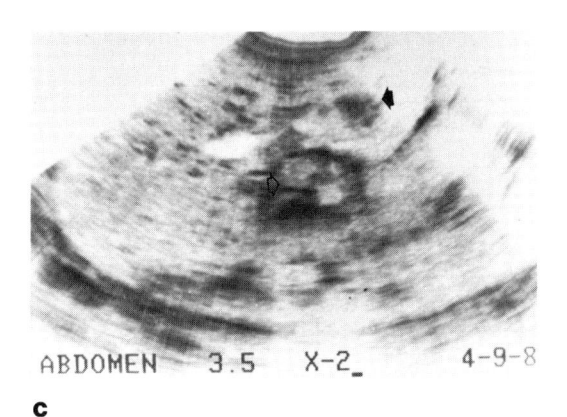

Figure 3-3. *A.* Patient with stomach carcinoma. Ultrasound shows extent of disease and varied appearance of hepatic metastases. Longitudinal sonogram through the right lobe of the liver shows a 3-cm hypoechoic metastasis (open arrows) in the region of the dome of the liver. *B.* Sagittal sonogram shows a retroperitoneal (black arrow) lymph node located anterior to the aorta (A) and posterior to the superior mesenteric artery (S). A celiac node (open arrow) is also noted. *C.* Transverse sonogram shows a hyperechoic metastasis in the left lobe of the liver (black arrow) and retrocrural nodes (open arrow).

3. Anechoic masses, 2 percent
4. Diffuse altered architecture of the liver with mixed echogenicity or echo-free areas with no discrete masses, 35 percent
5. A combination of types 1–4, 10 percent

Scheibel *et al.* (13) classified liver metastasis in 76 patients into four ultrasound categories:

1. Dense, 37 percent
2. Lucent, 18 percent
3. Bulls eye, 17 percent
4. Mixture, 28 percent

In both studies, there was no correlation between the histologic make-up of a lesion and ultrasound findings (Figure 3–3). However, calcified liver metastases demonstrate acoustical shadowing, and a diagnosis of metastatic disease from a primary carcinoma of the colon (mucinous variety) may be suggested. Mucinous cystadenocarcinoma of the ovary, adenocarcinoma of the stomach, islet cell carcinoma of the pancreas, and rarely adenocarcinoma of the breast and melanoma may also give rise to calcified liver metastases (14) (Figures 3–4, and 3–5).

In evaluating the oncologic patient, incidental cysts may be discovered. Weaver *et al.* demonstrated that metastatic sarcomas, having undergone necrosis, may be difficult

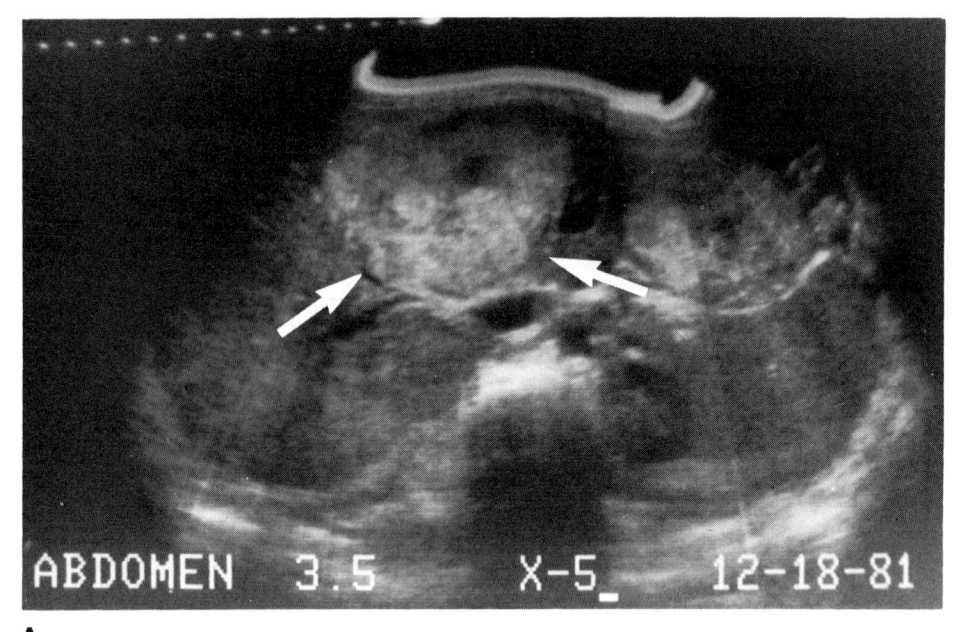

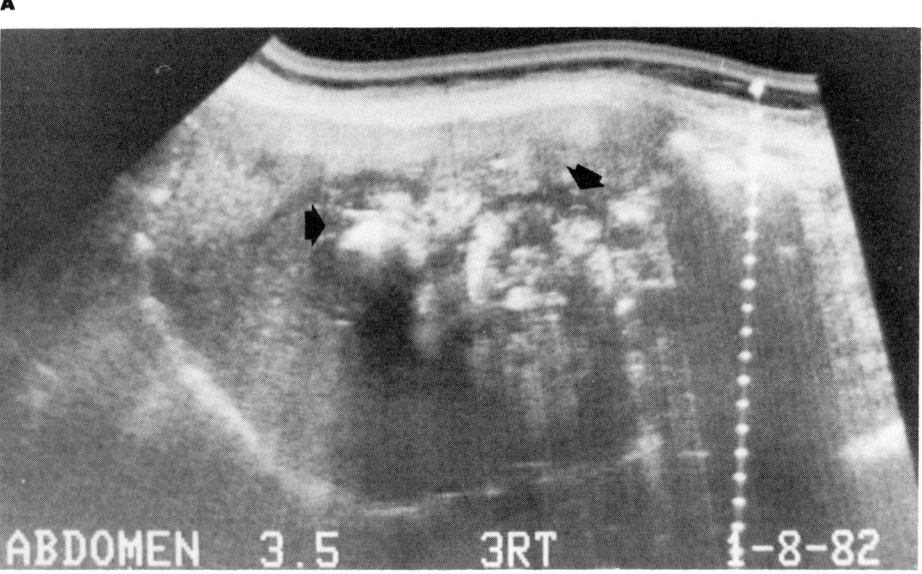

Figure 3-4. *A.* Transverse sonogram through the liver shows a large calcified metastasis from mucinous adenocarcinoma of the colon (arrows). *B.* A longitudinal scan through another patient shows multiple calcified metastases in the right hepatic lobe (arrows).

to distinguish from simple cysts (15). Barnes *et al.*, in evaluation of seven patients with CT evidence of hepatic lesions, showed that CT was unable to reliably distinguish benign hepatic cysts from other intrahepatic and extrahepatic cystic lesions (16). The CT density of cystic liver masses such as necrotic metastases, lymphangioma, and late-stage abscesses may have attenuation coefficients near zero (17). Thus the finding of "0" attenuation values does not indicate the nature of a cystic liver lesion (Figure 3-6). Findings of a thick rim, irregular margins, mural nodules, and fluid-fluid levels may

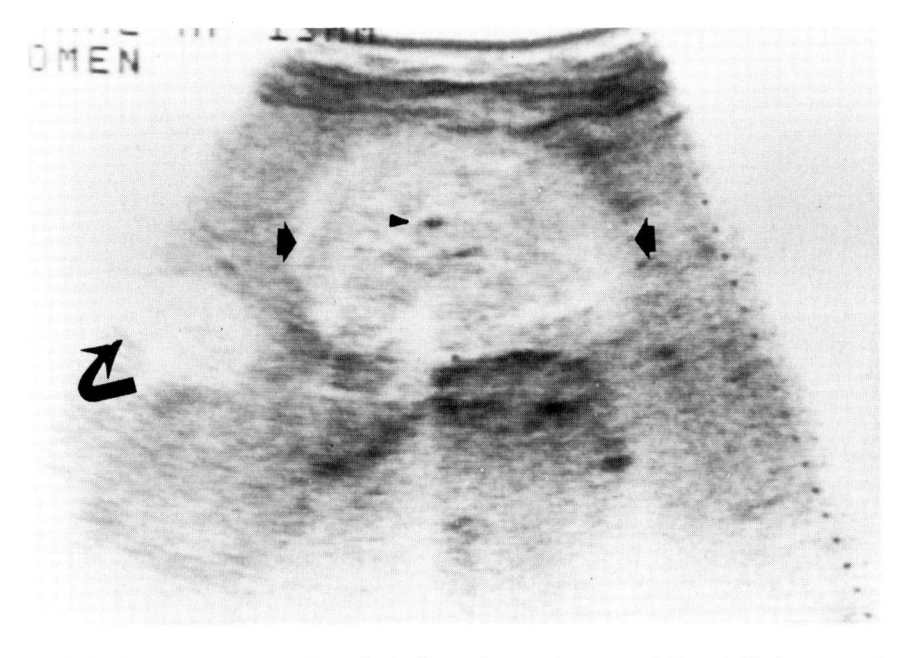

Figure 3-5. A transverse scan through the liver shows a large partially calcified metastasis from mucinous adenocarcinoma of the colon (black arrows). A central calcification with acoustical shadowing is demonstrated (black arrowhead). Just lateral to this lesion is a smaller hypoechoic metastasis (black curved arrow).

indicate a necrotic metastasis or an abscess (Figure 3-7). Usually, the clinical information will help distinguish these entities from a simple cyst, but if necessary, needle aspiration is advocated (Figures 3-8, 3-9, and 3-10). Unfortunately, a smooth margin is not a specific finding and may be seen with cysts, necrotic tumors, or abscesses.

Bernardino *et al.,* in evaluating 93 patients undergoing chemotherapy for metastatic lesions, found four patterns of ultrasound response (18). These responses included (1) no change, 46 percent, (2) improvement as manifested by a decrease in size or number of lesions or decrease in size of the liver, 18 percent, (3) progression of disease indicated by increase in size of the liver or size and/or number of lesions, 24 percent, and (4) change in the original sonographic pattern without definite progression or improvement, 12 percent (Figure 3-11). In groups 1, 2, and 3 there was essentially no variance with other imaging modalities (radionuclide, CT, and angiography) and the clinical findings. The changes in original sonographic pattern (group 4) included changes from echogenic to necrotic, echogenic to diffuse, echogenic to hypoechoic, and necrotic to septated. No lesions changed from a hypoechoic pattern to an echogenic pattern. In contrast to groups 1, 2, and 3, group 4 showed no correlation between the clinical response and ultrasound pattern changes. While a change representing necrosis is generally associated with clinical improvement, some patients undergoing necrosis of the metastatic lesions had clinical deterioration. Of note, the development of septation in necrotic lesions correlated well with clinical stability or improvement. Presently, useful clinical information is not obtained in those patients undergoing sonographic pattern changes. Computed tomography, scintigraphy, and angiography, however, also do not correlate with the patient's clinical condition in these cases. Technical factors must be given particular attention so that changes in the group 4 category are not simulated by changes

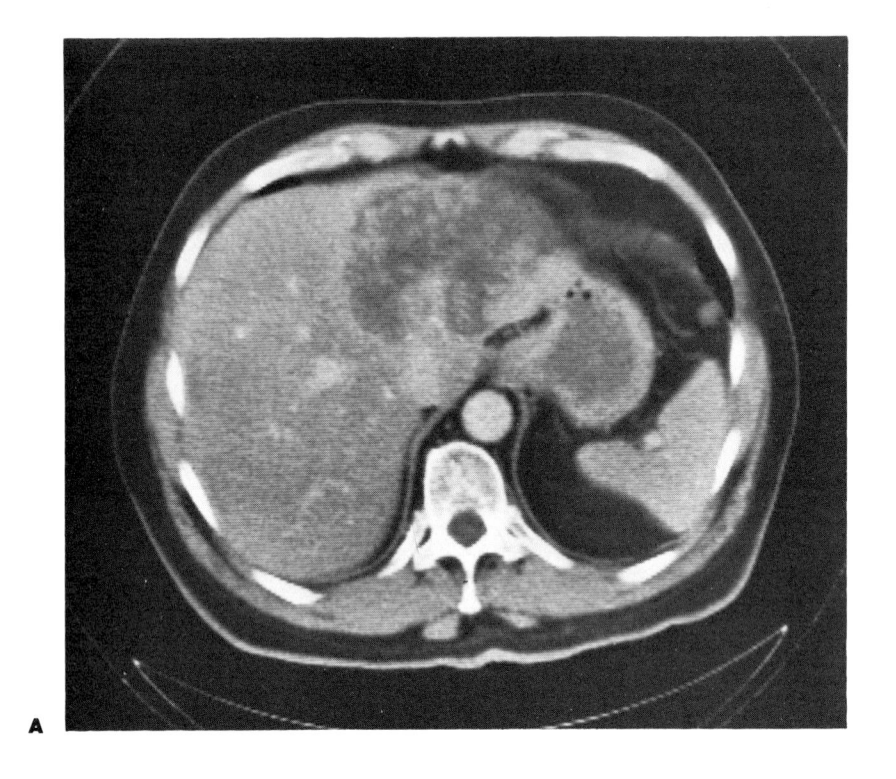

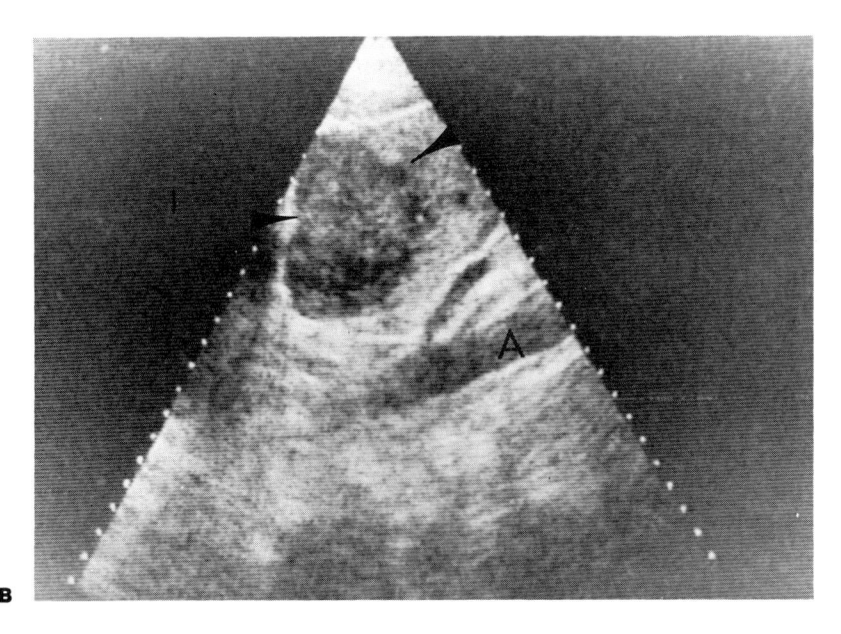

Figure 3–6. *A.* CT scan shows a large low-attenuation metastasis in the left lobe of the liver. *B.* A sagittal ultrasound section shows the same metastasis (arrows). A heterogeneous echo pattern is appreciated. A = aorta.

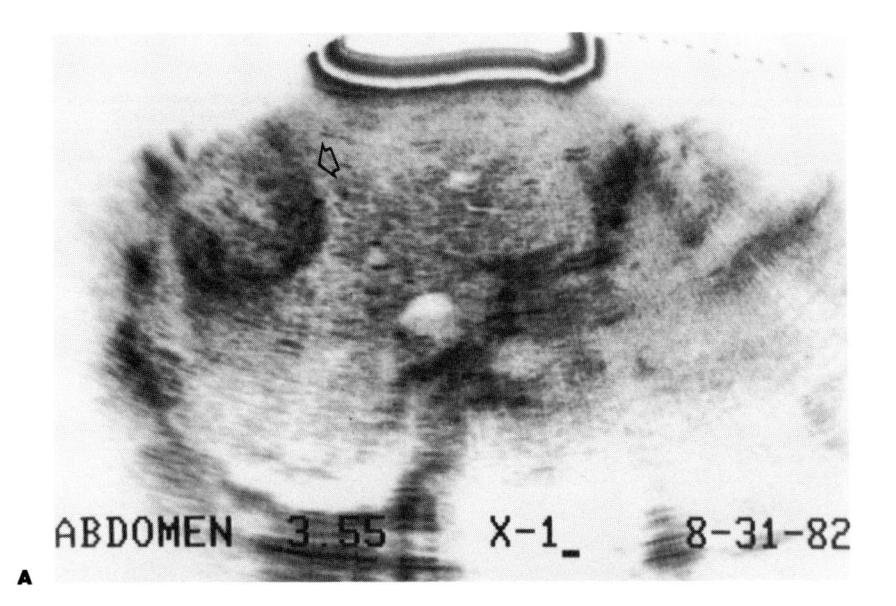

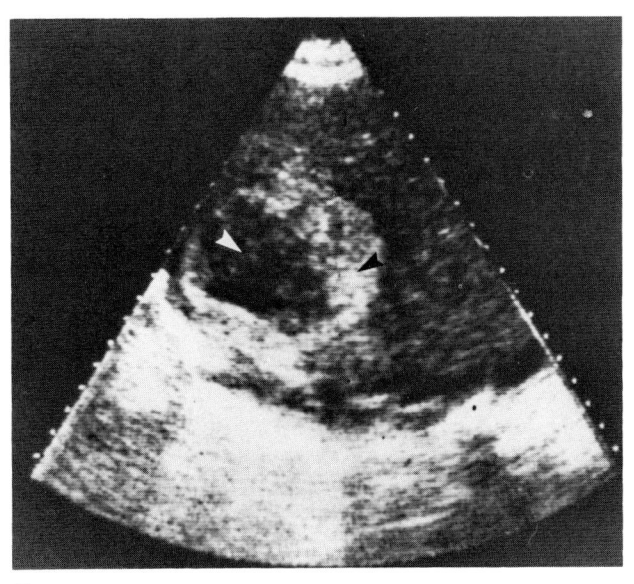

Figure 3-7. *A.* Transverse sonogram through a patient with known fibrosarcoma shows a large necrotic metastasis (open arrow) with a thick wall. *B.* In another patient with metastatic fibrosarcoma, a large metastasis within the liver exhibits a mural nodule (black arrowhead) and central necrosis (white arrowhead).

in transducer frequency or the time-gain compensation curves. In patients undergoing multiple examinations, technical factors must be kept constant.

Cysts

Cystic lesions of the liver are defined and characterized more readily by ultrasound than by other imaging modalities. Cystic lesions of the liver include congenital cysts, multiple cysts in association with polycystic liver disease and polycystic renal disease, and acquired cysts secondary to inflammatory or traumatic changes.

The most common benign cystic lesion of the liver is the congenital cyst (19). These lesions are relatively infrequent, with an incidence of 17/10,000 at exploratory lapro-

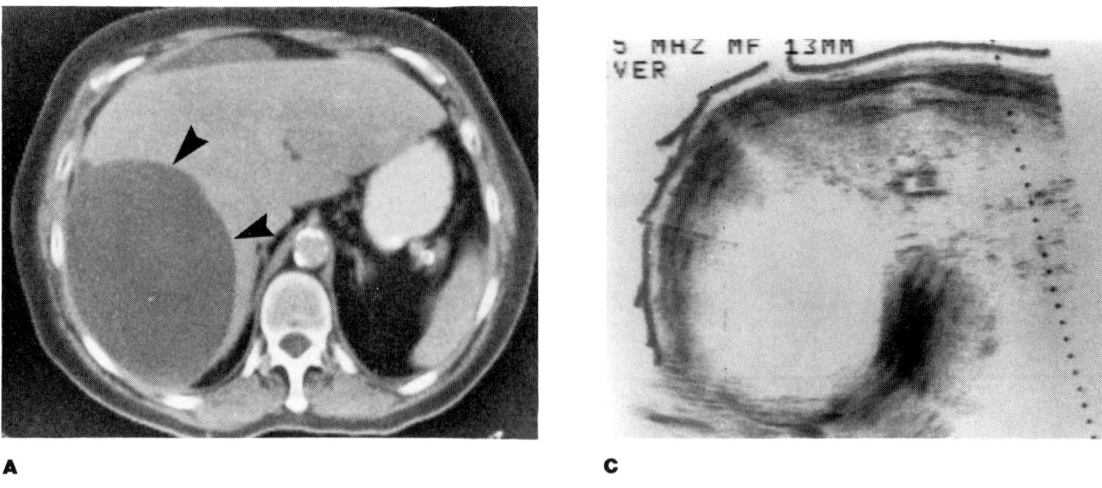

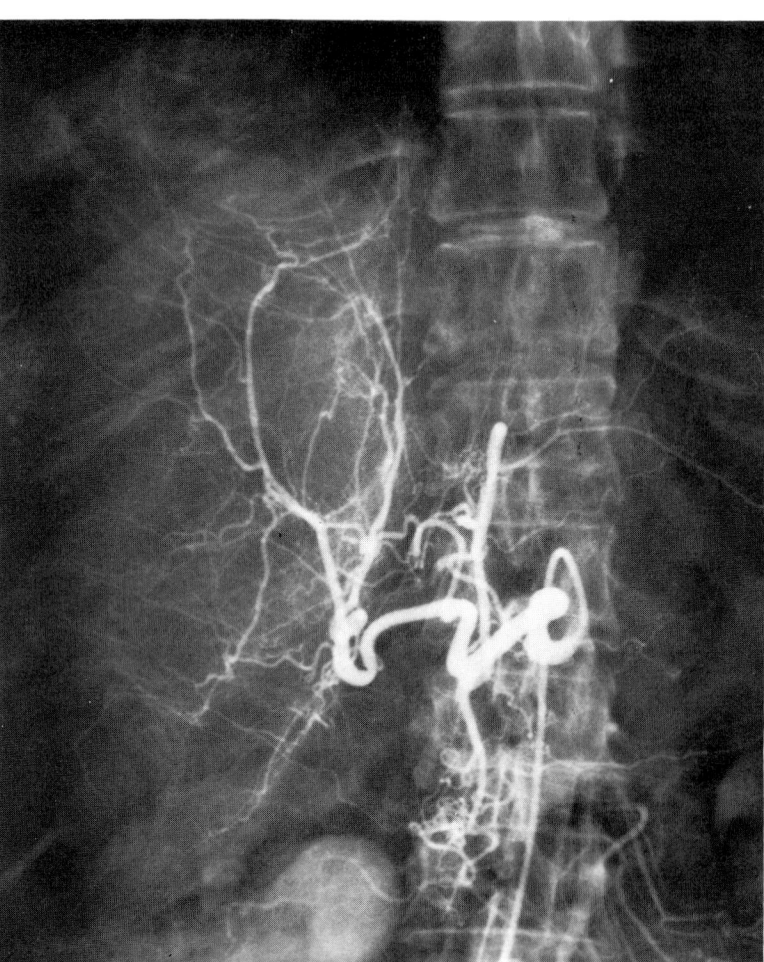

Figure 3-8. *A.* CT scan through the liver in a patient with ovarian carcinoma shows a cystic mass (black arrows) with the density of water. *B.* Selective hepatic arteriogram shows a hypovascular mass within the liver without evidence of tumor vascularity. *C.* A transverse sonogram through the same region of the liver shows a cystic mass meeting the characteristics of a benign cyst. Despite ultrasound, CT, and angiographic findings indicating benignity, because of the patient's clinical history, aspiration biopsy of the mass was performed under ultrasound and revealed cytology diagnostic of adenocarcinoma from the ovarian malignancy.

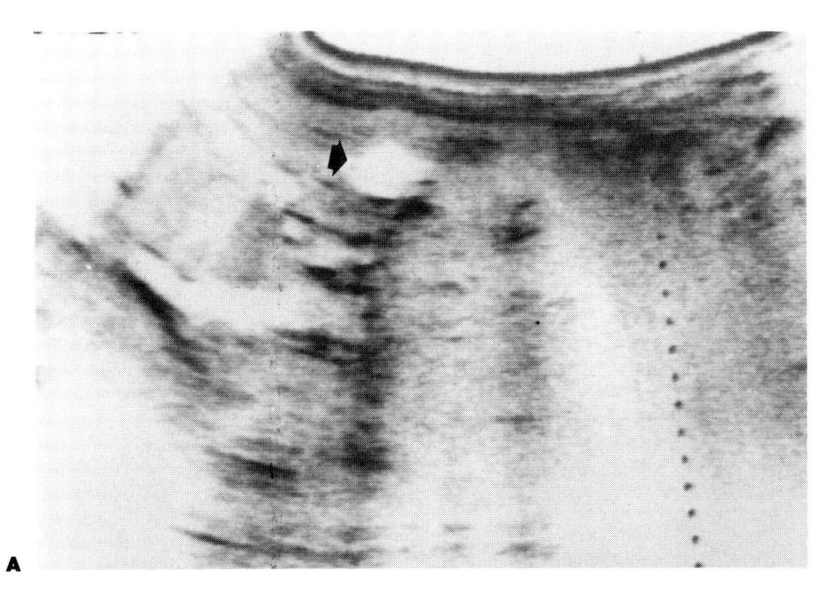

Figure 3-9. *A.* sagittal sonogram of the liver in a patient with known tumor shows a 2-cm anechoic lesion within the medial segment of the left lobe of the liver (black arrow).

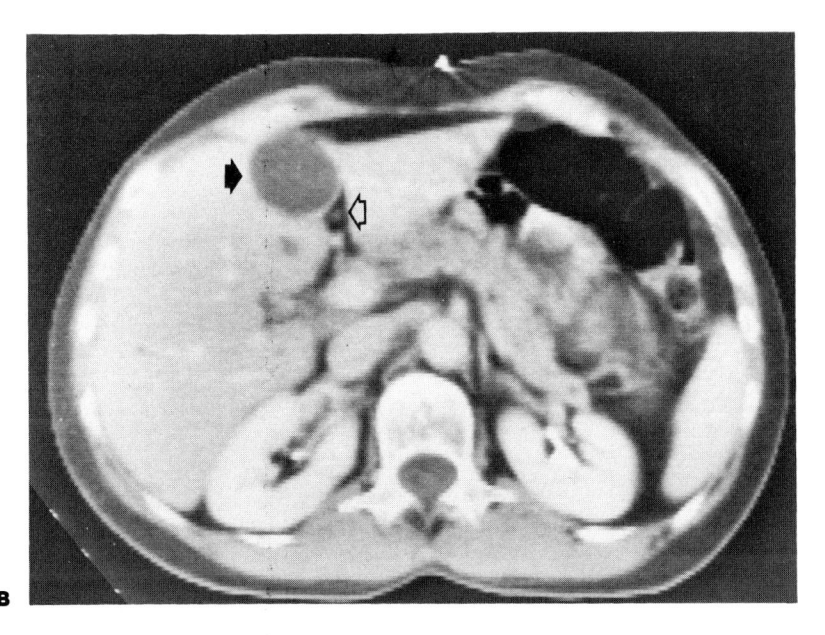

Figure 3-9. *B.* A corresponding CT scan through the liver again shows a mass lesion within the medial segment of the left lobe of the liver (black arrow). The falciform ligament is seen surrounded by fat (white arrow). The CT number of the lesion measured water, but because this was a patient with a known malignancy, needle aspiration was needed.

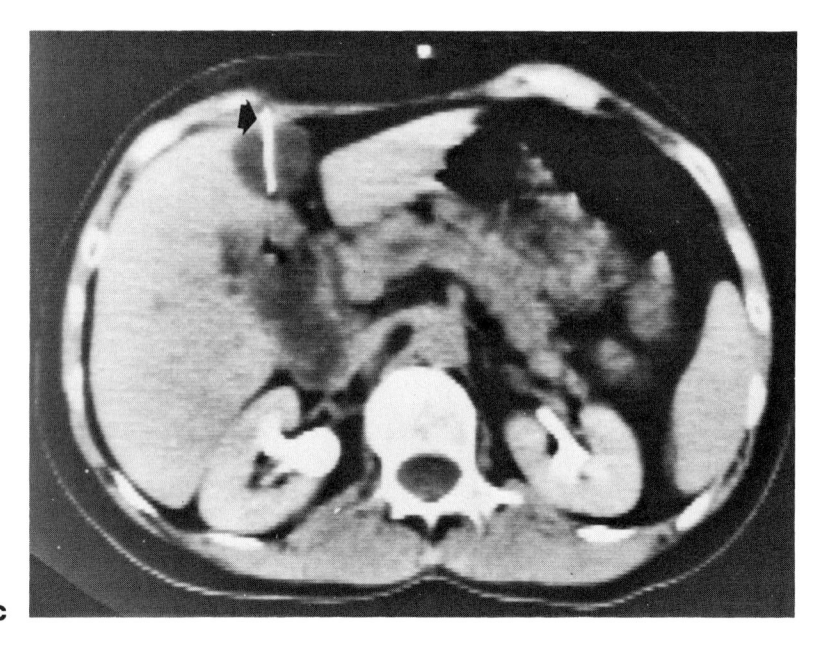

Figure 3–9. *C.* Under CT guidance, a biopsy needle is positioned within the lesion (black arrow).

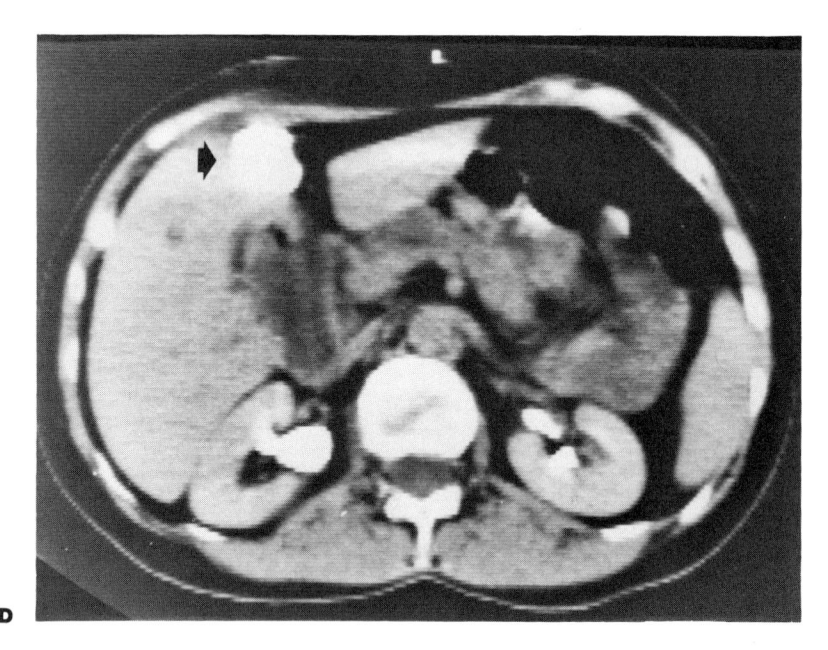

Figure 3–9. *D.* Following aspiration of clear fluid, contrast was injected through the needle, demonstrating the entire cavity of the cyst (black arrow). Cytology revealed clear fluid with no malignant cells.

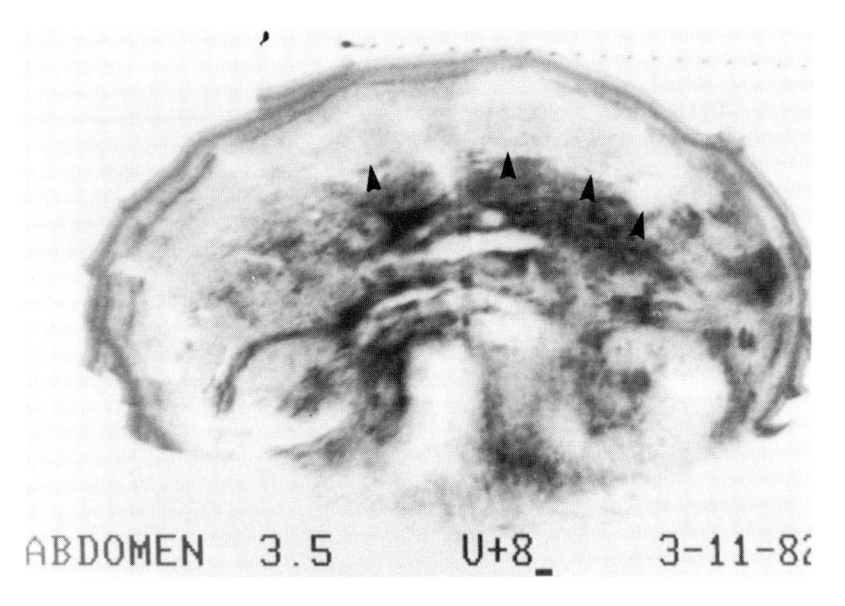

Figure 3-10. A transverse sonogram through the liver at the L2 level shows multiple hypoechoic metastases (black arrows) from a breast primary.

tomy. With the increasing use of computed tomography and ultrasound, however, incidental cysts are more frequently identified. Congenital cysts develop secondary to an excess of intrahepatic ductiles that fail to involute. There is an increase in incidence of congenital cysts in females, and these cysts are most frequently encountered in the fifth through seventh decades. While generally asymptomatic, hepatic cysts may grow to a large size and become infected or undergo hemorrhage. Thus, they may cause symptoms due to mass effect or abdominal pain. Rarely, cysts may cause obstructive jaundice due to their relationship to the common bile duct. The ultrasound characteristics of a liver cyst are similar to cysts in other regions of the body. They have a clearly defined thin wall surrounded by hepatic parenchyma. The internal structure of the cyst is anechoic, and there is clear definition of the posterior wall with enhanced through sound transmission.

Frequently, hepatic cysts are peripheral and may not be detected by radionuclide scans. Entities that may simulate a primary cyst of the liver include intrahepatic hematoma, echinococcal cyst, abscess, hepatic cystadenoma or cystadenocarcinoma, and necrotic primary or metastatic tumor. Infrequently, Caroli's disease, intrahepatic gallbladder, or enlarged intrahepatic vessels can simulate benign cysts. Scans in the longitudinal and oblique planes will identify these variations due to their nonuniform shape. Thus, the three-dimensional ability of ultrasound will clarify the etiology of otherwise misleading cystic structures as viewed on transverse images. Subcapsular hematomas tend to be elliptical in shape and are located peripherally, distinguishing them from simple cysts. Acquired cysts due to trauma or infection are generally not as well-defined as simple cysts. Hematomas may appear cystic, but are generally not as well defined. Abscesses can usually be differentiated from cysts by their thickened irregular walls and margins and by debris within the central portion.

Cyst aspiration is recommended (1) when a cystic lesion is noted in an oncologic patient, (2) when the clinical suspicion of tumor is high, or (3) when a history of trauma or sepsis is present.

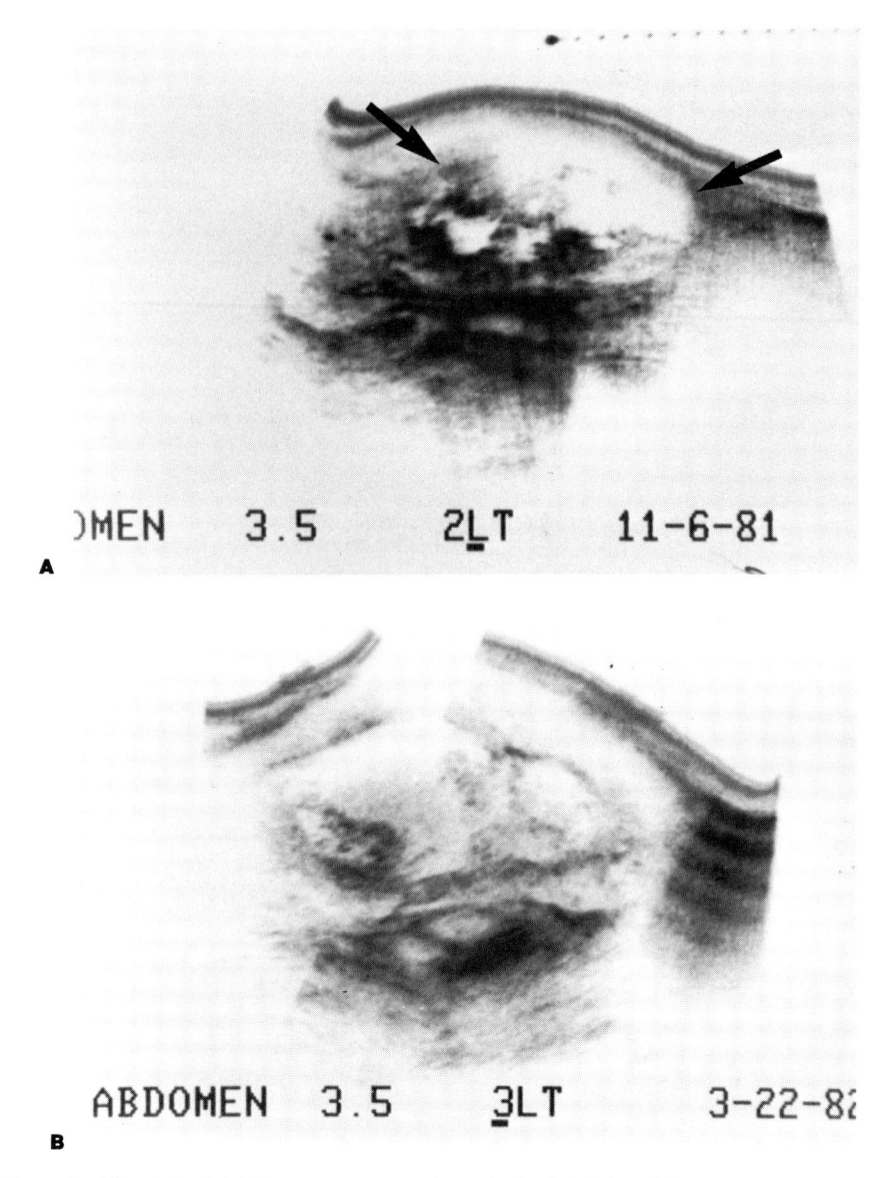

Figure 3-11. *A.* An initial transverse scan through the left lobe of the liver in a patient with known metastatic disease shows a hypoechoic metastasis (black arrows). *B.* A repeat scan 4 months later shows disease progression with increase in tumor size.

Hydatid Disease of the Liver

Echinococcus granulosus, a genus of tapeworm infecting man as an intermediate host, is endemic to large sheep-raising areas of Europe, Asia, the Mediterranean, South America, and Australia. The cystic fluid is highly antigenic, and in order to avoid the complications of anaphylaxis due to spreading of scolices into the peritoneal cavity or other body tissues, a prerequisite to needle aspiration should be a pertinent travel history. Gharbi (20) and Babcock (21) have described the ultrasound findings in hydatid disease of the liver. In analysis of 121 cases (20), five sonographic categories were found corresponding to evolutionary stages of the hydatid cyst. A purely fluid collection within the liver varying from 1 to 20 cm in size with localized thickening of the cyst wall was observed most commonly. Less frequent appearances included a fluid collection with a split wall or "floating membrane," fluid collections with septa, and a heterogeneous echo pattern. Rarely, the infestation may be manifested by highly reflective thick walls with a cone-shaped shadow. The authors noted compression of the inferior vena cava due to large cysts in the caudate lobe. The heterogeneous echo pattern (Type 4) is difficult to distinguish from a tumor. Echinococcal disease of the liver should be suspected when a multicystic mass is seen. This is particularly important in areas where echinococcal disease is endemic.

Cavernous Hemangioma

Cavernous hemangioma is the most common benign tumor of the liver. It is most frequently seen in women, with a five to one female-to-male ratio. Most hemangiomas are less than 5 cm in diameter and occur as single lesions, although multiple tumors occur in 10 percent of cases (22). The diagnosis of hepatic hemangioma is important in order to differentiate this lesion from metastatic disease or a primary tumor of the liver and to avoid biopsy that may cause massive or fatal hemorrhage. Freeney et al. (23), in evaluating five patients with cavernous hemangioma of the liver, found angiography

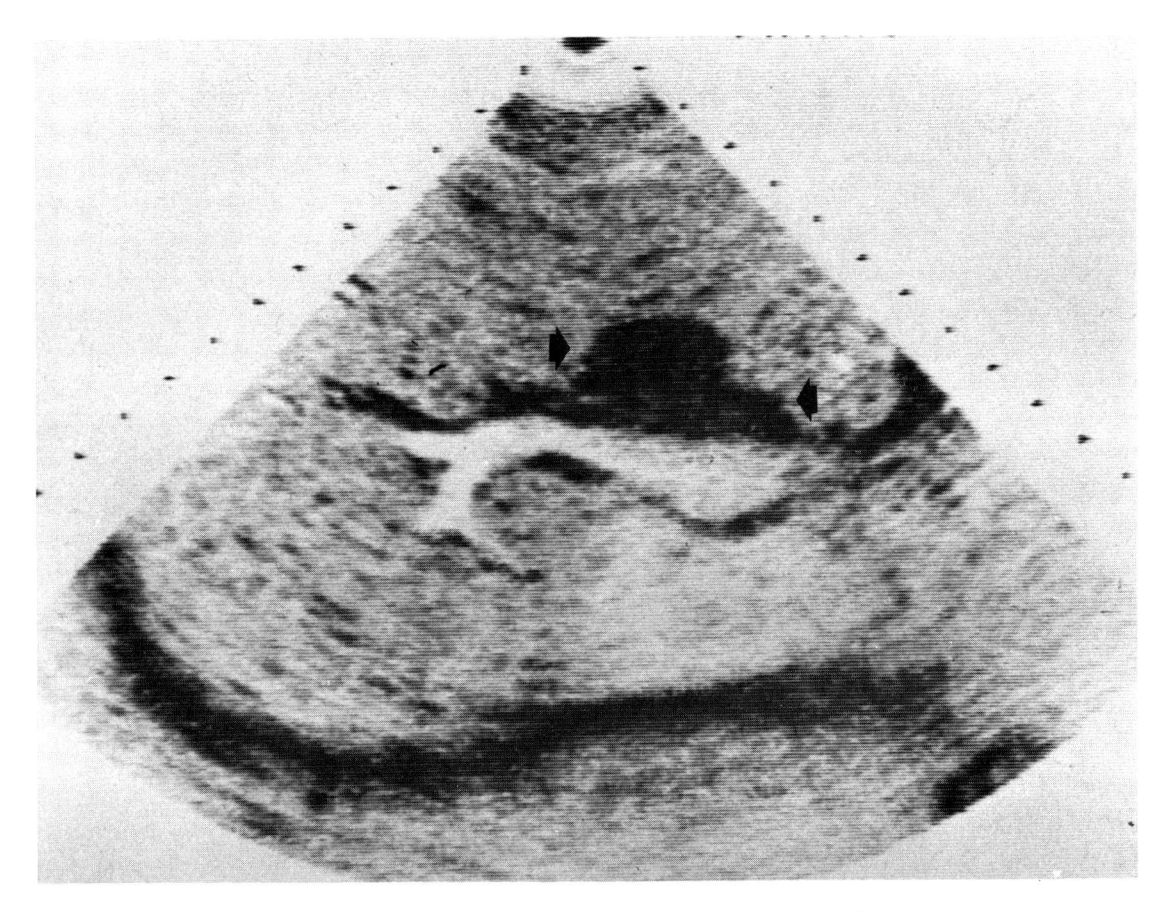

Figure 3-12. A transverse sector scan through the liver shows a densely echogenic lobulated hemangioma (black arrows).

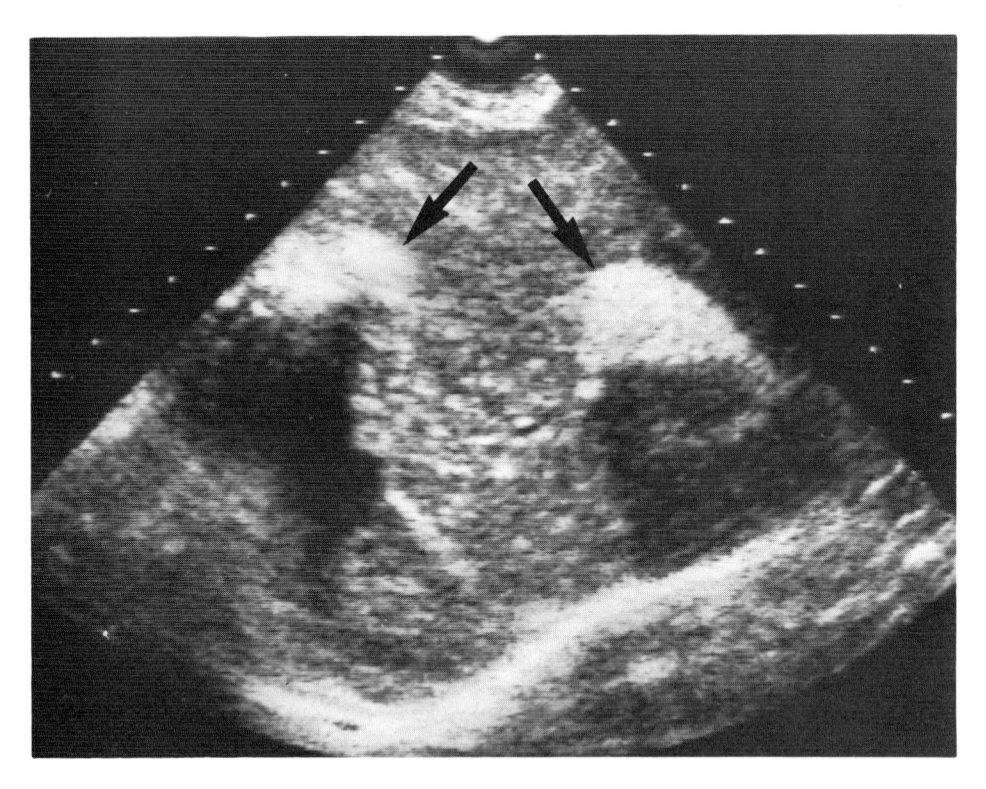

Figure 3-13. Transverse sector scan through the liver shows two calcified hemangiomas (black arrows). Notice the "shadowing" due to calcium.

to be the most specific diagnostic examination. Ultrasound showed areas of increased echogenicity compared with the surrounding hepatic parenchyma (Figures 3-12 and 3-13). The increased echogenicity of a hemangioma is due to the interfaces caused by the walls of the cavernous venous sinuses and the blood within these vessels. A slightly more irregular pattern develops as the hemangioma undergoes degeneration and fibrous replacement. Entities to be considered in the differential diagnosis of the solitary echogenic mass include liver cell adenoma, focal nodular hyperplasia, solitary metastasis and hepatocellular carcinoma. With age, hemangiomas enlarge and undergo fibrosis and calcification. Giant cavernous hemangiomas may present with hepatomegaly or symptoms of pressure on adjacent organs. Complications of hemangiomas include spontaneous rupture into the abdomen, thrombocytopenia, and hypofibrinogenemia. Bree *et al.* (24), in evaluating 26 asymptomatic patients with solitary cavernous hemangiomas, found that most of these masses were located in the posterior right lobe, were homogenous and smooth with increased echo texture, and were usually less than 3 cm in diameter. In evaluating 19 hemangiomas, Wiener *et al.* (25) found 9 to be hypoechoic, 3 complex, and 7 hyperechoic. These findings would be indistinguishable from malignant processes by an ultrasonographic appearance alone. A protocol (in asymptomatic patients without a known neoplasm) for evaluation of the echogenic "spot" in the liver would include dynamic CT after sonography. If the CT findings are characteristic of hemangioma, follow-up sonography could be obtained in 6 months to 1 year (Figure 3-14). If the CT examination does not have the characteristics of hemangioma, biopsy or

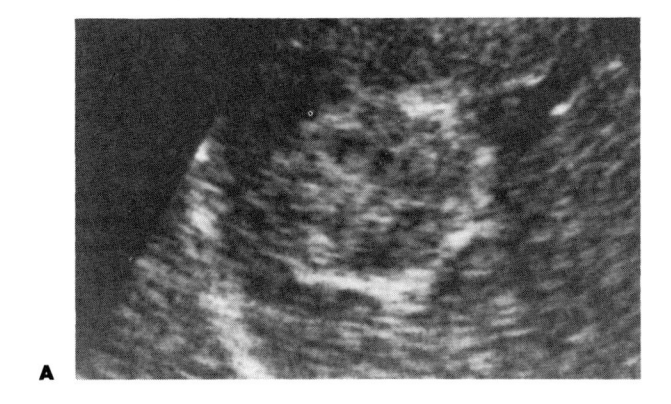

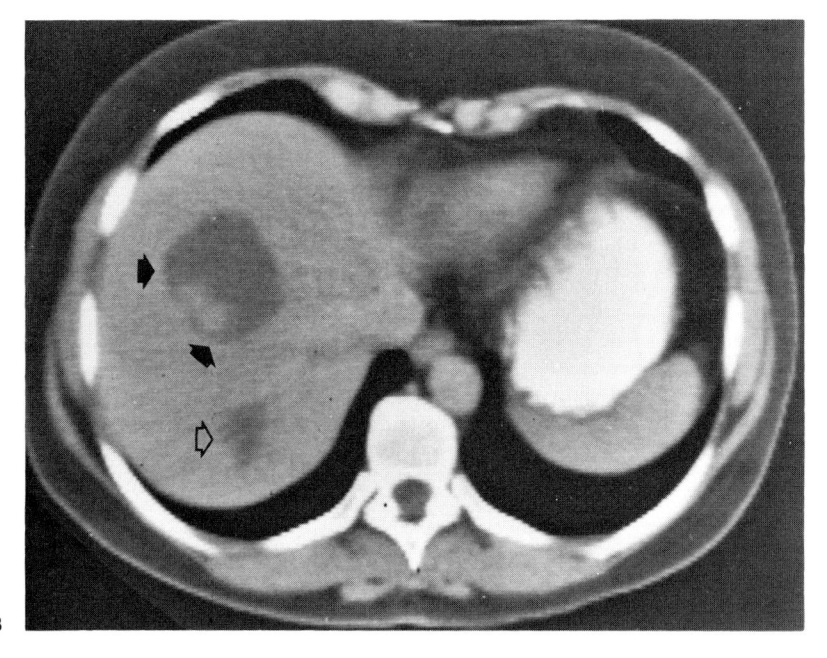

Figure 3-14. *A.* A transverse sonogram through the right lobe of the liver shows an echogenic 5-cm lesion within the right lobe of the liver. *B.* CT scan with contrast enhancement shows the typical CT appearance of hemangioma with peripheral enhancement (black arrows). A second hemangioma is seen in the posterior portion of the right lobe of the liver (open arrow). Ultrasonographically, this lesion is not as densely echogenic as others we have observed.

angiography is suggested. In patients with a primary malignancy, in order to be certain that the lesion is a hemangioma, either biopsy or arteriography may be necessary.

Focal Nodular Hyperplasia and Liver Cell Adenoma

Focal nodular hyperplasia and liver cell adenoma are benign liver tumors that present diagnostic difficulties to the radiologist. Liver cell adenoma usually causes symptoms of an abdominal mass, acute right upper quadrant abdominal pain, or vascular collapse due to rupture of the lesion with hemoperitoneum and bleeding within the tumor. In contrast, focal nodular hyperplasia is usually asymptomatic and an incidental finding. Liver function tests are generally normal in both entities. Focal nodular hyperplasia and liver cell adenoma can be distinguished pathologically. Liver cell adenomas are solitary encapsulated lesions with normal or slightly atypical hepatocytes. Occasionally, they may be multiple. They lack bile ducts. Focal nodular hyperplasia occurs in all age groups and in both sexes, while liver cell adenoma is seen predominantly in women and is linked to oral contraceptives (26). Focal nodular hyperplasia exhibits normal hepatocytes with disruption of the hepatic lobular architecture. Focal nodular hyperplasia appears as a 1 to 20 cm mass with a central fibrous band and radiating septa subdividing the mass (27); in approximately 13 percent of cases, multiple lesions are seen (28).

No definite sonographic features distinguish liver cell adenoma from focal nodular hyperplasia (Figure 3–15). Both lesions may appear as solid masses of increased or decreased echogenicity. Sonolucent areas, due to necrosis or hemorrhage, may be seen in adenomas. Pedunculated masses have also been observed with focal nodular hyperplasia. This appearance, or the appearance of a solid mass with a normal sulphur colloid scan, would be relatively specific for focal nodular hyperplasia (29). The only other lesion that concentrates sulphur colloid is a regenerating cirrhotic nodule. In the evaluation of focal nodular hyperplasia, hepatic scintigraphy is the pivotal examination. In evaluating focal nodular hyperplasia, Rogers *et al.* (30) found sonography most sensitive (100 percent, while scintigraphy demonstrated normal colloid uptake in 55 percent of 11 lesions. In their series, in the patients in whom the colloid scans showed decreased or absent uptake, arteriography showed findings diagnostic of focal nodular hyperplasia

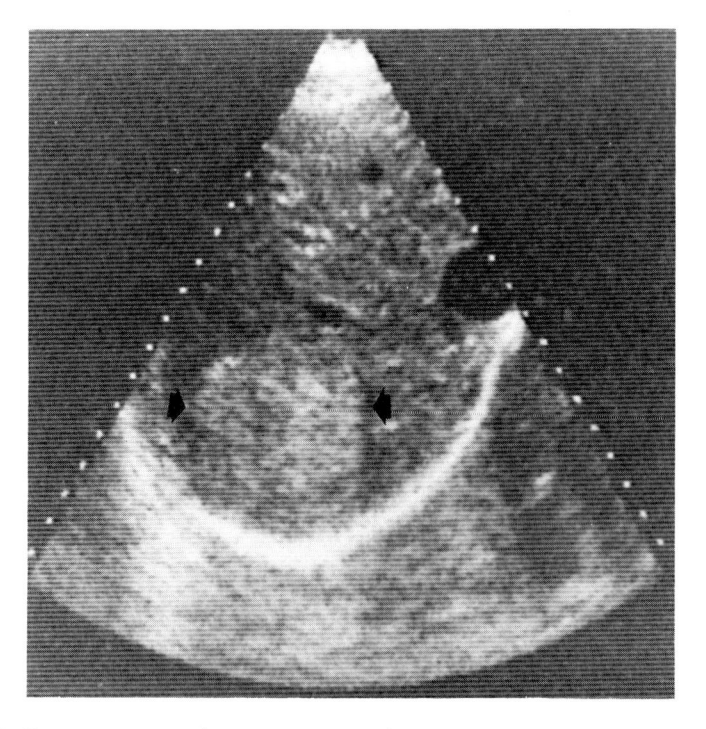

Figure 3–15. Sector sonogram demonstrates an echogenic lesion (black arrows) adjacent to the diaphragm. This lesion is due to focal nodular hyperplasia, but a hepatic adenoma could have a similar appearance.

in 75 percent of cases. Casarella *et al.* reported cases of focal nodular hyperplasia where the lesions showed decreased concentrations of radionuclide (27). When both radionuclide studies and ultrasound studies are abnormal, the differential diagnosis includes focal nodular hyperplasia with hemorrhage or necrosis, metastatic disease, liver cell adenoma, or other hepatic masses.

Hepatic Abscess

The early diagnosis and treatment of hepatic abscess is essential in order to reduce the high rate of mortality seen with this disease process (31, 32). Etiologic factors in hepatic abscesses include seeding from the portal vein, hepatic artery, biliary tree, or via direct extension from an adjacent affected organ. In earlier series, appendicitis was a common cause of liver abscess. Predisposing factors include diabetes mellitus, cirrhosis, or urinary tract infection. Trauma, biliary tract surgery, and biliary obstruction may lead to hepatic abscesses. Hepatic abscesses occur most commonly in the right lobe of the liver and are usually solitary. The most common organism isolated is *E. coli*. Unless careful aspiration technique is performed with attention to anaerobic bacteria, it is not infrequent to obtain pus without identifying the organism.

The walled-off chronic abscess is more easily diagnosed than an early liver abscess. In the acute stage, hepatic abscess consists of a focal accumulation of polymorphonuclear leukocytes in an area of parenchymal liquefaction necrosis. The early sonographic findings in liver abscess may be focal or diffuse areas of increased or decreased parenchymal echoes. In the subacute phase, small anechoic foci may be seen. The more chronic stage appears as a well-defined cavity with varying degrees of internal echogenicity and a well-defined, thickened, irregular wall. The walls of an hepatic abscess tend to be more ragged than abscesses elsewhere in the abdomen (33). Microabscesses of the liver may appear as "targets" with sonolucent peripheries and echogenic centers (34). Highly echogenic liver abscesses may be due to a high protein and lipid content or to small gas bubbles from gas-forming organisms. If the abscess has an echogenic solid appearance, it may be confused with other focal lesions.

The differential diagnostic considerations with hepatic abscesses include neoplasm, hematoma, complicated (hemorrhagic) cyst, and amebic abscess. An individual metastatic lesion with a necrotic center may simulate an abscess. Simple hepatic cysts have a higher degree of sonolucency and thin walls, and their margins are regular and smooth. In general, abscesses have walls thicker than do complicated cysts. Microabscesses, because of their relative sonolucency and small size, may be difficult to diagnose. Amebic abscesses are generally located more peripherally and are contiguous with the liver capsule (35). In the ultrasonic analysis of 42 hepatic amebic abscesses, all but one were contiguous with the liver capsule and exhibited slight distal sonic enhancement. A predominantly homogeneous, fine, low-level echo pattern suggested hepatic amebic abscess.

DIFFUSE LIVER DISEASE

In contrast to the diagnosis of focal hepatic liver disease, the role of ultrasound in evaluation of diffuse hepatic disease processes such as fatty infiltration, cirrhosis, hepatitis, lymphomas, storage diseases, and some hepatomas has been less valuable. Ultrasonic diagnosis of diffuse liver disease is complex, and liver biopsy, although more invasive, is frequently preferred to ultrasound evaluation (Figure 3–16).

A normal ultrasound examination does not preclude the presence of diffuse hepatic disease; frequently, gross disease must be present before detectable. The ultrasound

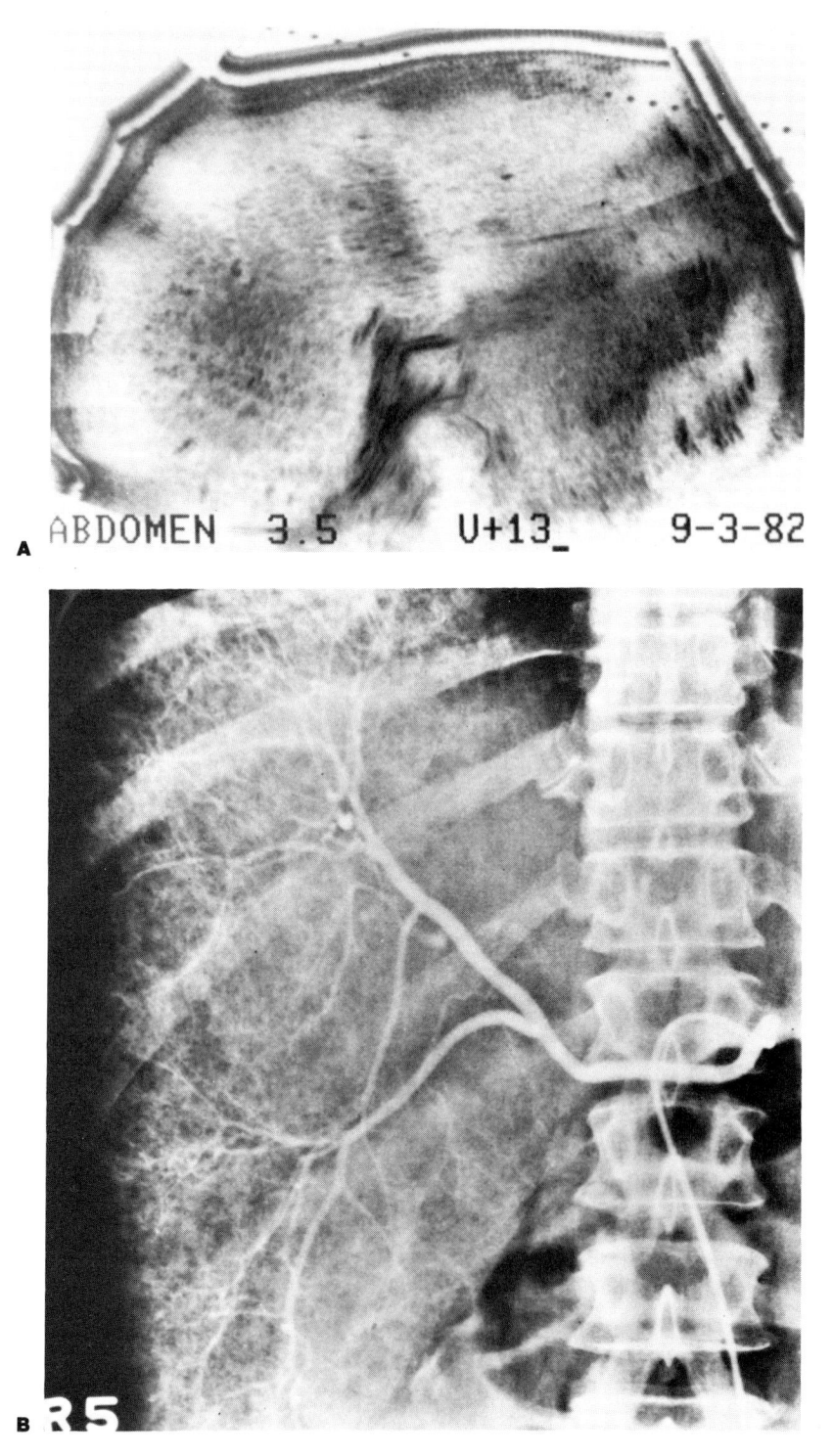

Figure 3-16. *A.* Transverse sonogram in a patient with melanoma. There is a subtle, diffuse, increased echogenicity of the liver that may represent diffuse metastases. *B.* A selective hepatic arteriogram shows diffuse hypervascular metastases throughout the entire liver. While the angiogram is diagnostic, diffuse disease of this magnitude may not be possible to identify by ultrasound. The diffuse heterogeneous pattern of malignancy is easily overlooked.

findings in diffuse hepatic disease are manifested by changes in liver contour, size, echogenicity, and penetration characteristics. Not all contour changes and enlargements or distortions of the normal anatomy indicate definite disease. Further complicating evaluation of diffuse liver disease are the technical factors that can result in increased or decreased echogenicity of the liver (36–38), such as errors in setting of the time-gain compensation curve or improper transducer choices that can mimic diffuse disease processes.

Hepatitis

Kurtz *et al.* (39) described two distinct ultrasound patterns in hepatitis. The predominant sonographic findings of acute hepatitis were accentuated echogenicity of the portal vein walls and an overall decreased echogenicity of the liver due to swollen liver cells. In chronic hepatitis, the parenchymal echo pattern was coarsened. They felt this was due to periportal fibrosis and inflammatory cells. The acute hepatitis pattern correlates with the clinical symptomatology and pathologic findings, but may also be seen in other intralobular processes such as leukemia. The sonographic examination may be normal in mild, acute, and chronic hepatitis. The severe chronic hepatitis pattern correlates clinically and pathologically, but is nonspecific as it may be seen in other abnormalities.

Fatty Liver

Fatty infiltration may result from hyperalimentation, bypass surgery for obesity, corticosteriod therapy, protein malnutrition, malignancy, and diabetes mellitus. However, the most frequent cause is excessive alcohol consumption. Fatty infiltration, the accumulation of excess fat within hepatocytes, is entirely reversible, but may be part of a common pathway to cirrhosis. The sonographic appearance of the fatty-infiltrated liver is characteristic (40). The liver is enlarged and sound transmission is markedly diminished. Because of the lack of penetration, the right hemidiaphragm and vascular structures within the liver are poorly visualized. The overall echo pattern is increased (Figure 3–17).

However, increased echogenicity may be due to fibrosis as well as to fatty infiltration. It may be difficult to differentiate the coarse, irregular echo pattern of cirrhosis from the finer uniform pattern of fatty change. Fatty infiltration may be nonuniform (41) and may lead to diagnostic dilemmas, causing confusion between metastasis and fat deposition (40). Since fatty infiltration can be focal, one may adjust the scanning technique so that the abnormal liver is the "normal" degree of echogenicity. This will cause the true normal liver to appear as hypoechoic focal defects. CT will more reliably indentify fat-infiltrated areas and alleviate confusion between metastases and fat deposition.

Cirrhosis

Cirrhosis results from severe and chronic injury to hepatocytes, resulting in cell necrosis with deposition of fibrous tissue within the liver. The echo texture is coarse with areas of less echogenicity and focal enlargement due to regenerating nodules. In cirrhosis, the overall liver size is decreased. However, the caudate lobe and lateral segment of the left hepatic lobe become prominent, while the remainder of the liver contours become bizarre and irregular due to scarring, fibrosis, and regenerating nodules. Harbin *et al.* (42), in evaluating the relationship between the caudate lobe and the right

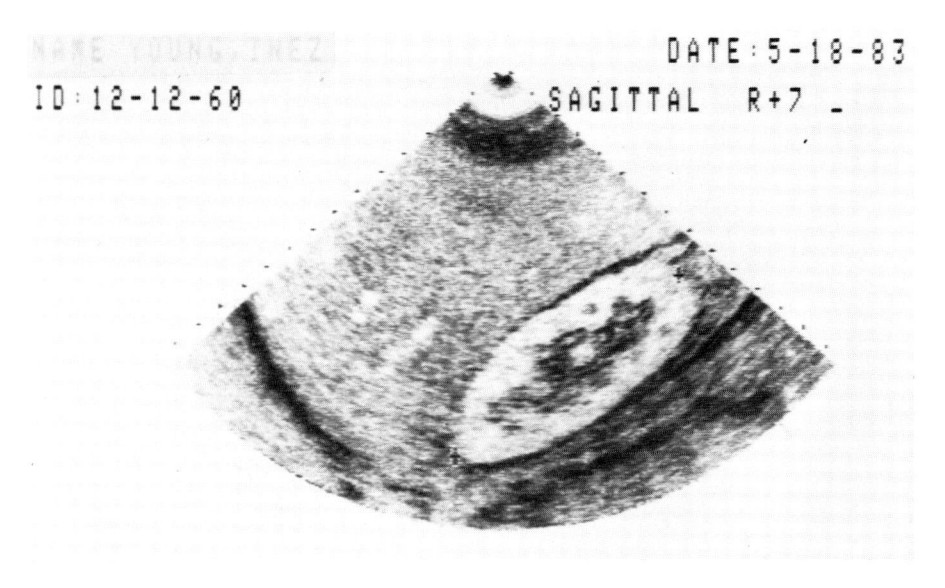

Figure 3-17. Longitudinal scan through the right lobe of the liver shows diffusely increased echogenicity of the liver in relation to the renal cortex. This increased echogenicity was due to fatty infiltration of the liver.

lobe of the liver, established a normal caudate-lobe/right-lobe ratio of less than 50%. In patients with cirrhosis, enlargement of the caudate lobe relative to the right lobe of the liver was 100 percent specific for cirrhosis. When severe cirrhosis ensues, manifestations of portal hypertension such as enlarged portal vein and recanalization of the umbilical vein may be observed. Ancillary signs include splenomegaly and ascites as well as visualization of collateral vessels. The splenic and extrahepatic portal veins become enlarged and tortuous.

Hepatic Lymphoma

Ginaldi *et al.* (43), in studying the hepatic sonograms of 443 patients with lymphoma, detected disease in 5.2 percent of the total population (43). The basic patterns included hypoechoic lesions, which were the most common (43 percent) (Figure 3-18), echogenic lesions (13 percent), target lesions (8.7 percent) with single hyperechoic central foci surrounded by an area of low-level echoes, and a diffuse alteration of the hepatic architecture (34.8 percent). Hypoechoic and diffuse disease patterns were seen in both types of lymphoma. The echogenic and target lesions were seen only in non-Hodgkins lymphomas. While marked hepatomegaly was seen with diffuse disease, liver size was a poor parameter for determining the degree of hepatic involvement. In addition, a normal liver size did not indicate a disease-free liver. The findings of lymphomatous involvement of the liver by sonography are nonspecific and may be difficult to distinguish from metastatic disease, primary hepatocellular carcinoma and cirrhosis.

Storage Disease

Type I glycogen storage disease is inherited as an autosomal recessive trait. The enzyme glucose 6-phosphatase is impaired, preventing glycogenolysis and release of glucose. With improvements in supportive therapy, infants may survive into childhood and

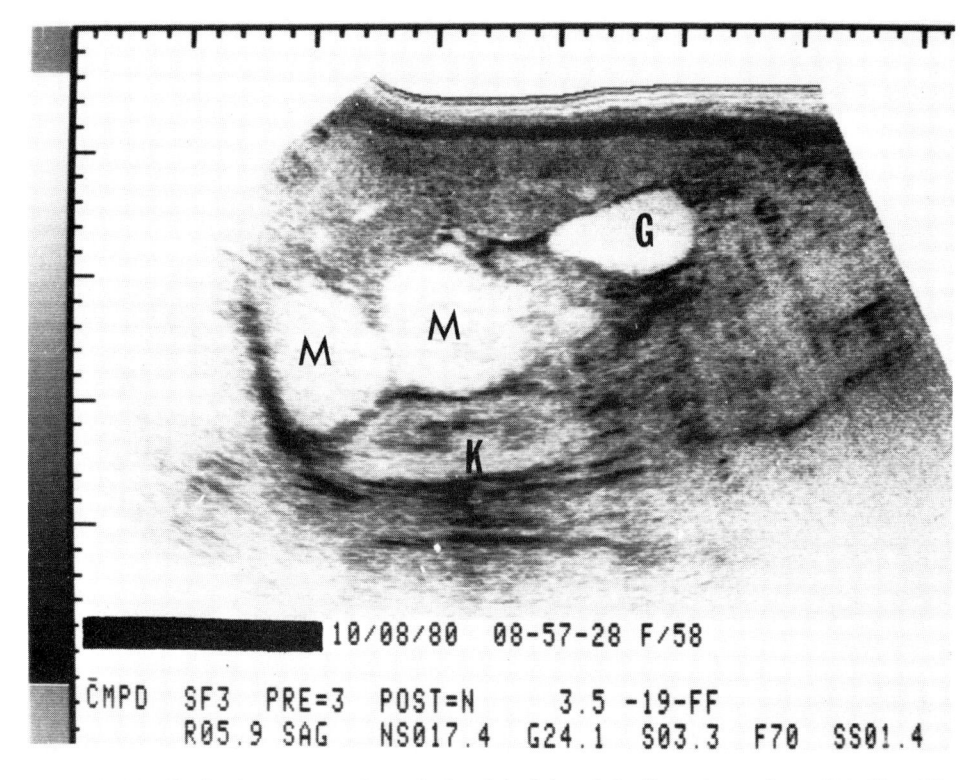

Figure 3–18. Sagittal sonogram through the right lobe of the liver shows the gallbladder (G), kidney (K), and two relatively anechoic masses (M) within the right lobe of the liver due to metastatic lymphoma.

young adulthood. Adenomas as well as hepatomas are seen frequently in these patients. In patients with preexisting glycogen storage disease, hepatic adenomas appeared predominantly hypoechoic when compared to the surrounding increased hepatic echogenicity. Grossman *et al.* (44) found hepatic ultrasonography to be an accurate and safe method of following the progression of liver disease in patients with von Gierke's disease who subsequently developed adenomas and/or hepatocellular carcinoma.

ACCURACY AND DIAGNOSTIC CAPABILITIES OF ULTRASOUND

Over the past 10 years there have been multiple comparative studies of radionuclide scintigraphy, ultrasound, and CT in the evaluation of focal hepatic abnormalities. Also during this period, remarkable improvements in both ultrasound and CT equipment have occurred, making the older reports obsolete. Sullivan *et al.* demonstrated the usefulness of ultrasound in evaluating equivocal areas identified on hepatic scintigraphy with an accuracy rate of 93 percent for ultrasound, compared to 74 percent for scintigraphy (45). Spiegel *et al.* demonstrated ultrasound to be the most accurate technique for visualizing and establishing the cystic nature of benign cysts of the liver (19). More recent reports have demonstrated that CT is the most sensitive method in evaluation of focal hepatic disease. Radionuclide liver imaging resolves masses 2 to 3 cm in size. Since sonography can detect lesions as small as 1 cm, this modality is at least as sensitive as radionuclide scanning when used as a screening procedure for focal liver lesions.

Ultrasound has a high degree of accuracy, is readily available, is cost effective, and utilizes no ionizing radiation. When suboptimal sonograms are eliminated from statistical evaluation, the accuracy of hepatic sonography approaches that of CT and is greater than that of radionuclide scanning. Perhaps the major limitation of sonography is that in 5 to 25 percent of patients, inadequate scans occur secondary to obesity, bowel gas, and body habitus. With persistence and aggressive scanning technique, the number of suboptimal examinations can be decreased.

In addition to clarifying questionable radionuclide scans, ultrasound is useful in evaluation of equivocal CT hepatic masses. Recent articles have demonstrated the difficulty in differentiating cystic from solid masses by CT (46). Also, sonography is helpful in the diagnosis of hemangiomas that do not have the classical CT appearance. These lesions are focal, lobulated, echogenic lesions in nononcologic, asymptomatic patients.

Clinical evaluation of active chemotherapy programs requires frequent evaluation of response. Computed tomography may be prohibitively expensive, while ultrasound represents an easy and inexpensive imaging modality for this purpose. Ultrasound offers the added advantage of visualizing other areas such as the retroperitoneum, porta hepatis, peripancreatic area, kidneys, and adrenal glands when compared to radionuclide imaging.

FUTURE DEVELOPMENTS

Present-day transducers lack stability. Higher frequency transducers with deeper focal zones are needed. Further advances in quantitative data display, eliminating purely subjective visual image analysis, may enable more specific tissue evaluation and definitive identification of some hepatic lesions. Another area of future advancements may occur with the addition of organ-specific ultrasound contrast agents. As with CT, these agents would provide selective alteration of the normal hepatic echogenicity and provide increases in contrast between normal and abnormal hepatic parenchyma. These changes may be relatively small and thus would require a highly sensitive system for evaluation (larger computers). The development of agents that would be specifically localized in abnormal liver parenchyma is less promising, since many agents for the different types of tumors would be needed. It is unlikely that a single agent would be appplicable for all tumors and diffuse disease processes.

Mattrey *et al.* (47) have evaluated perfluorocytlbromide (PFOB) as a liver/spleen specific ultrasound contrast material for tumor imaging in rabbits. They found that PFOB administered intravenously increased the echogenicity of livers at 48 hours. In addition, rabbits with VX2 liver tumors showed echogenic rim enhancement around the tumor following PFOB infusion. Further studies are required prior to application in humans, but this agent and similar agents show promise.

REFERENCES

1. Bernardino ME, Sones PJ, Price RB, Berkman WA: Focal liver lesions. Clin Ultrasound 1983, in press.
2. Prando A, Goldstein HM, Bernardino ME, et al.: Ultrasonic pseudo lesions of the liver. Radiology 1979;130:403–407.
3. Bernardino ME: Liver parenchyma-focal and diffuse disease. In Syllabus for the Categorical Course in Ultrasonography, San Francisco: American Roentgen Ray Society, 1981, pp. 91–106.
4. Bernardino ME, Thomas JL, Mays GB: An initial experience with post data processing in hepatic sonography. AJR 1981;136:521–525.

5. Kane RA: Ultrasonographic anatomy of the liver and biliary tree, Semin Ultrasound, 1980;1:87–95.
6. Carlsen EN, Filly RA: Newer ultrasonographic anatomy in the upper abdomen. 1. The portal and hepatic venous anatomy. J Clin Ultrasound 1976;4:85–90.
7. Callen PW, Filly RA, DeMartini WJ: The left portal vein: possible source of confusion on ultrasonograms. Radiology 1979;130:205–206.
8. Parulekar SG: Ligaments and fissures of the liver: sonographic anatomy. Radiology 1979;130:409–411.
9. Hillman BJ, D'Orsi CJ, Smith EH, Bartram RJ: Ultrasonic appearance of the falciform ligament. AJR 1979;132:205–206.
10. Kamin PD, Bernardino ME, Green B: Ultrasound manifestations of hepatocellular carcinoma. Radiology 131:459–461.
11. Akuda K, Obatn H, Jinnonchi S, et al.: Angiographic assessment of gross anatomy of hepato cellular carcinoma: comparison of celiac angiograms and pathology in 100 cases. Radiology 1977;123:21–29.
12. Green B, Bree RL, Goldstein HM, Stanley C: Gray scale ultrasound evaluation of hepatic neoplasms: patterns and correlations. Radiology 1977;124:203–208.
13. Scheibel W, Gosink BB, Leopold GR: Gray scale echographic patterns of hepatic metastatic disease. AJR 1977;129:983–987.
14. Katragadda CS, Goldstein HM, Green B: Gray-scale ultrasonography of calcified liver metastases. AJR 1977;129:591–593.
15. Weaver RM Jr, Goldstein HM, Green B, Perkins C: Gray scale ultrasonic evaluation of hepatic cystic disease. AJR 1978;130:849–852.
16. Barnes PA, Thomas JL, Bernardino ME: Pitfalls in diagnosis of hepatic cysts by computed tomography. Radiology 1981;141:129–133.
17. Callen PW: Computed tomographic evaluation of abdominal and pelvic abscesses. Radiology 1979;131:171–175.
18. Bernardino ME, Green B: Ultrasonic evaluation of chemotherapeutic response in hepatic metastases. Radiology 1979;133:437–441.
19. Spiegel RM, King DL, Green WM: Ultrasonography of primary cysts of the liver. AJR 1978;131:235–238.
20. Gharbi HA, Hassine W, Brauner MW, Depuch K: Ultrasound examination of the hydatid liver. Radiology 1981;139:459–463.
21. Babcock DS, Kaufman L, Kosno I: Ultrasound diagnosis of a hydatid disease (echinococcosis) in two cases. AJR 1978;131:895–897.
22. Ishak KG, Rabin L: Benign tumors of the liver. Med Clin North Am 1975;59:995–1013.
23. Freeney PC, Vimont TR, Barnett TC: Cavernous hemangioma of the liver: ultrasonography, arteriography and computed tomography. Radiology 1979;132:142–148.
24. Bree RL, Schwab RE, Neiman HL: Solitary echogenic spot in the liver: is it diagnostic of a hemangioma? AJR 1983;140:41–45.
25. Wiener SN, Parulekar SG: Scintigraphy and ultrasonography of hepatic hemangioma. Radiology 1979;132:149–153.
26. Baum JK, Holtz F, Bookstein JJ, et al.: Possible association between benign hepatomas and oral contraceptives. Lancet 1973;2:926–929.
27. Casarella WJ, Knowles DF, Wolf M, et al.: Focal nodular hyperplasia and liver cell adenoma: radiologic and pathologic differentiation. Am J Roentgenol 1978;131:393–402.
28. Knowles DM, Wolf M: Focal nodular hyperplasia of the liver. A clinical pathologic study and review of the literature. Hum Pathol 1976;7:545–553.
29. Sandler MA, Petrocelli RD, Marks DS, et al.: Ultrasonic features and radionuclide correlation in liver cell adenoma and focal nodular hyperplasia. Radiology 1980;135:393–397.
30. Rogers JV, Mack LA, Freeney PC, et al.: Hepatic focal nodular hyperplasia: angiography, CT, sonography, and scintigraphy. AJR 1981;137:983–990.
31. Setiani B, Davidson ED: Hepatic abscess: improvement in mortality with early diagnosis and treatment. Am J Surg 1978;135:647–650.

32. Gerzoff SG, Robbins AH, Birkeh DH, et al.: Percutaneous catheter drainage of abnormal abscesses guided by ultrasound and computed tomography. Am J Roentgenol 1979;133:1-8.
33. Newlin N, Silver TM, Stuck KJ, Sandler MA: Ultrasonic features of pyogenic liver abscesses. Radiology 1981;139:155-159.
34. Callen PW, Filly RA, Marcus FS: Ultrasonography and computed tomography in the evaluation of hepatic microabscesses in the immuno-suppressed patient. Radiology 1980; 136:433-434.
35. Rawls PW, Myers HI, Lappen SA, et al.: Gray scale ultrasonography of hepatic amebic abscess. Radiology 1979;132:125-129.
36. Black EB, Ferucci JT, Wittenburg J, et al.: Acoustic contrast enhancement: value of several system gain variations and gray scale ultrasonography. AJR 1979;133:689-693.
37. Jaffe CC, Harris DJ: Sonographic tissue texture: influence of transducer focusing pattern. AJR 1980;135:343-347.
38. Jaffe CC, Taylor KJW: The clinical impact of ultrasonic beam focusing patterns. Radiology 1979;131:469-472.
39. Kurtz AB, Rubin CS, Cooper HS, et al.: Ultrasound findings in hepatitis. Radiology 1980;136;717-723.
40. Scott WW Jr, Sanders RC, Siegelman SS: Irregular fatty infiltration of the liver: diagnostic dilemmas. AJR 1980;136:67-71.
41. Mulherne CB Jr, Arger CH, Coleman BG, et al.: Non-uniform attenuation in computed tomography: study of the cirrhotic liver. Radiology 1979;132:399-402.
42. Harbin WP, Robert NJ, Ferucci JT: Diagnosis of cirrhosis based on regional changes in hepatic morphology. Radiology 1980;135:273-283.
43. Ginaldi S, Bernardino ME, Jing B-S, Green B: Ultrasonographic patterns of hepatic lymphoma. Radiology 1980;136:427-431.
44. Grossman H, Rahm P, Coleman R, et al.: Hepatic ultrasonography in Type I glycogen storage disease (von Gierke disease): detection of hepatic adenoma and carcinoma. Radiology 1981;141:753-756.
45. Sullivan DC, Taylor KJW, Gottschalk A: The use of ultrasound to enhance the diagnostic utility of the equivocal liver scintigraph. Radiology 1978;128:727-732.
46. Federle MP, Filly RA, Moss AA: Cystic hepatic neoplasms: complementary roles of CT and sonography. AJR 1981;136:345-348.
47. Mattrey RF, Scheible FW, Gosink BB, et al.: Perfluorocytlbromide: A liver/spleen-specific and tumor imaging ultrasound contrast material. Radiology 1982;45:759-769.

4
Hepatic Computed Tomography

MICHAEL E. BERNARDINO

INTRODUCTION

Since the mid-1970's, hepatic computed tomography (CT) has undergone vast changes. Initially, the abdomen and liver were scanned with 2-½-minute scanners. Thus, there was significant motion artifact and poor resolution. These scanners imaged the liver with wide slices (13 mm). The resolution of the equipment increased with scan times below 20 seconds and then below 10 seconds. Now most new CT equipment has scan times below 5 seconds. Also, the slice thickness can be varied from 1.5 to 10.0 mm. Thus, both our techniques and our understanding of hepatic disease have increased and changed with the advances in CT equipment. This chapter will develop an understanding of proper technique in scanning the liver, knowledge of normal anatomy, knowledge of focal liver masses, and ways of differentiating these masses. This chapter will also deal with diffuse liver disease and its varying CT patterns. Its role with regard to other diagnostic imaging and its sensitivity will be discussed. Also, some insight into future developments, such as hepatic-specific contrast agents and dual energy scanning will be demonstrated.

TECHNIQUE

Initial Scan Point

When studying the liver by computed tomography, the first slice should have at least two-thirds lung and one-third liver demonstrated (1) (Figure 4–1). If more liver is noted on the initial slice, masses at the dome of the diaphragm could be missed. Fifteen to 25 percent of the liver, predominately the right hepatic lobe, may be located under the diaphragm (depending on the patient's anatomy). An added reward from this technique

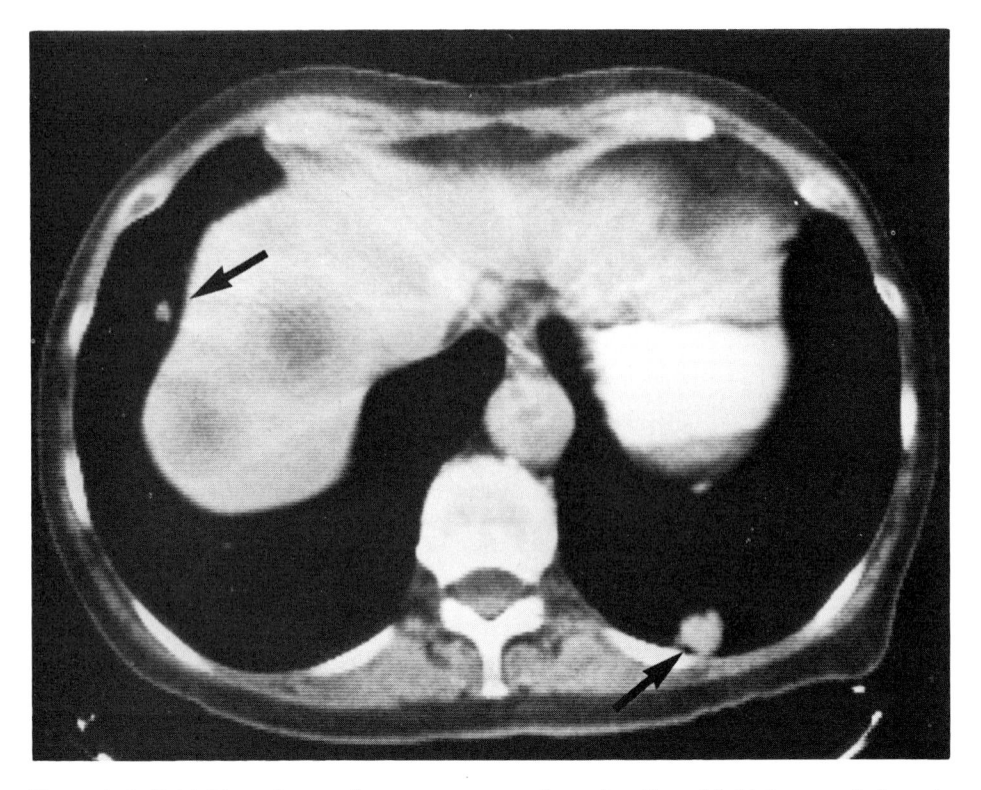

Figure 4-1. Initial hepatic scan demonstrates more lung than liver. Multiple necrotic hepatic metastases are noted under the diaphragm. Also, two lung metastases (arrows) are seen. The latter may be difficult to detect by chest x-ray due to their location.

is that both lower lung fields are imaged. They should be visualized with lung windows, since many lung metastases are noted in the lower lung fields due to the increased blood flow in this region.

Collimation

Most advanced CT equipment allows the radiologist to decide between various collimators. When surveying the liver for disease, 8- or 10-mm collimation is usually sufficient. In more detailed types of examinations, the physician may wish to switch to a smaller collimator such as 5 mm, 4 mm, or smaller. The thinner sections may give more detail. However, unless one increases the radiographic technique, they may be grainier due to photon deficiency.

Slice Spacing

The most accurate way to evaluate the liver would be with adjacent slices throughout the organ. This would leave no gap and thus decrease the incidence of missing small lesions. However, the spacing between slices may be dependent on factors other than optimum technique. It may be dependent on patient load at the institution and whether other organs in the body are to be examined. In a report comparing CT scans taken every 2 cm through the liver and scans taken every 1 cm through the liver, only two more hepatic lesions were detected by the more detailed examination (2). However, the finer detailed examination missed many lesions outside of the liver because more organs were evaluated in the survey type (2 cm) examination. Thus, one has to determine whether a survey or a detailed examination is needed for the type of patient being examined. It may be more appropriate to do a survey examination in an oncologic patient because there is a higher probability of serendipitous lesion detection elsewhere in the abdomen (3). In a patient where a questionable hepatic defect is the only reason for the CT study, a more detailed, focused examination is indicated.

Window Widths and Levels

When evaluating the liver, it is important to use at least two window widths and various density levels. A wide window is sufficient to give soft-tissue density and bone density. However, many small or subtle lesions may not be detected by a wide window. Thus, a narrow window is needed to detect lesions that are minimally less dense than the surrounding normal hepatic parenchyma (Figure 4–2). The narrow window accentuates the contrast between normal liver and the subtle abnormality.

Iodinated Contrast

One of the areas of greatest controversy in hepatic CT is *if* and *when* to use intravenous iodinated contrast (4–9). Early data performed on a second generation CT scanner using a drip infusion of iodine (42 grams) demonstrated that more lesions were masked by intravenous contrast than seen only with intravenous contrast (6). This early paper demonstrated that some lesions were better seen after intravenous contrast. Also, in roughly 50 percent of the cases it did not matter whether intravenous contrast was or was not used (Figure 4–3). Recent literature has supported the use of high doses of iodine (50 to 60 grams) with scanning performed rapidly after the contrast injection. In this particular study, more information was obtained and more lesions were noted after the iodinated scans (10). Foley *et al.* in a prospective study, using 50-gram iodine bolus with rapid scanning (entire liver in less than 5 minutes) demonstrated no false negative lesions (11). The noncontrasted liver studies on the same patients demonstrated two false negative studies. The focal masses not detected on the noncontrast studies were less than 1 cm in size. Using this contrast technique, the liver increased more than 60-Hounsfield units (Hu) in density, thus creating a significant density difference between normal and abnormal tissue. Also, a lesion that was made isodense was detected because it displaced the surrounding hepatic vessels.

Others have reported that due to the dual blood supply of the liver, focal liver masses may have various appearances. Most primary tumors and metastases receive their blood supply from the hepatic artery. Therefore, after a rapid bolus, their periphery may be hyperdense. However, in the portal phase of hepatic blood flow, the lesions may be hypodense. The portal vein is rarely the blood supply to hepatic masses. Thus, the appearance of a lesion is dependant upon when it was scanned after the iodinated contrast load (12). Some lesions begin hyperdense and become isodense. Other lesions may start hyperdense and become hypodense. Some may remain hyperdense, isodense, or hypodense throughout the scanning sequence. Also multiple metastases from the same tumor may have a varied hepatic CT appearance (Figure 4–4). Another key factor to note in any discussion of the use of iodine is that almost all the literature has reported the detection of a lesion or lesions either precontrast or postcontrast. However, very little data have pointed out that the detection of lesions does not mean that these are the only

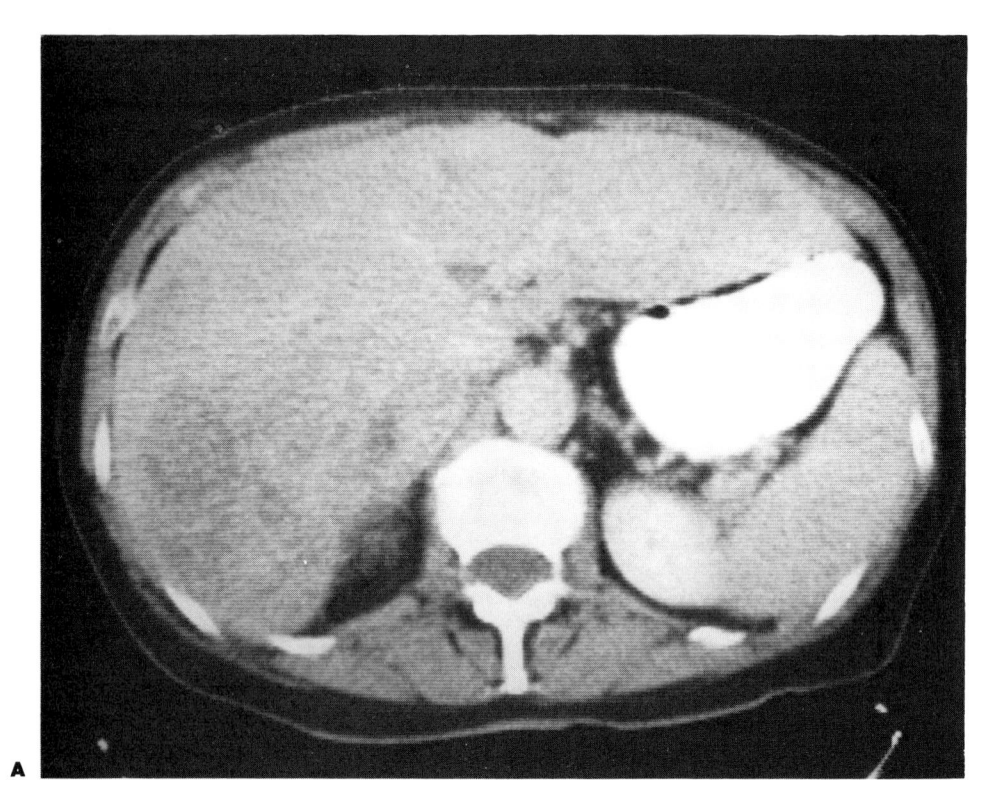

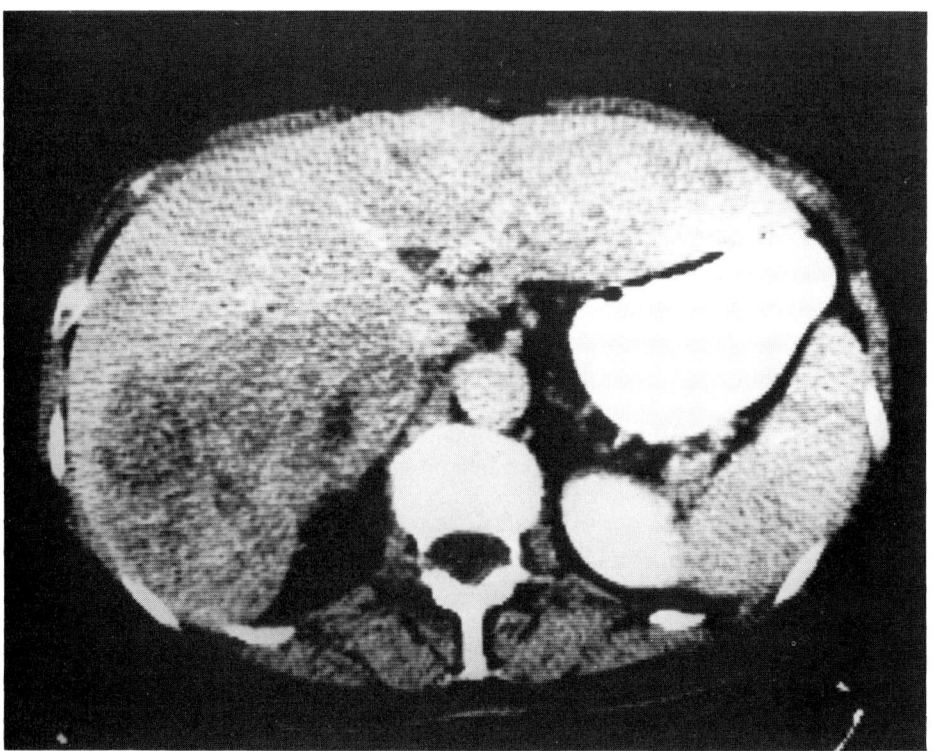

Figure 4-2. *A.* CT scan photographed at a wide window demonstrates the multiple hepatic lesions with great difficulty. *B.* Narrower windows increase the contrast. The masses are easily seen.

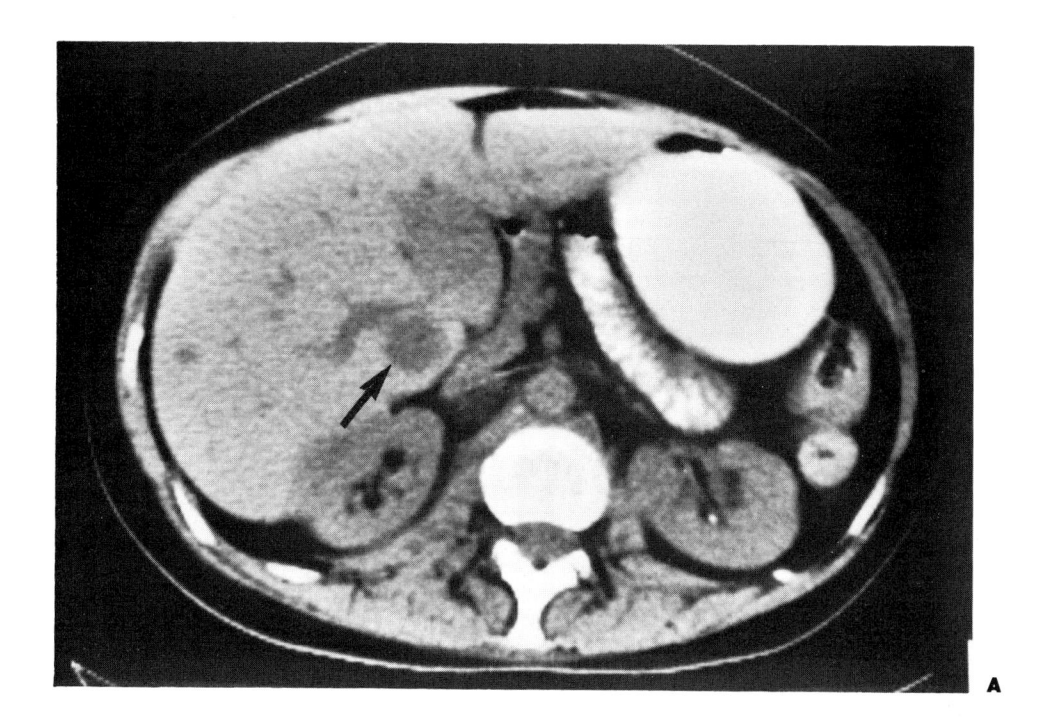

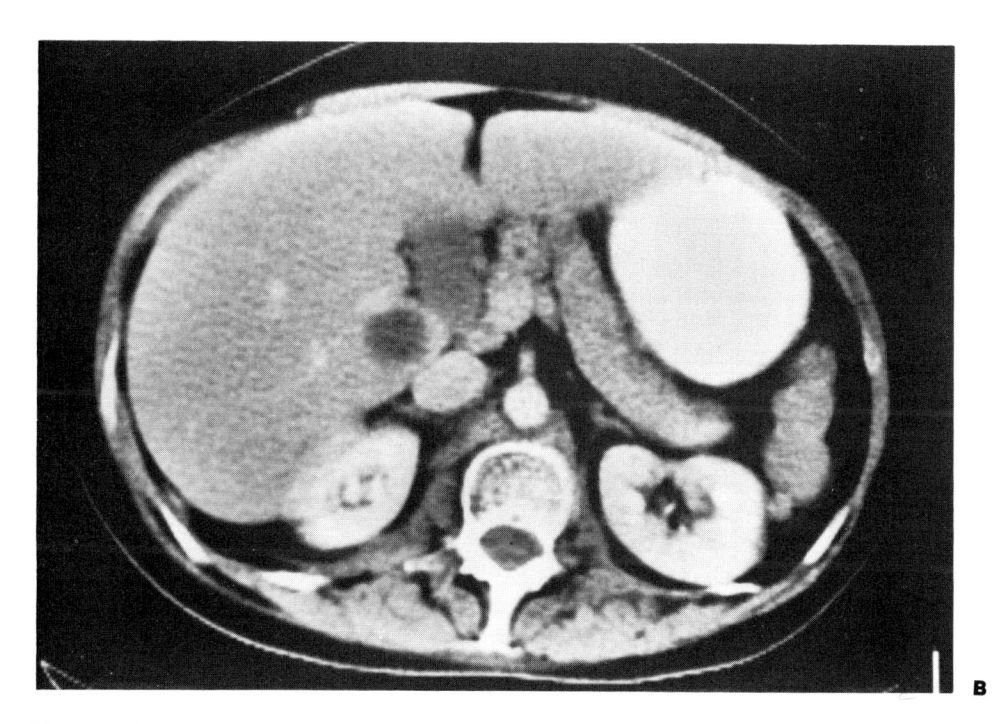

Figure 4-3. *A.* Precontrast study demonstrates a solitary lesion (arrow) in the liver. *B.* Postcontrast study shows no improvement in the visualization of the metastasis.

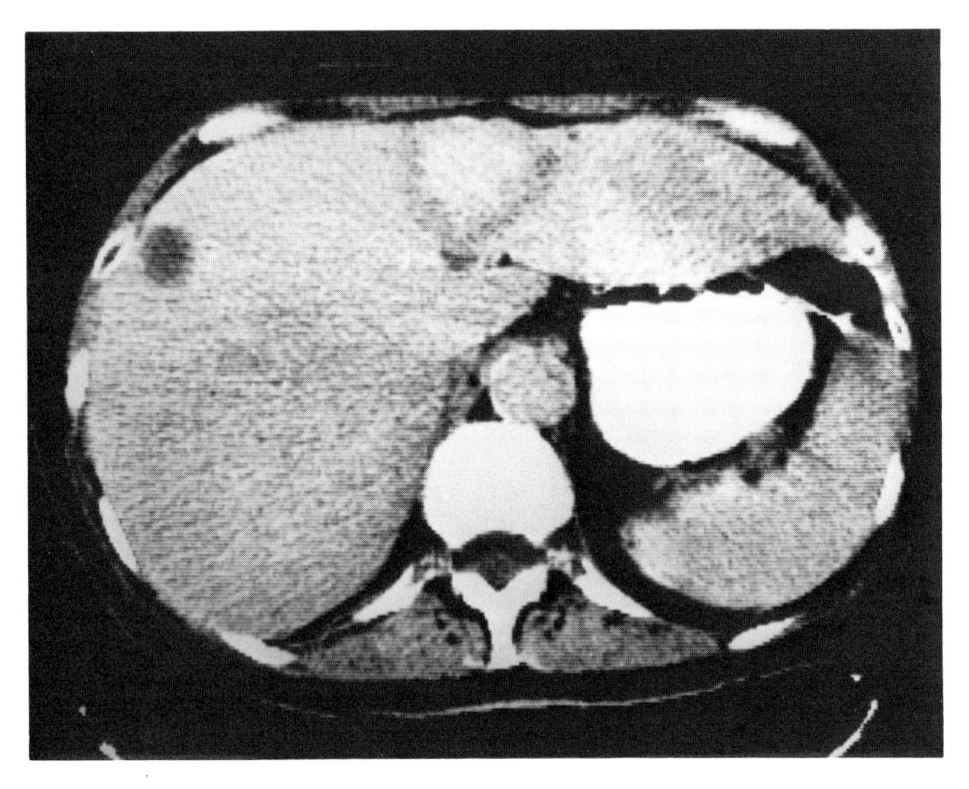

Figure 4-4. Multiple hepatic lesions from colon carcinoma are noted after intravenous contrast administration. One appears hyperdense and the other hypodense.

masses within the liver. None of the literature dealing with the use of intravenous iodine discusses the "true extent" of disease within the liver (13).

Computed Angiotomography

Computed angiotomography is a technique whereby a catheter is placed in either the hepatic artery or superior mesenteric artery and iodine is infused through the catheter while the CT scan is done. In performing such scans, about 3 ml of diluted intravenous iodine should be administered per second. The dilution is dependent on the sensitivity of the CT scanner. Less sensitive scanners may need 60 percent iodinated contrast during the infusion, while more sensitive CT scanners need only 20 to 25 percent iodinated solution. Higher concentrations on more sensitive CT scanners may cause beam-hardening artifacts. In the previous reports of these techniques, more focal masses have been detected when compared to routine computed tomography (with or without intravenous iodine), selective angiography, or even hepatic-specific contrast agents (14) (Figure 4-5). The majority of new lesions detected when compared to angiography are in the left hepatic lobe and the subcapsular area.

Hepatic Artery Computed Tomography

In the technique utilizing hepatic artery catheterization, the lesions are detected due to their hypervascularity and to the fact that the majority of the tumor blood supply is from the hepatic artery. Therefore, the lesion's periphery is usually much more dense

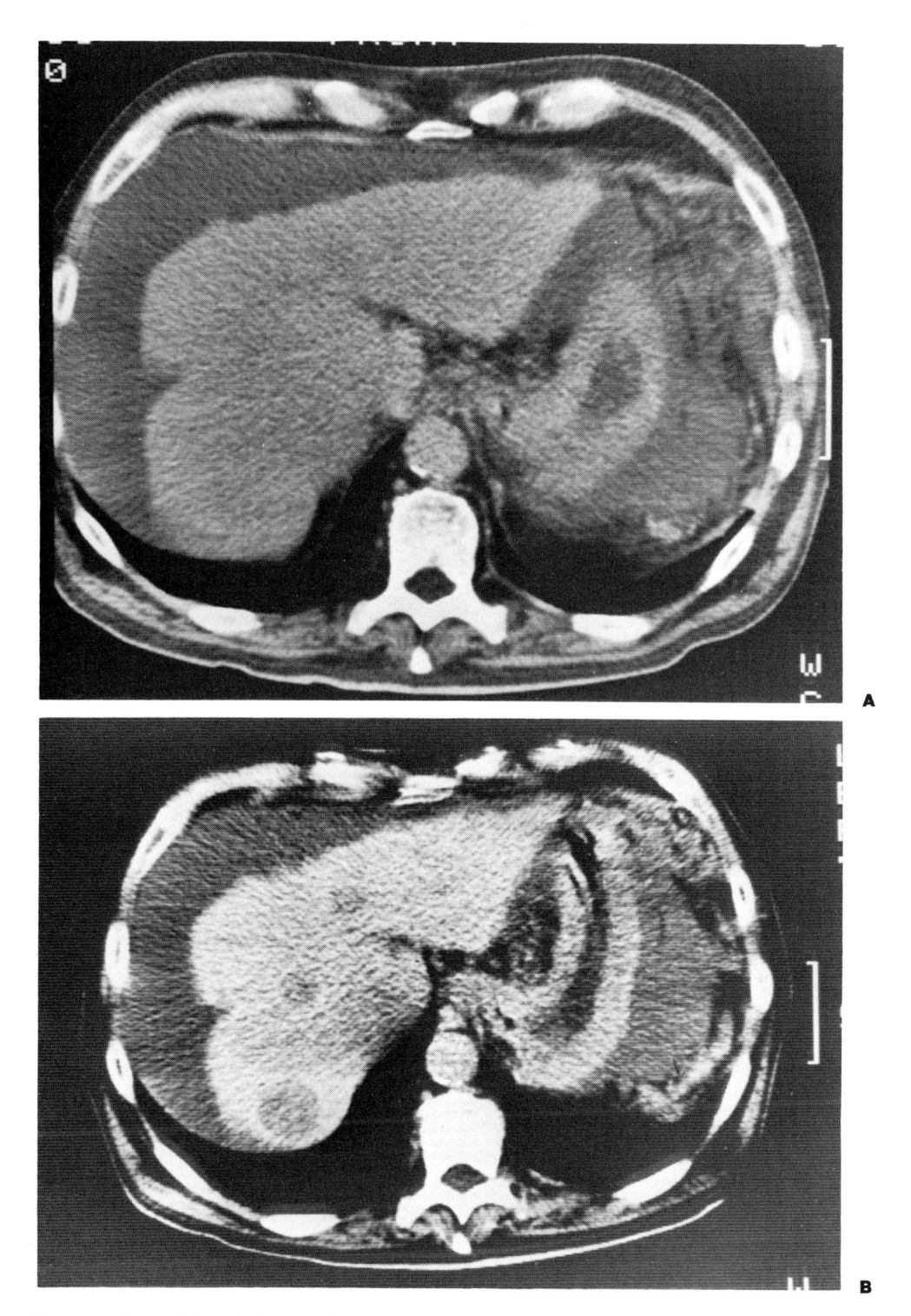

Figure 4–5. *A.* CT study in a patient with portal hypertension due to cirrhosis demonstrates neither focal lesions, ascites, nor varices. *B.* Computed angiotomogram study shows three focal masses (multifocal hepatoma). Note the increased density of the liver due to the hepatic artery injection.

115

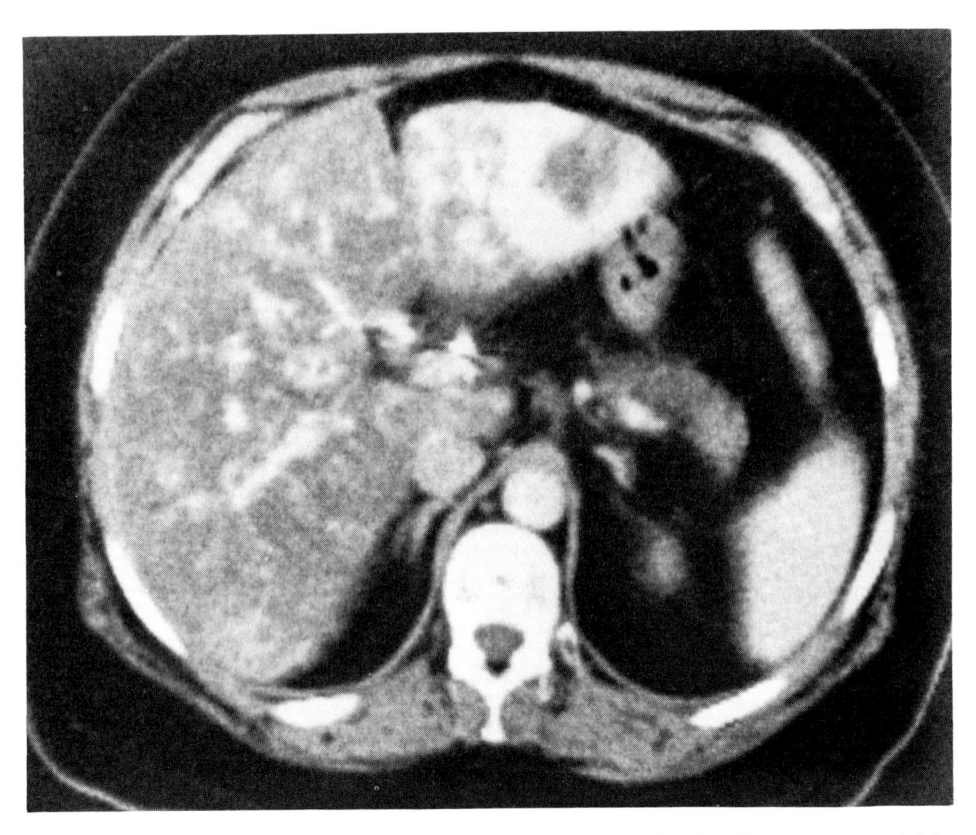

Figure 4-6. Computed angiotomogram from a hepatic artery injection demonstrates multiple hepatic metastases. Their peripheries are hypervascular and dense.

than the surrounding hepatic parenchyma (Figure 4-6). Freeny and Marks reported that this technique detected 12 more hepatic masses in 22 patients than did conventional methods (15).

Superior Mesenteric Artery CT

In this computed portography technique, the injection is into a superior mesenteric artery catheter. The lesions are less dense than the surrounding hepatic parenchyma since the portal vein is the main blood supply of the liver. Also, the portal vein is rarely the vascular supply to hepatic tumors. Thus, only the normal liver increases in density. Matsui *et al.* found this method detected more hepatic masses in 13 of 17 patients (16). Because of the time-consuming nature of selective hepatic artery catheterization, the superior mesenteric technique may be easier to perform. However, this type of examination should not be performed on everyone. The best candidates for such a study are those patients who may benefit from a partial hepatectomy for localized or isolated primary or metastatic hepatic malignancies. Freeny and Marks felt that this amounted to about 3 percent of their oncologic population (15).

ANATOMY

It is very easy to divide the liver up into its various lobes and segments with axial CT sections (17) (Figure 4-7). The right hepatic lobe is divided from the left hepatic lobe

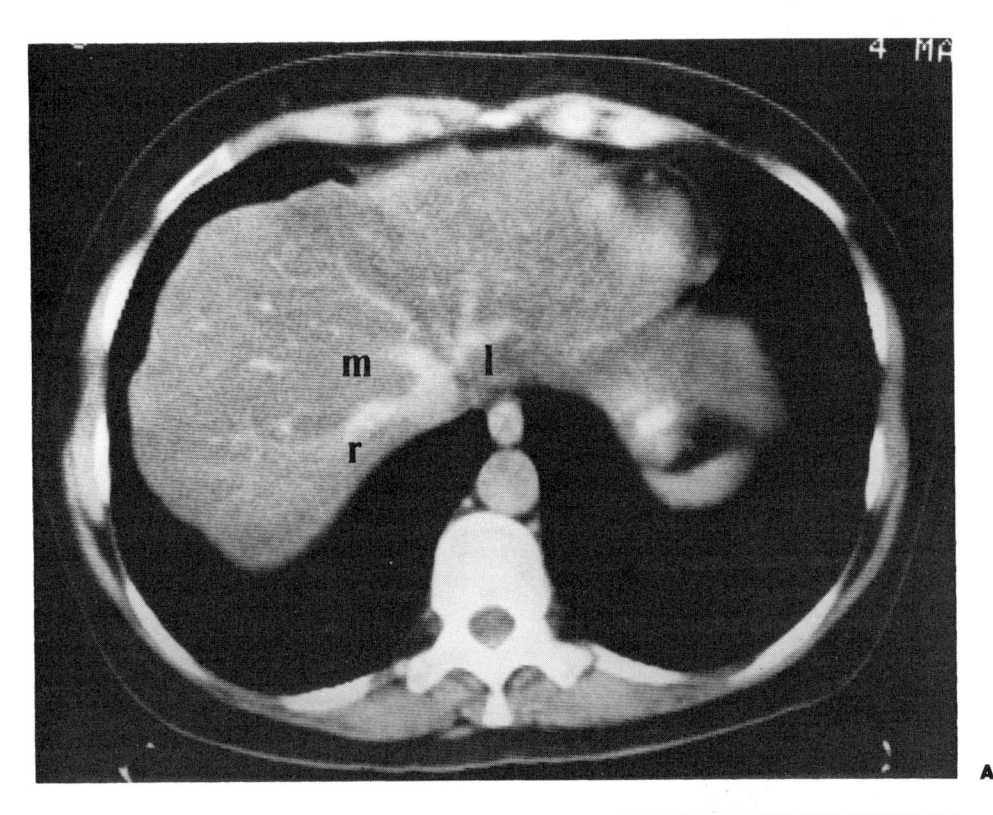

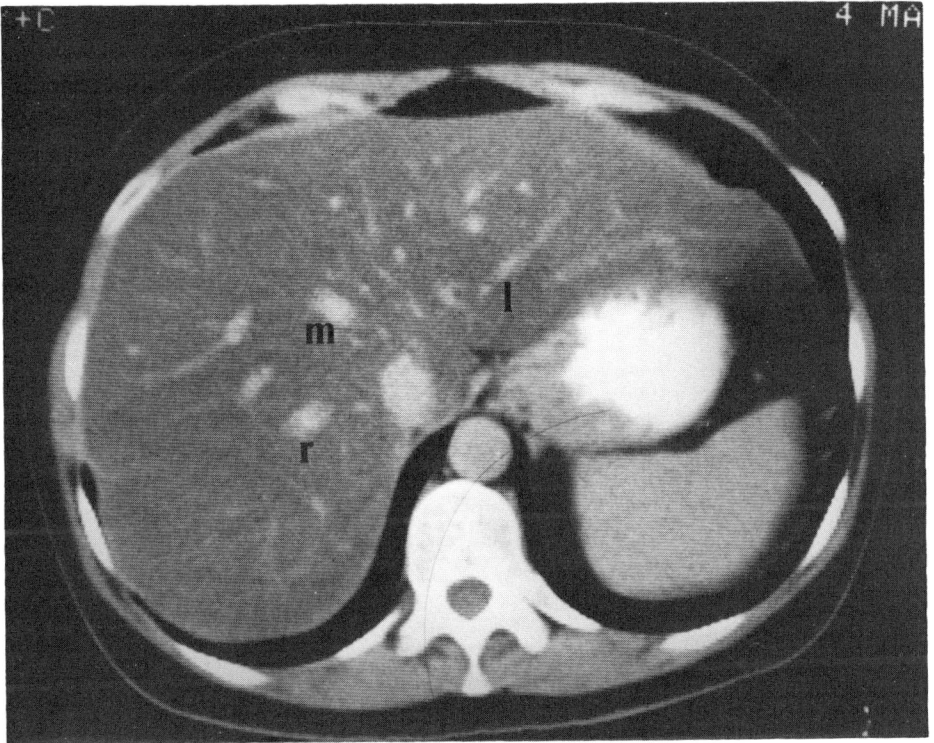

Figure 4–7. Normal hepatic CT anatomy. *A.* Scan near the diaphragm shows the IVC, left hepatic vein (l), right hepatic vein (r), and middle hepatic vein (m). *B.* Scan 2 cm lower than *A* demonstrates the same vessels.

117

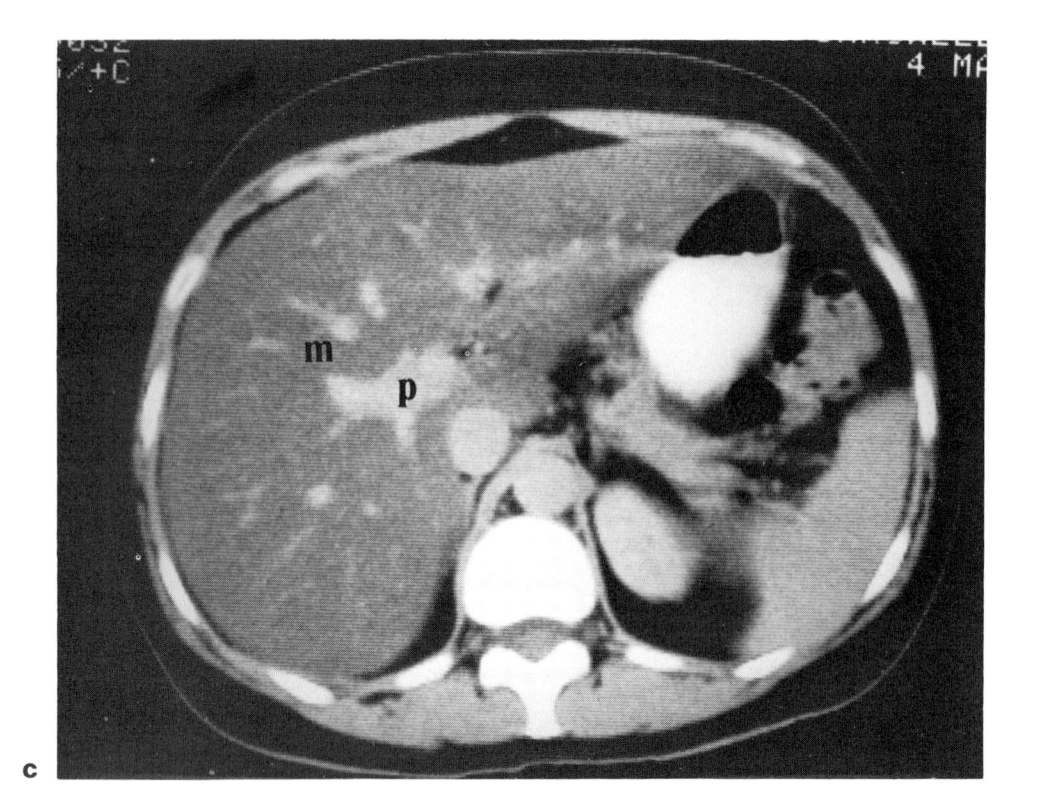

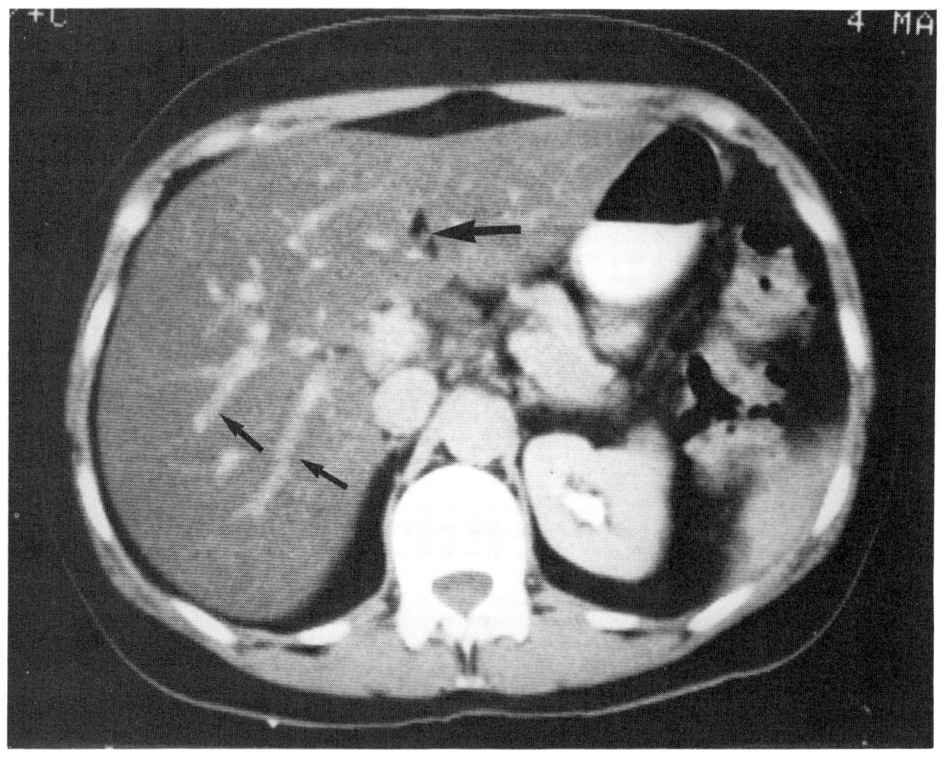

Figure 4–7. *C.* Scan 2 cm lower than *B* shows the main portal vein (p). The left hepatic lobe is divided from the right hepatic lobe by the middle hepatic vein or an imaginary line from the gallbladder fossa to the IVC. *D.* Scan 2 cm lower than *C* shows the right portal vein (small arrow) branches in the right hepatic lobe. The falsiform ligament (large arrow) divides the medial from the lateral segment of the left hepatic lobe.

by an imaginary line from the gallbladder fossa to the inferior vena cava. The middle hepatic vein is also located in this fissure. The right hepatic lobe is divided into anterior and posterior segments by the right hepatic vein. The left hepatic lobe is divided into the medial and lateral segments by the falciform ligament and left hepatic vein. Also, a portion of the left portal vein is noted in this ligament. The major portal vein lies anterior to the caudate lobe, which lies anterior to the inferior vena cava. As the portal vein bifurcates into its left main and right main branches, the portal vein then travels intralobar and intrasegmental.

The hepatic vessels can be detected because of the inherent density difference with the liver or immediately after bolus injection of iodine. The portal vessels are usually seen much lower in the liver-scanning sequence, while the hepatic veins are noted more frequently on the more superior sections. These veins converge toward the inferior vena cava.

Normally, the right hepatic lobe occupies 70 to 80 percent of the hepatic volume. The left hepatic lobe hypertrophies only after injury or surgery to the right hepatic lobe (Figure 4–8). It usually has a triangular shape with a flat anterior border. The right hepatic lobe usually has a smooth capsular border and occasionally will have a defect medially due to an anatomically high positioned kidney.

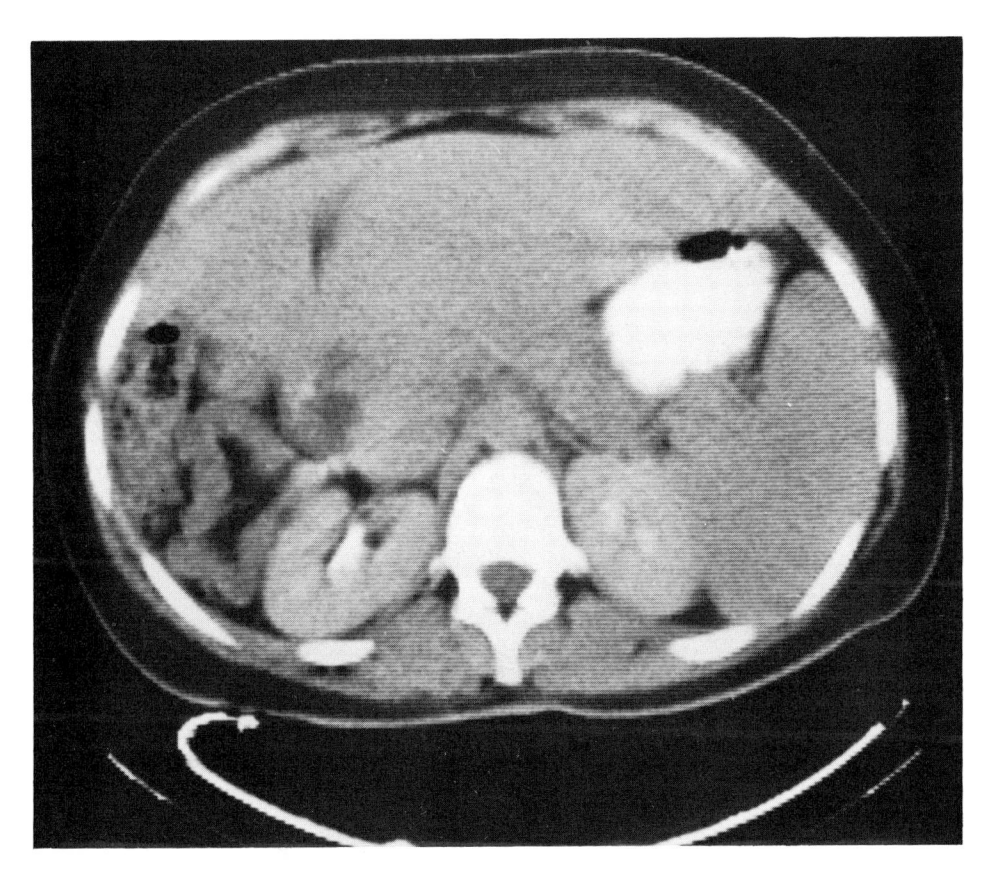

Figure 4–8. After a partial hepatectomy involving the right hepatic lobes, the left lobe hypertrophies. The majority of the hyperplasia is noted in the lateral segment.

FOCAL LIVER MASSES

Hepatomas

Hepatomas can be seen as areas of decreased attenuation within the liver. They may be focal, diffuse, or multifocal. Their tissue density may be so similar to the surrounding liver that they are difficult to detect by conventional methods. The key to the diagnosis of hepatomas is to determine whether there is involvement of either the portal vein, hepatic vein, or inferior vena cava (18–24).

The detection of hepatomas may be difficult in those patients who already have diseased livers, such as the cirrhotic patient. In such patients, the liver is shrunken, lobulated, and of less than normal density. There may be an increase in fibrosis or regenerating nodules present in the same patient (19). Thus, subtle density changes within such a liver may be difficult to observe. Also, the tumor (especially if well-differentiated) may have similar tissue density and vascular characteristics when compared to the surrounding liver. In one series, only 80 percent of 47 hepatomas were detected by CT. The authors suggested that precontrast and postcontrast scans be used in possible hepatoma patients because three lesions were seen only after intravenous contrast, while two tumors were noted only on the precontrast satellite scans. Hepatoma nodules below 2 cm are difficult to detect. Takashima *et al.* have shown that more lesions are detected by conventional selective hepatic angiography than by computed tomography (25).

As part of the CT examination, it is important to look for vascular involvement of either the portal or hepatic veins (Figure 4–9). This can be done with bolus-iodinated

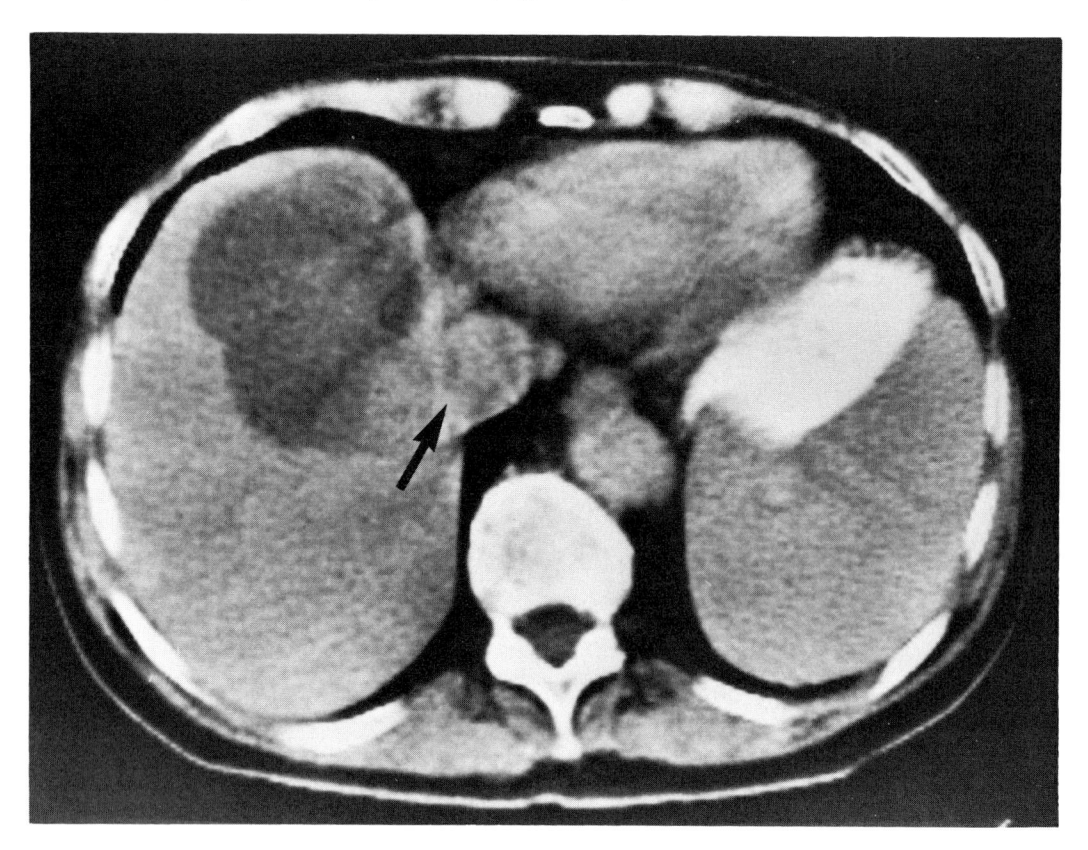

Figure 4–9. Hepatoma invades the hepatic veins and IVC (arrow).

examinations. However, it may be necessary to perform a computed angiotomogram to determine portal or hepatic venous involvement. If the portal vein is obstructed by tumor, the area of low attenuation seen by CT will be larger than the tumor (26). This may be secondary to poor perfusion of the obstructed vascular territories and a lack of glycogen. Glycogen is the molecule that makes up a significant amount of the liver's CT density.

Metastases

Metastatic lesions, like primary hepatic tumors, are detected due to the decrease in tissue density of the lesion with regard to the surrounding normal liver (28) (Figure 4–10). The tumor vascular enhancement pattern (whether by drip infusion, bolus, or a combination of both methods) is not related to the tumor's histologic origin. Many of the metastases develop necrotic areas as they grow (28–30). In such cases, they may have a thin rim of tissue that is less dense than the surrounding liver, and then a central area of low attenuation that is either circular or eccentric. This central area has a density similar to that of water. The central area usually corresponds to an area of necrosis and/or hemmorhage. Some necrotic lesions have mural nodules. The mural nodule is an area of necrotic tissue that protrudes into the central portion of the cystic region. Necrotic lesions may also have fluid-fluid layers. This is due to debris. Fluid-fluid layers may also be noted in patients who have infected cysts or hemorrhagic cysts.

Rarely, a hepatic metastasis may appear entirely cystic on CT (Figure 4–11). In such cases, they may have the density of water with sharp margins that do not enhance

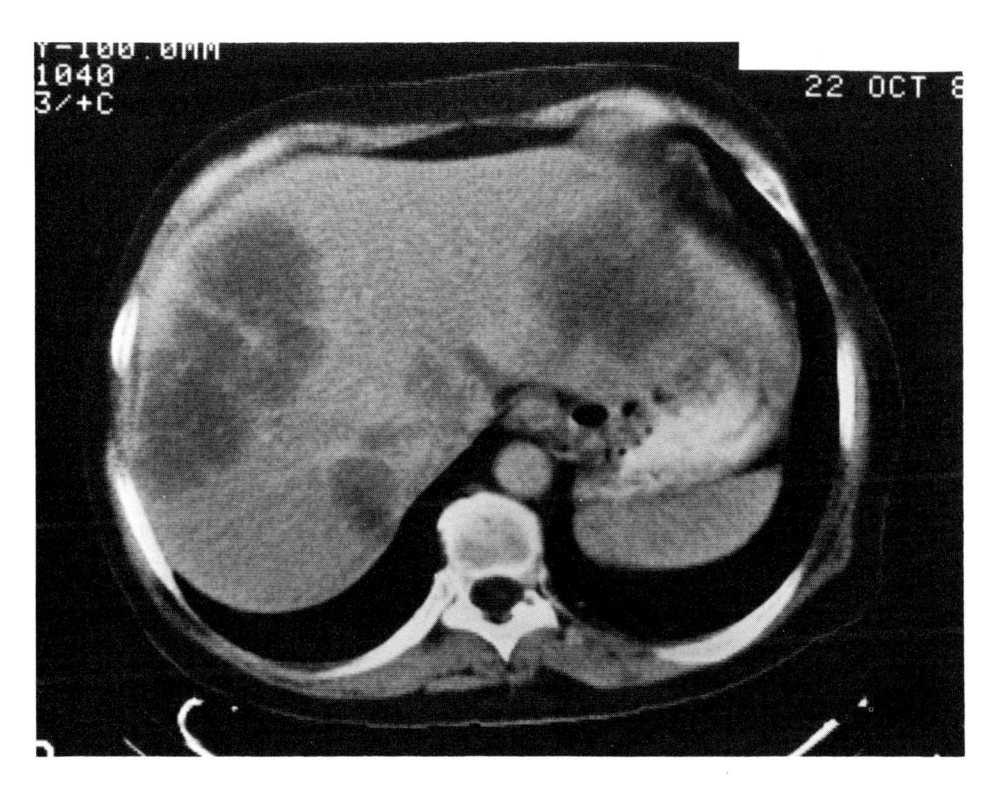

Figure 4–10. Multiple hepatic metastases are noted. They are less dense than the surrounding hepatic parenchyma.

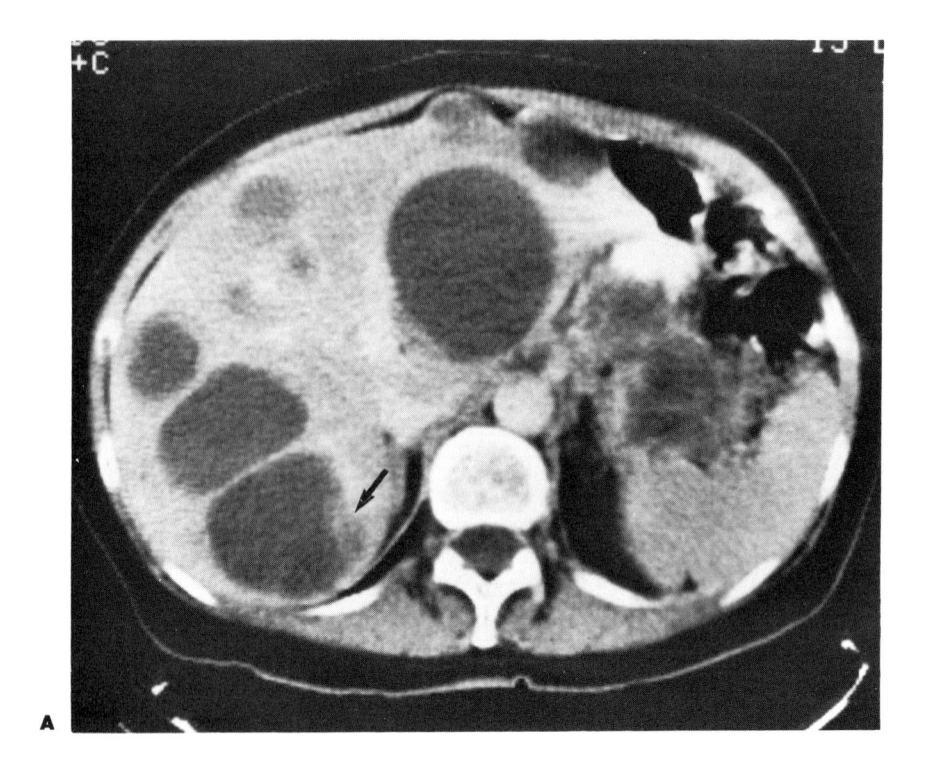

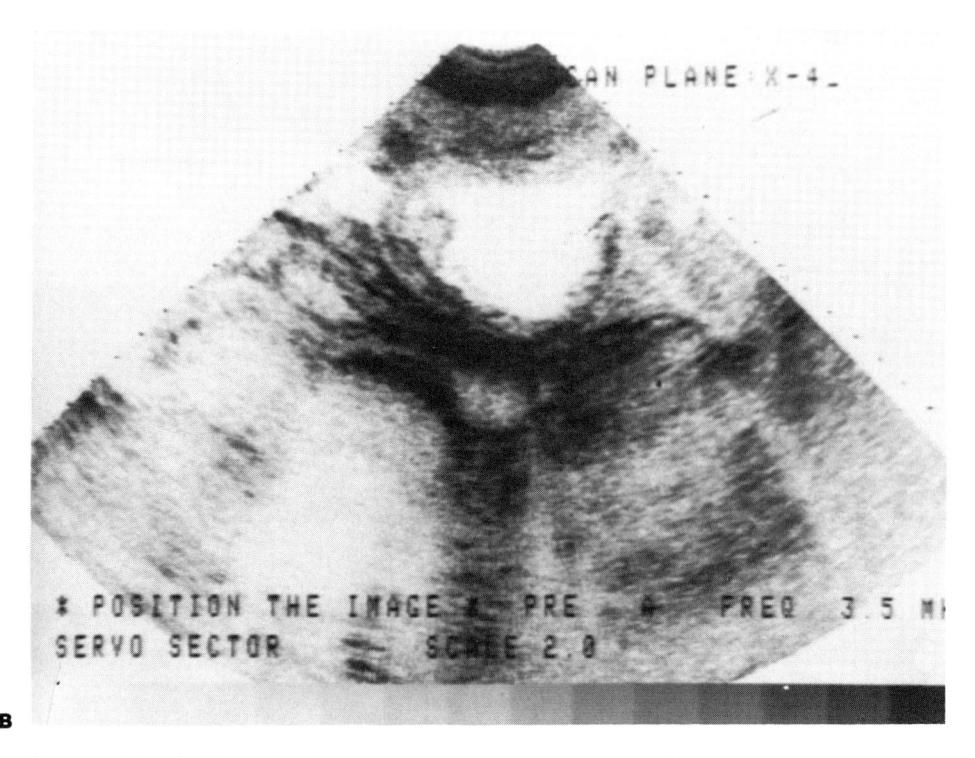

Figure 4–11. *A.* CT section demonstrates cystic-appearing hepatic metastases. At least one has a mural nodule (arrow). *B.* Sonogram from the same patient demonstrates the mural nodules and tumor rind more easily.

(29). No mural nodules are present. Tumors most likely to have this pattern are ovarian carcinomas and some leiomyosarcomas. In cases where there is a high degree of suspicion for metastases, further diagnostic studies are suggested, such as ultrasound (looking for the mural nodule or thickened rind of the tumor) or a more interventional procedure, such as percutaneous needle aspiration and biopsy.

Occasionally, neoplastic deposits may have areas of increased density within the focal masses. These areas of increased density are rarely due to vascular tumor enhancement by intravenous iodine. They are more often noted in patients with hepatoma or metastases from mucinous adenocarcinoma of the colon, upper gastrointestinal tract cancer, or ovarian carcinoma. The areas of increased density usually correspond to calcifications within the tumor (31–32). Most of the calcifications are eccentrically located within the central area of decreased attenuation (Figure 4–12). This calcification is different from benign calcifications, which are usually "fleck-like" single densities without areas of decreased attenuation noted around them (Figure 4–13). Benign calcifications are the result of previous granulomatous disease. Occasionally, calcifications in areas of decreased attenuation are noted in cavernous hemangiomas, which is the main differential diagnosis from malignant calcification.

Metastatic deposits may cause focal obstruction of the biliary tree (33, 34). The obstructed duct is noted distal to a metastatic deposit. This is in contrast to an obstructed duct due to a stone, fibrosis, or sclerosing cholangitis. In the latter conditions, the obstructed duct may end in a calcification, without a low-density metastasis (Figure

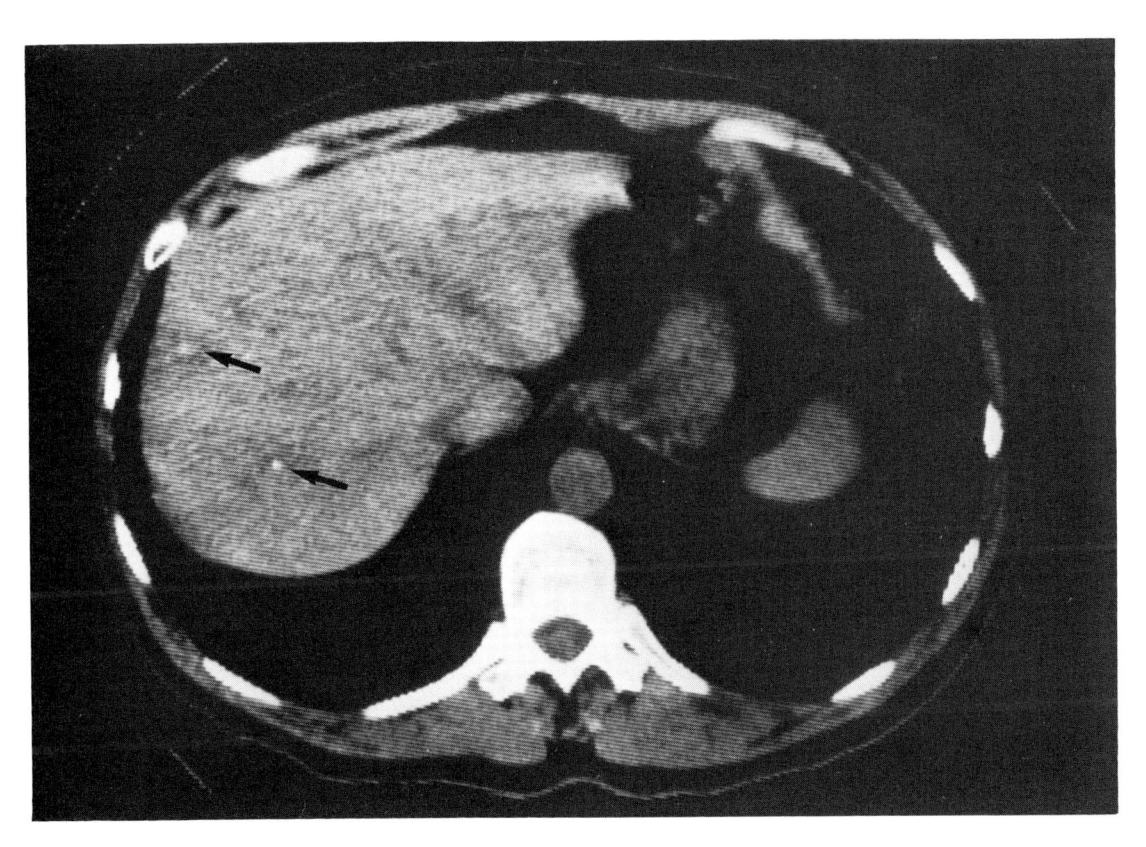

Figure 4-12. Calcified metastases (arrows) from colon carcinoma are seen. The calcifications are noted in areas of decreased density.

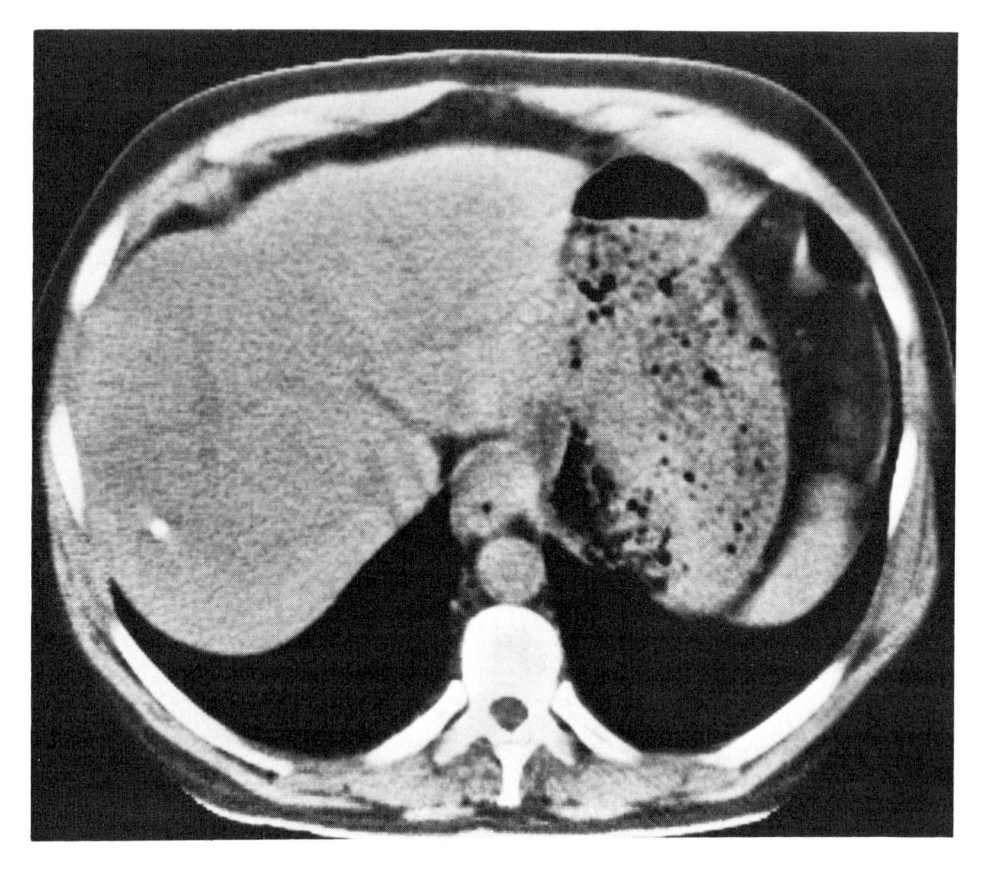

Figure 4–13. A single calcification from benign granulomatous disease is illustrated. It is not surrounded by a low-density metastatic area.

4–14) or have an intermittent beaded appearance. Segmental biliary obstruction is seen more in oncologic patients than has been suspected previously. Usually on initial CT study, the patient is asymptomatic and may have no or minimal elevation of the bilirubin and/or alkaline phosphatase.

Adenoma

The hepatocellular adenoma is seen more frequently in women who have been taking birth control pills. They are prone to hemorrhage and may have some malignant potential. The latter seems to be more a problem in the initial diagnosis of the tumor. Was it really a low-grade malignancy versus a benign adenoma at diagnosis? These lesions may be isodense or slightly less dense than the surrounding liver (35). Occasionally, in those adenomas that have hemorrhaged, there may be cystic areas (Figure 4–15). These cystic areas are usually eccentrically located. After a fresh hemorrhage, the cystic component might have an increased CT density due to the fresh blood. Lesions are isodense usually due to the similar vascularity or tissue cell type when compared to the surrounding normal liver. Also, they may be multifocal within the same liver.

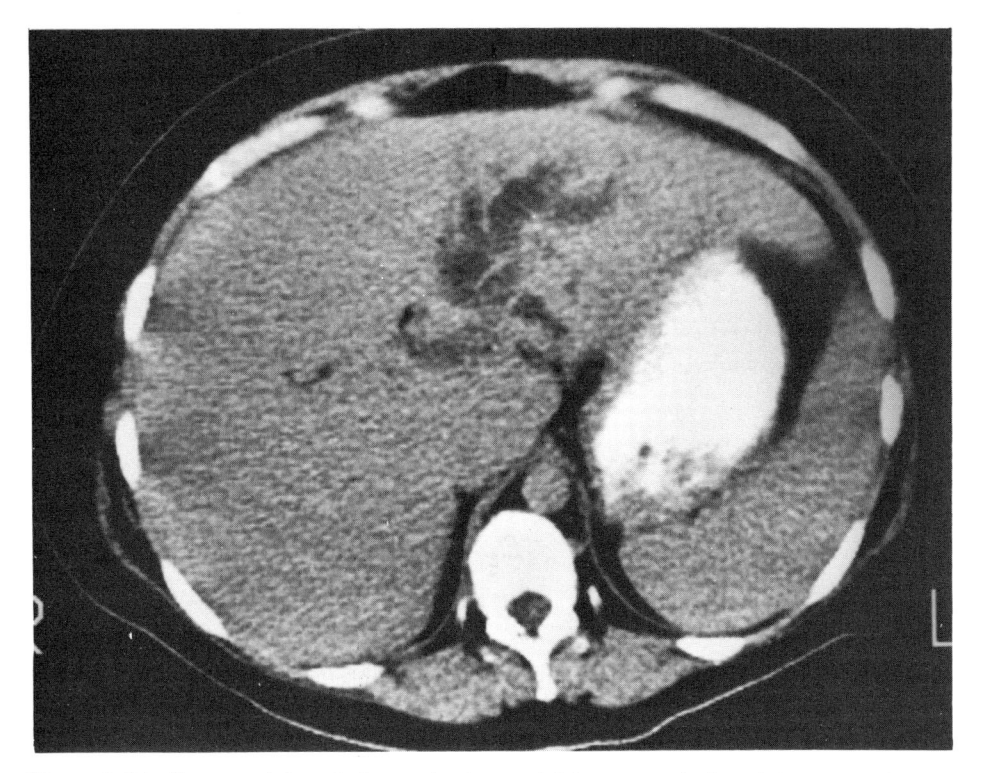

Figure 4-14. Segmental ductal obstruction is noted. No metastatic deposit is seen at the obstruction site. This obstruction was due to a benign stricture.

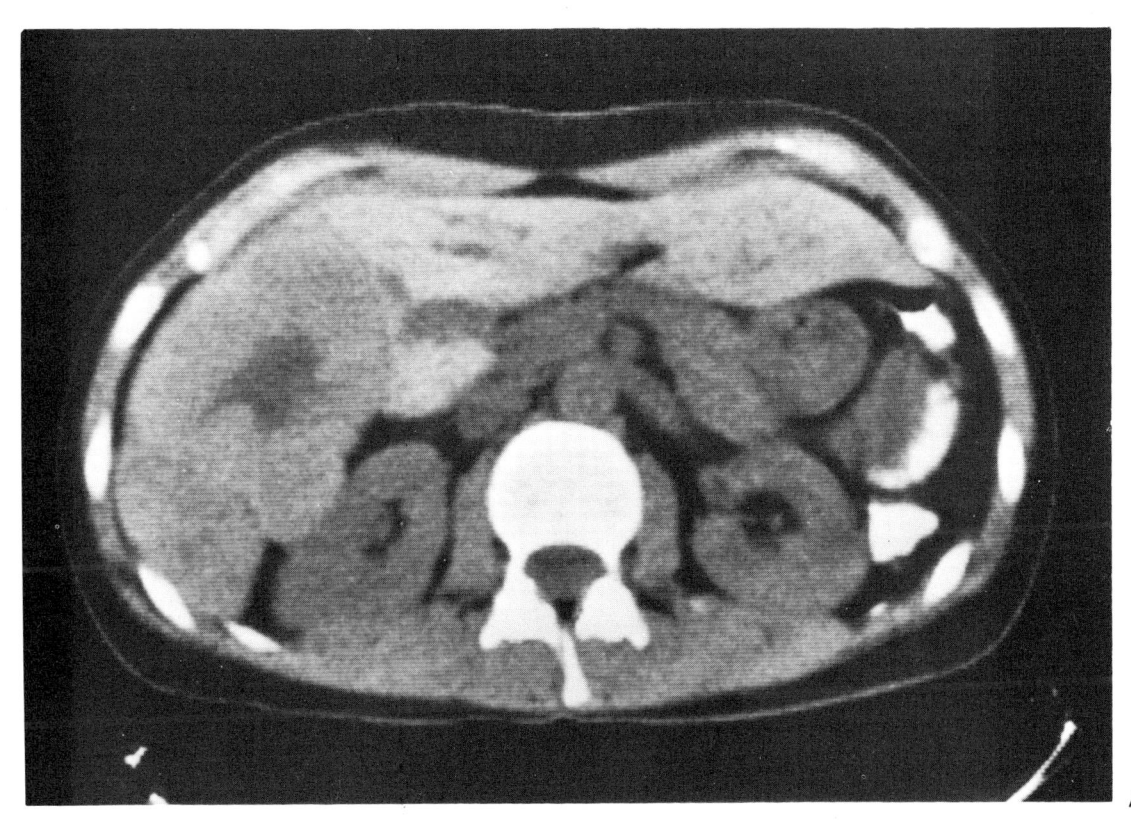

Figure 4-15. *A.* A CT section demonstrates multiple adenomas in the right hepatic lobe. One of these adenomas has a central low density area due to hemorrhage.

125

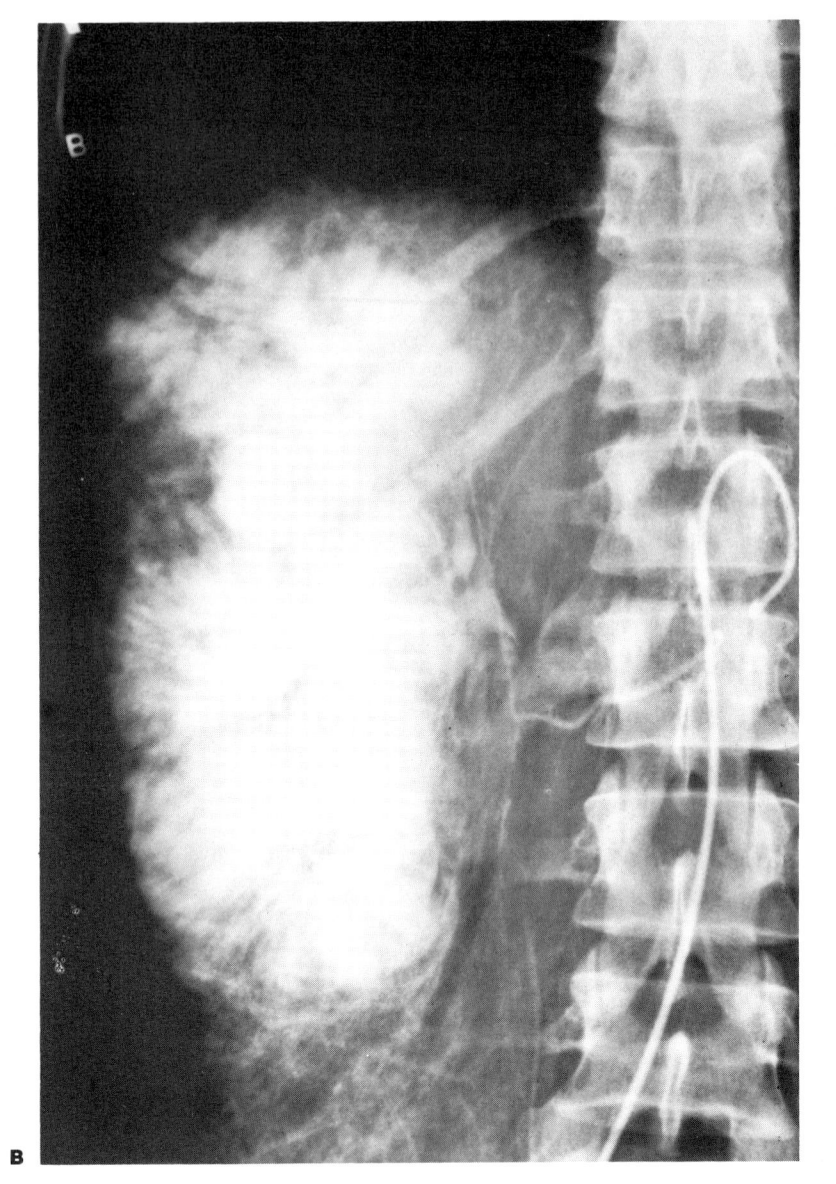

Figure 4-15. *B.* Hepatic angiogram shows the hypervascular nature of the lesions.

Focal Nodular Hyperplasia

Focal nodular hyperplasia is a lesion that has no malignant potential. It rarely hemorrhages and is usually an incidental finding. It may have a variable degree of RE system. Thus, it may have minimal or a great deal of uptake on a radionuclide scan. When detected by CT, it is well-circumscribed and slightly less dense than the surrounding liver. Occasionally, this lesion may be isodense with the liver due to similar tissue density or vascularity (Figure 4-16). Thus rarely it may not be detected. It may have a central scar that is similar to its angiographic appearance (35-37). However, care should be taken not to call a central area of necrosis the central scar. Also, it may be difficult to distinguish focal nodular hyperplasia from other hepatic lesions without knowing the patient's clinical history or without obtaining histology.

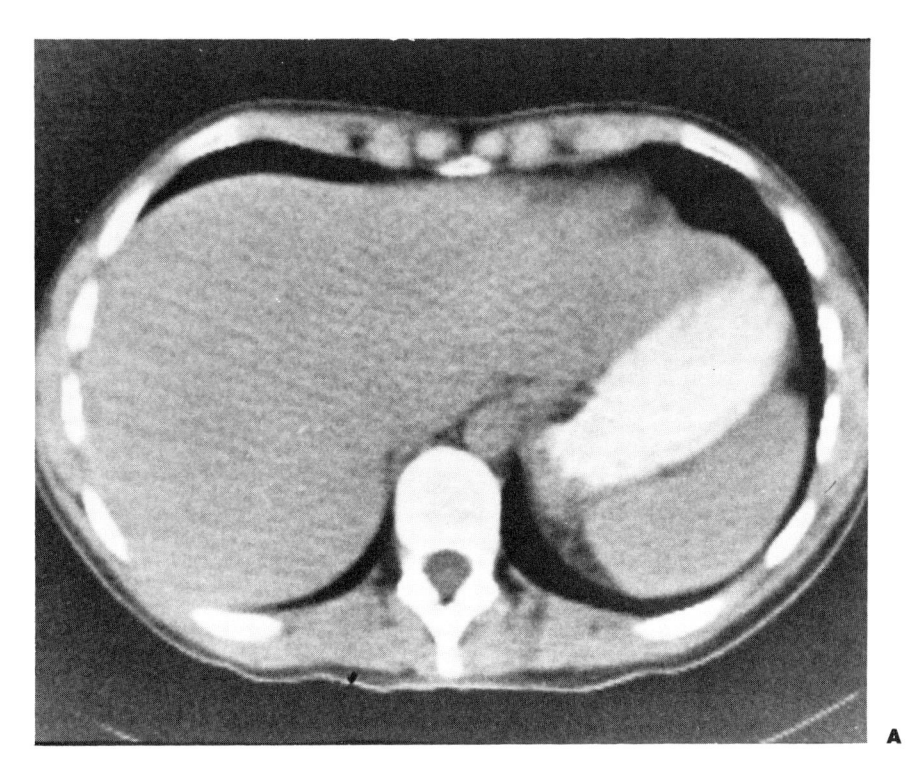

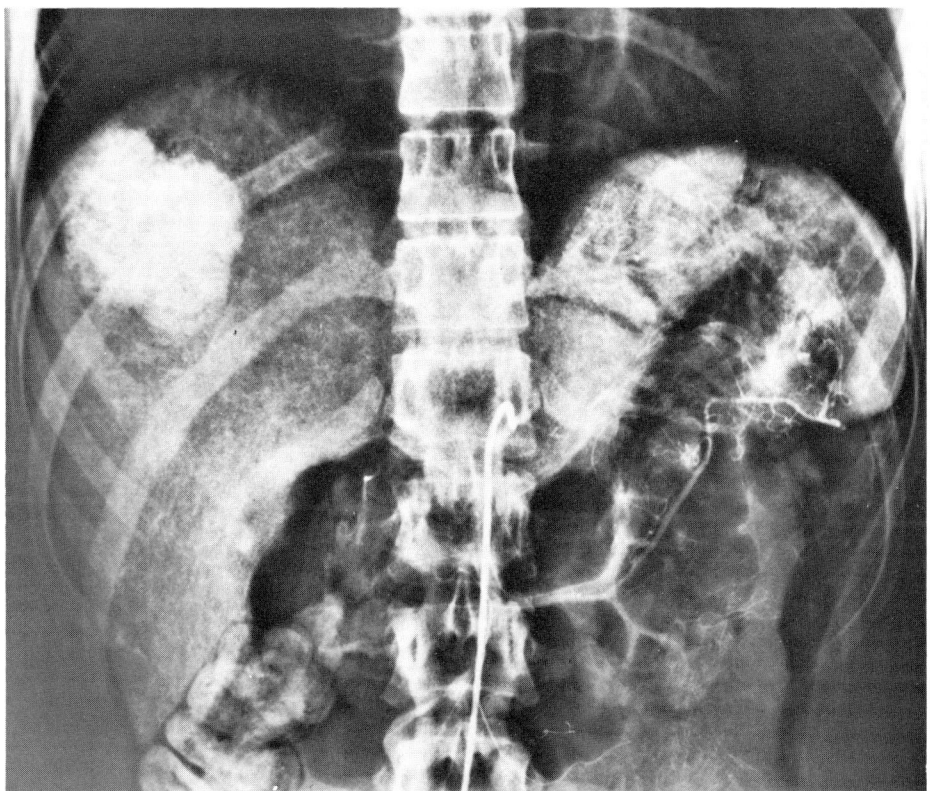

Figure 4–16. *A.* CT scan through the liver shows no abnormality. *B.* Angiogram demonstrates a hypervascular mass due to focal nodular hyperplasia.

Abscess

Abscesses can have a variable appearance (38–41). They may be small, large, focal, or multiple. If they are tiny and punctate, they may be clinically difficult to distinguish from other hepatic lesions. However, the patient's clinical history usually leads the clinician to the correct diagnosis. The larger focal lesions may have a variable appearance (Figures 4–17 and 4–18). The density of an abscess depends upon the evolution of the inflammatory process within the liver. They may be from water density to slightly less dense than the surrounding hepatic parenchyma. Thus, they may mimic cysts, metastases, or focal fatty infiltration. If a bolus-dose-iodinated CT examination or computed angiotomography is performed, the regional blood flow may vary around the abscess. The abscess may not be hypervascular, but may have shunting of blood away from the abscess cavity. The exact reason for this finding is not known. Abscesses may also have debris or more necrotic tissue densities in their most dependent portions. Thus, fluid-fluid layers may be seen (9).

Cysts

Cysts are a very common finding on hepatic CT. They are far more common than was previously believed (42, 43). In autopsy series, 2 to 7 percent of the population have

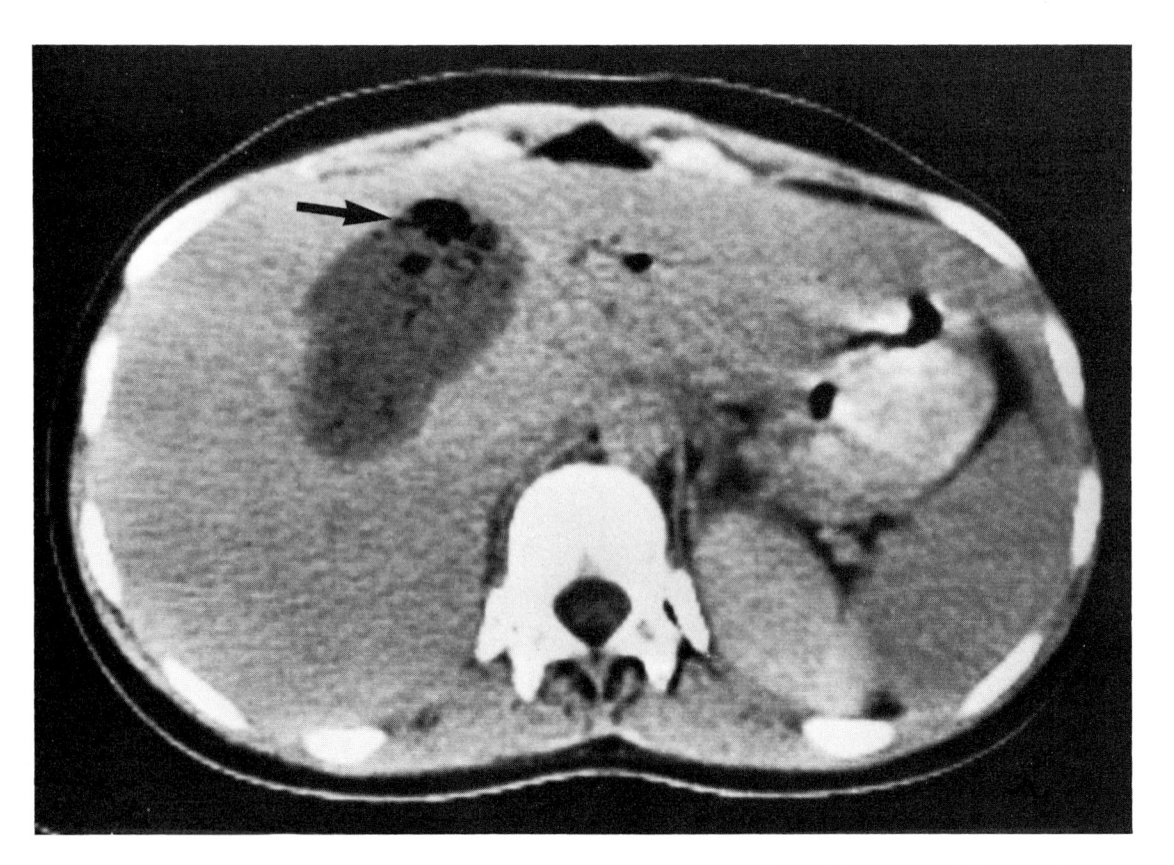

Figure 4–17. CT scan demonstrates a hepatic abscess. Part of the abscess is low density while gas bubbles (arrow) are also noted.

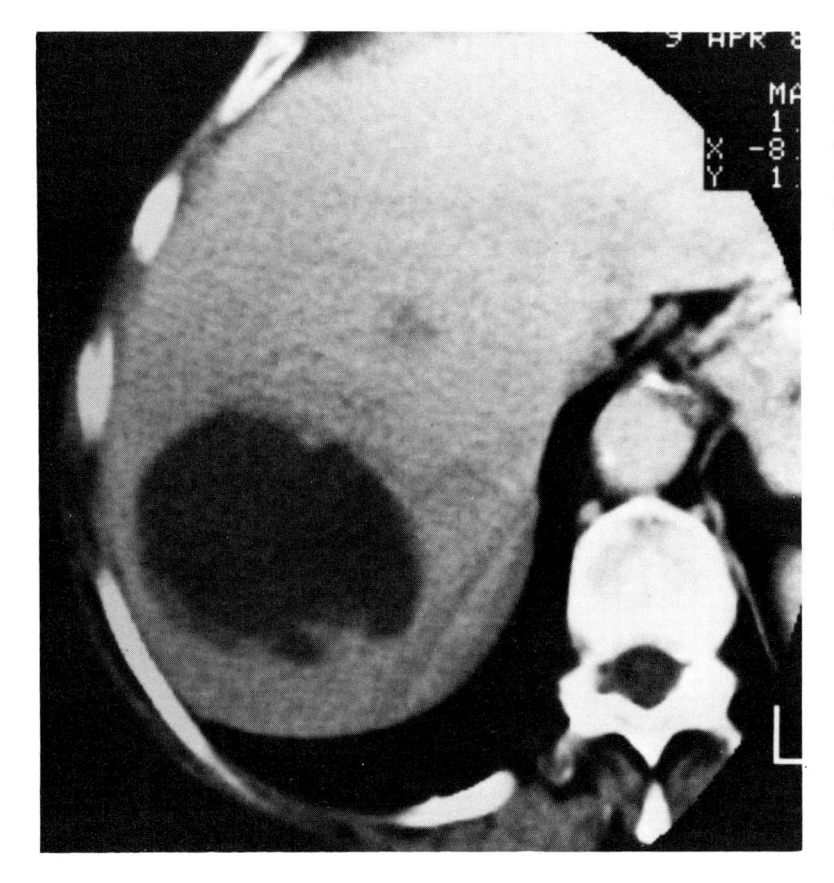

Figure 4-18. This amebic abscess mimics an irregular cyst. It has a density similar to water, but was filled with "paste-like" material.

hepatic cysts. These cysts may vary in size from less than 1 cm to greater than 5 cm. They are usually well-circumscribed without enhancing margins. They have homogeneous densities that are roughly 0 ± 15 Hounsfield units (Hu, water density) (Figure 4-19). Occasionally, cysts can hemorrhage or have debris within them (44). In such cases, they may have fluid-fluid levels present. Some cysts have slight irregularities of the wall due to septations. The routine cyst is usually very easy to distinguish from unusual types of cysts such as echinococcal, in which the daughter cysts lie within the mother cyst in a spoke-wheel, multiseptated pattern (45). Also in an echinococcal cyst, the periphery of a single cyst may be calcified.

In a review of 1,000 consecutive CT scans of the abdomen, we detected 68 patients who had at least one focal lesion less than 1.5 cm in size. The majority of these small lesions were cysts. In nononcologic patients, no single small focal hepatic lesion was due to cancer. In greater than 40 percent of the patients with cancer, the newly found multiple lesions (at least one < 1.5 cm) were cysts. Thus, the incidence of hepatic cysts detected by CT is greater than reported in the pathology literature. This is due to the increased sensitivity of computed tomography in detecting small hepatic masses. It is also important to note that in cancer patients, the newly found small focal masses may be cysts and not metastases. Thus, a more invasive procedure (i. e., needle biopsy) may be necessary before the patient is properly staged (46). If the patient has metastatic disease elsewhere in the abdomen or chest, the etiology of the focal hepatic mass(es) is probably not needed.

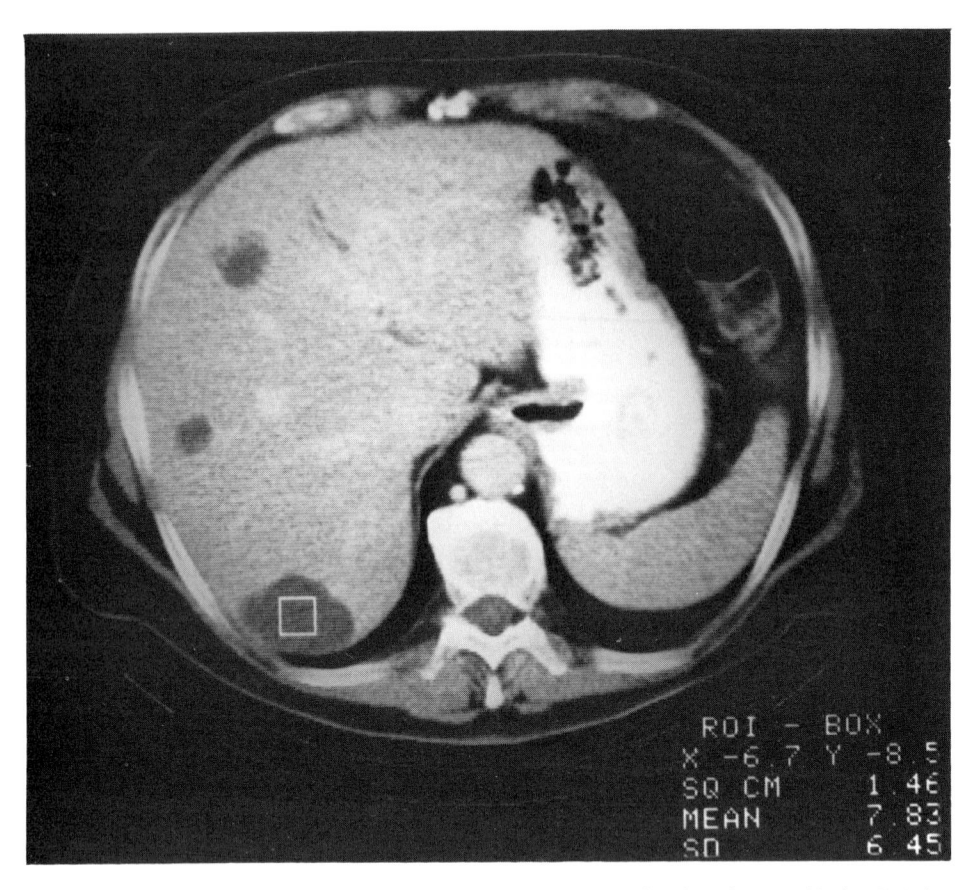

Figure 4-19. Multiple hepatic cysts are noted. They have the density of water (0 ± 15 Hu).

Hemangioma

Hemangiomas are noted in up to 9 percent of the population. Most hemangiomas are located in the right hepatic lobe and are subcapsular. They are seen far more often in females than in males. They can hemorrhage. Their CT appearance may be that of small focal low-density areas that could mimic cysts or metastases. They may be large, lobulated lesions with central areas of decreased attenuation. The central low-density areas may measure close to water density. Occasionally, hemangiomas may have calcifications within them.

Much has been written in the literature about the characteristic appearance of a hemangioma after a bolus of intravenous contrast. The typical appearance after a bolus injection of iodine is that of a lesion that has eccentric peripheral enhancement. This enhancement slowly migrates toward the center of the lesion (Figure 4-20). The lesion may become isodense over a long period of time or may remain hyperdense as on an angiogram (47-52). However, it should be noted that at least 15 percent of hemangiomas will not show this characteristic pattern. The characteristic pattern is usually seen in the larger lesions, but may not be seen in the smaller lesions less than 2 cm in size. In such cases, a definitive diagnosis of hemangioma cannot be made by CT alone, and reliance on other diagnostic modalities such as ultrasound or angiography may be necessary.

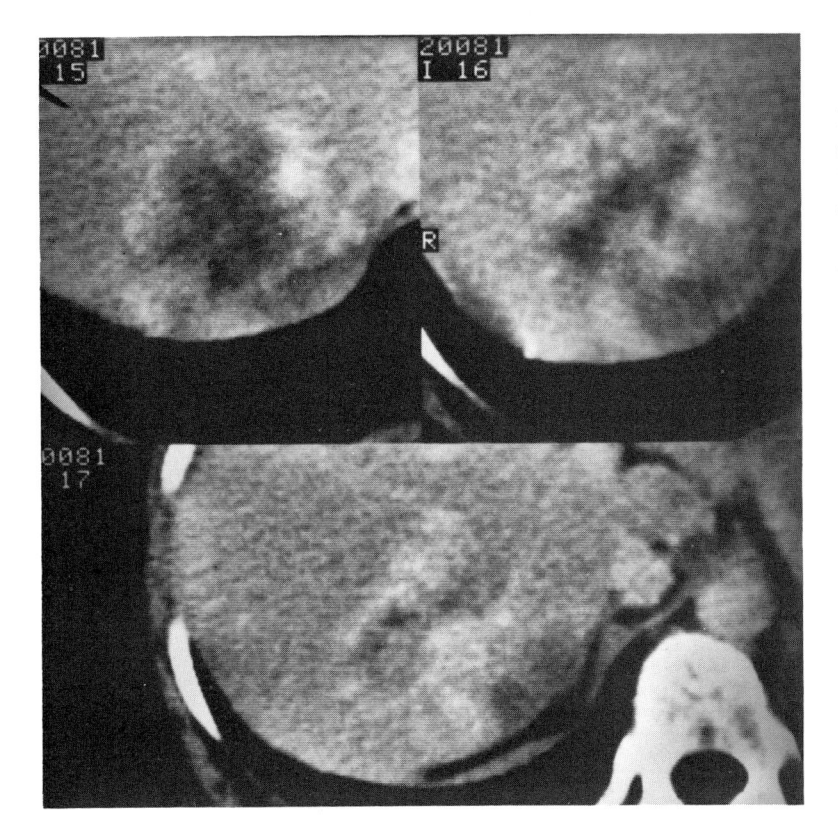

Figure 4-20. Multiple CT sections through a hemangioma demonstrate a density-enhancing lesion after intravenous contrast. The enhancement slowly migrates toward the center of the mass.

DIFFUSE LIVER DISEASE

Fatty Infiltration of the Liver

Fatty infiltration of the liver is due to the increased deposition of triglycerides within the liver. This is usually seen in chronic alcoholism, hyperalimentation, Cushing's disease, iatrogenic corticosteroids, diabetes, Reye's syndrome, protein deprivation, after ileojejunal bypass, and morbid obesity. It is noted by CT when the density of the liver decreases from normal. Usually, the liver is about 8 ± 4 Hounsfield units greater than the spleen in density (53). Thus, if the liver decreases in density, the difference between it and the spleen becomes less. In many instances, the liver is significantly less dense than the spleen. One can actually calculate the number of milligrams of fat per gram of liver by knowing the density of the spleen and the density of the liver. If a liver measures 25 and a spleen measures 30, the liver should normally measure 38. Thus, the difference between 38 and 25 is 13 Hounsfield units. This number is then multiplied by 1.6 (1.6 = the change in Hounsfield units per milligram of triglyceride deposited within a gram of liver) to obtain the number of milligrams of fat per gram of liver (54). This quantitation is relatively useful estimation for indicating the degree of severity of the underlying liver process. It can be followed to determine whether the liver has worsened or improved after the institution of therapy.

Diffuse fatty infiltration is detected by CT when the liver has decreased density attenuation throughout (Figure 4-21). The vascular structures, such as the hepatic veins, portal veins, and inferior vena cava, "stand out" against the low-density hepatic background. The liver is usually not abnormally shaped. Occasionally in alcoholics or

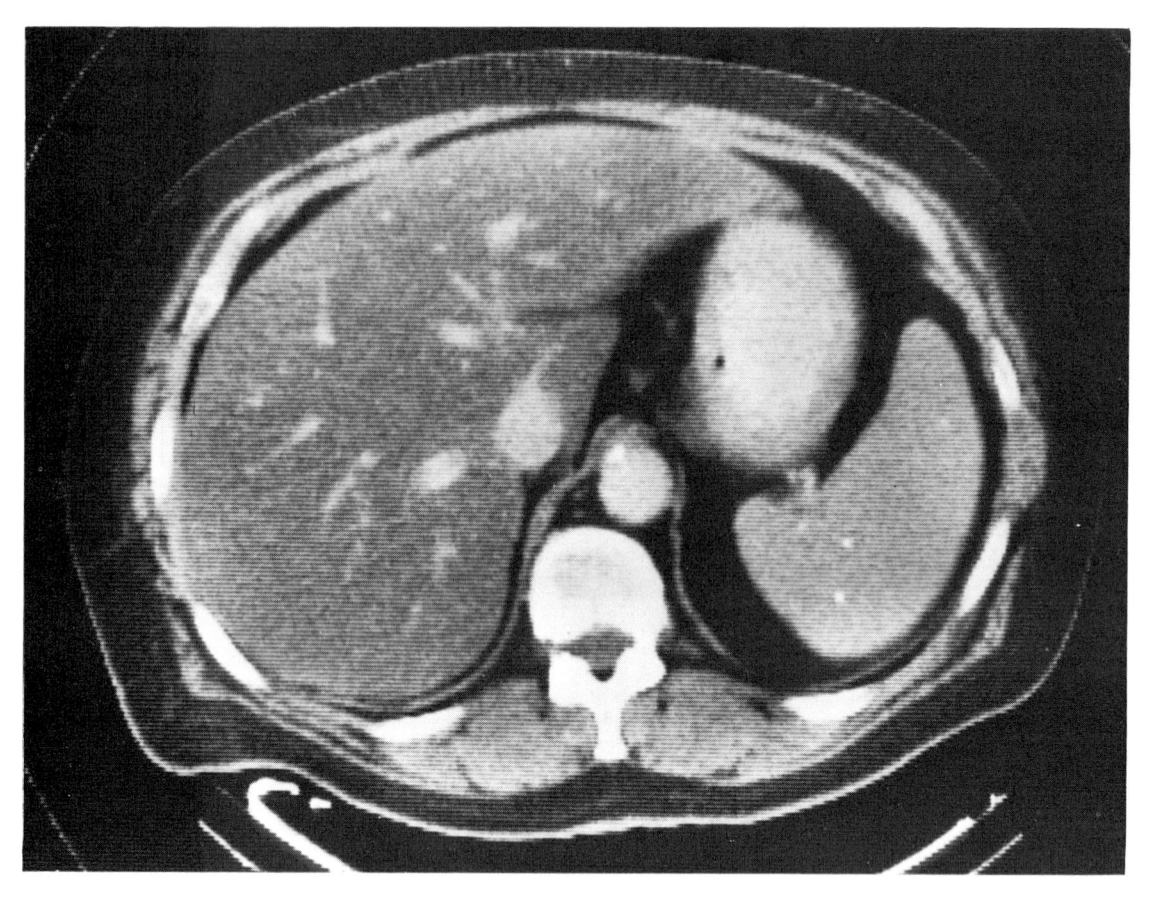

Figure 4-21. Diffuse fatty infiltration shows a liver that is less dense than the spleen. Note how well the hepatic vessels are detected due to the decreased hepatic density.

diabetics, there may be focal areas of decreased attenuation within the liver that may be difficult to distinguish from metastatic deposits (54–57) (Figure 4-22). A detailed clinical history is beneficial in such cases. However, a xenon[133] scan or a CT-directed biopsy of the questionable area for definite histologic analysis may be needed. Xenon[133], when inhaled, is deposited in fat. If the xenon[133] scan matches the CT defect, then focal fatty infiltration is the cause (58).

In patients with diffuse hepatic fatty infiltration, the possibility of detecting metastatic disease by computed tomography may be difficult (14). Also, detection of the true extent of metastatic disease by computed tomography is hampered. This is because the liver is lower in density than normal. Its density approaches density of the metastasis. Thus, metastatic deposits blend imperceptibly into the surrounding fatty liver. In order to obtain the proper diagnosis in such cases, it may be necessary to proceed to a more invasive procedure, such as selective angiography or computed angiotomography.

Hemosiderosis

Hemosiderosis has just the opposite CT appearance from triglyceride deposition within the liver. In this disease, iron is either stored in the recticuloendothelial system of the liver and spleen or in the hepatocytes (Figure 4-23). This may be a primary or

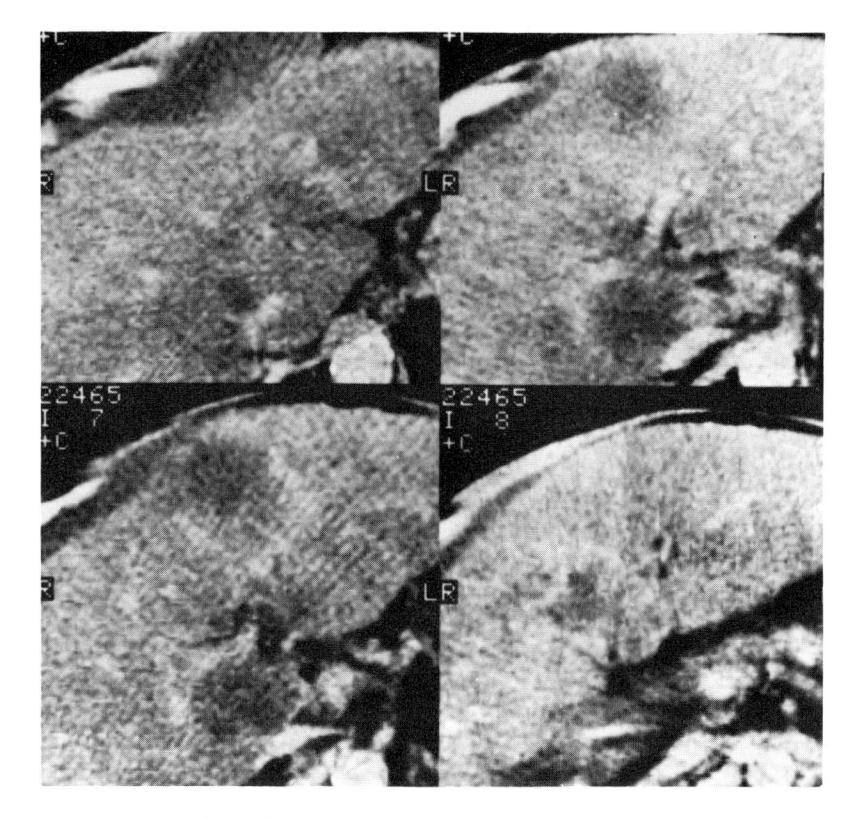

Figure 4-22. Multiple focal defects due to focal fatty infiltration are noted. They could be mistaken for other hepatic lesions, such as metastases.

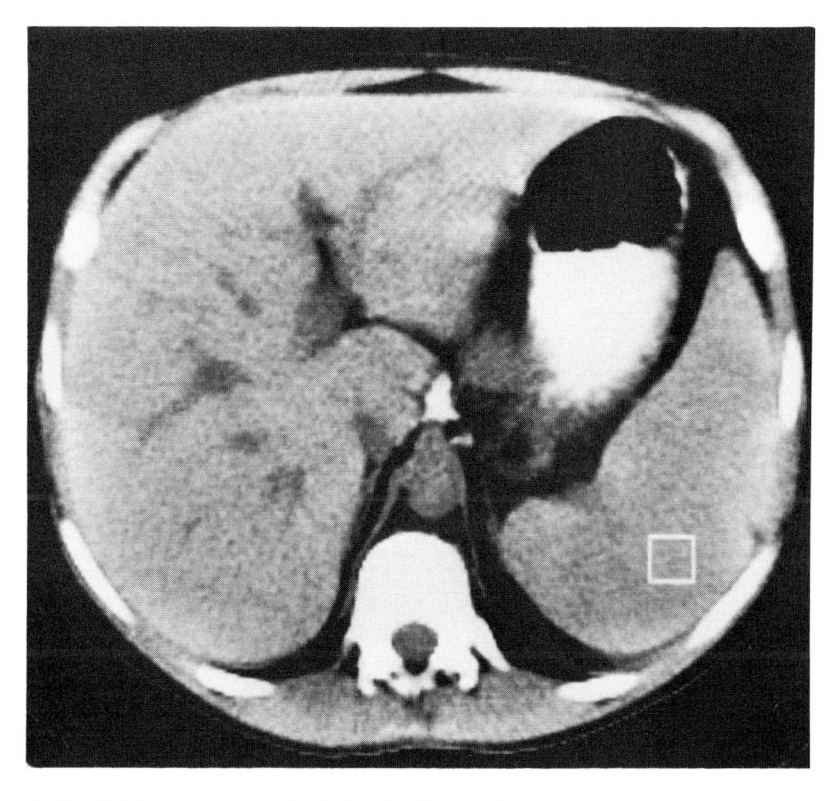

Figure 4-23. CT demonstrates a high-density liver and spleen due to iron deposition. Note that the hepatic vessels are visualized easily.

secondary disease. When secondary, it is usually due to multiple blood transfusions. The latter is seen in patients with blood dyscrasias or in chronic bleeders such as cirrhotics. In this particular disease, the liver density increases significantly over normal (59–61). If no contrast is used, the intrahepatic vessels "stand out" against the increased background density of the liver. They appear as lucent areas within the liver, which has an almost white appearance. It is possible to quantitate the amount of iron deposited with dual energy scanning. In dual energy scanning, a single slice of the liver may be scanned at a low kilovolt (kV) such as 80 to 90, and a high kV, such as 120 (62). By determining the density differences at the different kV levels, it is possible to determine the number of milligrams of iron per gram of liver. The determination is gross and has an accuracy of roughly 10 ± 5 percent.

Wilson's Disease—Biliary Cirrhosis

Little has been written about the use of CT in Wilson's disease (63,64). In patients with biliary cirrhosis, there is increased intrahepatic copper deposition. However, the amount of copper deposited usually causes no change in hepatic density measurements. Thus, CT is of little use in determining the amount of copper deposited in the liver in patients with biliary cirrhosis.

Glycogen Storage Disease

In glycogen storage disease, the liver may have a dense appearance since glycogen is one of the dense substances in the liver detected by computed tomography. However, it may also have a diffuse fatty-infiltrated appearance. The liver itself may take on an enlarged bulbous appearance and the kidneys may be involved. A key in examining a liver with glycogen storage disease is to search carefully for liver tumors, since this particular entity is associated with an increased incidence of liver tumors such as adenomas (65). Some of these tumors may be malignant.

Lymphoma

Although lymphoma involves the liver and spleen, it is rarely detected by CT. In one study performed with a second-generation scanner and using the drip infusion method of intravenous iodine administration, CT detected hepatic disease in only 50 percent of the patients (66). The reason for the poor detectability is that lymphoma is usually a microscopic process, with diffuse hepatic involvement of the liver rather than a focal mass. It is hypovascular and of similar tissue density to the surrounding liver (even when focal). Thus, unless hepatic-specific contrast agents or computed angiotomography are performed, its detection by CT will probably remain low in the future.

Radiation

CT can detect changes in the liver due to radiation. These changes usually take place within weeks of the radiation exposure and correspond to the therapy ports (67). The irradiated liver has low density due to fatty change from hepatic injury. The demarcation of damaged from normal tissue is sharp and linear. If the liver is scanned 1 year to 18 months later, there may be total or partial resolution of the process.

Cirrhosis

Cirrhotic livers may demonstrate areas of focal fatty infiltration, regional fatty infiltration, or diffuse areas of decreased beam attenuation (68). In late stage disease, the outer margins of the liver become quite lobulated, and nodular regeneration may be noted (Figure 4–24). The right lobe of the liver may shrink dramatically and thus the gallbladder will rotate posteriorly, assuming an extremely lateral position. The medial segment of the left lobe of the liver does not usually hypertrophy. The lateral segment of the left lobe of the liver may show a bulging appearance and gross hypertrophy. Also, the caudate lobe may hypertrophy in 50 percent of the cases. With the shrinkage of the liver lobes, the fissures between the lobes take on a relative increased size. Ascites may be noted. The portal vein may be quite prominent and the spleen enlarged (Figure 4–25). If boluses of intravenous iodine are used, varices may be noted. The most common varices detected by CT are the coronary vein, retrogastric varices, parasplenic varices, and the umbilical vein.

SENSITIVITY, ROLES, AND FUTURE DEVELOPMENTS

Sensitivity

Most previous studies comparing computed tomography to other diagnostic imaging modalities, such as ultrasound or radionuclide imaging, show that computed tomogra-

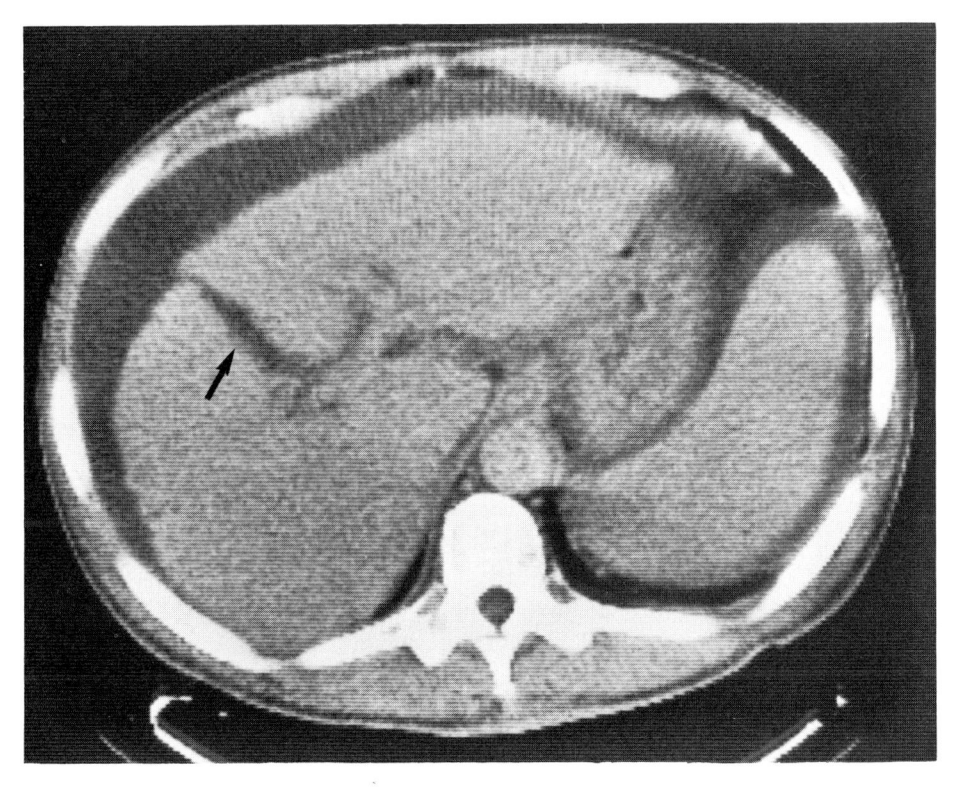

Figure 4–24. In cirrhotic livers, the lateral segment of the left lobe enlarges. Ascites is noted. Also, the fissure (arrow) between the right and left lobe appears larger due to shrinkage of the right lobe.

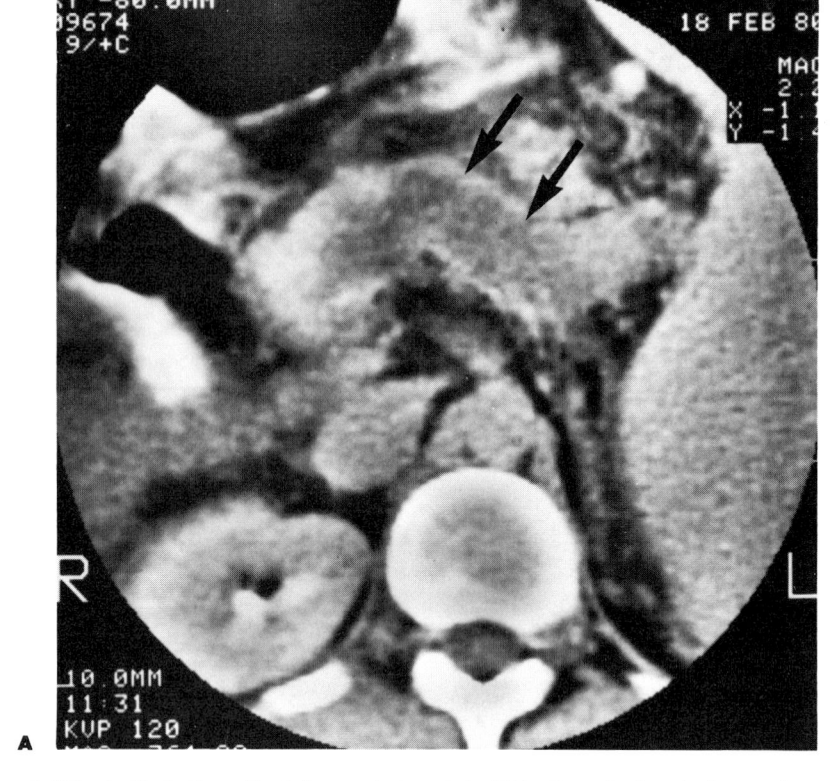

Figure 4–25. *A.* Cirrhotic patient demonstrates clot within the splenic vein (arrows).

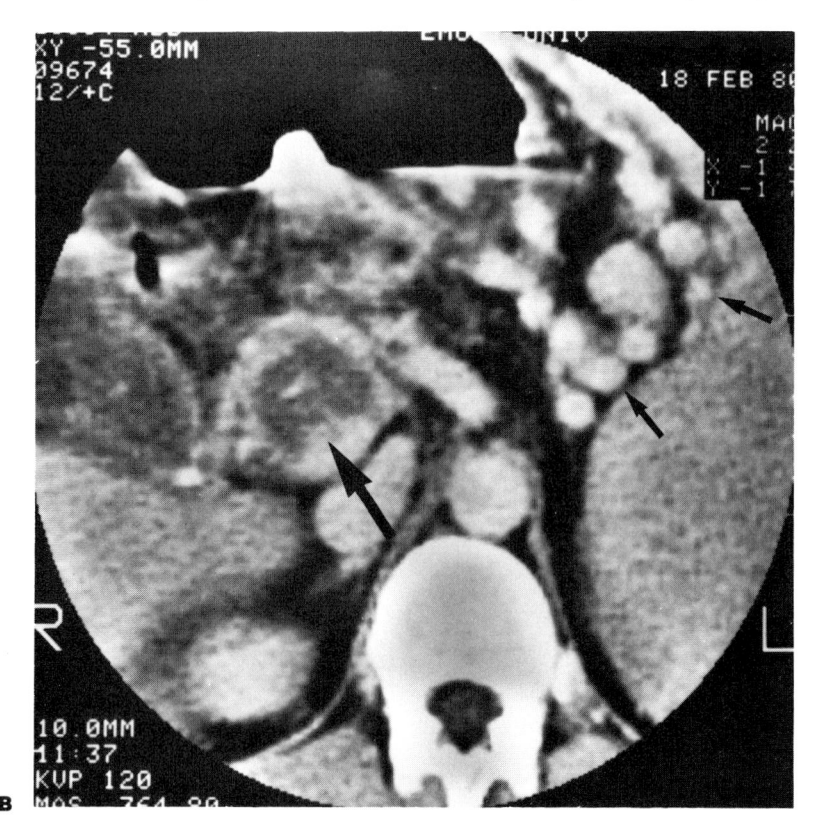

Figure 4–25. *B.* The clot extends into the proximal portal vein (large arrow). Also noted are splenic and gastric varices (small arrows).

phy is more accurate than the other conventional imaging techniques at detecting focal lesions of 1 cm or greater in size (2, 69–73). Many of these studies were done on early generation CT scanners or were comparing poor quality radionuclide imaging and/or ultrasound. None of the studies compared state of the art equipment in all three modalities. However, it is my feeling that computed tomography is the most accurate way to image a focal liver lesion noninvasively. It is possible to have a true negative radionuclide liver scan and still have disease in the adrenal glands or retroperitoneum. These are areas that are covered routinely during a hepatic CT study. The advantage of CT cross-sectional imaging over other invasive and noninvasive diagnostic techniques is that many other areas of the abdomen are imaged as well as the liver. It is my opinion that the liver should be evaluated by computed tomography as a screening procedure. However, CT is not infallible, and there are many instances when lesions are either masked or only a single lesion is detected when multiple masses are present. Thus, in the oncologic patient or the patient who is a possible surgical (partial hepatectomy) candidate, more invasive techniques such as angiography or computed angiotomography may be needed to determine the true extent of hepatic disease. In addition to its diagnostic role, CT has a role in monitoring therapy, especially in patients who are receiving chemotherapy or radiation. Its role in interventional procedures will be discussed in another chapter.

LIVER-SPLEEN VOLUMES

Henderson *et al.* have demonstrated the usefulness and reliability of calculating the total volume of the liver by CT (74). In this process, CT sections are obtained through the entire liver and spleen. The organ area of each section is then outlined and the square centimeters calculated by the CT computer. The number is then multiplied by the slice thickness for a slice volume (75). Then all the slice volumes are added together for a total organ volume.

Calculations of liver volumes have their greatest advantage in monitoring the course of cirrhotic patients (preshunt and postshunt procedure). Variations of this technique can be applied to monitoring the response of hepatic neoplasms to therapy.

FUTURE DEVELOPMENTS

One of the greatest areas of controversy in hepatic CT is the area of intravenous contrast administration. Radiologists worry about masking lesions with contrast and not seeing lesions well enough without intravenous contrast. Thus, agents will be developed along the lines of EOE-13. This is a hepatic specific contrast agent developed by Vermess that is phagocytized by the reticuloendothelial system and raises the inherent density of a normal liver from 40 to 60 Hounsfield units, depending upon the dose. It also raises the density of the spleen (76–79). Most tumors do not have a reticuloendothelial system and thus appear as negative defects on the CT scan. The material's greatest asset is that it is rapidly excreted with few side-effects and targets roughly 5 grams of iodine to the liver. This is in contrast to the usual intravenous dose of iodine that may be from 40 to 60 grams and is untargeted. In CT studies using EOE-13, more hepatic lesions have been seen than were noted on the pre-EOE-13 study (Figure 4-26). One study demonstrated an increase in hepatic mass detection of greater than 37 percent, with the predominant increase in lesions that were less than 3 cm in size (80). However, the increased sensitivity of this material, or similar materials that might be developed, must be balanced against the decrease in specificity. Not all the new lesions detected are malignant (Figures 4–27 and 4–28). Many of the new lesions detected may be small cysts and/or hemangiomas. Others may be benign lesions, such as focal nodular hyperplasia or liver cell adenomas.

Other materials being developed similar to EOE-13 that hold a great deal of promise are liposomes, iodinated starch, and other iodinated emulsions (81–84). Heavy metals that significantly increase the hepatic CT density are not prime candidates for future development because they remain in the liver and are not excreted. Their long-term biologic side-effects are not known.

In a diffuse-liver disease patient, dual energy scanning may hold future benefits. This will depend upon machine standardization and an increase in the reliability of the density measurements. Under such conditions, better quantitation of the amount of fat and/or iron or other heavy metals within the liver may provide a quick and easy basis to follow therapy without resorting to a more invasive procedure, such as a liver biopsy.

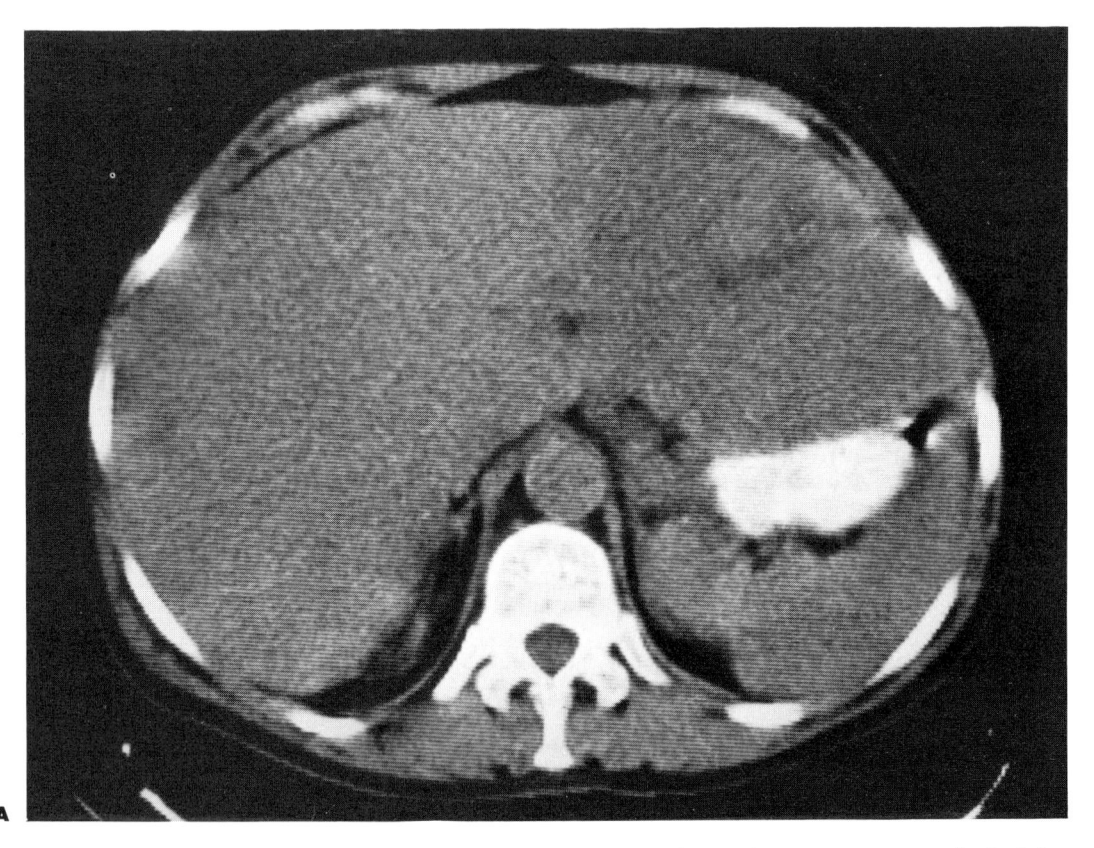

Figure 4–26. *A.* CT study in a patient with colon carcinoma demonstrates a mass in the left hepatic lobe.

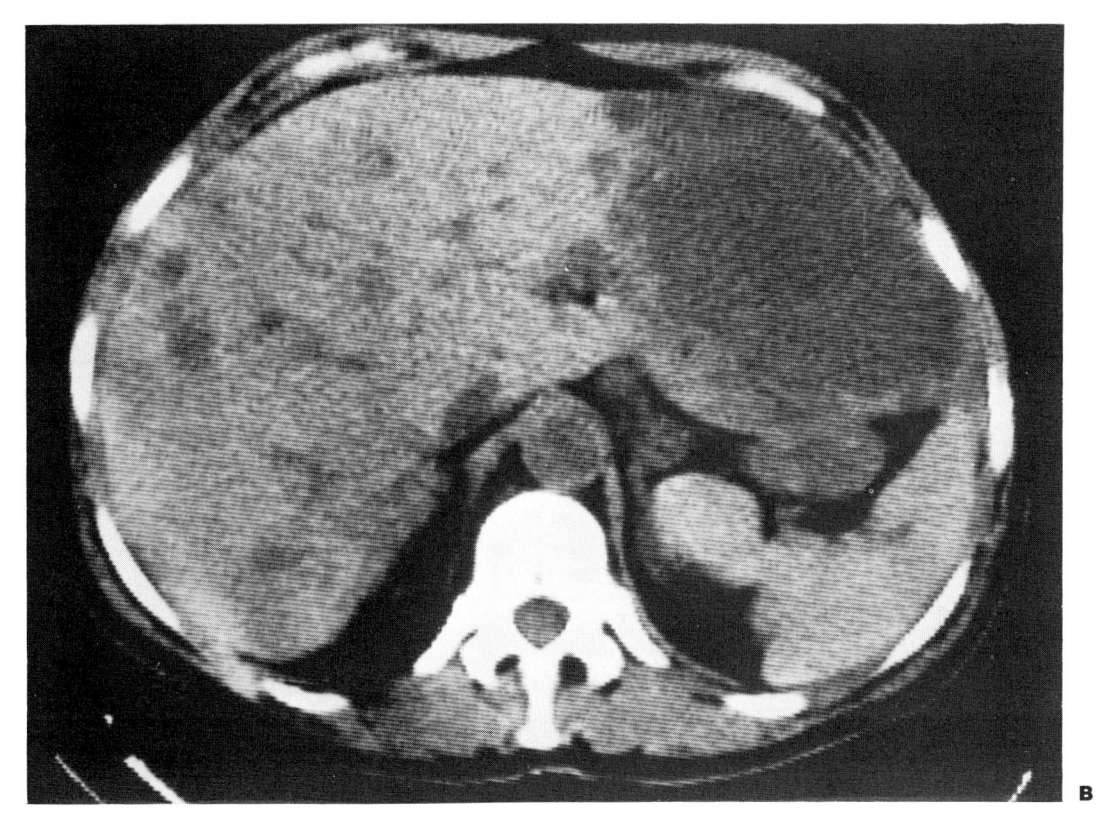

Figure 4-26. *B.* After EOE-13, many lesions less than 3 cm are noted in the right hepatic lobe. Both images were taken at the same window width and level.

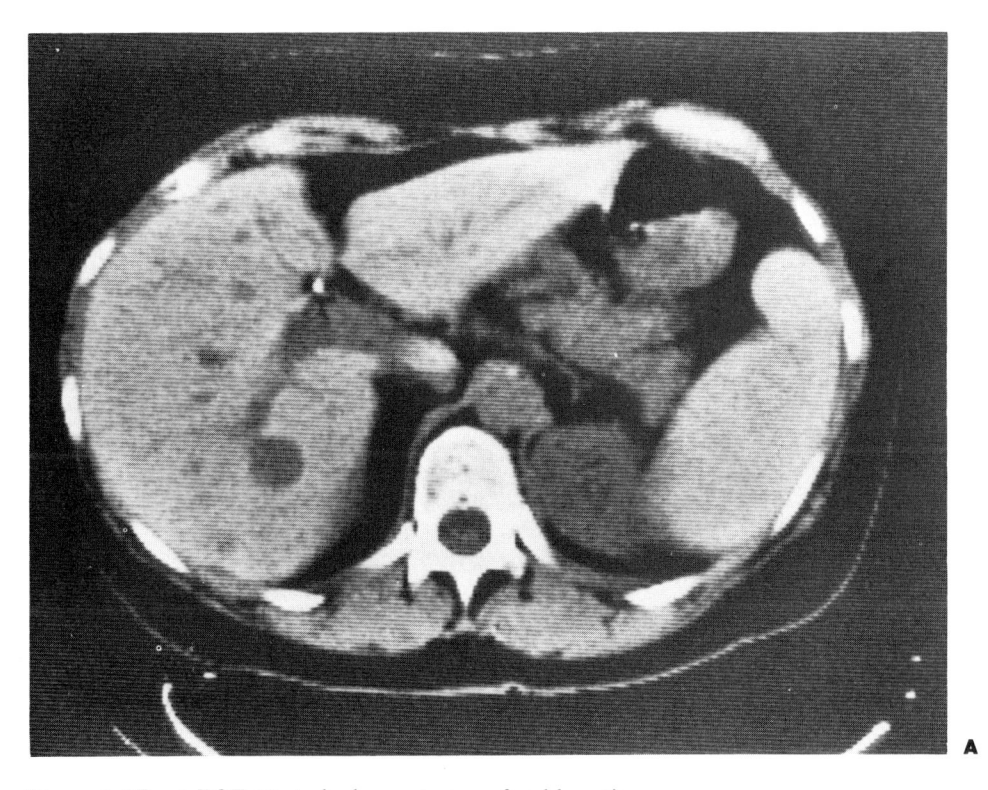

Figure 4-27. *A.* EOE-13 study demonstrates a focal hepatic mass.

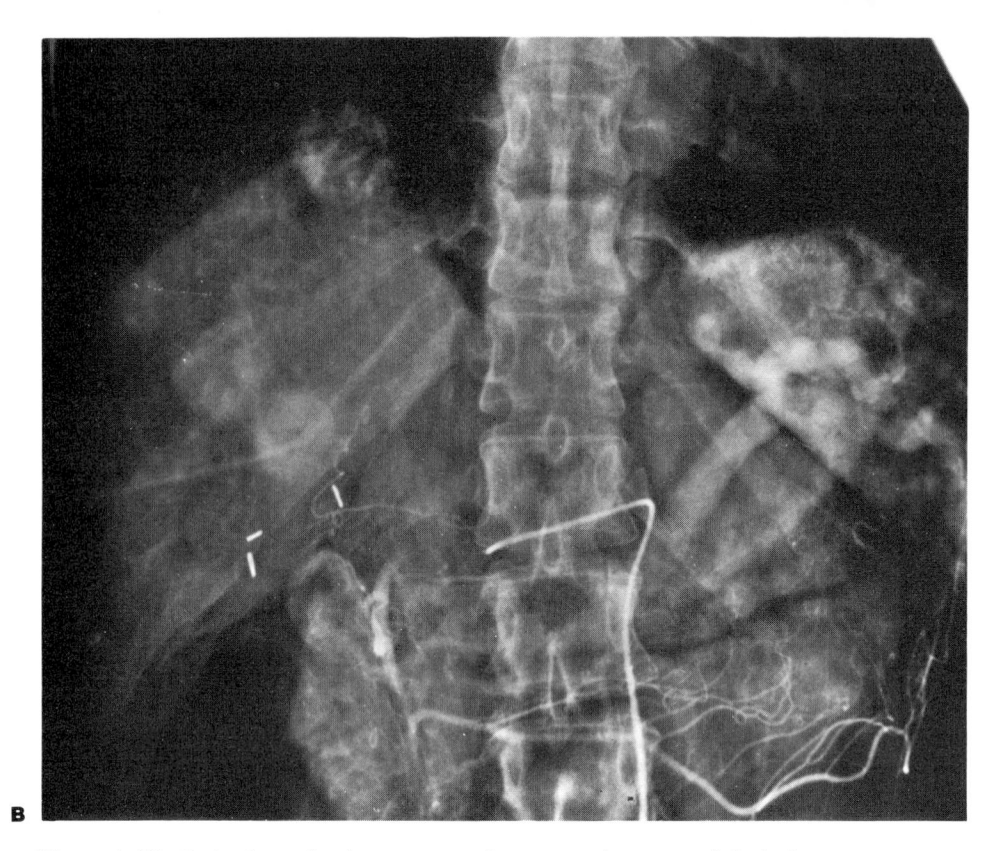

Figure 4–27. *B*. Angiography demonstrates the metastatic nature of the lesion.

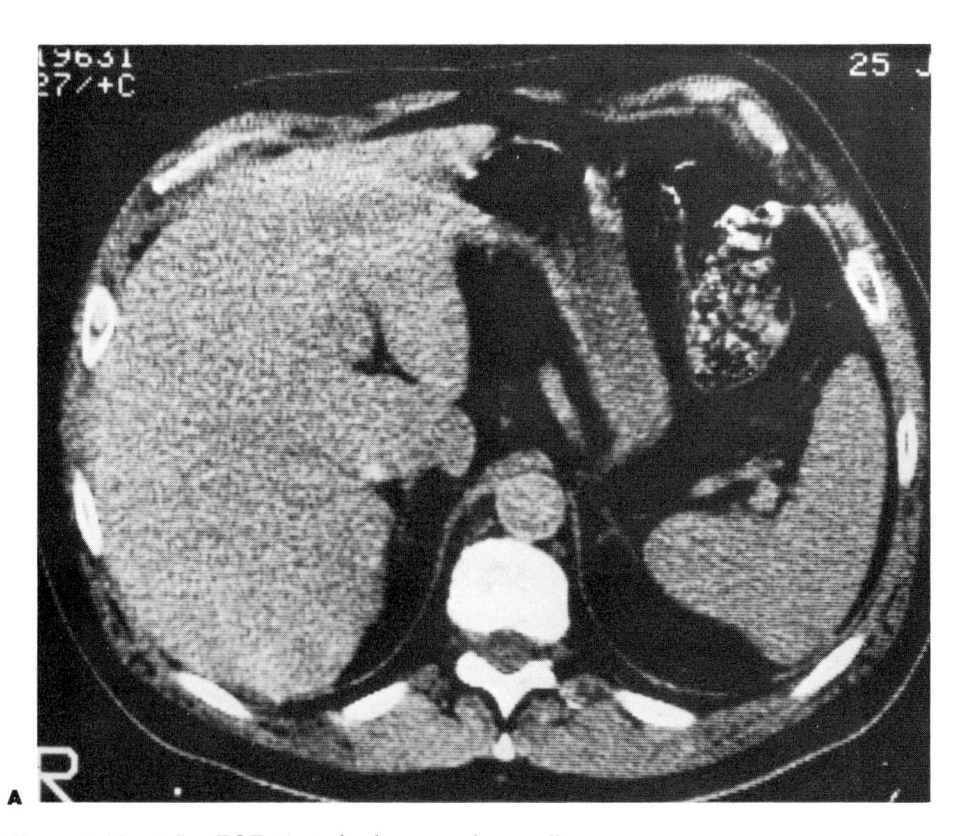

Figure 4–28. *A*. Pre-EOE-13 study shows no abnormality.

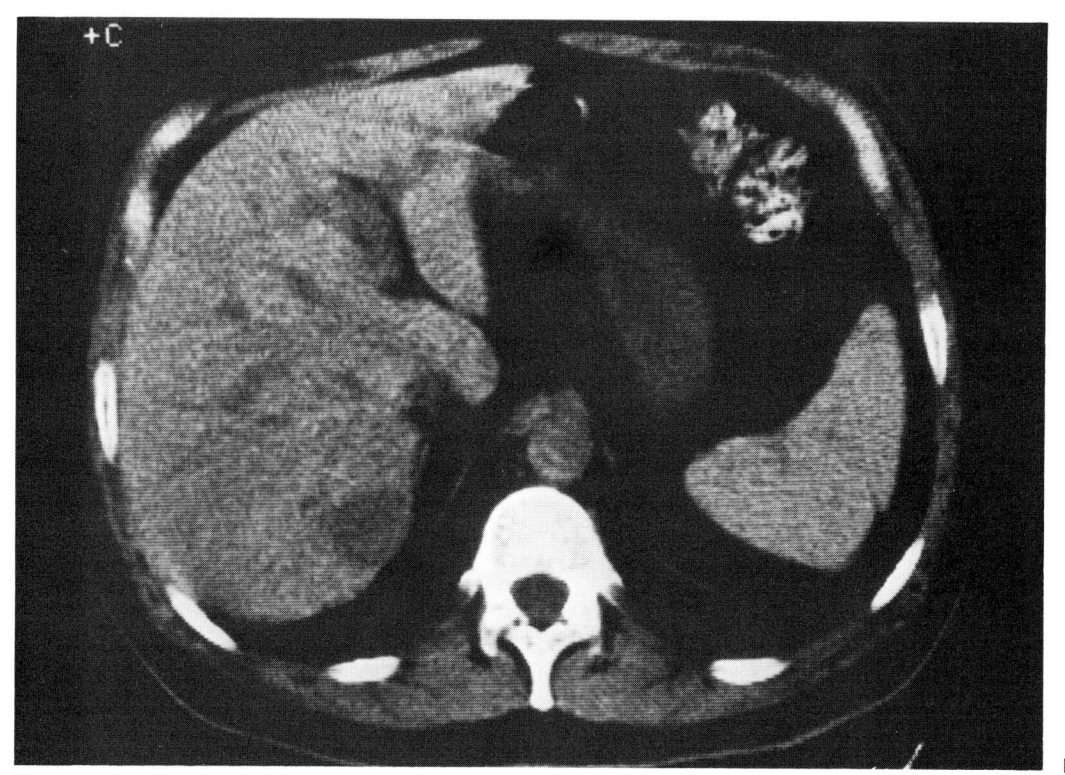

Figure 4–28. *B.* After EOE-13, a single lesion is noted. Is it benign or malignant?

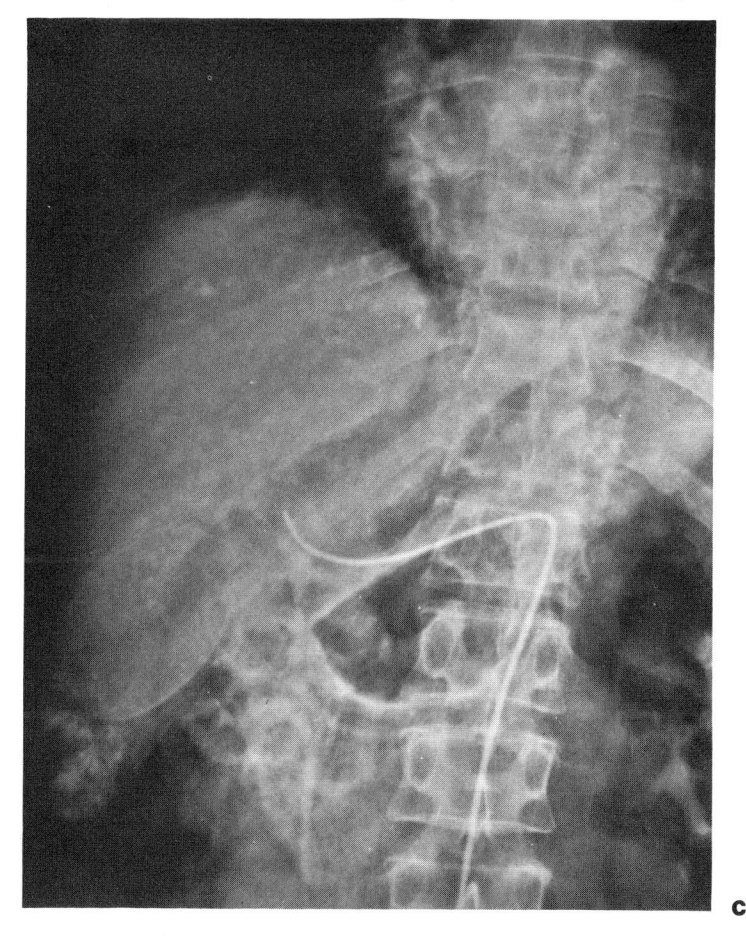

Figure 4–28. *C.* An angiogram demonstrates that it is a hemangioma.

REFERENCES

1. Bernardino ME: The computed tomographic diagnosis of hepatic metastases. In R Weiss and HA Gilbert (eds): Liver Metastasis. Boston: GK Hall 1982, pp. 187–209.
2. Knopf DR, Torres WE, Fajman WJ, Sones PJ Jr: Liver lesions: comparative accuracy of scintigraphy and computed tomography. AJR 1982;138:623–627.
3. Pagani JJ, Bernardino ME: Incidence and significance of serendipitous CT detections in the oncologic patient. J Comput Assist Tomogr, 1982;6:268–275.
4. Burgener FA, Hamlin DJ: Contrast enhancement of focal hepatic lesions in CT: effect of size and histology. AJR 1983;140:297–301.
5. Itai Y, Moss AA, Goldberg HI: Transient hepatic attenuation difference of lobar or segmental distribution detected by dynamic computed tomography. Radiology 1982;144:835–839.
6. Marchal GJ, Baert AL, Wilms GE: CT of noncystic liver lesions: bolus enhancement. AJR 1980;135:57–65.
7. Araki T, Itai Y, Furui S, Tasaka A: Dynamic CT densitometry of hepatic tumors. AJR 1980;135:1037–1043.
8. Burgener FA, Hamlin DJ: Contrast enhancement of hepatic tumors in CT: comparison between bolus and infusion techniques. AJR 1983;140:291–295.
9. Bernardino ME, Thomas JL, Barnes PA, Lewis E: Diagnostic approaches to liver and spleen metastases. Radiol Clin North Am 1982;20:531–544.
10. Berland LL, Lawson TL, Foley WD, et al.: Comparison of pre- and postcontrast CT in hepatic masses. AJR 1982;138:853–858.
11. Foley WD, Berland LL, Lawson TL, et al.: Contrast enhancement technique for dynamic hepatic computed tomographic scanning. Radiology 1983;147:797–803.
12. Moss AA, Dean PB, Axel L, et al.: Dynamic CT of hepatic masses with intravenous and intraarterial contrast material. AJR 1982;138:847–852.
13. Lewis E, Bernardino ME, Barnes PA, et al.: The fatty liver: pitfalls in the CT and angiographic evaluation of metastatic disease. J Comput Assist Tomogr 1983;7:235–241.
14. Prando A, Wallace S, Bernardino ME, Lindell MM: Computed tomographic arteriography of the liver. Radiology 1979;130:679–701.
15. Freeny PC, Marks WM: Computed tomographic arteriography of the liver. Radiology 1983;148:193–197.
16. Matsui O, Kadoya M, Suzuki M, et al.: Work in progress: dynamic sequential computed tomography during arterial portography in the detection of hepatic neoplasms. Radiology 1983;146:721–727.
17. Pagani JJ: Intrahepatic vascular territories shown by computed tomography. Radiology 1983;147:173–178.
18. Vigo M, De Faweri D, Biondetti PR Jr, Benedetti L: CT demonstration of portal and superior mesenteric vein thrombosis in hepatocellular carcinoma. J Comput Assist Tomogr 1980;4:627–629.
19. Itai Y, Nishikawa J, Tasaka A: Computed tomography in the evaluation of hepatocellular carcinoma. Radiology 1979;131:165–170.
20. Inamoto K, Sugiki K, Yamasaki H, et al.: Computed tomography and angiography of hepatocellular carcinoma. J Comput Assist Tomogr 1980;4:832–839.
21. Inamoto K, Sugiki K, Yamasaki H, Miura T: CT of hepatoma: effects of portal vein obstruction. AJR 1981;136:349–353.
22. Kunstlinger F, Federle MP, Moss AA, Marks W: Computed tomography of hepatocellular carcinoma. AJR 1980:134:431–437.
23. Hosoki T, Chatani M, Mori S: Dynamic computed tomography of hepatocellular carcinoma. AJR 1982;139:1099–1106.
24. Harter LP, Gross BH, Hilaire JS, et al.: CT and sonographic appearance of hepatic vein obstruction. AJR 1982;139:176–178.
25. Takashima T, Matsui O, Suzuki M, Ida M: Diagnosis and screening of small hepatocellular carcinomas. Radiology 1982;145:635–638.

26. Nishikawa J, Itai Y, Tasake A: Lobar attenuation difference of the liver on computed tomography. Radiology 1981;141:725-728.
27. Bernardino ME, Lewis E: Imaging hepatic neoplasms. Cancer 1982;50:2666-2671.
28. Barnes PA, Thomas JL, Bernardino ME: Pitfalls in the diagnosis of hepatic cysts by computed tomography. Radiology 1981;141:129-133.
29. Wooten WB, Bernardino ME, Goldstein HM: Computed tomographic features of necrotic hepatic masses. AJR 1978;131:839-842.
30. Bernardino ME, Chuang VP, Wallace S, et al.: Therapeutically infarcted tumors: CT findings. AJR 1981;136:527-530.
31. Bernardino ME: Computed tomography of calcified liver metastasis. J Comput Assist Tomogr 1979;3:32-35.
32. Scatarige JC, Fishman EK, Saksouk FA, Siegelman SS: Computed tomography of calcified liver masses. J Comput Assist Tomogr 1983;7:83-89.
33. Thomas JL, Bernardino ME: Segmental biliary obstruction: its detection and significance. J Comput Assist Tomogr 1980;40:155-158.
34. Itai Y, Araki T, Furui S, et al.: Computed tomography and ultrasound in the diagnosis of intrahepatic calculi. Radiology 1980;136:399-405.
35. Fishman E, Farmlett E, Kadir S, Siegelman S: Computer tomography of benign hepatic tumors. J Comput Assist Tomogr 1982;6:472-481.
36. Rogers JV, Mack LA, Freeny PC, et al.: Hepatic focal nodular hyperplasia: angiography, CT, sonography, and scintigraphy. AJR 1981;137:983-990.
37. Atkinson GO Jr, Kodroff M, Sones PJ, Gay BB Jr: Focal nodular hyperplasia of the liver in children: a report of three new cases. Radiology 1980;137:171-174.
38. Greenwood LH, Collins TL, Yrizarry JM: Percutaneous management of multiple liver abscesses. AJR 1982;139:390-392.
39. Haaga JR, Alfidi RJ, Havrilla TR, et al.: CT detection and aspiration of abdominal abscesses. AJR 1980;135:1187-1194.
40. Rubinson HA, Isikoff MB, Hill MC: Diagnostic imaging of hepatic abscesses: a retrospective analysis. AJR 1980;135:735-740.
41. Callen PW, Filly RA, Marcus FS: Ultrasonography and computed tomography in the evaluation of hepatic microabscesses in the immunosuppressed patient. Radiology 1980;136:433-434.
42. Sanfelippo PM, Beahrs OH, Weiland LH: Cystic disease of the liver. Ann Surg 1974;179:922-925.
43. Taylor KJW, Viscomi GN: Ultrasound diagnosis of cystic disease of the liver. J Clin Gastroenterol 1980;2:197-204.
44. Federle MP, Filly RA, Moss AA: Cystic hepatic neoplasms: complementary roles of CT and sonography. AJR 1981;136:345-348.
45. Choliz JD, Olaverri FJL, Casas TF, Zubieta SO: Computed tomography in hepatic echinococcosis. AJR 1982;139:699-702.
46. Roemer CE, Ferucci JT Jr, Mueller PR, et al.: Hepatic cysts: diagnosis and therapy by sonographic needle aspiration. AJR 1981;136:1065-1070.
47. Johnson CM, Sheedy PF, Stanson AW, et al.: Computed tomography and angiography of cavernous hemangiomas of the liver. Radiology 1981;138:115-121.
48. Itai Y, Furui S, Araki T, et al.: Computed tomography of cavernous hemangioma of the liver. Radiology 1980;137:149-155.
49. Freeny PC, Vimont TR, Barnett DC: Cavernous hemangioma of the liver: ultrasonography, arteriography, and computed tomography. Radiology 1979;132:143-148.
50. Barnett PH, Zerhouni EA, White RI Jr, Siegelman SS: Computed tomography in the diagnosis of cavernous hemangioma of the liver. AJR 1980;134:439-447.
51. Bree RL, Schwab RE, Neiman HL: Solitary echogenic spot in the liver: is it diagnostic of a hemangioma? AJR 1983;140:41-45.
52. Olmsted WW, Stocker JR: Cavernous hemangioma of the liver. RPC from the AFIP. Radiology 1975;117:59-62.

53. Piekarski J, Goldberg HI, Royal SA, et al.: Difference between liver and spleen CT numbers in the normal adult: its usefulness in predicting the presence of diffuse liver disease. Radiology 1980;137:727–729.
54. Bashist B, Hecht HL, Harley WD: Computed tomographic demonstration of rapid changes in fatty infiltration of the liver. Radiology 1982;142:691–692.
55. Scott WW, Sanders RC, Siegelman SS: Irregular fatty infiltration of the liver: diagnostic dilemmas. AJR 1980;135:67–71.
56. Cunningham DG, Churchill RJ, Reynes CJ: Computed tomography in the evaluation of liver disease in cystic fibrosis patients. J Comput Assist Tomogr 1980;4:151–154.
57. Halvorsen RA, Korobkin M, Ram PC, Thompson WM: CT appearance of focal fatty infiltration of the liver. AJR 1982;139:277–281.
58. Patel S, Sandler CM, Rauschkolb EN, McConnell BJ: [133]Xe uptake in focal hepatic fat accumulation: CT correlation. AJR 1982;138:541–544.
59. Chapman RWG, Williams G, Bydder G, et al.: Computed tomography for determining liver iron content in primary haemochromatosis. Br Med J 1980;280:440–442.
60. Mills SR, Doppman JL, Nienhaus AW: Computed tomography in the diagnosis of disorders of excessive iron storage in the liver. J Comput Assist Tomogr 1977;1:101–104.
61. Long JA, Doppman JL, Nienhaus AW, Mills SR: Computed tomographic analysis of beta-thalassemic syndromes with hemochromatosis: pathologic findings with clinical and laboratory correlations. J Comput Assist Tomogr 1980;4:159–165.
62. Moss AA, Goldberg HI: Interventional Radiologic Techniques: Computed Tomography and Ultrasound. New York: Academic Press 1981, pp. 265–274.
63. Smevik B, Ritland S, Nilsen T, Johansen O: Liver attenuation values at computed tomography related to liver copper content. Scand J Gastroenterol 1982;17:461–463.
64. Harik SI, Post MJD: Computed tomography in Wilson disease. Neurology 1981;31:107–110.
65. Doppman JL, Cornblath M, Dwyer AJ, et al.: Computed tomography of the liver and kidneys in glycogen storage disease. J Comput Assist Tomogr 1982;6:67–71.
66. Zornoza J, Ginaldi S: Computed tomography in hepatic lymphoma. Radiology 1981;138:405–410.
67. Jeffrey RB, Moss AA, Quivey JM, et al.: CT of radiation-induced hepatic injury. AJR 1980;135:445–448.
68. Harbin WP, Rober NJ, Ferrucci JT: Diagnosis of cirrhosis based on regional changes in hepatic morphology. Radiology 1980;135:273–283.
69. Snow JH, Goldstein HM, Wallace S: Comparison of scintigraphy, sonography, and computed tomography in the evaluation of hepatic neoplasms. AJR 1979;132:915–918.
70. Grossman Z, Wistow B, Bryan P, et al.: Radionuclide imaging, computed tomography and gray scale ultrasonography of the liver: a comparative study. J Nucl Med 1977;18:327–333.
71. MacCarty R, Heinz W, Stephens D, et al.: Retrospective comparison of radionuclide scans and computed tomography of the liver and pancreas. AJR 1977;129:23–28.
72. Doiron MJ, Bernardino ME: A comparison of noninvasive imaging modalities in the melonoma patient. Cancer 1981;47:2581–2584.
73. Kemeny MM, Sugarbaker PH, Jones AE, et al.: Prospective study of hepatic imaging in the detection of metastatic disease. Ann Surg 1982;446–491.
74. Henderson JM, Heymsfield SB, Horowitz J, Kutner MH: Measurement of liver and spleen volume by computed tomography. Radiology 1981;141:525–527.
75. Moss AA, Griedman MA, Brito AC: Determination of liver, kidney, and spleen volumes by computed tomography: an experimental study in dogs. J Comput Assist Tomogr 1981;5:12–14.
76. Vermess M, Doppman JL, Sugarbaker PH, et al.: Computed tomography of the liver and spleen with intravenous lipoid contrast material: review of 60 examinations. AJR 1982;138:1063–1071.
77. Vermess M, Doppman JL, Sugarbaker P, et al.: Clinical trials with a newly developed

intravenous liposoluble contrast material for computed tomography examination of the liver and spleen. Radiology 1980;137:217–222.
78. Vermess M, Bernardino ME, Doppman JL, et al.: Use of intravenous liposoluble contrast material for the examination of the liver and spleen in lyphoma. J Comput Assist Tomogr 1981;5:709–713.
79. Thomas JL, Bernardino ME, Vermess M, et al.: EOE-13 in the detection of hepatosplenic lymphoma. Radiology 1982;145:629–634.
80. Lewis E, AufderHeide JF, Bernardino ME, et al.: CT detection of hepatic metastases with ethiodized oil emulsion 13. J Comput Assist Tomogr 1982;6:1108–1114.
81. Havron A, Seltzer SE, Davis MA, Shulkin P: Radiopaque liposomes: a promising new contrast material for computed tomography of the spleen. Radiology 1981;140:507–511.
82. Seltzer SE, Adams DF, Davis MA: Hepatic contrast agents for computed tomography: high atomic number particulate material. J Comput Assist Tomogr 1981;5:370–374.
83. Mattrey RF, Long DM, Multer F, et al.: Perfluorocytlbromide: a reticuloendothelial-specific and tumor-imaging agent for computed tomography. Radiology 1982;145:755–758.
84. Marincek B, Young SW, Enzmann DR: Time-density evaluation of the liver after iosulamide meglumine: a tissue-specific CT contrast agent. Invest Radiol 1982;17:90–94.

5

Magnetic Resonance Imaging of the Liver

THOMAS L. LAWSON • MICHAEL E. BERNARDINO

INTRODUCTION

It is beyond the scope of this chapter to delve into the details of nuclear magnetic resonance. Several excellent articles in the literature are available for those interested in further reading (1–14). However, a very brief and basic description of the technique is appropriate.

The existence of nuclear spins, the entity essential to nuclear magnetic resonance (NMR), was known long before the first NMR experiments were reported by Felix Bloch and his co-workers at Stanford University and independently by Edward Purcell at Harvard in 1946. The nuclear spins of specific nuclei with odd numbers of electrons or neutrons provide them with magnetic moments so that the nuclei act like small magnets. When these spinning nuclei are subjected to an external static magnetic field, the randomly oriented magnetic dipoles respond to the force of the external magnetic field by aligning with it. For these spinning nuclei, two basic states are allowable: one, a parallel orientation to the external magnetic field, or spin up; and second, a higher energy state termed antiparallel, or spin down. There are slightly more nuclei oriented in a parallel, spin-up parallel, and antiparallel position than the reverse, providing a net nuclear magnetization that is parallel and aligned to the external magnetic field. There is a dynamic balance between the two basic energy states, which is determined by the energy strength of the external magnetic field and temperature. Shift of the spinning nuclei from a lower to a higher energy state can be initiated by energizing the nuclei by a resonant radio-frequency field. When the resonant radio-frequency field has been turned off, nuclei decay to the lower energy state, reemitting energy in the form of a radio-frequency wave. By the use of gradient magnetic fields and selective radio-frequency signal reception, a two-dimensional magnetic resonance image can be produced.

Both two-dimensional imaging data and chemical shift, spectroscopic information can be obtained from the emitted radio-frequency energy.

The electromagnetic energy delivered by the radio waves interacts with the spinning nuclei, or proton in the case of hydrogen. Therefore, energy absorption is proportional to the number of nuclei per unit volume (i.e., nuclear density). Nuclear density is one of the factors that makes up signal intensity and contrast in a magnetic resonance image. The proton, the principal isotope of hydrogen, is the best signal source in magnetic resonance imaging because it is abundant in biologic tissues and its magnetic moment is the largest among all naturally occurring nuclei. Therefore, virtually all current clinical magnetic resonance images are proton images. In addition to nuclear density or proton density, relaxation times of the proton contribute to the signal and contrast in an image. There are two basic relaxation times, longitudinal or spin-lattice relaxation time (T_1) and transverse or spin-spin relaxation time (T_2). The T_1, or spin-lattice, relaxation time is an exponential time constant that measures the time required for the proton to return to equilibrium (i.e., return to its original position longitudinal to the external magnetic field) after it has been shifted or flipped by an applied radio frequency. The transverse of T_2, or spin-spin, relaxation time is an exponential time constant that measures the interaction of protons with one another (the loss of coherence) in the plane perpendicular to the external magnetic field. The strength of the NMR signal and image contrast in a magnetic resonance image is dependent, in part, on proton density and the T_1 and T_2 relaxation times within a tissue sample. The appearance of the image itself depends on the pulsing sequence and the time intervals between radio-frequency excitations, as well as on the delay between each pulse sequence. For a complete discussion of contrast, relaxation times, and imaging methods, the reader is referred to the literature (9–13).

The most critical component of an NMR unit is the magnet for generating the static magnetic field required for polarization of the nuclei. Magnets may be of three basic designs: permanent, resistive electromagnetic, and superconductive electromagnetic. There are advantages and disadvantages for each system. The major disadvantages of the permanent magnet are its very high weight and relatively limited field strength. Electromagnets have the advantage of lower weight and smaller size than permanet magnets; however, their magnetic fields extend for several feet outside the confines of the magnet, which may pose hazards. Resistive electromagnets have relatively high electric requirements and relatively limited field strength because of high heat generation at the higher field strength. This problem has been largely eliminated by the use of superconductive electromagnets. The superconductivity allows extremely high field strengths to be generated. However, relatively expensive cryogens to supercool the magnet are required.

There are four critical criteria for the magnet performance: field strength, temporal stability, homogeneity, and bore size. While optimal field strength for imaging and spectroscopy is controversial, it appears that high field-strength magnets, of greater than 1 to 2 tesla, will be necessary for medical imaging and spectroscopic studies of nuclei other than hydrogen. Stability and homogeneity of the magnetic field are also important factors in high-resolution imaging. Bore size is also important, since the opening needs to be large enough to admit the human body, but not so large that the magnetic field is dissipated. Additional components of the system include the radio-frequency coils for transmitting and receiving the radio-frequency waves and the gradient system required for spatial localization. Very powerful computers with large memories are necessary for computation and image reconstruction. A display console with television monitors and a system for recording the image are the final components.

NMR has two major applications: imaging and spectroscopy. Because of the inherent high contrast in NMR imaging, high-resolution images of the body can be attained. In the field of spectroscopy, NMR has the potential to probe body chemistry *in vivo* and provide information about metabolic processes occurring inside cells and organs. For example, it has been shown that *in vivo* NMR spectroscopy of phosphorous 31 monitors and concentrations of the energy metabolites: ATP, ADP, phosphocreatinine, and inorganic phosphates, which play critical roles in the production of energy and cellular metabolism. Thus, NMR spectroscopy may have a major impact on medical diagnosis.

SAFETY

Potential risks related to the use of an NMR imager are related to three factors: magnetic torque forces, induced electrical currents, and heating effects. Recognizing these factors, the Bureau of Radiologic Health has published guidelines for NMR imaging. These guidelines suggest upper limits for the operating parameters in human NMR imaging. The guidelines for maximum exposure are:

1. Static magnetic fields: whole or partial body exposures of a maximum of 2 tesla.
2. Time: varying magnetic fields (dB/dt); whole or partial exposures of 3 tesla/second.
3. Radio-frequency electromagnetic fields: exposure to radio-frequency fields that result in a specific absorption rate that exceeds 0.4 watts per kilogram (W/kg) as averaged over the whole body, or 2.0 W/kg as averaged over any 1 gram of tissue.

Most NMR units in clinical use today are operating at static magnetic fields of less than 2 tesla. Some experimental and animal units, however, are operating at well above this level.

Most units in clinical use today are operating at a rate of change of the magnetic field (dB/dt) that exceeds the Bureau of Radiologic Health guideline of 3 tesla/second. However, in the Bureau of Radiologic Health guidelines, the length of exposure to this time-varying magnetic field is not specified. The maximum rate of change of a magnetic field in a 1-tesla system is approximately 6 tesla/second over a duration of approximately 400 microseconds. A similar rate of magnetic field strength changes are projected for a 1.5-tesla system. It should be noted that these gradient fields are applied for only a fraction of a second. Rates of magnetic field change considerably larger than 3 tesla/second are required to produce biologic effects if the duration is short and less than 10 milliseconds. All current information indicates that NMR as currently utilized is safe, with no biologic hazard in the patient not using a pacemarker, a large metallic prosthesis, or ferromagnetic clips placed on strategic blood vessels. Patients with these devices may be at risk from both the time-varying magnetic fields and the static magnetic fields. These risks have been discussed in the medical literature (15–18).

The strength of the radio-frequency electromagnetic fields and the exposure to these radio-frequency fields used in magnetic resonance imaging are well within the Bureau of Radiologic Health guidelines.

PULSE SEQUENCES

Three basic pulsing sequences are used commonly in magnetic resonance imaging: partial saturation, inversion recovery, and spin echo, as well as a variant of spin echo called

A. PARTIAL SATURATION

B. INVERSION RECOVERY

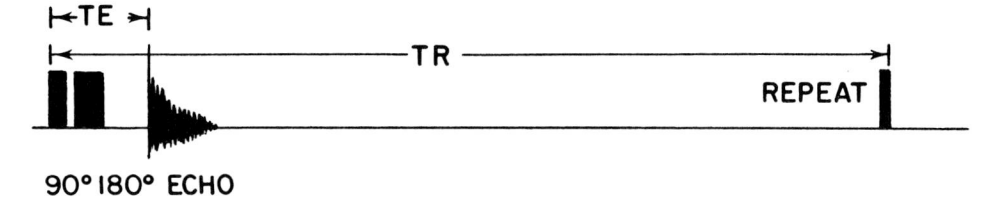

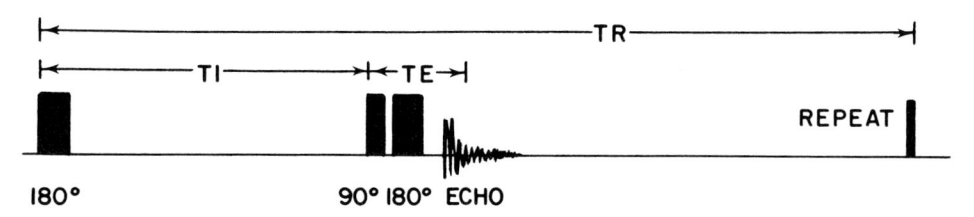

C. SPIN ECHO

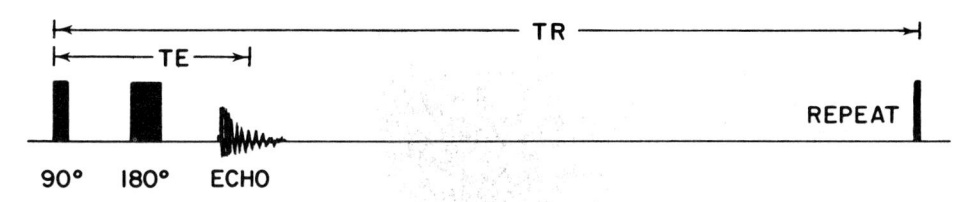

D. MULTIPLE SPIN ECHO

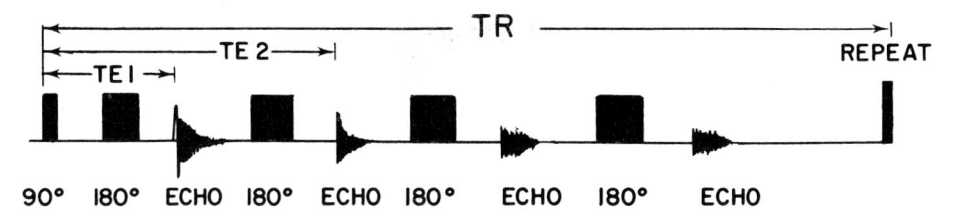

Figure 5–1. *Representation of magnetic-resonance-imaging pulse sequences. A.* Partial saturation: A 90° inversion radio-frequency pulse is follwed by 180° inversion pulse. There is a time delay, or echo time (TE), of from 5 to 25 milliseconds before the echo, or reemitted, radio-frequency signals are recorded. The repetition time (TR) is usually from 0.1 to 0.4 second. This pulse sequence produces a T_1-weighted image. *B.* Inversion recovery: An initial 180° inversion pulse is followed by a 90° inversion radio-frequency pulse with a delay between the pulses, or an inversion time (TI), that varies from 100 to 900 milliseconds. The 90° inversion radio-frequency pulse is followed by a 180° inversion radio-frequency pulse with subsequent reception of the echo, or reemitted radio signal. The repetition time (TR) is usually from 1 to 2 seconds. This pulse sequence produces a T_1-weighted image. *C.* Spin echo: This sequence uses a 90° followed by a 180° inversion radio-frequency pulse. The echo time is from 20 to 100 milliseconds before reemitted radio-frequency signals are received. The repitition time is usually 1 or 2 seconds. This pulse sequence produces a T_2-weighted image. *D.* Multiple spin echo: The multiple spin echo sequence is similar to the single echo, except that a series of 180° inversion pulses follow the 90° pulse, with a series of diminishing echoes being recorded. The echo times vary from 20 to 100 milliseconds and are termed TE-1, TE-2, etc. This pulse sequence produces a T_2-weighted image.

multiple spin echo (Figure 5-1). In all of these imaging sequences, the proton is energized by sets of radio-frequency electromagnetic energy pulses activated with varying time delays between pulses. In most scanning sequences, the time of reception of reemitted radio-frequency energy, or echo time (TE), varies from 10 to 60 milliseconds. The repetition time (TR), or time period of each pulse sequence, varies from 0.2 second to 2.0 seconds. With inversion recovery pulse sequences, usually a series of inversion times (TI) is used, and these may vary from 100 to 900 milliseconds. In spin-echo imaging sequences, the echo times usually vary from 20 to 100 milliseconds. Commonly, multiple spin-echo sequences are employed as a time-saving device, with a series of echo-delay time intervals between echoes that vary from 20 to 30 milliseconds (19).

Following excitation or absorption of radio-frequency energy by the proton, there is reemission of the energy in the form of radio-frequency electromagnetic energy. However, the reemission of energy decreases over time, and the received echo signals decay over time. Depending on the time of echo sampling, weak to strong signals will be obtained. Strong signals are by convention displayed as white or near white on NMR images. Weak or absent signals are displayed as black, and intermediate strength signals displayed in various shades of gray.

The T_1 (spin-lattice) and the T_2 (spin-spin) relaxation times are the primary determinants of relative contrast in magnetic resonance imaging. It is possible to highlight inherent contrast between tissues with different T_1 and T_2 relaxation times by varying the timing and duration of the radio-frequency pulses and the pulse sequences used. The T_1 relaxation time is always longer than the T_2 relaxation time. Fat has a short T_1 relaxation time, while water has a longer T_1 relaxation time. In pulse sequences that are T_1 weighted, such as partial saturation and inversion recovery, fat with a short T_1 relaxation time will be light colored, indicating an intense signal. With this same pulse sequence, water with a long T_1 relaxation time will be dark, indicating a low signal intensity (Figure 5-2). The signal strength or appearance of an organ or a lesion is in part determined by the variables of pulse sequence and the different pulse times used. Selection of the optimal echo time and repetition time is critical in accurate identification of pathology.

One of the major hopes for NMR is its ability to provide a specific diagnosis based on the tissue-specific intrinsic NMR parameters, T_1 and T_2 relaxation times and proton density. The *in vivo* determination of these intrinsic NMR parameters requires the performance of a variety of pulsed sequences, usually inversion recovery and/or spin echo with multiple delay times to provide adequate samples (Figure 5-3). While the ability of T_1 and T_2 relaxation times and proton density to provide a specific diagnosis has been intriguing, to date it is an elusive promise of NMR. There are several technical difficulties with *in vivo* determination of decay times, and this includes the necessity of obtaining both inversion recovery and spin-echo sequences with long enough echo-delay times or inversion times to provide sufficient data points for an accurate plot of the decay curve. The measurements made to perform the calculations are intensity measurements, and errors in the intensity measurements themselves or technical problems or artifacts on the images will be reflected in errors in the T_1 and T_2 measurements. An important potential use of the *in vivo* T_1 and T_2 measurements is the calculated relative contrast curves based on these relaxation times. These calculated relative contrast curves can provide information in determining optimal pulse sequences in the scanning of a particular organ or disease (Figure 5-4). This type of analysis may shorten examination time in the future.

One of the major disadvantages of magnetic resonance imaging compared to computed tomography is the relatively long scanning time for each slice or series of slices,

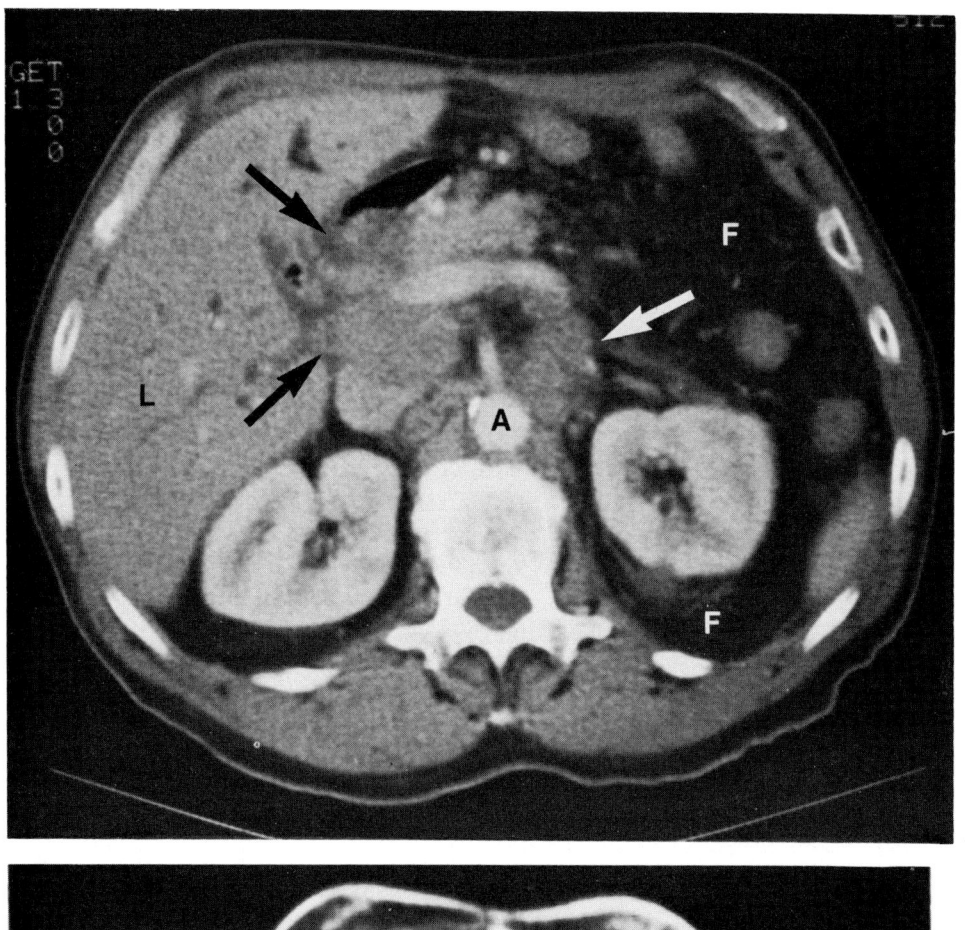

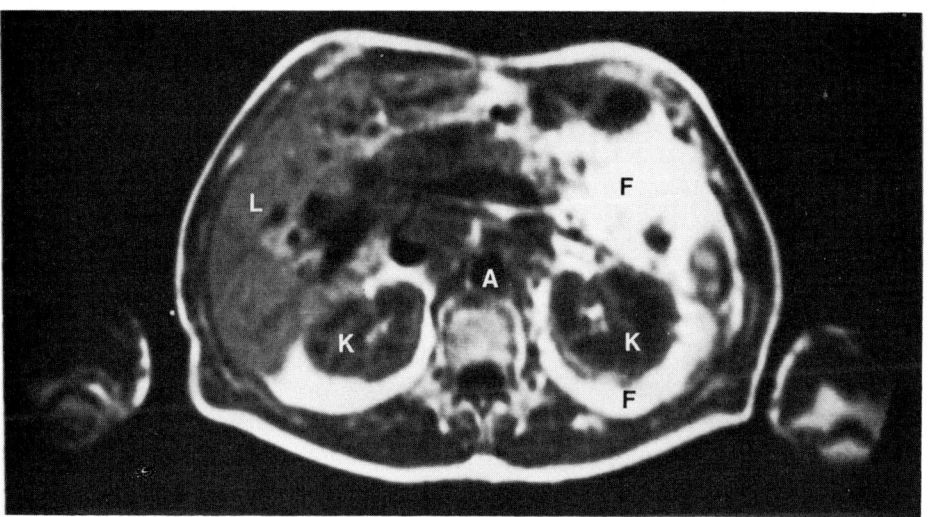

Figure 5-2. Metastases to the liver and portal hepatis. 0.5 T, partial-saturation pulse sequence. Computed tomogram (*A*) demonstrates metastatic disease to the porta hepatis and retroperitoneum (arrows). *B.* A magnetic resonance image of this patient at the same level performed with a partial-saturation pulse sequence demonstrates the peritoneal and retroperitoneal fat as white, the fluid within the aorta, inferior vena cava, and portal vein as black, and the liver and infiltrating tumor as intermediate shades of gray. K = kidney; L = liver; F = Fat.

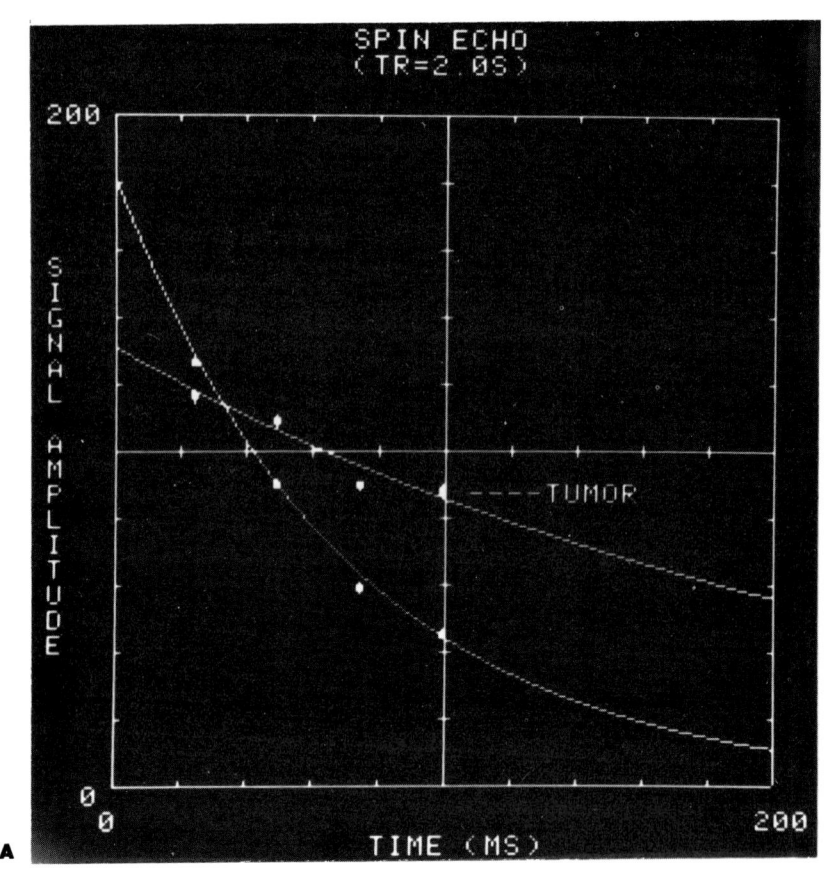

Figure 5-3. Decay curves of signal intensity versus time. Spin-echo (*A*) and inversion-recovery (*B*) pulse sequences in a patient demonstrate the signal intensity decay of normal liver versus a tumor over time. *In vivo* calculation of T_1 and T_2 relaxation times may be obtained with a plot such as this. Signal intensity values from pixels in a selected region of interest for various echo-delay times form a decay curve. The relaxation times are then computed as a best fit using regression analysis to the calculated decay curves, which are based on or generated from the Bloch equation. This manipulation yields a numerical relaxation time. Improved accuracy in the calculation of T_1 and T_2 can be achieved by increasing the number of sampling points.

if volume imaging or multiple-slice imaging is not performed. This relatively long scanning time, in the range of 1 to 30 minutes per image or set of images, results in motion blurring of organs and tissues that move as a response to cardiac motion, vascular pulsation, peristaltic action and, respiratory motion. Motion degrades images and blurs margins; however, unlike computed tomography, anatomic information is still present, and there is not total degradation of the image.

MAGNETIC RESONANCE IMAGING

Normal Anatomy

The potential of magnetic resonance imaging in hepatic diagnosis has not yet been defined fully. NMR has the ability to accurately define the normal liver, to identify

B

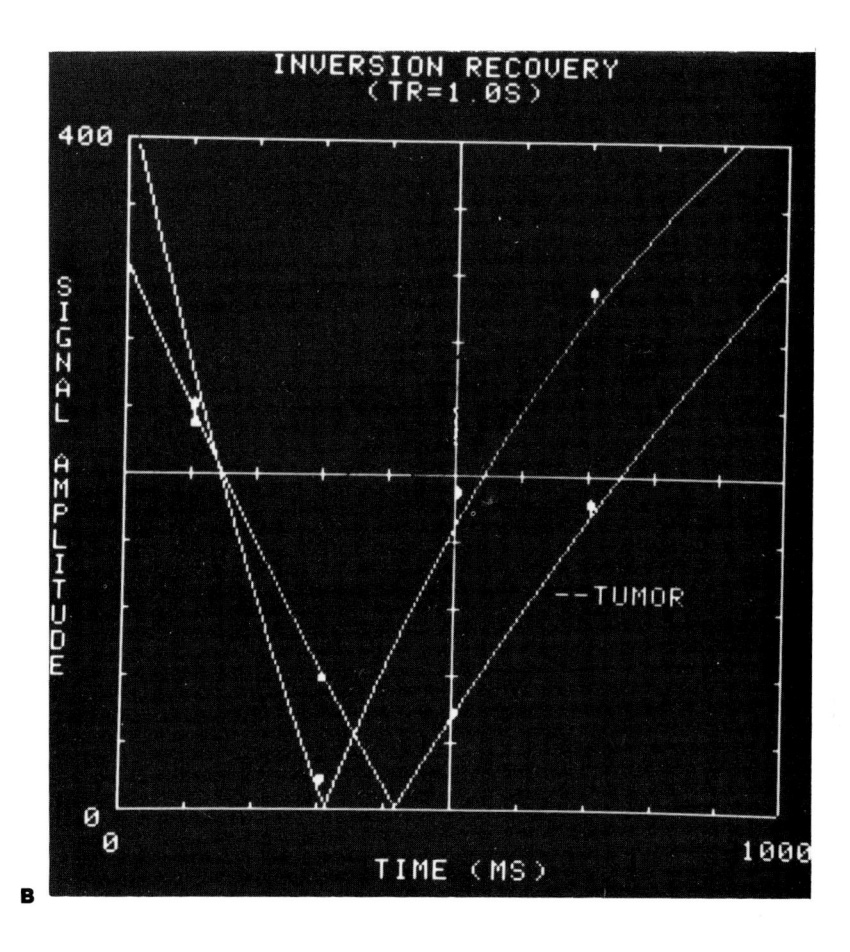

morphologic changes in the liver, and to define the various lobes and segments of the liver (Figure 5-5). The high inherent tissue contrast in the NMR signal allows accurate definition of the liver and differentiation of the normal blood vessels from the liver parenchyma without the use of intravenous contrast agents. Magnetic resonance imaging of the liver may be obtained in the axial, coronal, and sagittal anatomic planes (Figure 5-6). The ability for multiplanar imaging may be an advantage, particularly the use of coronal imaging.

Hepatic Masses

Benign and malignant hepatic masses can be identified by magnetic resonance imaging because of a difference in signal intensity of a mass compared to the adjacent normal liver (Figure 5-7) (20-25). However, specific signal intensities or specific NMR tissue parameters have not yet been able to distinguish benign masses and neoplasms from malignant tumors.

In vivo estimation of T_1 and T_2 relaxation times may be determined based on plots of signal amplitude versus time. However, because of the difficulty in accurate measurement of these relaxation times and the wide variation in decay times, analysis of relaxation times to provide a specific histologic diagnosis has not been accomplished to

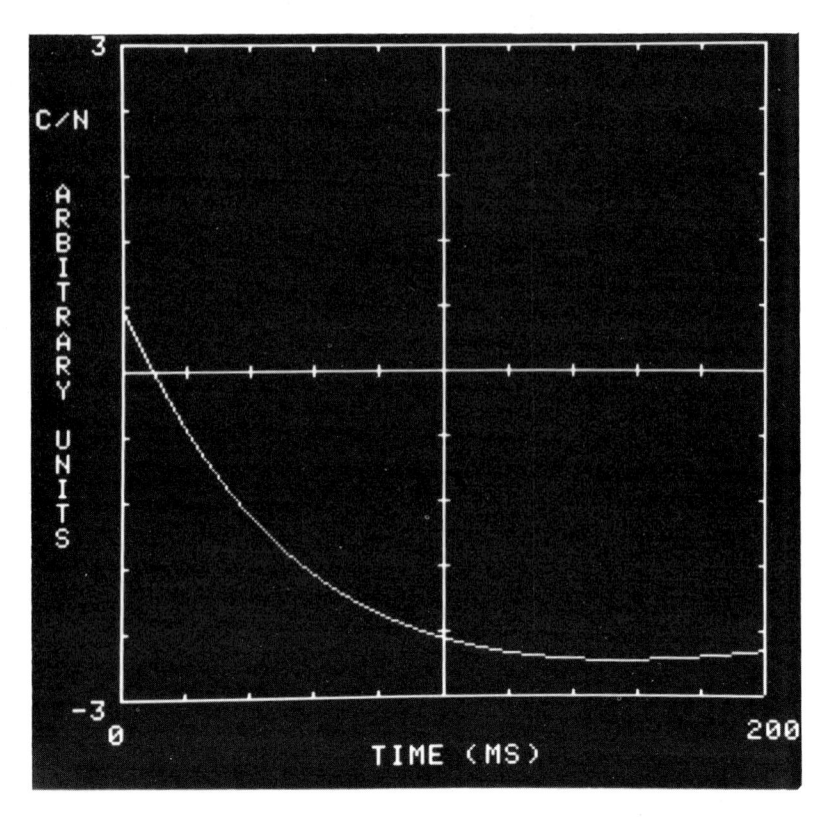

Figure 5-4. Plot of contrast differences versus time. Using *in vivo* calculations of T_1 and T_2 values for normal liver versus a hepatic mass, a computer-generated contrast curve for a spin-echo pulse sequence indicates the best times for echo recovery to maximize inherent tissue contrast. In this patient, the spin-echo pulse sequence would provide excellent contrast with an echo time of approximately 90 milliseconds, but almost no contrast at 20 milliseconds. Curves such as these may be helpful in determining correct pulse sequences, echo times, and repetition time for patient imaging.

date. The average T_1 and T_2 relaxation times for normal hepatic tissue do differ significantly from the normal liver, however, allowing the masses to be clearly identified by magnetic resonance imaging (Figure 5-8). In one report, the mean T_1 time of tumors was increased 40 percent over normal, and the T_2 time increased an average of 20 percent (23). In all cases, both T_1 and T_2 values were longer than the normal adjacent tissue. However, T_1 and T_2 values varied among tumors of different types, among tumors of the same histologic type in different patients, among tumors of the same histology in the same patient, and in different regions of a single tumor (23). Therefore, a specific relaxation time or specific NMR tissue parameter could not be given for any specific solid hepatic neoplasm.

The signal intensity of a hepatic neoplasm compared to the normal liver varies, depending upon the time parameters and pulse sequence used (Figure 5-9). Variations in the appearance of the tumor can be seen with different pulse sequences.

Care must be taken in the selection of pulse sequences, and a complete examination must be performed, as some lesions are isointense with the normal liver and are detected only on a single or particular pulse sequence. It is uncommon for a primary or meta-

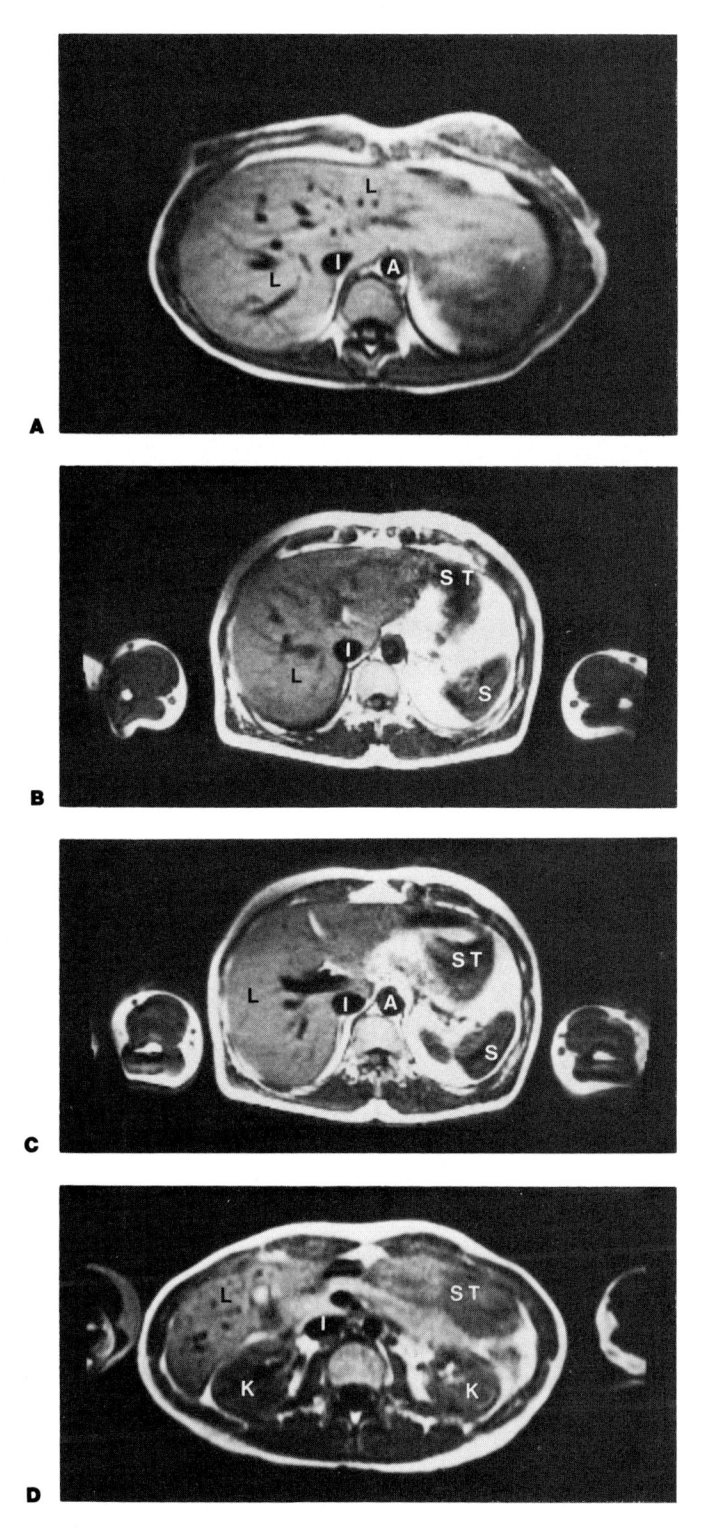

Figure 5-5. Normal magnetic resonance images of the liver. 1.0 T, partial-saturation pulse sequence. A series of normal axial images of the liver are arranged from cranial (*A*) to caudal (*D*). A = aorta; ST = stomach; K = kidney; L = liver; I = inferior vena cava; S = spleen.

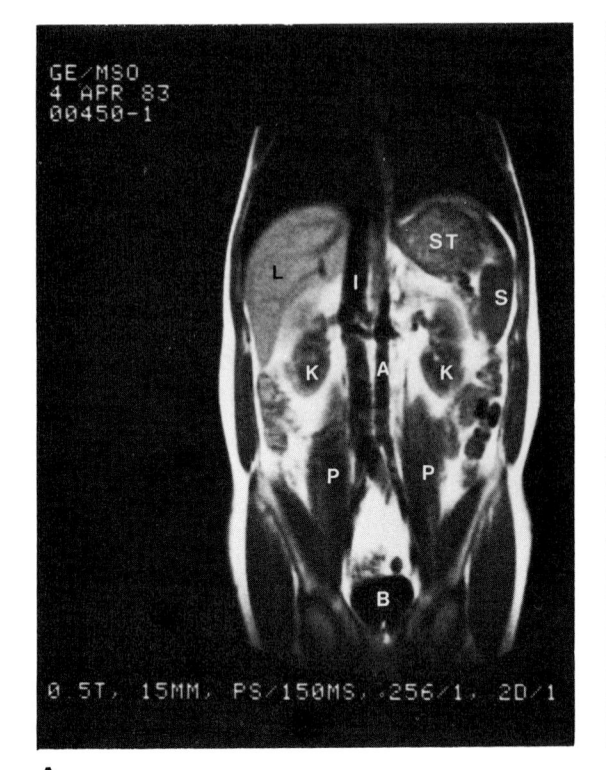

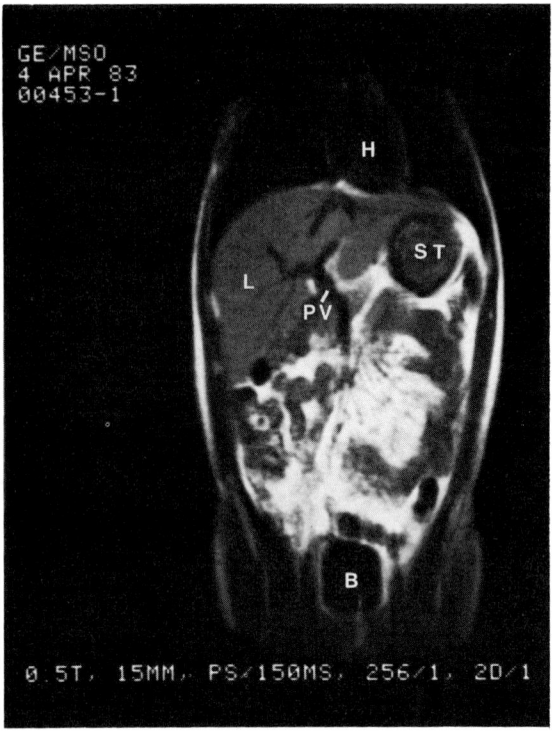

Figure 5-6. Normal magnetic resonance images of the liver. 0.5 T, partial-saturation pulse sequence. Magnetic resonance imaging is not limited to the transverse plane, but direct coronal and sagittal anatomic images can be obtained. The ability for multiplanar imaging may be an advantage. Coronal hepatic images at the level of the aorta and inferior vena cava (*A*) and slightly more ventral at the level of the portal vein (*B*) demonstrate regional anatomy. L = liver; A = aorta; I = inferior vena cava; ST = stomach; S = spleen; K = kidney; B = urinary bladder; P = psoas muscle; PV = portal vein; H = heart.

static hepatic mass to be detected with equal certainty or clarity on all pulse sequences; conversely, they are almost never detectable on all pulse sequences when a complete examination is performed. In these cases, it may be valuable to use contrast curves to anticipate the best pulse sequence and delay times that will accentuate contrast difference between the suspected mass and normal liver.

The ideal method and pulsing sequence to image the liver by NMR is yet to be determined. Because tumors have prolonged T_1 and T_2 values when compared to normal liver—even though the degree of prolongation varies among patients and lesions, and even within various portions of the same patient and lesion—it nevertheless appears that pulse sequences using relatively long echo times and inversion times will be beneficial. However, a complete pulse sequence in each examination would appear prudent. It is suggested that techniques that are both relatively T_1-dependent (inversion recovery and partial saturation) and T_2-dependent (spin-echo) be used, with varying inversion times and echo times. If a complete sequence and careful examination are performed, the degree of detection of primary and metastatic hepatic neoplasms and masses certainly approaches the degree of accuracy of high-resolution computed tomography (Figure 5-10) (23).

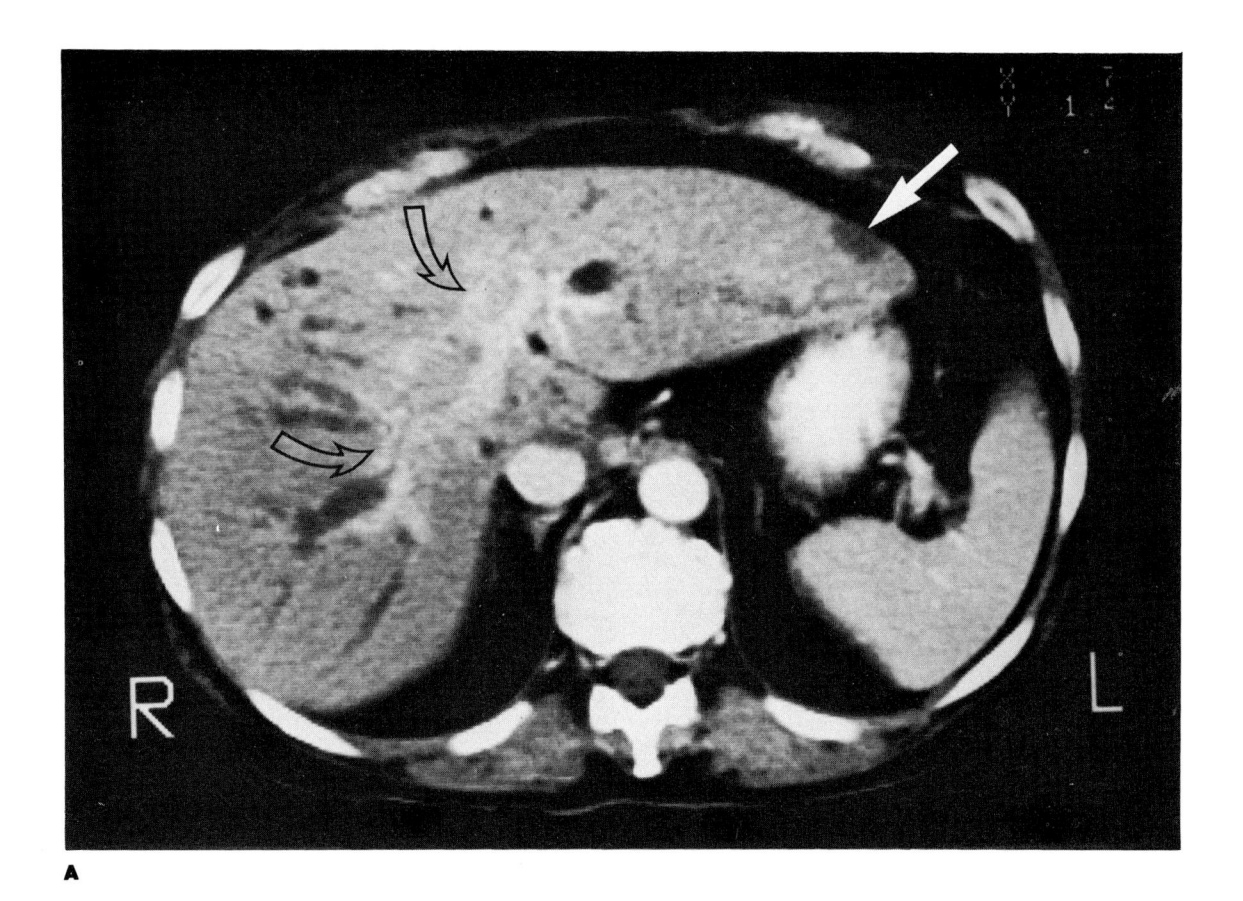

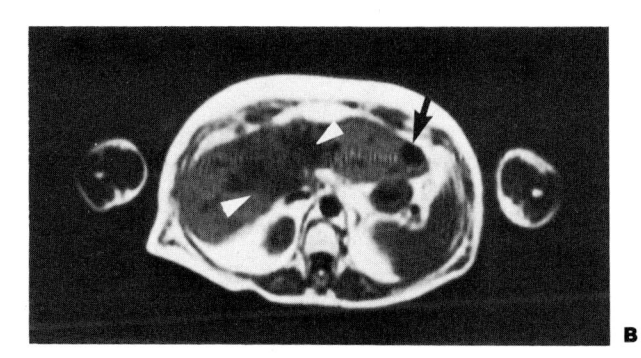

Figure 5-7. Benign and malignant hepatic masses. 0.5 T, partial-saturation pulse sequence. Benign and malignant hepatic masses can be identified because of signal intensity that is different from the adjacent normal liver. However, specific signal intensities or specific NMR tissue parameters have yet to be encountered that distinguish benign masses from malignant neoplasms. Contrast-enhanced hepatic computed tomogram (*A*) and hepatic magnetic resonance image (*B*) demonstrate a mass (arrow) in the lateral segment of the left lobe of the liver of low signal intensity. This represents a hepatic cyst. This patient also has an infiltrating cholangiocarcinoma seen in the porta hepatis, which enhances on the computed tomogram (curved arrow) and is of low signal strength on the magnetic resonance image (arrowhead).

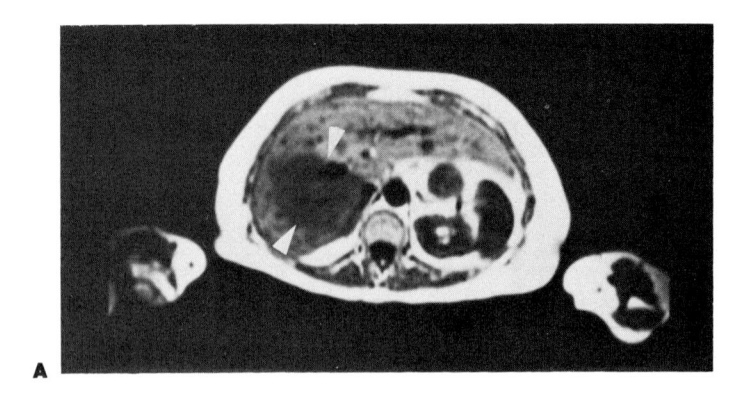

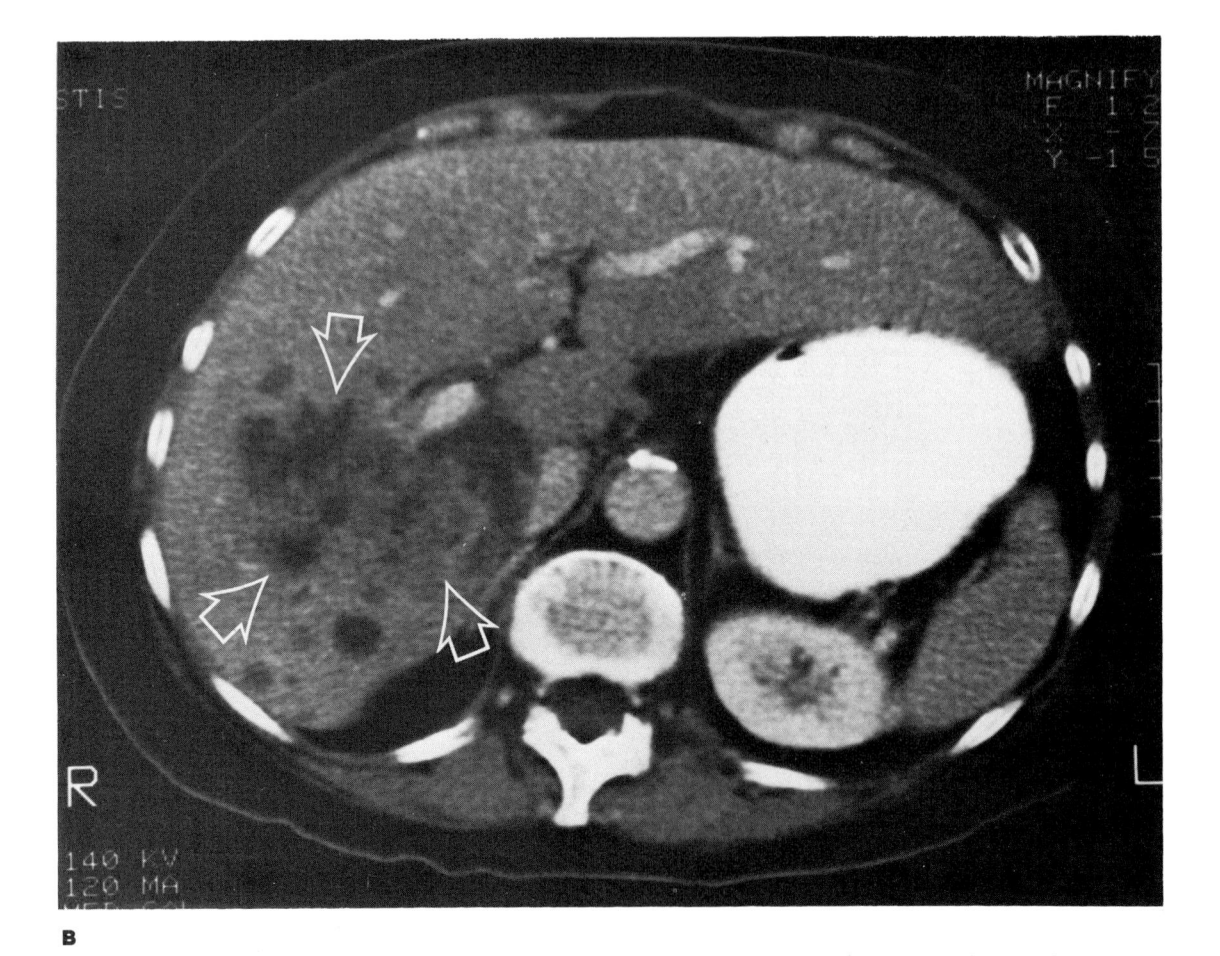

Figure 5-8. Metastatic carcinoma of the colon. 0.5 T, partial-saturation pulse sequence. Magnetic resonance image (*A*) and computed tomogram (*B*) of the liver in a patient with metastatic carcinoma of the colon. To optimally visualize the metastasis by computed tomography (arrows), intravenous contrast was employed. The inherent high difference in signal intensity between the normal liver and the metastasis allows easy identification by magnetic resonance imaging (arrowhead).

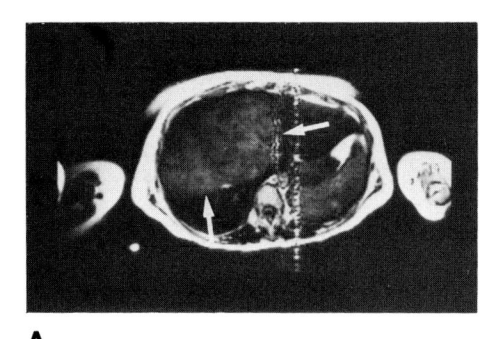

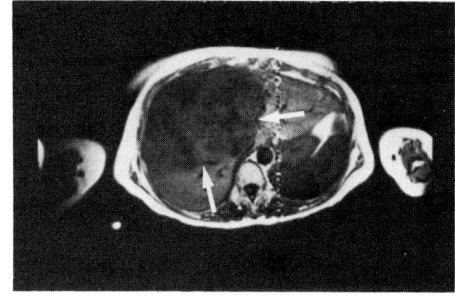

Figure 5-9. Metastatic carcinoma of the cervix. 1.0 T, inversion-recovery pulse sequence. Two inversion-recovery images in a patient with metastatic carcinoma demonstrate the change in the appearance of the lesion with different inversion times (arrows). Signal intensity and appearance of normal parenchyma and neoplasms will vary depending on time parameters and pulse sequences used.

Infiltrative Disease

Characterization of infiltrative or diffuse diseases using inherent tissue-specific NMR parameters has been limited by poor reproducibility of *in vivo* measurements of T_1 and T_2 relaxation times. While accurate morphologic images can be obtained, current pulses sequences designed to create the anatomic images are not optimal for precise or accurate tissue characterization. *In vivo* calculation of T_1 and T_2 suffers from variations caused by technical problems, artifacts, variations in radio-frequency amplifier gain, radio-frequency attenuation in homogeneity, and difficulty in obtaining accurate and reproducible spin flip angles. However, use of signal intensities from various portions of the liver, either simply on a subjective basis or compared to adjacent known normal tissues or to reference standards such as solutions of fat and water imaged at the same time as the patient, may provide clues to infiltrative diseases of the liver (Figure 5-10) (26,27). Preliminary reports have suggested that hepatitis, fatty infiltration, increased deposits of metal, such as iron or copper, and glycogen may be detected by NMR imaging (26-28). It has been suggested that T_1 relaxation time is prolonged in hepatitis, but only minimally altered in fatty liver (26,27). However, variations will occur depending on the influence on relaxation times of the amount of free water, fat, and other deposits within the liver.

NMR SPECTROSCOPY

Data concerning *in vivo* chemical analysis of human liver tissue by spectrographic analysis is quite limited. This is due to the lack of proper equipment for such analysis. However, spectroscopy has been applied to liver tissue *in vitro*. The relaxation-time results from such analysis have been promising and may be helpful in discriminating disease in the future without invasive techniques.

In vitro analysis of relaxation times (T_1 and T_2) can be performed reliably, assuming that the tissue samples have been properly processed (29). Measurements of T_1 values from livers and spleens in rats demonstrate T_1 stability for 6 hours, if the sample is untreated and kept at room temperature. After this time, the sample T_1 values are degraded. However, if this same sample is placed in some fixative, the T_1 stability may

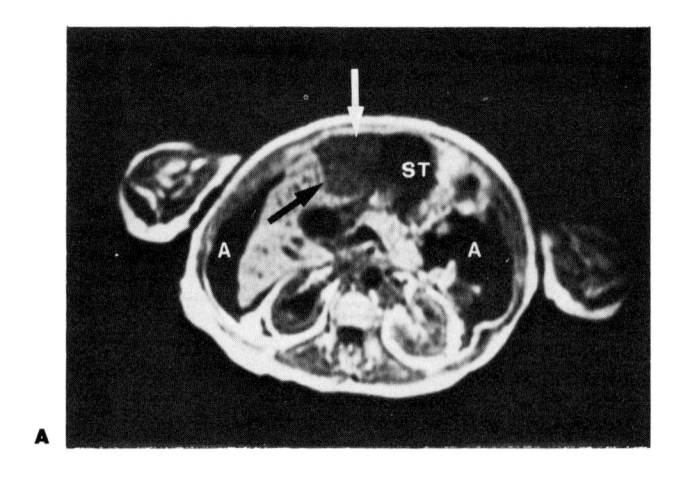

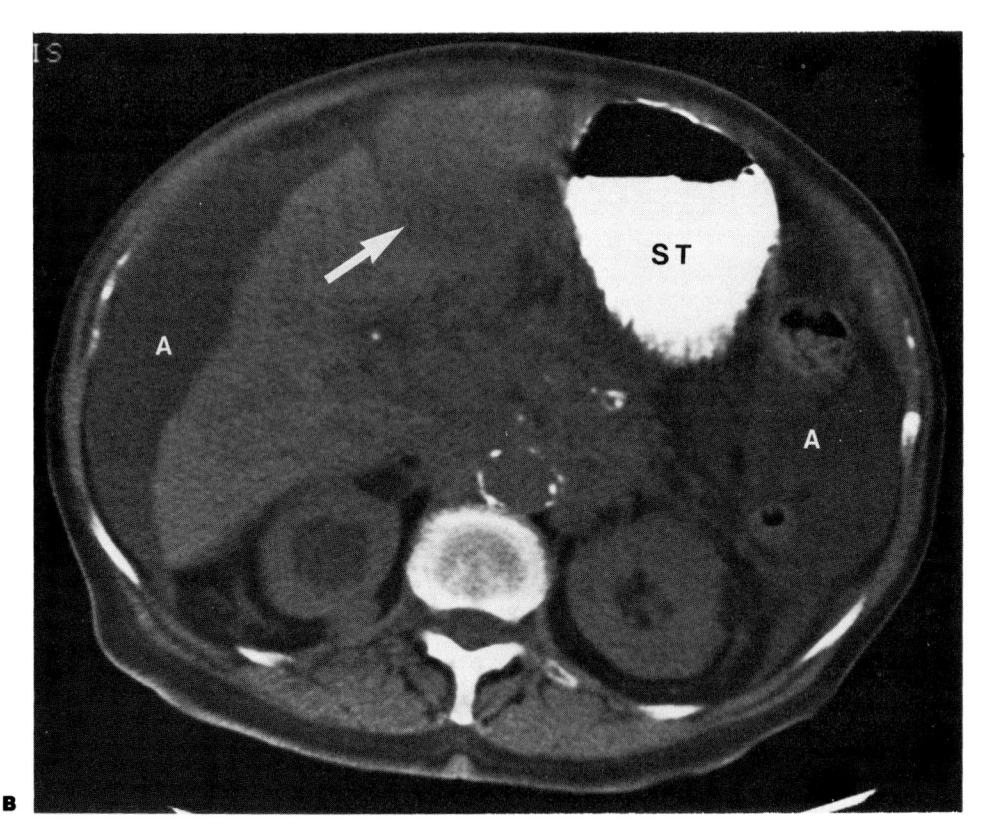

Figure 5–10. Metastatic hepatic disease: computed tomography, magnetic resonance imaging comparison. Magnetic resonance image (*A*) demonstrates a hepatic lesion (arrows) because of the marked difference in signal intensity of the metastatic deposit versus the adjacent liver. Baseline, noncontrast (*B*) and contrast-enhanced (*C*) computed tomogram does not demonstrate the metastasis (arrow) as well. Ascites (A), right hydronephrosis, and retroperitoneal metastases are also present. In another patient, hepatic metastasis is demonstrated by magnetic resonance imaging (*D*) (arrows).

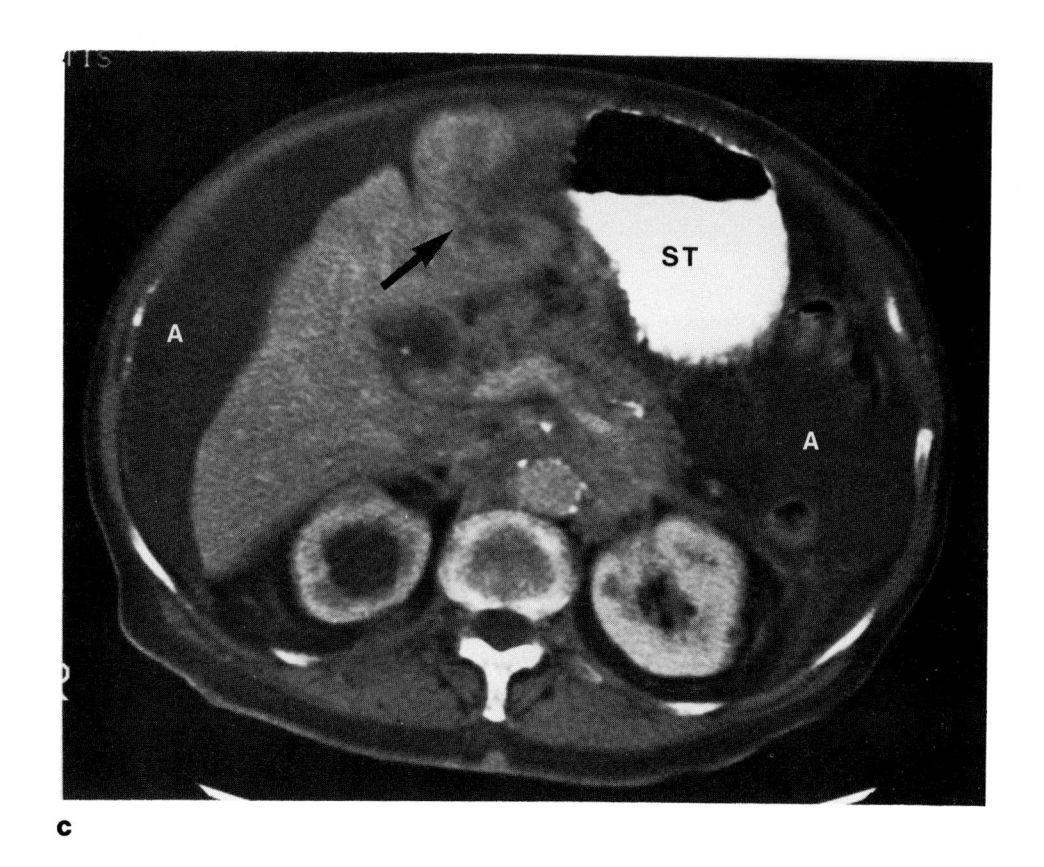

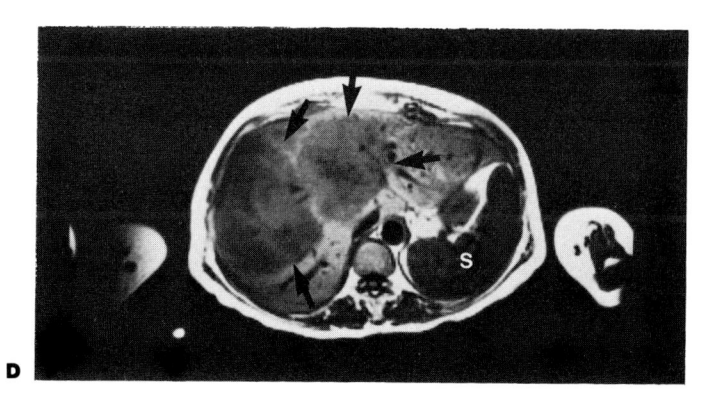

Figure 5-10. (*Continued*)

161

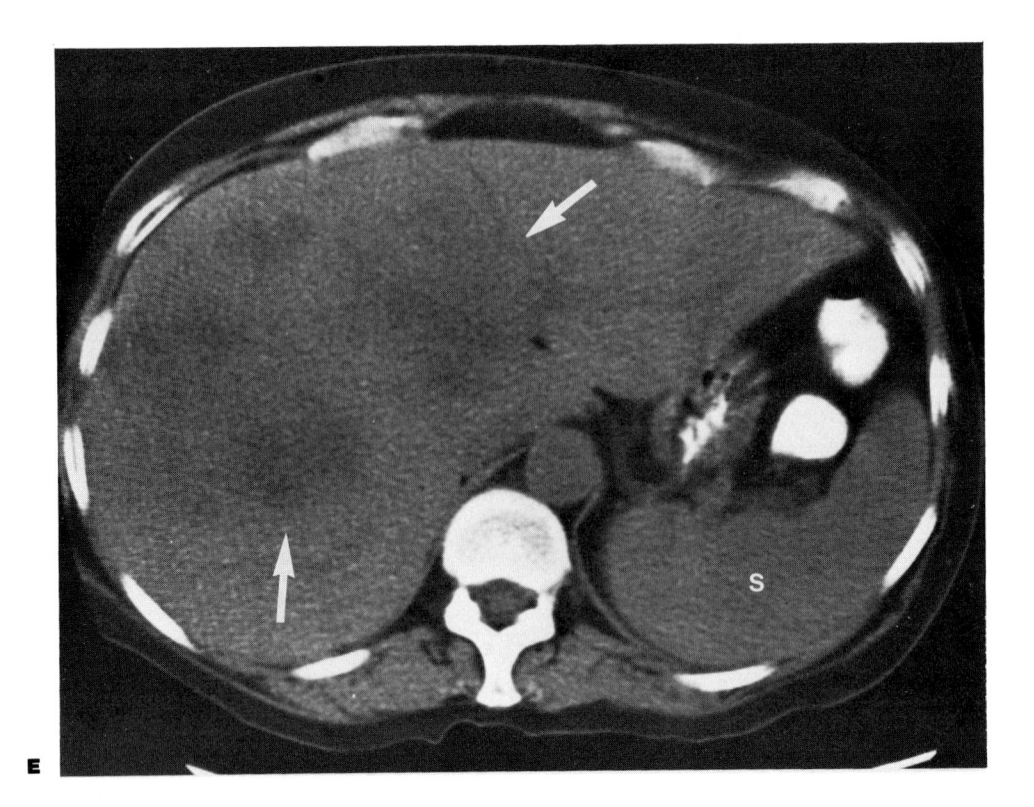

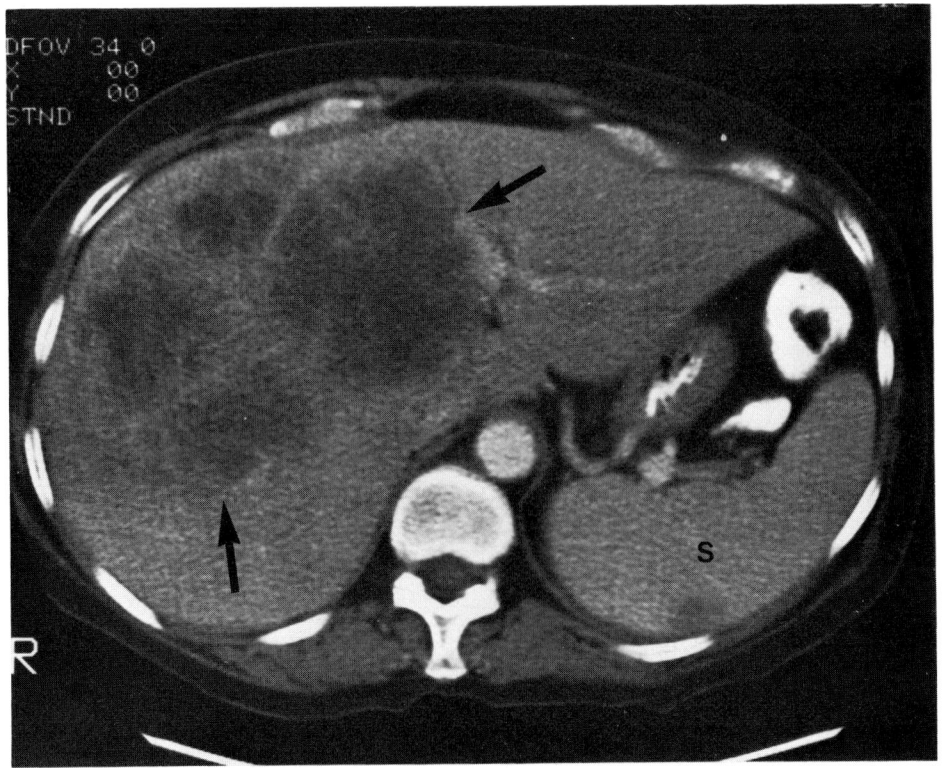

Figure 5-10. (*Continued*) The extent and size of the metastatic disease is poorly defined on the non-contrast-enhanced computed tomogram (*E*) (arrows), although somewhat better defined on the contrast-enhanced computed tomogram (*F*) (arrows). ST = stomach; S = spleen.

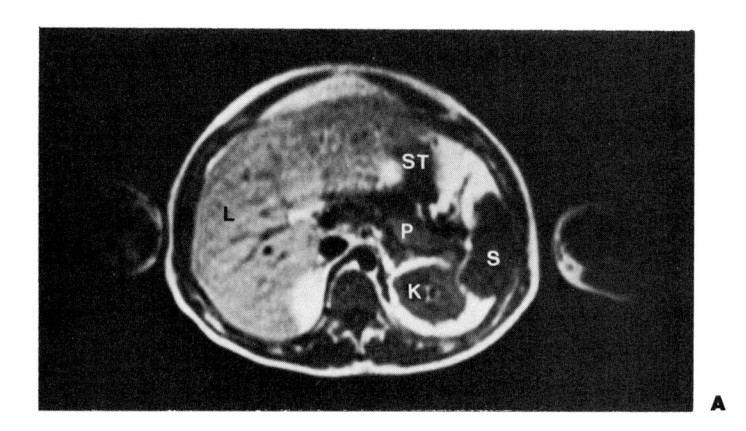

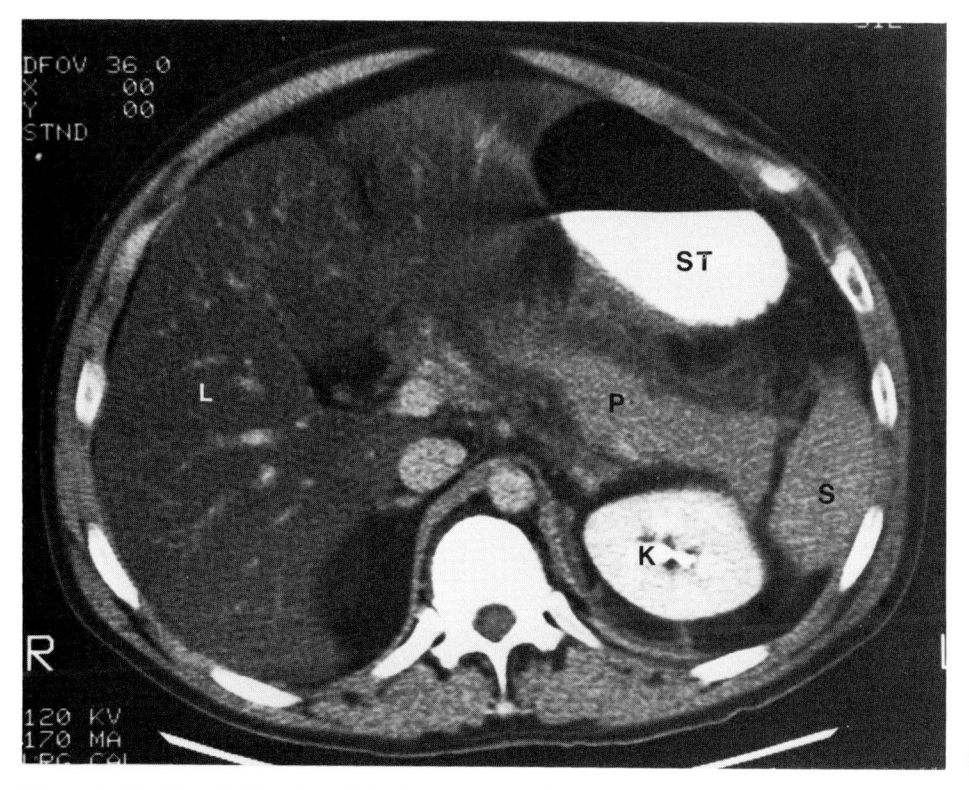

Figure 5-11. Fatty infiltration of the liver: computed tomography, magnetic resonance imaging comparison. Patient with extensive fatty infiltration of the liver, as well as acute pancreatitis and peripancreatic fluid collections. Note the high signal intensity of the liver on the magnetic resonance image (*A*) as compared to the more normal-appearing spleen. Computed tomograph (*B*) in this patient also demonstrates the relatively low attenuation of the liver, indicating extensive fatty infiltration. K = kidney; P = pancreas; ST = stomach; L = liver; S = spleen.

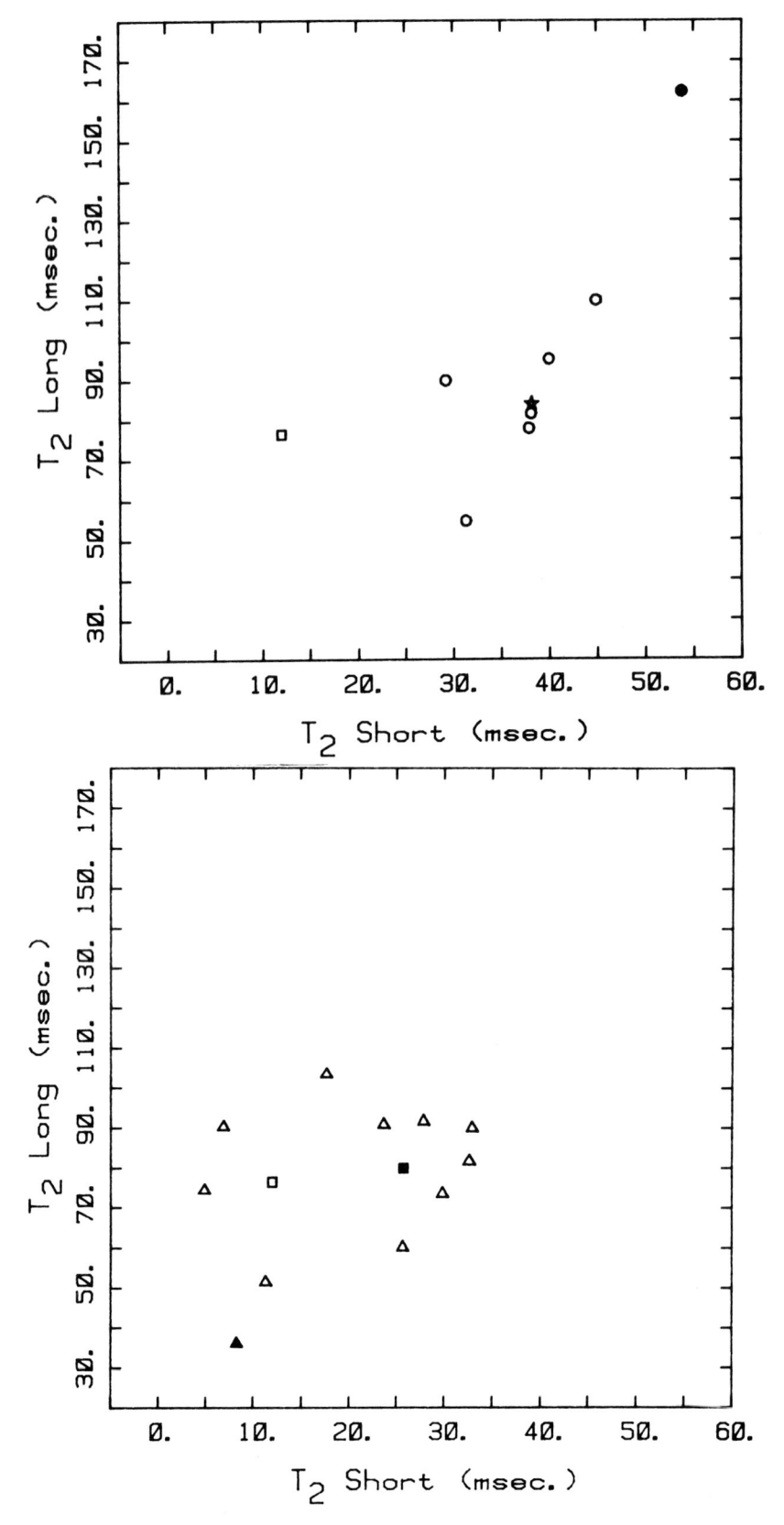

Figure 5–12. T_2 long and short values from human hepatic tissue samples demonstrate a good demarcation between malignant and diffuse hepatic disease. Tumor with necrosis (solid circle); tumor (open circle); normal (open square); normal sample from malignant liver (star); diffuse disease (open triangle); iron deposition (solid triangle); abscess (solid square).

be as small as one-half hour. T_2 values, when kept at room temperature and unfixed, are stable up to 48 hours. These same values are stable at less than one-half hour when the sample is placed in fixative. The degradation of the values seems to be related to water loss in the samples.

In vitro analysis of human liver samples is extremely limited at present. In one report, multiple T_2 values, instead of a single T_2 value, were found for each liver sample (30). Both a T_2 long and T_2 short were noted. It is possible that human liver tissue may actually have a third T_2 value. The different T_2 values correspond to different types of water and fat present. Thus, the molecular binding of water within different tissues may cause specific T_2 values. Further work in this area is needed before this statement can be considered definitive.

There is a good demarcation by T_2 *in vitro* analysis of diffuse hepatic disease from malignant hepatic disease (Figure 5-12). There also seems to be a correlation between the short T_2 values and the degree of cancer cellularity within the tissue specimens. There is minimal correlation between the longer T_2 value and the amount of fat within the tissue, with no correlation between either of the T_2 values and the amount of inflammation or fibrosis noted within the tissue specimens. The latter were predominantly in cirrhotic livers.

It is of note that the amount of iron within the specimens significantly influenced the T_2 values, as well as the amount of necrosis. Also, one of the specimens from this report was from a section of normal liver in a patient who had diffuse hepatic metastases. This particular specimen (although normal) demonstrated T_2 values in the range demonstrated by the malignant tissue samples. This is consistent with previous reports that have shown that significantly altered relaxation times are noted in normal tissue coming from abnormal organs (31-33). Most of these reports conclude that there is a critical threshold that must be crossed before this phenomenon is noted. This threshold might be finite involvement of the organ by malignancy. How much malignancy is not known at present. Thus, spectroscopy offers not only the ability to distinguish the chemical changes within the liver and relaxation times related to these changes, but also the possibility of determining malignant disease, either noninvasively or earlier than by present diagnostic techniques. This may have more significance in patients who have diffuse hepatic neoplastic processes such as lymphoma which are the most difficult to detect by present radiographic means.

REFERENCES

1. Shaw D: Fourier Transform NMR Spectroscopy. Amsterdam: Elsevier, 1976.
2. Farrar TC, Becker ED: Pulse and Fourier Transform NMR. New York: Academic Press, 1971.
3. Pykett IL, Newhouse JH, Buonanno FS, et al.: Principles of nuclear magnetic resonance imaging. Radiology 1982;143:157.
4. Abragam A: The Principles of Nuclear Magnetism. London: Oxford University Press (Clarendon), 1961.
5. Fullerton GD: Basic concepts for nuclear magnetic resonance imaging. Magnetic Resonance Imaging 1982;1:39-55.
6. Rosen BR, Brady TJ: Principles of nuclear magnetic resonance for medical applications. Semin Nucl Med 1983;13:308-318.
7. Mansfield P, Morris PG: NMR Imaging in Biomedicine. New York: Academic Press, 1982.
8. Kaufman L, Crooks LE, Margulis AR: Nuclear Magnetic Resonance Imaging in Medicine. New York, Tokyo: Igaku-Shoin, 1981, chaps. 1, 2.
9. Borromley PA: NMR imaging techniques and applications: a review. Rev Sci Instrum 1982;53:1319

10. Salles-Cunha SX, Halback RE, Battocletti JH, Sances A Jr: The NMR blood flowmeter—applications. Med Phys 1982;8(4):452–458.
11. Steiner RE: New imaging techniques: their relation to conventional radiology. Br Med J (Clin Res) 1982;284(6329):1590–1592 (review).
12. Taylor DG, Bore CF: A review of the magnetic resonance response of biological tissue and its applicability to the diagnosis of cancer by NMR radiology. Comput Tomogr 1981;5(2):122–173.
13. Wehrli FW, MacFall JR, Newton TH: Parameters determining the appearance of NMR images. In TH Newton, DG Potts (eds), Advanced Imaging Techniques. Clavadel Press, 1982.
14. Pukett IL: Instrumentation for nuclear magnetic resonance imaging. Semin Nucl Med 1983;13:319–328.
15. Budinger TF: Nuclear magnetic resonance in vivo studies: known thresholds for health effects. J Comput Assist Tomogr 1981;5:800–811.
16. New PFJ, Rosen BR, Brady TJ, et al.: Potential hazards and artifacts of ferromagnetic and nonferromagnetic surgical and dental materials and devices in nuclear magnetic resonance imaging. Radiology 1983;147:139.
17. Pavlicek W, Geisinger N, Castel L, et al.: The effects of nuclear magnetic resonance on patients with cardiac pacemakers. Radiology 1983;147:1489.
18. Davis PL, Crooks SL, Arakawa M, et al.: Potential hazards in NMR imaging: heating effects of changing magnetic fields and RF fields on small metallic implants. Am J Roentgenol 1981;137(4):857–860.
19. Axel L, Margulis AR, Meaney TF: Glossary of NMR Terms. Chicago: American College of Radiology, 1983.
20. Borokowski GP, Buonocore E, George CR, et al.: Nuclear magnetic resonance (NMR) imaging in the evaluation of the liver: a preliminary experience. J Comput Assist Tomogr 1983;7:768–774.
21. Smith RW, Mallard JR, Rein A, et al.: Nuclear magnetic resonance tomographic imaging in liver disease. Lancet 1981;1(8227):963–966.
22. Davis PL, Kaufman L, Crooks LE, et al.: Detectability of hepatomas in rat livers by nuclear magnetic resonance imaging. Invest Radiol 1981;16(5):354–359.
23. Moss AA, Goldberg HI, Stark DB, et al.: Hepatic tumors: magnetic resonance and CT appearance. Radiology 1984;150:141–147.
24. Higgins CB, Goldberg H, Hricak H, et al.: Nuclear magnetic resonance imaging of musculature of abdominal viscera: normal and pathologic features. AJR 1983;140:1217–1225.
25. Higgins CB, Hricak H, Gamsu G, et al.: Clinical nuclear magnetic resonance imaging of the body. Semin Nucl Med 1983;13:347–363.
26. Stark DD, Bass NM, Moss AA, et al.: Nuclear magnetic resonance imaging of experimentally induced liver disease. Radiology 1983;148:743–751.
27. Stark DD, Goldberg HI, Moss AA: Chronic liver disease: evaluation by magnetic resonance. Radiology 1984;150:149–151.
28. Runge VM, Clanton JA, Smith FW, et al.: Nuclear magnetic resonance of iron and copper disease states. AJR 1983;141:943–948.
29. Thickman DI, Kundel HL, Wolf G: Nuclear magnetic resonance characteristics of fresh and fixed tissue: the effect of elapsed time. Radiology 1983;148:183–185.
30. Bernardino ME, Small B, Goldstein J, et al.: Multiple NMR T_2 relaxation values in human liver tissue. AJR 1983;141:1203–1208.
31. Hazelwood CF, Cleveland G, Medina D: Relationship between hydration and proton nuclear magnetic resonance relaxation times in tissues of tumor-bearing and non-tumor-bearing mice: implications for cancer detection. JNCI 1974;52:1849–1853.
32. Floyd RA, Yoshida T, Leigh JS: Changes of tissue water proton relaxation rates during early phases of chemical carcinogenesis. Proc Natl Acad Sci USA 1975;72:56–58.
33. Hollis DP, Saryan LA, Economou JS, et al.: Nuclear magnetic resonance studies of cancer v. appearance and development of a tumor systemic effect in serum and tissues. JNCI 1974;53:807–815.

6

Radiographic Evaluation of Hepatic Trauma

MICHAEL P. FEDERLE

INTRODUCTION

The incidence of significant abdominal trauma continues to rise and accounts currently for approximately 10 percent of the annual 130,000 trauma-related deaths in the United States. Over 60 percent of patients are from 10 to 40 years of age, with a striking predominance of males. Children are mostly victims of blunt trauma, while some large reviews of liver trauma in adults show a prevalence of penetrating injuries.

Injury to the liver is second only to the spleen in incidence of intraperitoneal injuries. Morbidity and mortality from hepatic trauma are related to the mechanism and extent of injury. Penetrating injuries generally have a lower mortality, about 5 percent, especially if they are due to stab wounds or low velocity gunshot wounds. Shotgun and high velocity gunshot wounds may cause massive fragmentation of the liver and are associated with proportionately greater mortality. The mortality from blunt trauma is from 15 to 45 percent in many large series (1–3). Death from isolated liver injury is uncommon, but is usually due to uncontrolled hemorrhage. Injury to other abdominal organs is associated in many cases, as are injuries to the head, chest, and limbs. The extraabdominal injuries are frequently more apparent clinically, but may mask potentially life-threatening abdominal visceral injuries.

Types of Injury

Knowledge of the various types of hepatic injuries that may result from penetrating or blunt trauma is useful in understanding the variety of radiographic findings that may be found and also in assessing the clinical implications. These include subcapsular and central parenchymal hematomas with intact hepatic capsule, lacerations of the capsule and parenchyma, and "bursting" injuries with massive capsular and parenchymal disruption.

Hepatic injuries with an intact capsule have been regarded as uncommon, but are now recognized more frequently with the availability of ultrasonography and computed tomography. Such injuries probably account for about 10 percent of hepatic traumatic lesions. They are not associated with intraperitoneal hemorrhage and are not detected by peritoneal lavage nor even, on occasion, at surgical exploration. There is growing evidence that such injuries are best managed nonoperatively in many cases, unless there are signs of expanding hematoma (4).

Lacerations of the hepatic parenchyma and capsule are the most frequent type of injury but vary in type and severity. Simple linear or stellate ("bear-claw") lacerations often result from a direct blow. If the capsule is minimally disrupted, little peritoneal hemorrhage may result, even with substantial parenchymal damage. Proper diagnosis and management of this type of injury is controversial and will be discussed further in the section on computed tomography in hepatic trauma.

More severe hepatic injuries result from high velocity gunshot wounds or massive blunt trauma, often crushing injuries. These result in massive laceration and devitalization of hepatic parenchyma. Such injuries are usually obvious clinically, and there is little role for radiography in the preoperative evaluation of such patients.

Both blunt and penetrating trauma can avulse or lacerate the gallbladder or biliary tree. If bile and blood are extravasated into the peritoneal cavity, marked peritonitis usually results with early surgical intervention. However, injuries to the biliary tree may be missed because of more compelling or obvious injuries to adjacent structures, such as hepatic parenchyma or major blood vessels. If diagnosis is delayed, there may be continued bile leakage or stenosis at the site of ductal injury. This may result in bile pseudocyst (biloma), fistulas (biliary-cutaneous, arteriobiliary), or jaundice.

RADIOGRAPHIC EVALUATION

A variety of imaging techniques are available for evaluation of hepatic trauma. All have their proponents and all may be useful or essential in specific settings. The sequence of radiographic evaluation is often dictated by the availability, interests, and expertise of the physicians involved in the care of traumatized patients. Recent experience suggests that computed tomography (CT) is emerging as the examination of choice in most cases of major or multiple trauma, but these data must be compared with other established techniques, including conventional radiography, angiography, radionuclide scintigraphy, and ultrasonography.

Conventional Radiography

Technique The standard series of films obtained in cases of abdominal trauma should include supine and erect (or left decubitus) abdominal films and an upright chest film whenever possible. Upright or decubitus films are essential in diagnosis of free intraperitoneal or intrathoracic gas or fluid and are useful in distinguishing mechanical and "adynamic" ileus.

Signs The radiographic signs of hepatic injury are often nonspecific or absent, but should be carefully sought. A combination of plain film findings, when positive, and clinical evaluation may be all that is necessary to indicate the need for laparotomy.

Hepatic injuries are frequently associated with fractures of the right lower ribs or lumbar transverse processes, and these findings should prompt careful clinical and

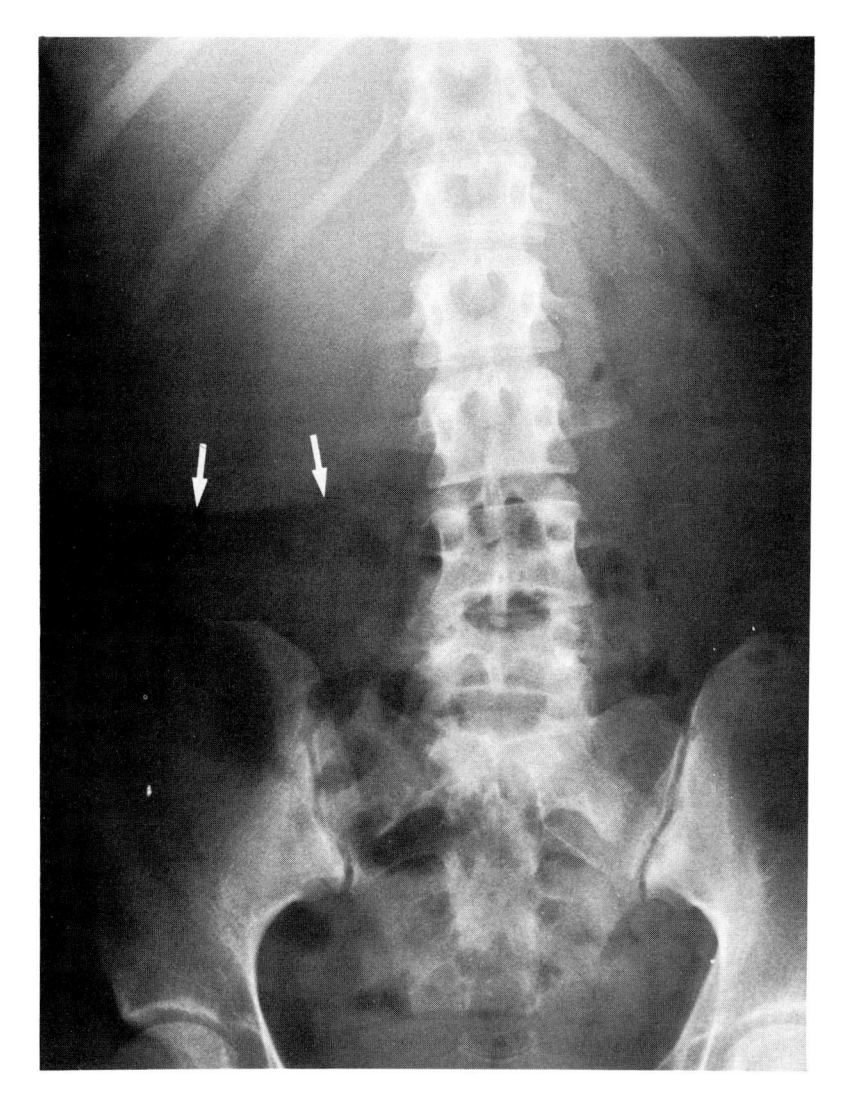

Figure 6-1. Large subcapsular hematoma; convex inferior margin of liver (arrows) displaces kidney and hepatic flexure of colon caudally.

radiographic evaluation of the liver. Intraparenchymal and subcapsular hematomas with an intact liver capsule may be manifested as hepatomegaly. Unfortunately, the liver has a wide range of normal shapes and sizes, limiting the utility of this sign. Hepatomegaly may be suggested by elevation of the right hemidiaphragm, lateral displacement of the stomach, or inferior displacement of the hepatic flexure and transverse colon (5) (Figure 6-1).

Capsular lacerations are associated with variable amounts of intraperitoneal hemorrhage, which may be detected on abdominal radiographs. Normal hemostatic forces may effectively control the bleeding with surface clotting at the laceration site. More extensive bleeding consumes clotting factors and results in free-flowing blood that collects in peritoneal recesses of the abdomen and pelvis. Morrison's pouch (hepatorenal fossa) is the most dependent recess of the upper abdomen and the most common site of blood accumulation in liver trauma. Morrison's pouch is continuous superiorly with the right subphrenic space and inferiorly with the right paracolic gutter. Important plain

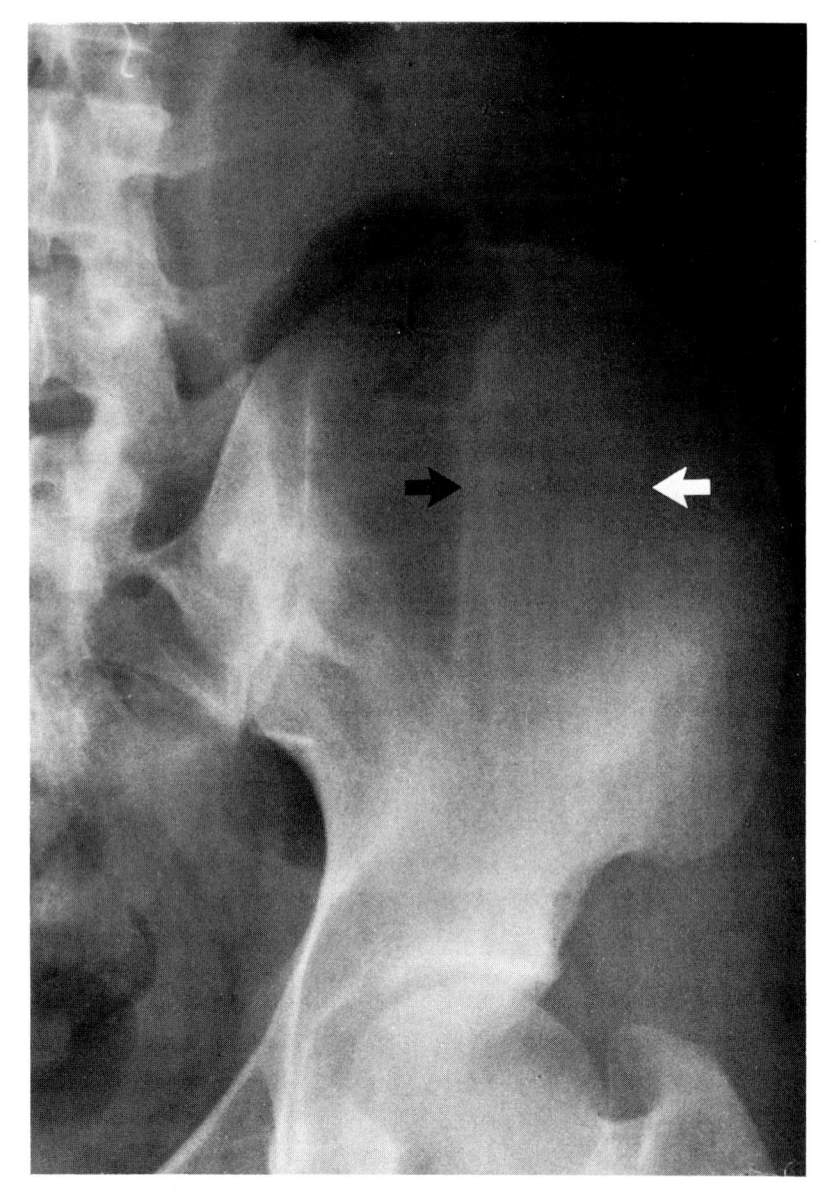

Figure 6-2. Flank-stripe sign. The gas-filled descending colon is displaced from the properitoneal fat by a water-density band of tissue (blood, arrows). Note the sharp lateral convex margin formed by parietal peritoneum.

film findings of hemorrhage in these areas are the "hepatic angle" and "flank stripe" signs.

Parietal peritoneum is reflected over the vertical retroperitoneal colon segments, ascending and descending, to form dependent troughs known as the paracolic gutters. A thin layer of intraperitoneal fat ordinarily occupies the space between the colon and the peritoneum. Just outside the peritoneum and medial to the flank musculature (transversalis and oblique muscles) is a zone of properitoneal (extraperitoneal) fat. The flank stripe is that radiolucent zone comprised of intraperitoneal and extraperitoneal fat. Normally the medial border of the flank stripe is a poorly defined undulating line representing the lateral wall of the colon. With accumulation of fluid in the paracolic gutter, a water-density band with a sharp lateral margin formed by the peritoneum separates the properitoneal fat zone from the lateral margin of the colon (Figure 6-2). Some diagnostic pitfalls may be encountered. Fluid-filled small bowel lying lateral to the colon may cause a false positive flank stripe sign, particularly on the left side. If the colon is not visualized, owing to either contraction or intraluminal fluid, the flank stripe sign is unreliable. The flank stripe is often not visible in infants and in dehydrated, elderly, or cachetic adults (6-8).

The inferior and right lateral margins of the liver (hepatic angle) are commonly identified on plain films of the abdomen. This finding is dependent on the liver (and parietal peritoneum) being applied closely to the extraperitoneal fat laterally and the greater omentum and pericolic fat inferiorly. Intraperitoneal fluid interposed between the lower edge of the liver and the omental fat obscures the hepatic angle (9) (Figure 6-3). Unfortunately, the hepatic angle may also be obscured by overlying colon, respiratory motion, or retroperitoneal hematoma.

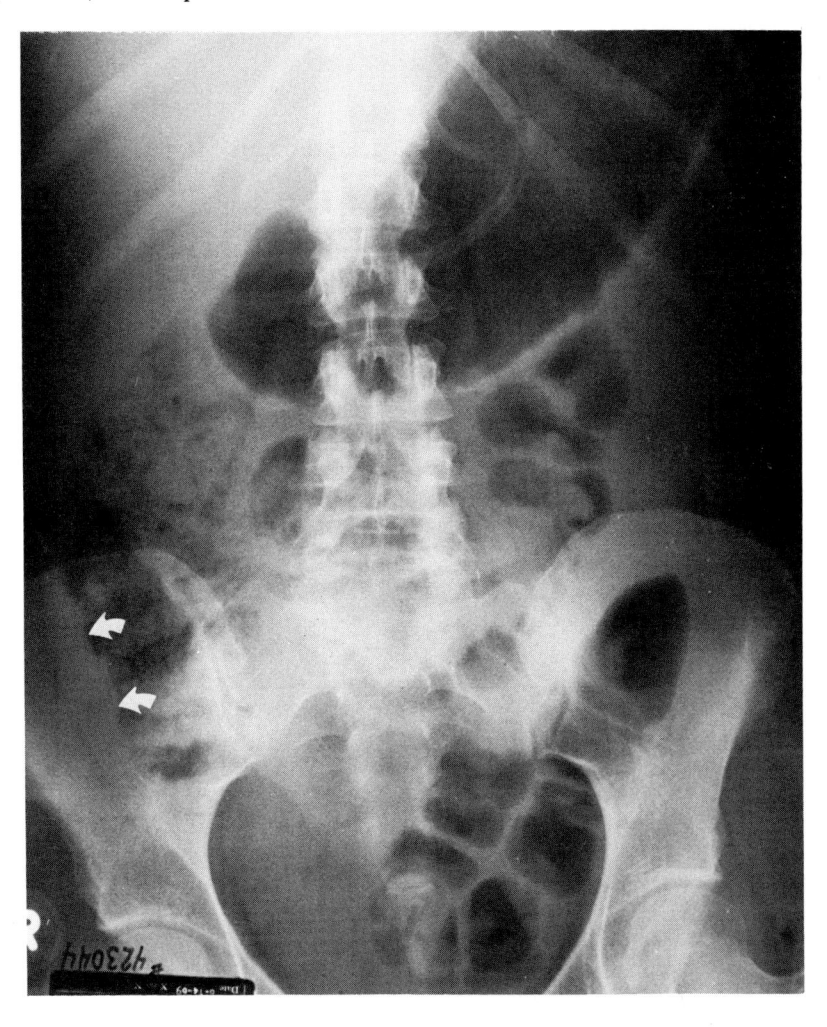

Figure 6-3. Hepatic laceration with hemoperitoneum. The right inferolateral margin of the liver (hepatic angle) is obscured. Also note blood in right paracolic gutter (arrows), a positive flank-stripe sign.

The pelvis is the most dependent portion of the peritoneal cavity in the supine or erect position and may constitute one third of its total volume. As such, large amounts of blood may accumulate in the pelvis following injury, although small amounts of blood may not be detectable on plain radiographs. Classic radiographic findings with larger accumulations of blood are due to the homogeneous density of the liquid blood displacing the gas, stool, and fluid-filled loops of bowel (8).

Blood in the perivesical spaces extending cephalad to the bladder may suggest the projecting ears of a dog, the "dog ears" sign, although rounded, pear-shaped, and other configurations may be assumed (Figure 6-4). The central homogeneous density has sharply defined convex lateral margins formed by the bulging pelvic peritoneum. Fluid-filled loops of bowel within the pelvis are a frequent source of error in diagnosing pelvic hemorrhage. Retroperitoneal hematoma, bladder diverticula, and uterine or ovarian masses may also resemble fluid collections. A characteristic that may help distinguish intraperitoneal from extraperitoneal hemorrhage is the preservation of margins of extraperitoneal pelvic structures, such as the bladder and obturator internus muscles with intraperitoneal bleeding.

Advantages and Limitations Conventional radiography is relatively inexpensive and available in virtually all emergency departments. In some cases, plain radiographs may provide sufficient information on which to plan management. For example, a blunt trauma victim with plain film findings of fractured right lower ribs and large amounts

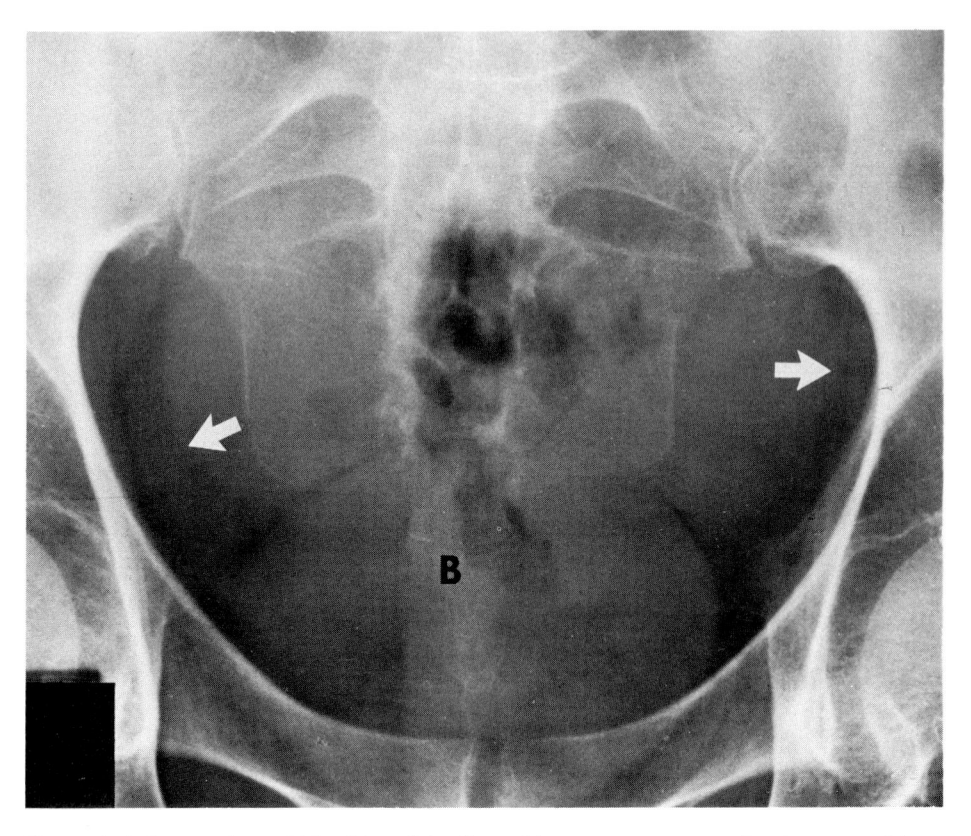

Figure 6-4. Intraperitoneal blood in pelvis. Central homogeneous water-density mass with sharply defined convex lateral margins formed by the bulging pelvic peritoneum (arrows). Note the intact fat plane between the blood and the urinary bladder (B).

of intraperitoneal fluid could be presumed to have a liver laceration. Plain radiographs, however, are usually not sufficiently sensitive or specific to plan therapy. Cadaver experiments have demonstrated that 800 mL of intraperitoneal fluid was the minimum amount that could be detected radiographically (10). Because of this, a negative plain film is of little value in excluding significant trauma.

Angiography

Technique Detailed descriptions of techniques for hepatic angiography can be found in Chapters 8–10. In the trauma setting, selective celiac or hepatic visceral injuries require, in most cases, selective catheterization of those specific arteries. Several injections of contrast material in frontal and oblique positions may be necessary to completely evaluate the liver.

Signs The angiographic findings of hepatic laceration include extravasation of contrast material, early venous filling, displacement of intrahepatic arteries due to hematoma, and mottled accumulation of contrast during the capillary phase (11–13). Subcapsular hematoma may be detected by displacement of a flattened parenchymal contour from the lateral abdominal wall (Figure 6–5). Perihepatic hemorrhage may also displace liver from the costal margin.

False-positive results are encountered due to congenital variation in the size and

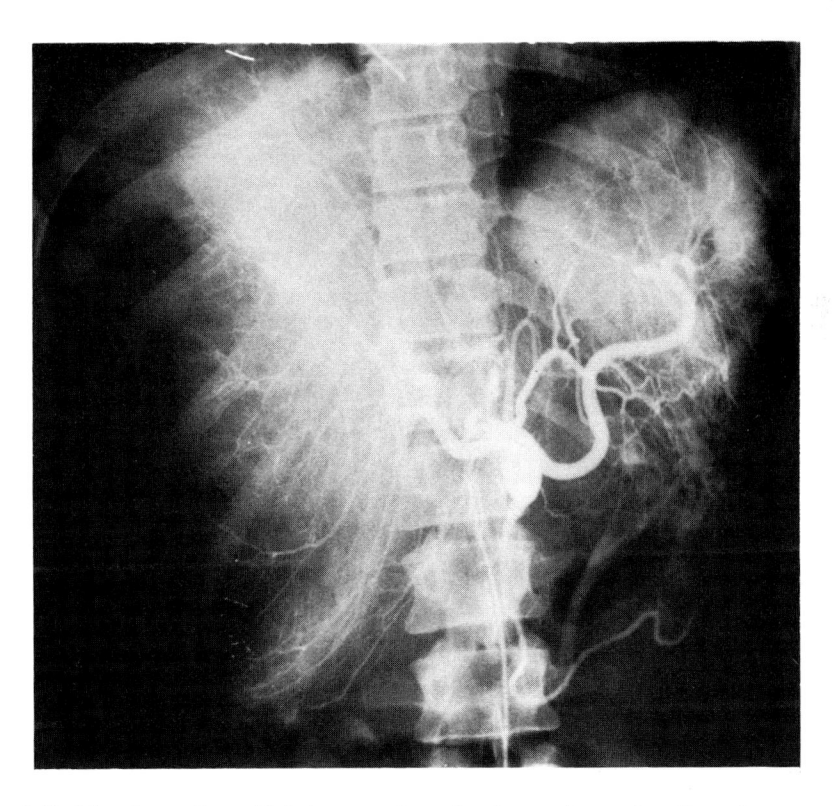

Figure 6–5. Liver laceration with intraparenchymal, subcapsular, and perihepatic hemorrhage. Intrahepatic hematoma manifested by curvilinear displacement of hepatic arteries, while subcapsular and perihepatic hemorrhage is detected by flattening and displacement of the liver edge from the abdominal wall.

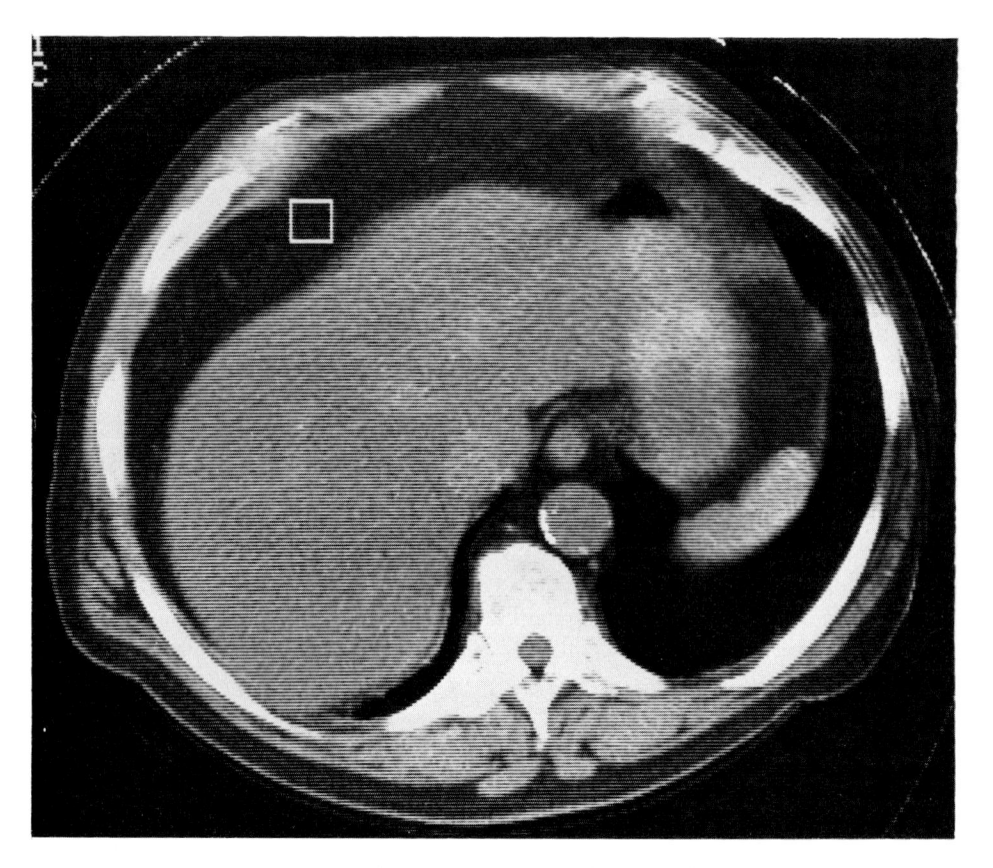

Figure 6-6. Extensive perihepatic fat (cursor box) may flatten and displace the liver margin, potentially resulting in a false-positive interpretation of an angiogram or radionuclide scan.

contour of the liver. Deep interlobar clefts may simulate parenchymal hematoma, and abundant intraabdominal fat may flatten and displace the lateral hepatic contour, simulating subcapsular hematoma (Figure 6-6). False-negative results may be caused by overlapping vessels, masking deep lacerations and hematomas; hematomas located along the superior or posterior hepatic margins are difficult to detect.

Advantages and Limitations Angiography is the most direct means of detecting arteriovenous fistulas (Figure 6-7), false aneurysms, or arteriobiliary fistulas. These conditions may result from blunt or penetrating trauma and are sometimes self-limited. If there is clinical suspicion of ongoing vascular injury, arteriography should be performed, usually as an elective procedure after a period of initial resuscitation and observation.

Angiography suffers many inherent limitations that markedly reduce its value in evaluation of acute hepatic trauma. A major limitation is the complexity of the examination itself, requiring patient transport to the angiography suite and often multiple selective contrast material injections in various projections. This is time-consuming and not without risk in a badly traumatized patient. Other limitations are due to the nontomographic nature of angiographic images and the reliance on indirect signs of injury, such as displaced blood vessels. Even when angiography successfully detects an hepatic parenchymal injury, it cannot detect the presence or amount of intraperitoneal hemorrhage, which is often a major criterion for operative versus nonoperative management.

Even though angiography was first reported to be of value in hepatic trauma more than 15 years ago, it has never gained widespread acceptance, and we rarely utilize angiography in evaluation of acute hepatic trauma.

Radionuclide Scintigraphy

Technique

Sulfur Colloid Liver-Spleen Scan Technetium^{99m} sulfur colloid is injected intravenously and the uptake of the radiocolloid in the hepatic reticuloendothelial cells is imaged on a gamma camera. Multiple (at least eight) projections are recorded on film.

Cholescintigraphy Tc^{99m} dimethyliminodiacetic acid and its derivative (HIDA and PIPIDA) are selectively taken up in the liver and excreted into the biliary tree. Gamma camera records of the flow of this radionuclide can be useful in demonstrating cystic duct obstruction in the setting of acute cholecystitis. Obstruction or laceration of the biliary tree from trauma can be detected similarily by serial scintigraphy over the liver and upper abdomen following intravenous injection of the radionuclide.

Signs Minor hepatic ruptures (subcapsular hematomas) may be manifested by flattening of the lateral organ contour and displacement from the lateral abdominal wall (Figure 6-8). Damaged parenchyma and hematomas appear as linear, wedge-shaped, or stellate defects within the organ. The defects, or areas of nonfunction ("photopenic areas"), may appear larger than the volume of the hematoma because the surrounding compressed tissue is often hypofunctioning (14–16).

Hepatic scintiscans must be interpreted with consideration of the numerous variations in shape and contour that the liver may exhibit normally. Deep gallbladder or renal fossae or interlobar fissures may simulate lesions. The photopenic defects are not specific for hematomas, but are seen with any space-occupying lesion, including cyst, tumor or abscess.

The detection of bile leakage by radionuclide cholescintigraphy will be discussed further in the section on cholangiography.

Advantages and Limitations Hepatic radionuclide sulfur colloid scans are simple to perform, relatively inexpensive, and widely available, though nuclear medicine departments are sometimes far removed from emergency departments. False-negative results are uncommon, though false-positive results occur in 7 to 10 percent of cases (14–16).

Disadvantages of radionuclide evaluation include the "organ specificity" of the exam and the lack of anatomical resolution. Sulfur colloid liver-spleen scans cannot evaluate other visceral injuries. Moreover, detection of a parenchymal laceration/hematoma alone is not sufficient to properly guide therapy, since the presence and amount of hemoperitoneum is at least as important a criterion for surgical intervention.

Cholangiography

Technique In the trauma setting, occlusion or laceration of the biliary system can be specifically diagnosed by direct injection of positive contrast material into the bile ducts or by radionuclide cholescintigraphy as previously described. Cholangiograms may be obtained by endoscopic retrograde injections (ERCP), percutaneous thin-needle transhepatic injection (PTC), or catheter injections of biliary-cutaneous fistulas.

Signs Injuries to the biliary tree that are not immediately detected and surgically corrected may lead to chronic bile leakage, bile duct stenosis, or both. Intrahepatic or extrahepatic bilomas (bile pseudocysts) result more commonly from penetrating rather

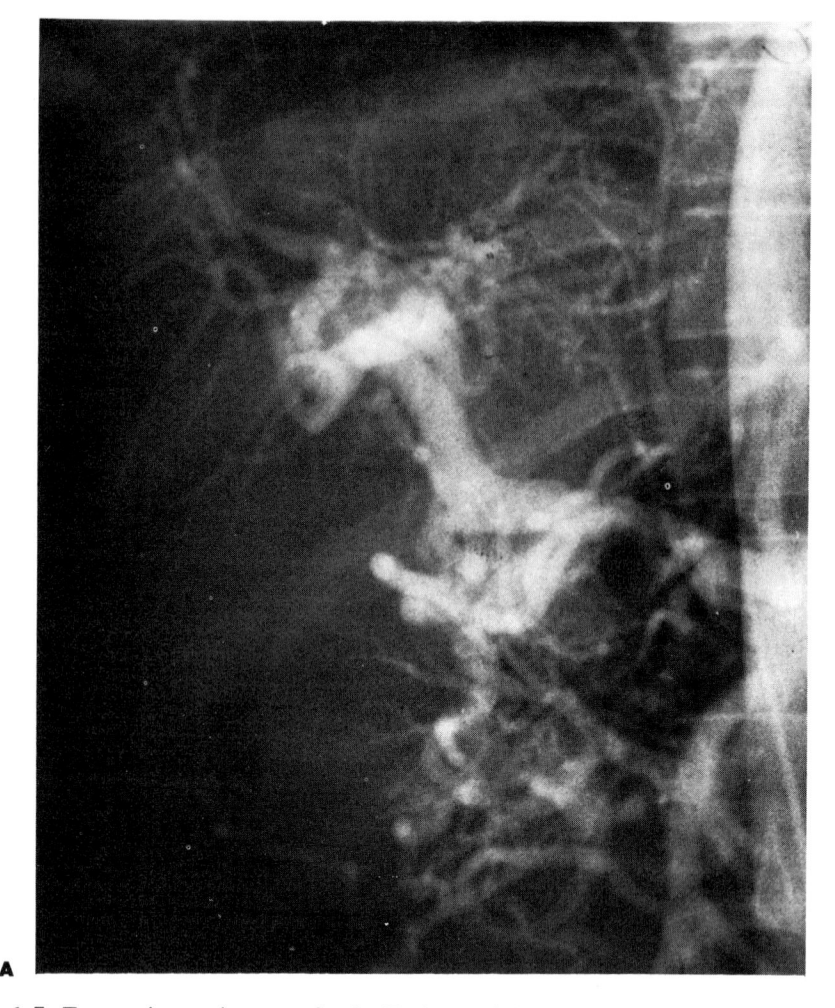

Figure 6-7. Traumatic arteriovenous fistula. Early arterial phase (*A*) and later arterial phase (*B*) show early opacification of the portal vein (arrows).

than blunt trauma (17,18). Diagnosis is often delayed by days to years after the initial injury. Symptoms occur as the biloma grows by continued bile leakage. Jaundice, hemobilia, or fever (due to secondary infection of the biloma) are often the presenting signs.

Bilomas are easily detected by ultrasonography (Figure 6-9) or computed tomography (18-21) (Figures 6-10, 6-11), but cannot be reliably distinguished from other fluid collections. Tc HIDA cholescintigraphy is useful in detecting bile leakage, seen as extravasation and progressive accumulation of radiotracer within predefined cavities on sequential images (22,23). Spontaneous resolution of bile leaks or biliary-cutaneous fistulas can also be demonstrated noninvasively by cholescintigraphy.

Direct cholangiography is most useful as a preoperative study to precisely define the site of bile leakage or stenosis (10,11).

Advantages and Limitations Tc HIDA cholescintigraphy is a noninvasive physiological means of demonstrating bile leakage or major obstruction. Its disadvantages are lack of anatomical resolution and a certain degree of operator dependency, since it may occasionally be difficult to distinguish accumulations of radiotracer in bilomas from those in gallbladder, gut, or other structures. Cholangiography is unsurpassed in its

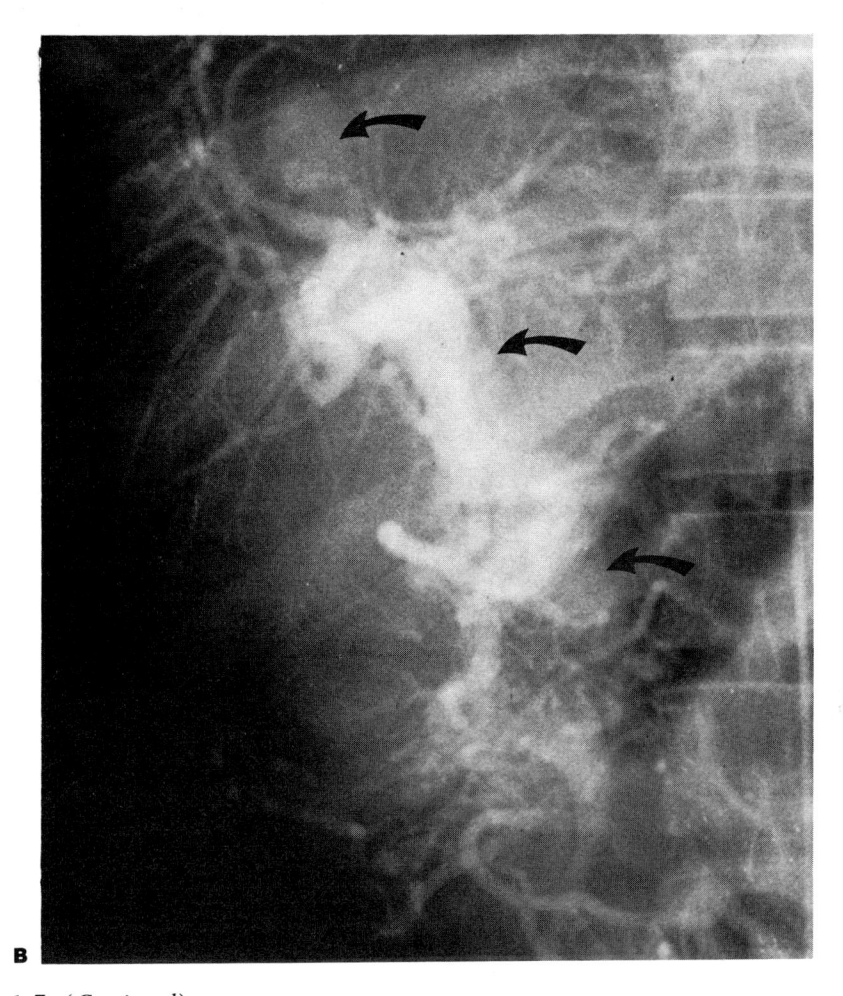

Figure 6-7. (*Continued*)

ability to directly visualize traumatic biliary injuries and is considered essential by our surgeons if operative intervention is being considered. It is an invasive and nonphysiological test, since contrast material is injected under pressure, limiting its usefulness in following a patient on conservative management for possible spontaneous resolution of a fistula.

Ultrasonography

Technique Patients with acute abdominal trauma are often difficult to adequately examine sonographically. The presence of spine, pelvic or rib fractures makes it difficult, painful or even dangerous to obtain necessary prone or decubitus views. Bandages, chest tubes, wounds, and ileus limit access to important structures. Splinting and inability to take and hold a deep inspiration limit visualization of the upper portions of the liver (and spleen). Real-time equipment is essential to maximize the area that can be scanned through small acoustic access points on the skin surface, such as between ribs.

Signs Sonographic criteria for diagnosing hepatic trauma have not been well-

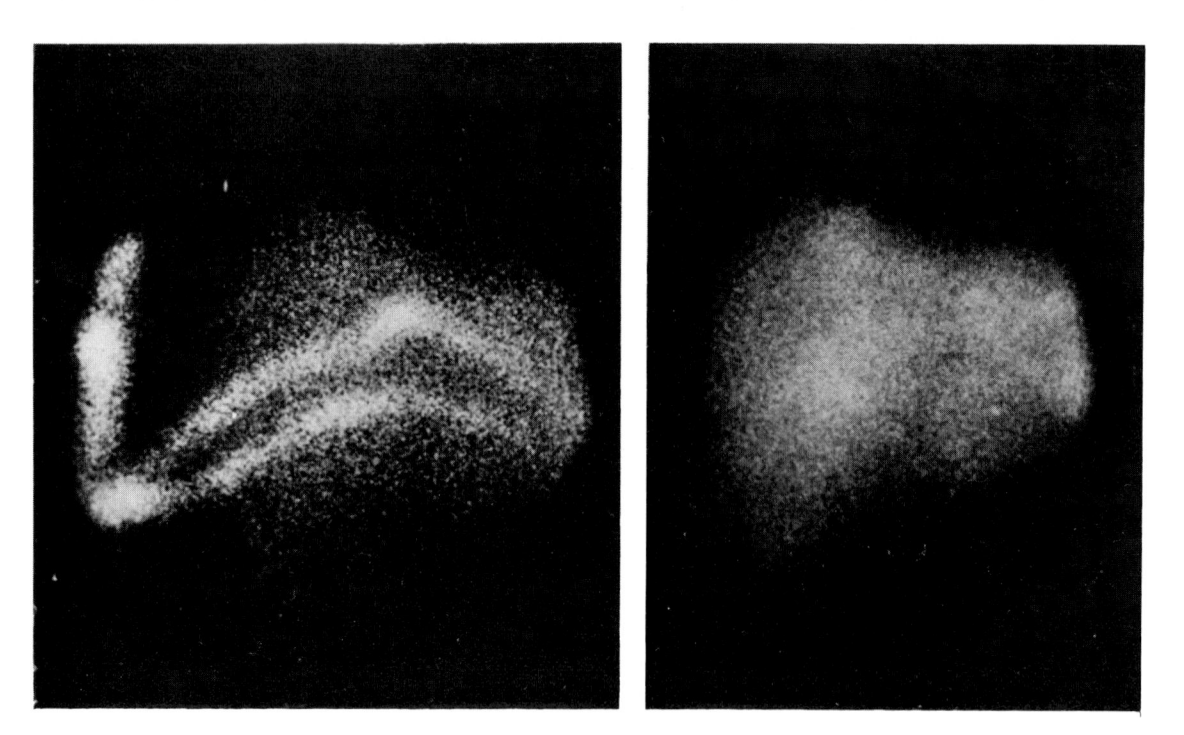

Figure 6-8. Subcapsular hematoma. Right lateral liver margin is displaced away from the lateral abdominal wall, marked by radioactive strips.

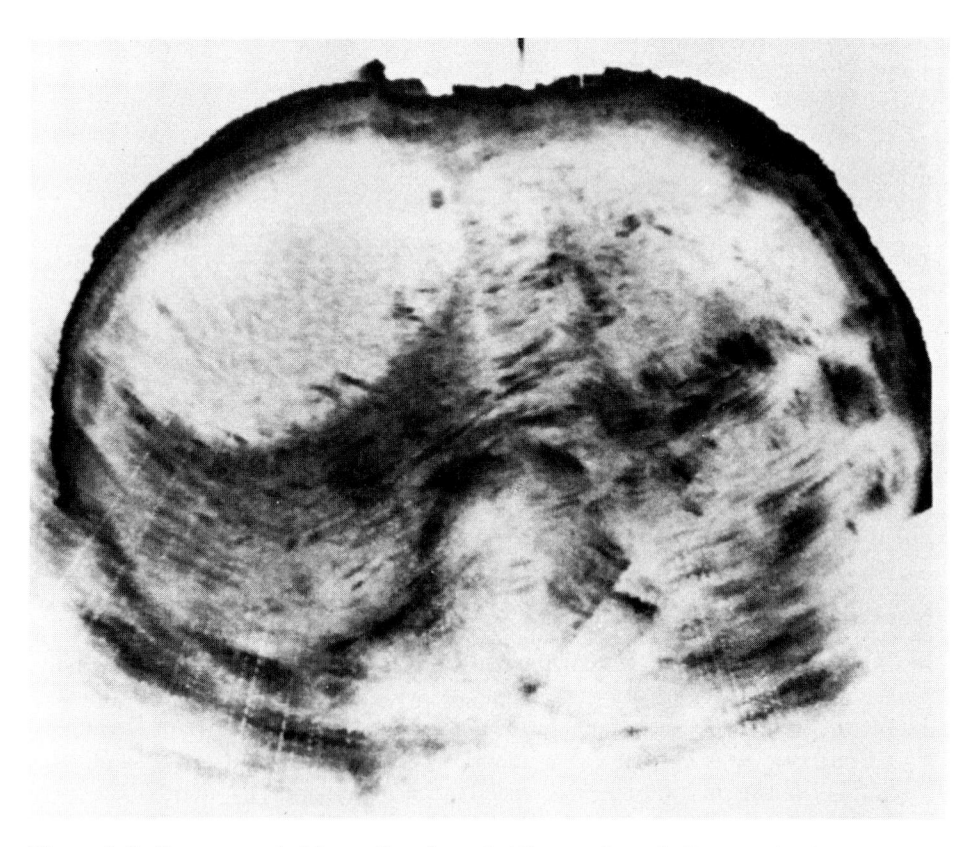

Figure 6-9. Posttraumatic biloma (intrahepatic bile pseudocyst). Sonography demonstrates poorly echogenic cystic mass with internal septations.

A

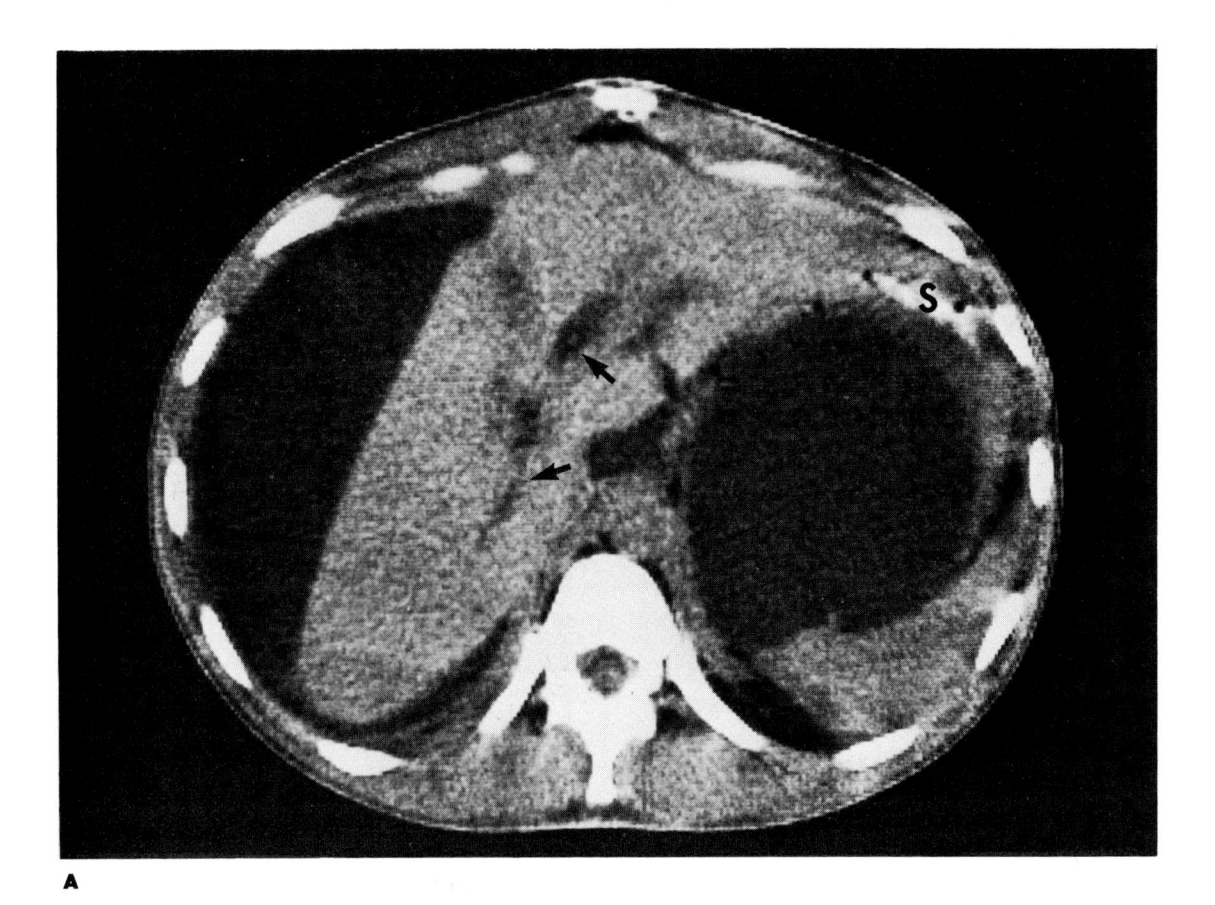

Figure 6-10. Patient presenting with increasing jaundice 1 week following laparotomy for stab wound to the epigastrium. *A.* CT scan demonstrates large fluid collections, one lateral to the liver and one in the lesser sac, displacing stomach (S) anteriorly. Intrahepatic bile ducts are also dilated (arrows). (From Federle MP, Goldberg HI, Kaiser JA, *et al.:* Evaluation of abdominal trauma by computed tomography. Radiology 1981;138:637.)

defined as experience is very limited. Signs that may be detected include linear or echogenic foci within the hepatic parenchyma (Figures 6-12, 6-13), irregular hepatic contour, and free intraperitoneal blood. Blood in or around the liver may have a variety of appearances (Figures 6-12, 6-13, 6-14) depending on the type of ultrasound transducer, the physical state of the blood (clotted or not), and age of the hematoma (16,24-26). Some hematomas may be nearly isoechoic with the liver and escape detection.

Advantages and Limitations Ultrasonography is an excellent means of detecting intraperitoneal fluid and may be accurate for parenchymal hematomas, although sufficient experience is lacking to establish the latter. The major limitation of sonography is the inability to obtain technically adequate scans in the acute trauma setting. Evaluation of blunt abdominal trauma requires the ability to image confidently all intraperitoneal and retroperitoneal viscera as well as intraperitoneal and retroperitoneal bleeding. In one recent study of sonography and radionuclide imaging for liver-spleen trauma, 19 percent of patients had inadequate sonographic exams, even for a single specific organ of interest (16). An interesting observation by the authors of this study was that some patients with left upper quadrant trauma and a clinical suspicion of

B   C

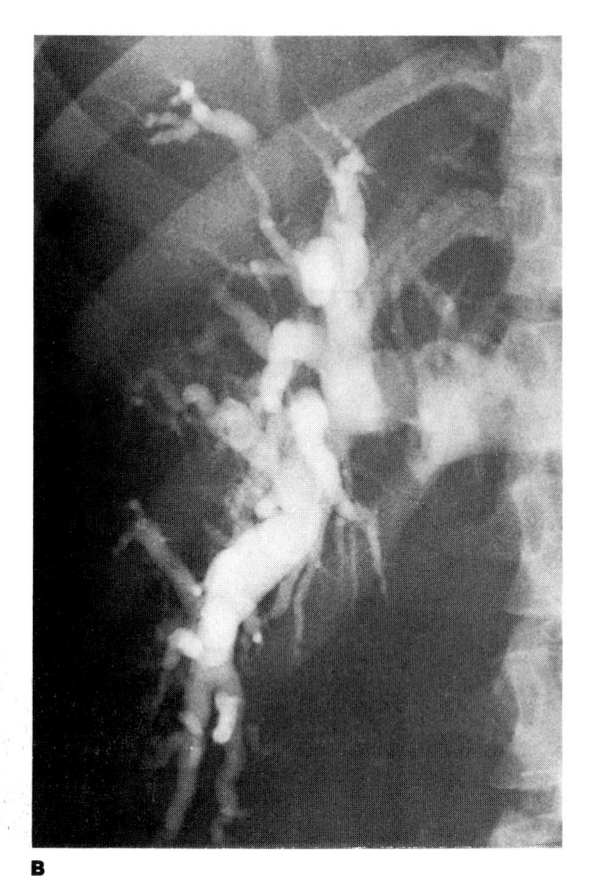

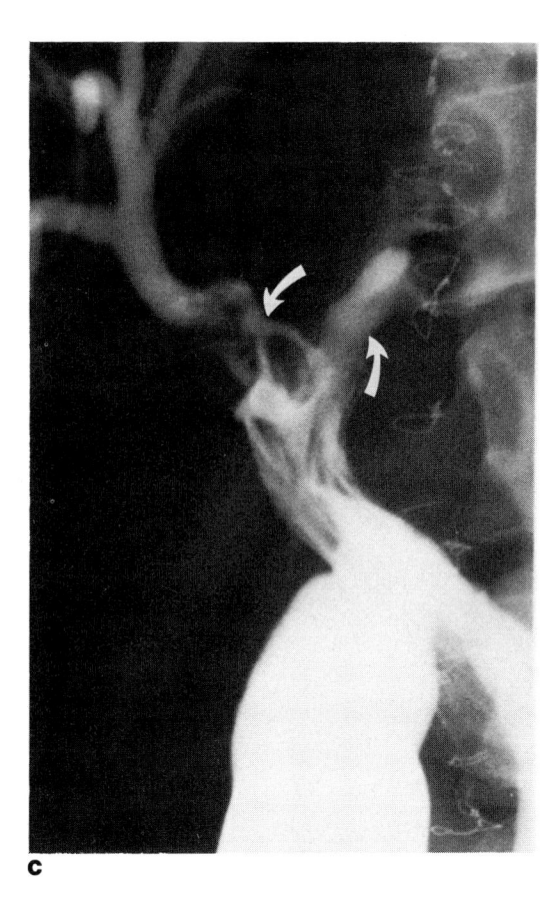

Figure 6–10. *B.* Transhepatic cholangiogram demonstrates complete obstruction of common duct. *C.* Endoscopic retrograde cholangiogram demonstrates irregular stenosis and extravasation from common hepatic duct (arrows). Reexploration confirmed these findings; bile duct injury had been overlooked at initial operation. (From Federle MP, Goldberg, HI, Kaiser JA, et al.: Evaluation of abdominal trauma by computed tomography. Radiology 1981;138:637.)

splenic trauma were found to have hepatic trauma. In Corica's review of 75 patients with liver trauma, 24 percent had concomitant splenic injuries, again emphasizing the need for comprehensive evaluation (27).

Computed Tomography

Perhaps the most dramatic new development in evaluation of hepatic (and other abdominal) trauma has been the recent application of computed tomography. Within the past few years, newer-generation high-resolution CT scanners have become available more widely in major trauma centers, with published studies totaling over 1,000 cases from various hospitals, and our own experience with over 600 cases of CT in acute blunt abdominal trauma documenting the impact of CT (19,28–32).

Technique At our trauma center, we use a standard technique for almost all cases of acute blunt abdominal trauma, regardless of a clinician's concern for a single organ of interest. Our criteria for obtaining a CT scan have been published before (33), but

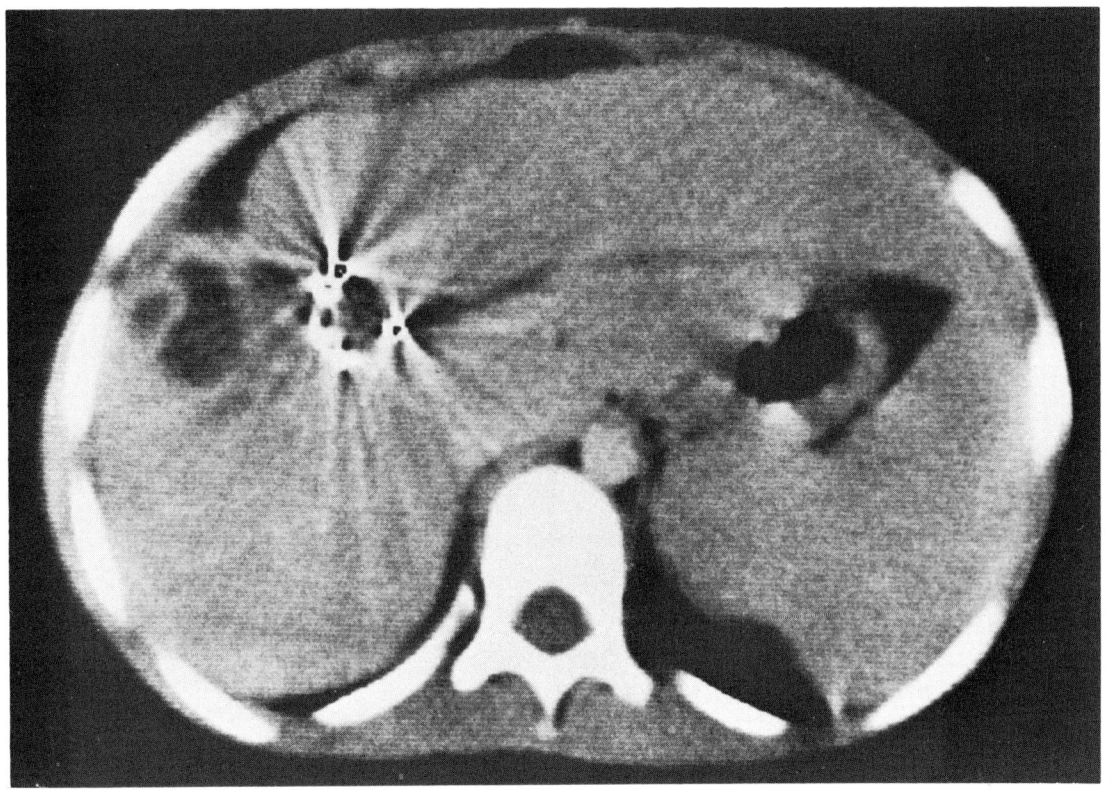

Figure 6-11. Ten-year-old girl with biliary-cutaneous fistula 2 weeks after surgery for blunt traumatic liver laceration. *A.* CT scan showing surgical clips and intrahepatic biloma.

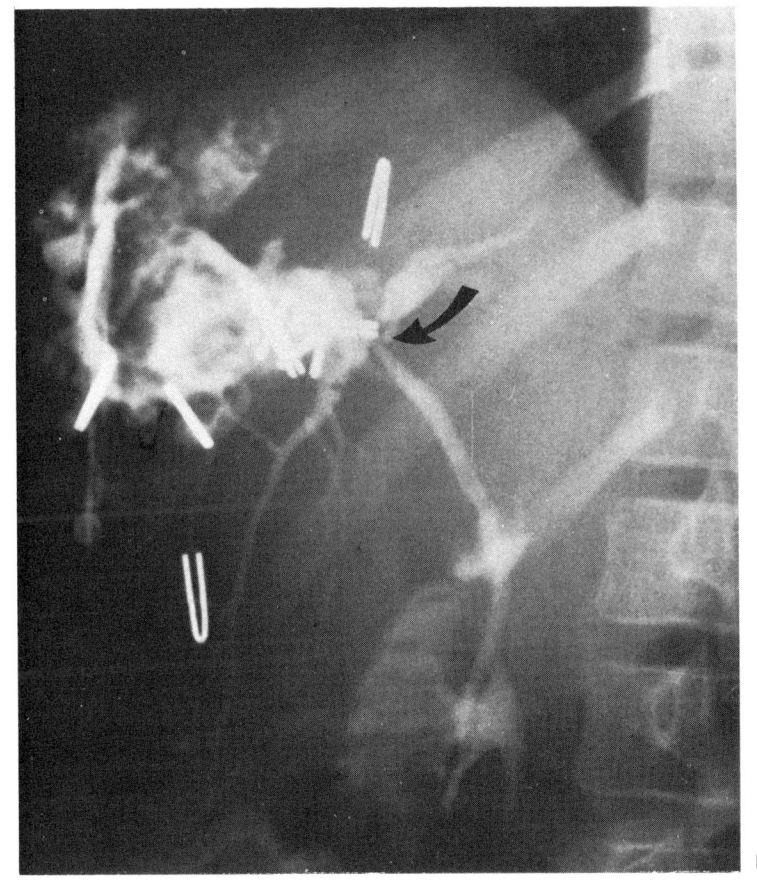

Figure 6-11. *B.* Cholangiogram performed via catheter injection of cutaneous fistula. Irregular cavity corresponds to biloma demonstrated by CT. Cholangiogram defines more accurately the point of biliary stenosis (arrow).

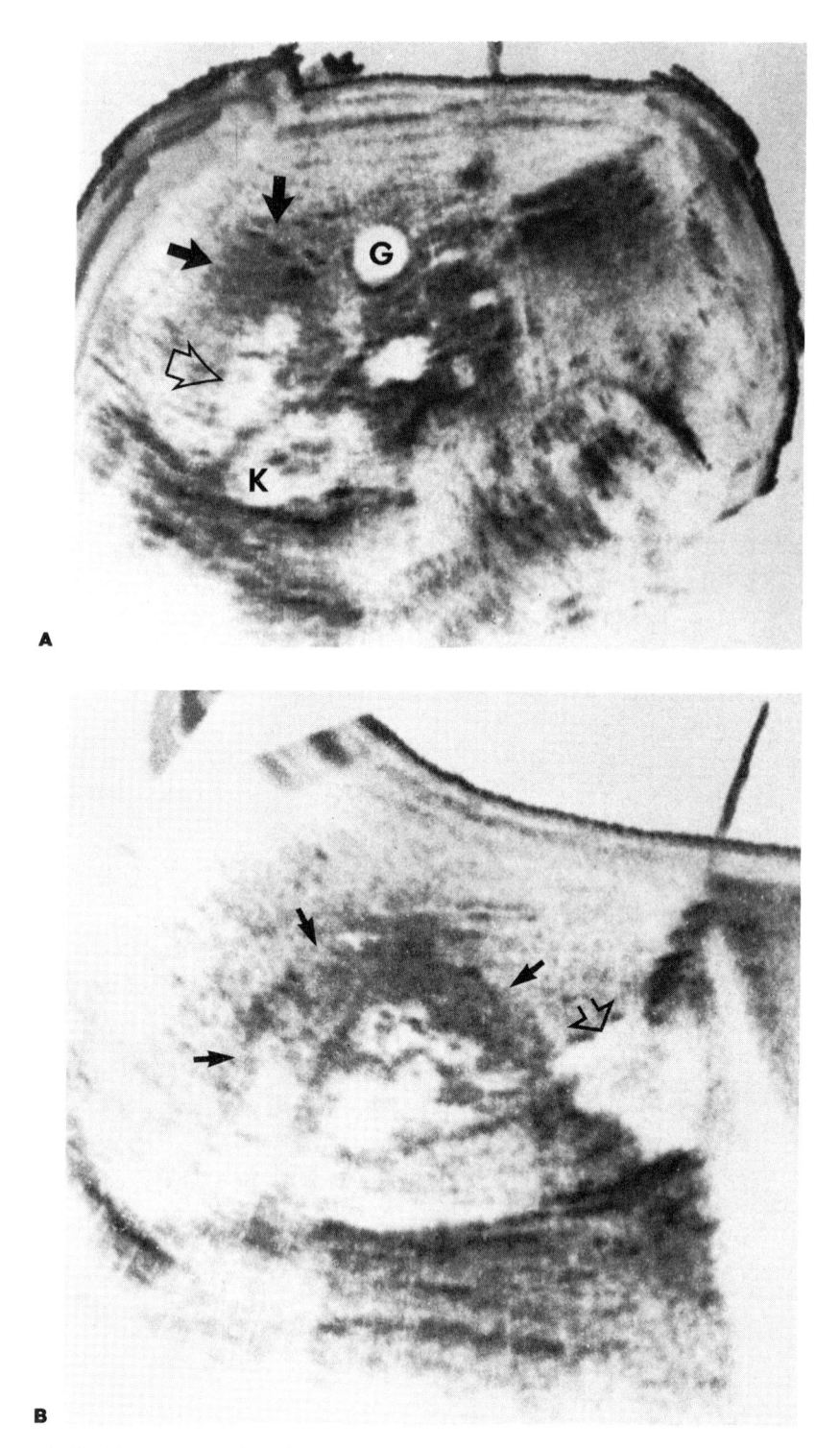

Figure 6–12. Transverse (*A*) and parasagittal (*B*) sonograms demonstrate a large irregularly echogenic hematoma in the posterior right lobe of the liver (arrows). Extrahepatic fluid collections (blood) also demonstrated near liver edge (open arrow), in flanks, and in pelvis (not shown). K = kidney; G = gallbladder.

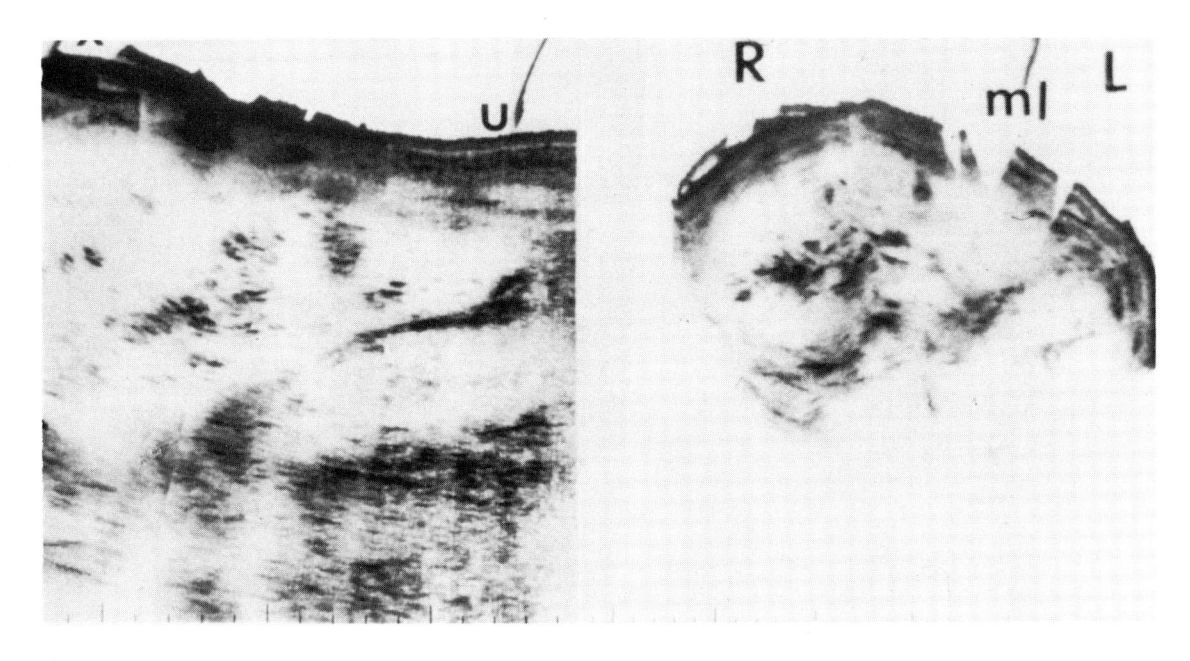

Figure 6-13. Parasagittal and transverse sonograms demonstrate irregular echogenic hematomas in the right lobe of the liver. R = right; L = left; x = xiphoid; u = umbilicus; ml = midline.

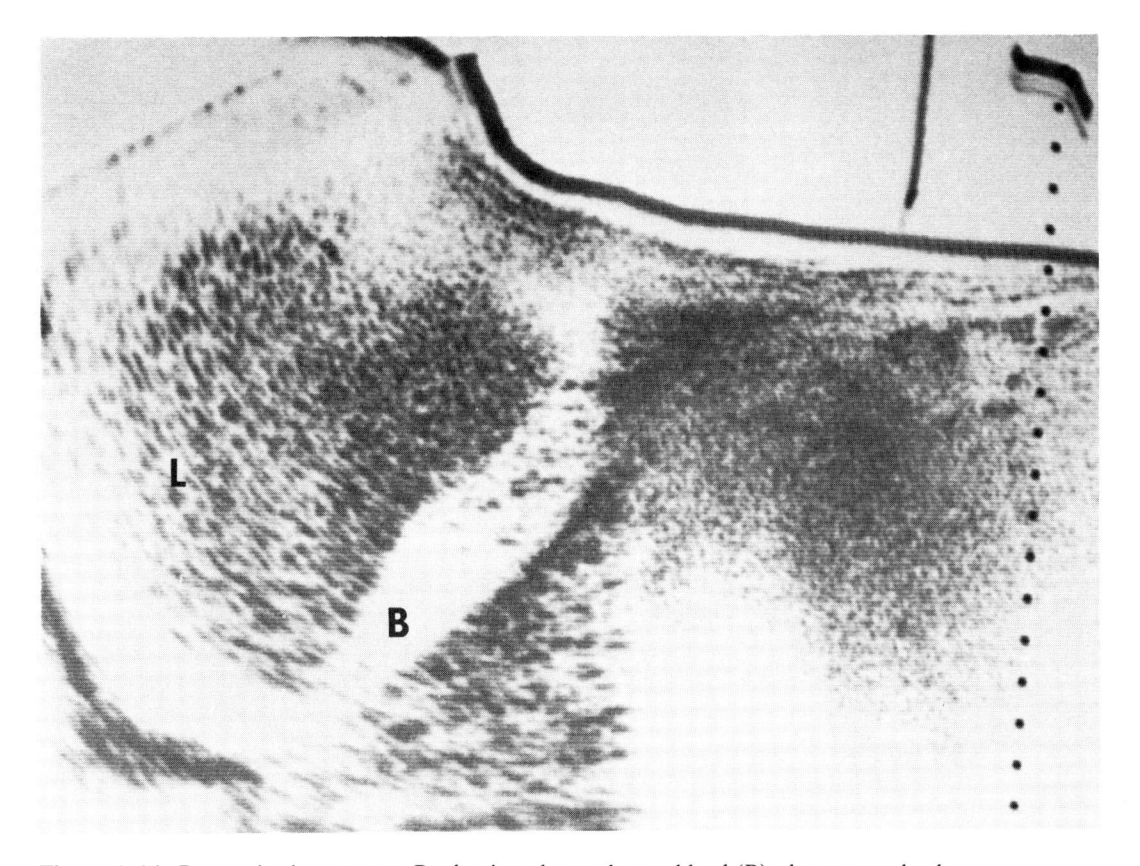

Figure 6-14. Parasagittal sonogram. Predominantly sonolucent blood (B) almost completely surrounds the right lobe of the liver (L). Decubitus views demonstrated no change in the position or appearance of the fluid, suggesting subcapsular hematoma.

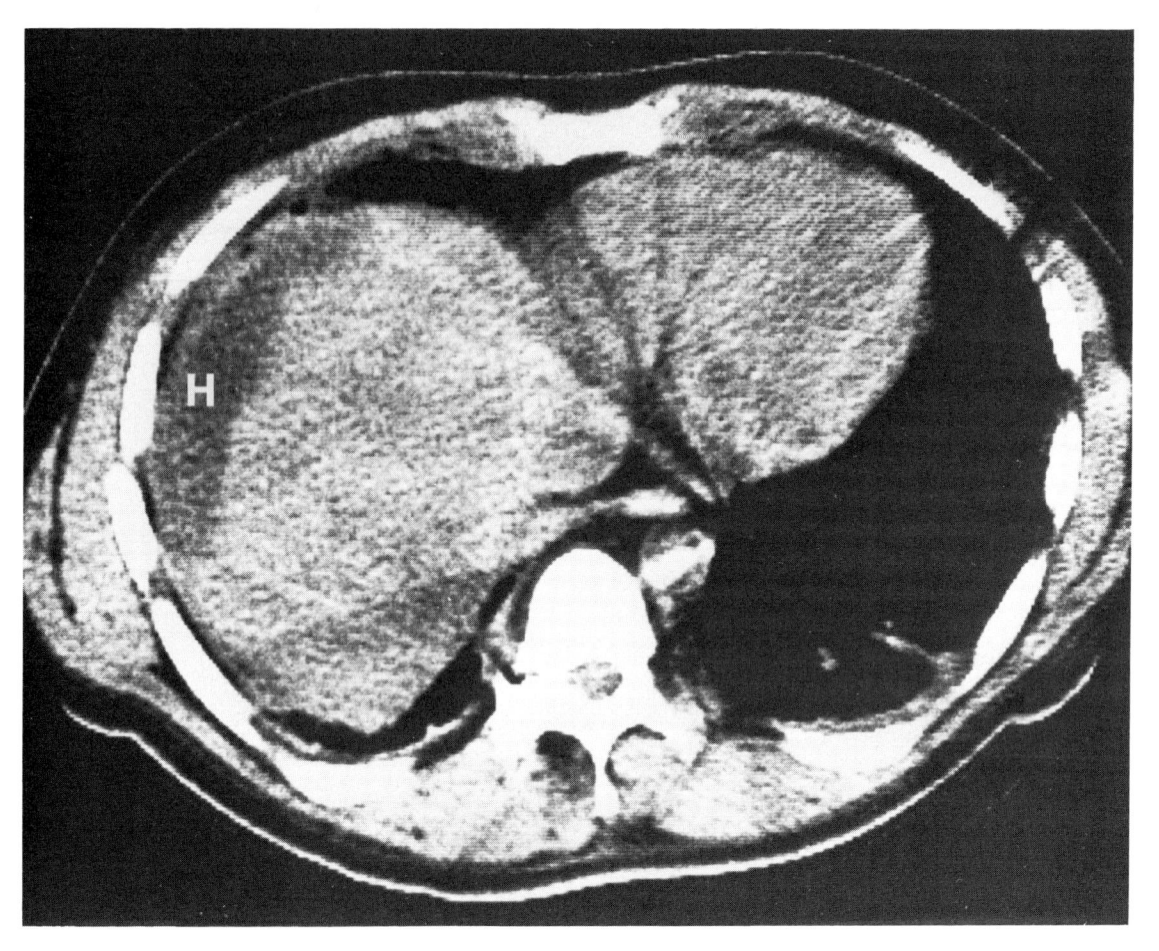

Figure 6–15. Small subcapsular hematoma (H) flattens underlying hepatic parenchyma. (From Federle MP, McCort JJ: Radiology—Abdominal trauma. In AR Margulis, HJ Burhenne (eds), Alimentary Tract Radiology, 3rd ed. St. Louis: Mosby, 1983, pp. 455–480.)

usually consist of substantial abdominal trauma with clinical, laboratory, or plain radiographic evidence suggesting visceral injury, or a suspicion of abdominal trauma in a patient for whom abdominal physical examination is unreliable (head trauma, intoxication, paraplegia, etc.). All patients receive intravenous contrast material (100 to 150 mL of 60 percent contrast) to help distinguish contrast-enhancing viscera from hematomas and to identify opacified urine that may be extravasated. All patients receive a dilute solution of GASTROGRAFIN (diatrizoate meglumine) either orally or by nasogastric tube, since unopacified bowel may be mistaken for abnormal fluid collections. CT sections are obtained at 1-cm intervals from the top of the diaphragm to the bottom of the kidneys, then at 2-cm intervals to the symphysis publis.

Signs Subcapsular hematomas typically appear as lenticular nonenhancing fluid collections that flatten or indent the underlying right lobe of liver and are limited by the hepatic capsule (Figures 6–15, 6–16). They usually occur along the anterolateral surface, often under fractured ribs, though we have seen posterior, medial, and left lobe hematomas in about 10 percent of cases.

Intraparenchymal hematomas may also occur without capsular disruption. Acute

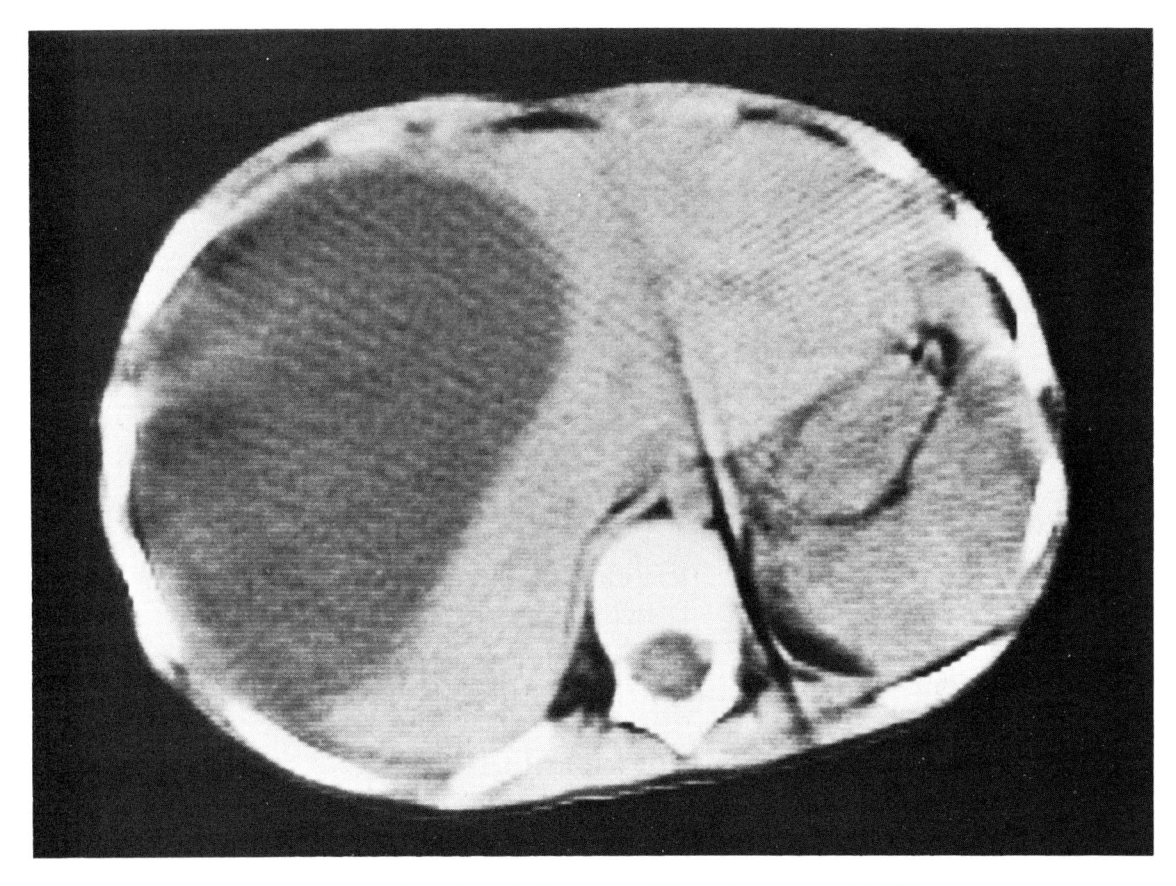

Figure 6-16. Large subcapsular and intrahepatic hematoma/biloma in a young girl. This lesion required surgical drainage, since the patient had progressive symptoms and sequential CT scans showed interval enlargement. (From Moon KL, Federle MP: Computed tomography in hepatic trauma. AJR 141:309, 1983.)

intrahepatic hematomas are typically oval or irregular in shape and heterogeneous in density (attenuation coefficient) (Figures 6-17 and 6-18). The CT appearance of hematoma depends on several factors, including the patient's hematocrit, the interval from the bleeding episode, and whether the blood is clotted. Blood extravasated into the peritoneal cavity is quickly lysed and appears relatively low in density, while hematoma within the hepatic parenchyma stays clotted for variable periods of time. Clotted blood is physically more dense and appears of higher attenuation on CT (Figure 6-18).

Hepatic lacerations with capsular disruption are manifested by free peritoneal hemorrhage in addition to the parenchymal abnormalities. The most common sites for identification of hemoperitoneum are the right subphrenic space, Morrison's pouch, right paracolic gutter and pelvis (34) (Figure 6-19). By CT, one can not only identify, but also quantify, the hemoperitoneum with important clinical implications discussed below.

Hepatic lacerations have a variety of appearances on CT. The most common is an irregular plane extending into the right lobe from the lateral surface (Figure 6-16). Fractures may have a stellate configuration, described by their appearance at surgery as "bear claw" lacerations (Figure 6-20). These may occasionally have a branching

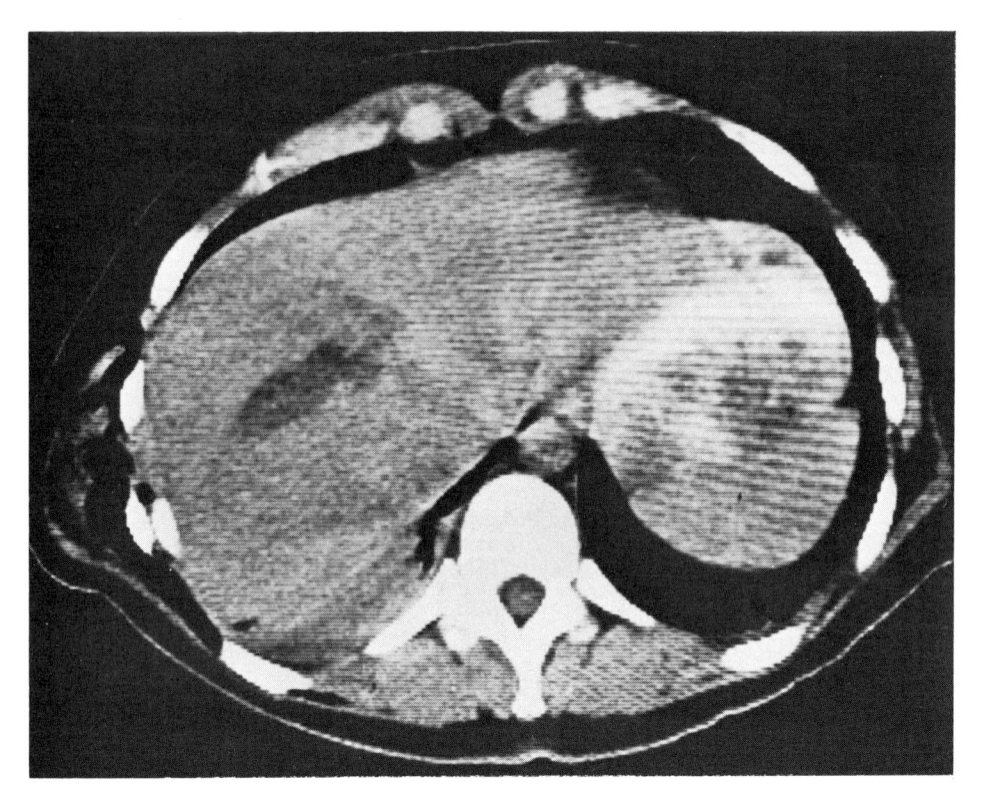

Figure 6-17. Small intrahepatic hematoma without capsular disruption. No intraperitoneal hemorrhage was identified. Note the adjacent rib fracture.

pattern that resembles a dilated biliary tree, but can be distinguished by knowledge of the expected position of bile ducts relative to other portal structures and the absence of normal arborization by parenchymal lacerations. Lacerations through the left lobe of the liver are uncommon but may present certain diagnostic problems on CT. An elongated left lobe of liver may appear separated from the right lobe by the heart on axial sections of the upper abdomen. Traumatic separation or laceration of the left lobe can be diagnosed only by careful attention to contiguous CT sections (Figure 6-21).

A final potential pitfall is CT identification of laceration or hematoma in a fatty liver (steatosis). While most hematomas are hypodense to the contrast-enhanced liver parenchyma, fatty infiltration may decrease liver density to the point of being nearly isodense or even hypodense to the hematoma (Figure 6-22). Careful attention to subtle inhomogeneities and viewing CT sections at narrow window widths permit diagnosis in such cases.

Injuries to biliary structures may be diagnosed indirectly by CT. Laceration or avulsion of the gallbladder or intrahepatic or extrahepatic bile ducts may result in intrahepatic collections of bile ("biloma" or "bile pseudocyst") or collections in the greater or lesser peritoneal cavities (Figure 6-10). While CT can reliably detect such fluid collections, differentiation from hematoma, abscess, or other collections may be difficult and require needle aspiration and fluid analysis. Radionuclide ("HIDA") scans or direct cholangiography are useful adjuncts to document continued bile leakage and to more precisely depict important surgical anatomy.

Posttraumatic hepatic arteriovenous fistulas and pseudoaneurysms may also be

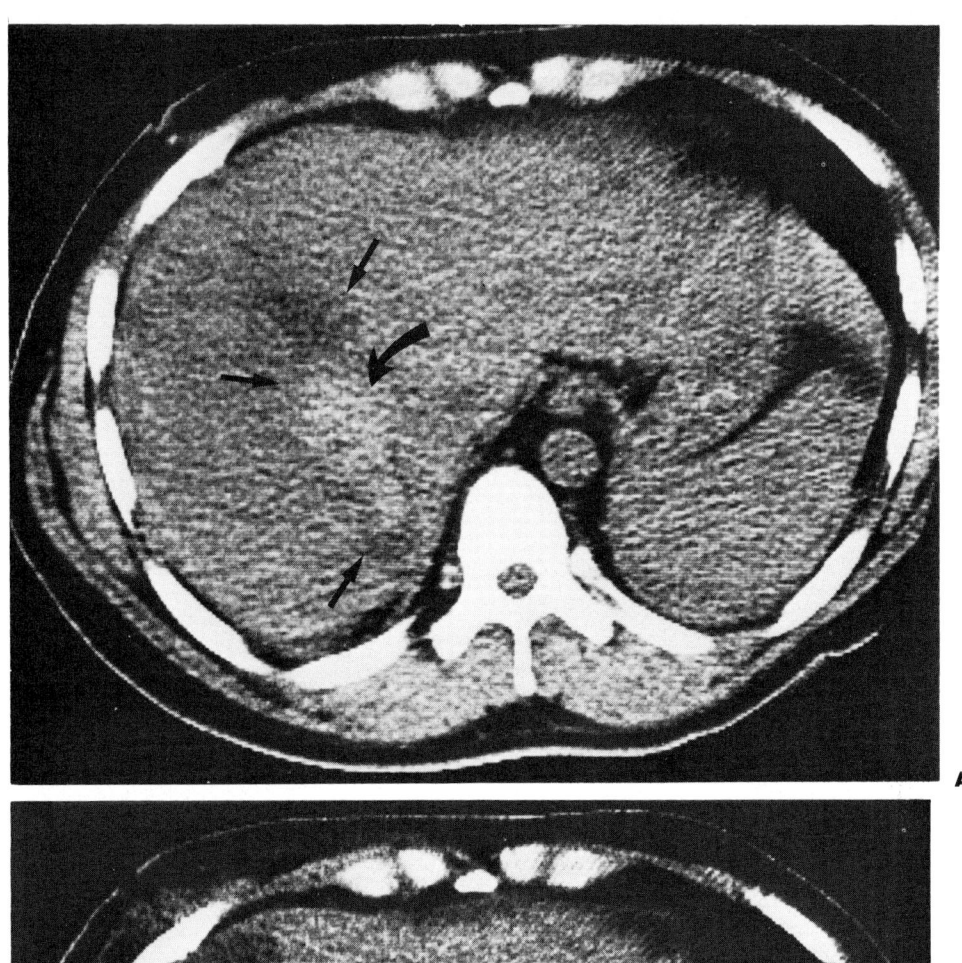

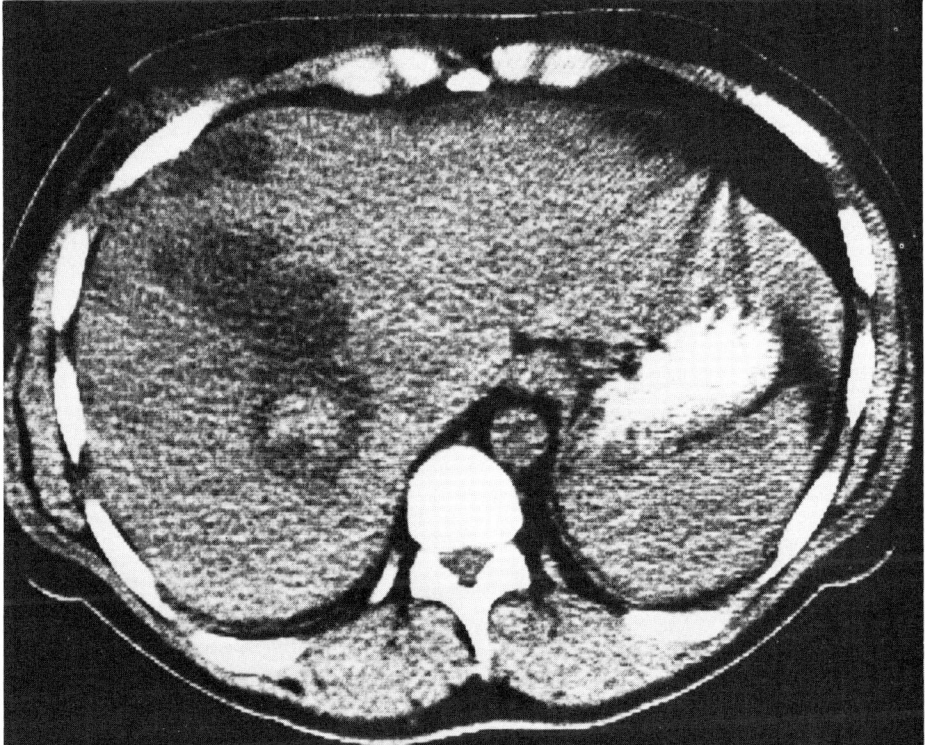

Figure 6-18. *A.* Initial CT scan shows heterogeneous oval laceration/hematoma in the right lobe (arrows). The higher-density center (curved arrow) is due to clotted blood, while the lower-density periphery consists of lysed blood clot. *B.* Repeat CT scan several days later demonstrates smaller dense residual blood clot in the dependent position and a somewhat larger area of lysed blood clot. (From Federle MP, McCort JJ: Abdominal trauma. In AR Margulis, HJ Burhenne (eds), Alimentary Tract Radiology, 3rd ed. St. Louis: Mosby, 1983, pp. 455–480.)

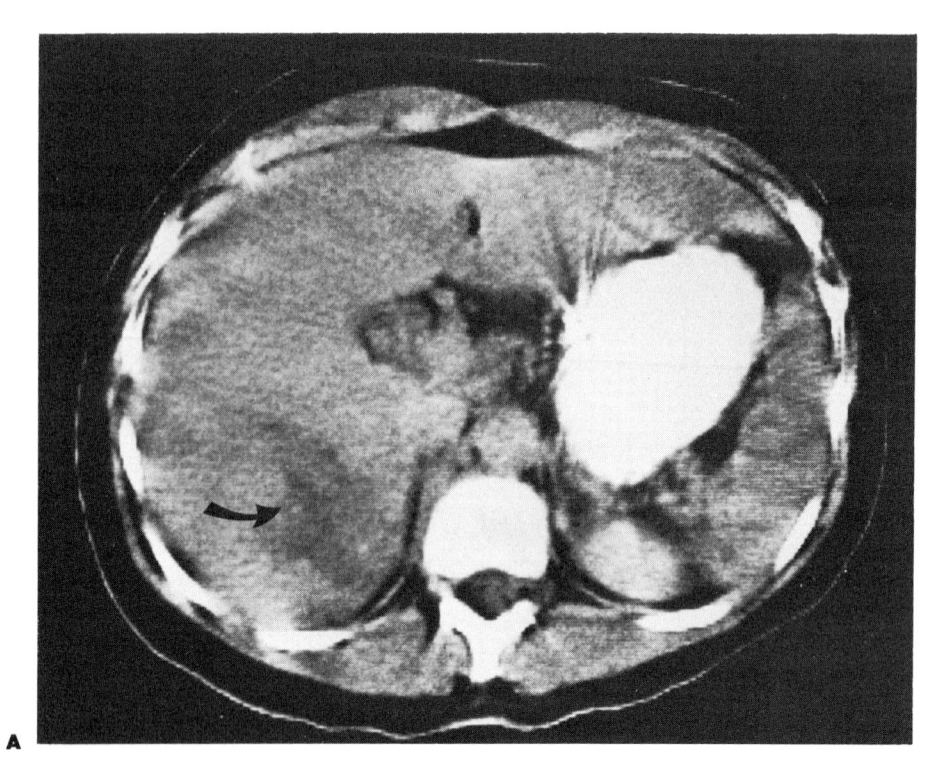

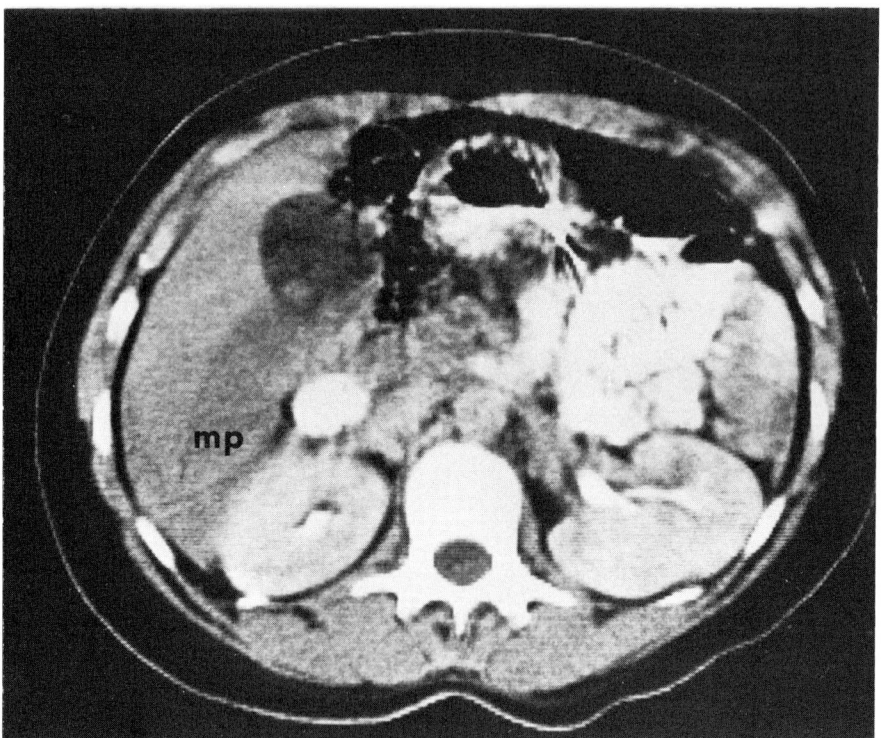

Figure 6–19. *A.* CT revealed multiple hepatic lacerations, including one in posterosuperior right lobe (arrow). *B* and *C.* Moderate hemoperitoneum, including collections in pouches of Morrison (mp) and Douglas (arrows). Findings confirmed at surgery. U = uterus. (From Moon KL, Federle MP: Computed tomography in hepatic trauma. AJR 141:309, 1983.)

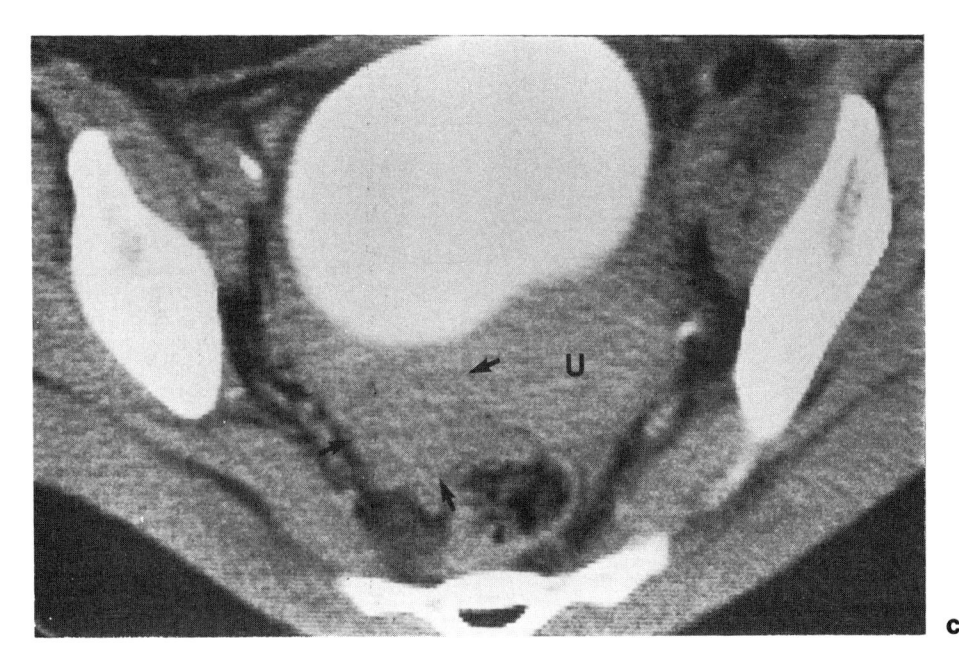

Figure 6-19. (*Continued*)

detected by CT using "dynamic scanning" adaptations available in most newer CT scanners (35,36). An intravenous bolus of contrast material is injected followed by rapid sequential CT sections through the area of interest. Early opacification of intrahepatic veins is indicative of traumatic fistula, though arteriography more precisely defines the nature of the lesion and may lead to transcatheter embolic therapy of the arteriovenous fistula.

Significance of Hemoperitoneum on CT and Effect on Management of Hepatic Trauma We recently reported our experience with 25 cases of hepatic injury from blunt trauma studied by CT (28). The size of the laceration and the associated hemoperitoneum were correlated with the mode of therapy employed in each case (operative vs. nonoperative). We found that while the need for surgery correlated roughly with the size of the hepatic laceration, the amount of hemoperitoneum was an important modifying factor (Figure 6-23). Fifteen patients (60 percent) with hepatic lacerations, but little or no hemoperitoneum, were successfully managed nonoperatively. The clinical and radiographic (CT) findings that have proved helpful in predicting successful nonoperative management include: limited or no hemoperitoneum; lack of significant extrahepatic injury; and stable vital signs after initial resuscitative therapy.

Reports from various children's medical centers similarly show excellent CT delineation of hepatic trauma in the pediatric population and successful nonoperative management of most cases (32). Whether similar success rates can be achieved in the adult population awaits further study.

Postoperative CT Evaluation of Liver Trauma Most patients who have undergone hepatic resection or extensive debridement will exhibit fever, increased output from abdominal drains, and abnormalities of liver function within 5 days postoperatively (37). Some, but not all, of these patients have abscesses that require surgical or catheter

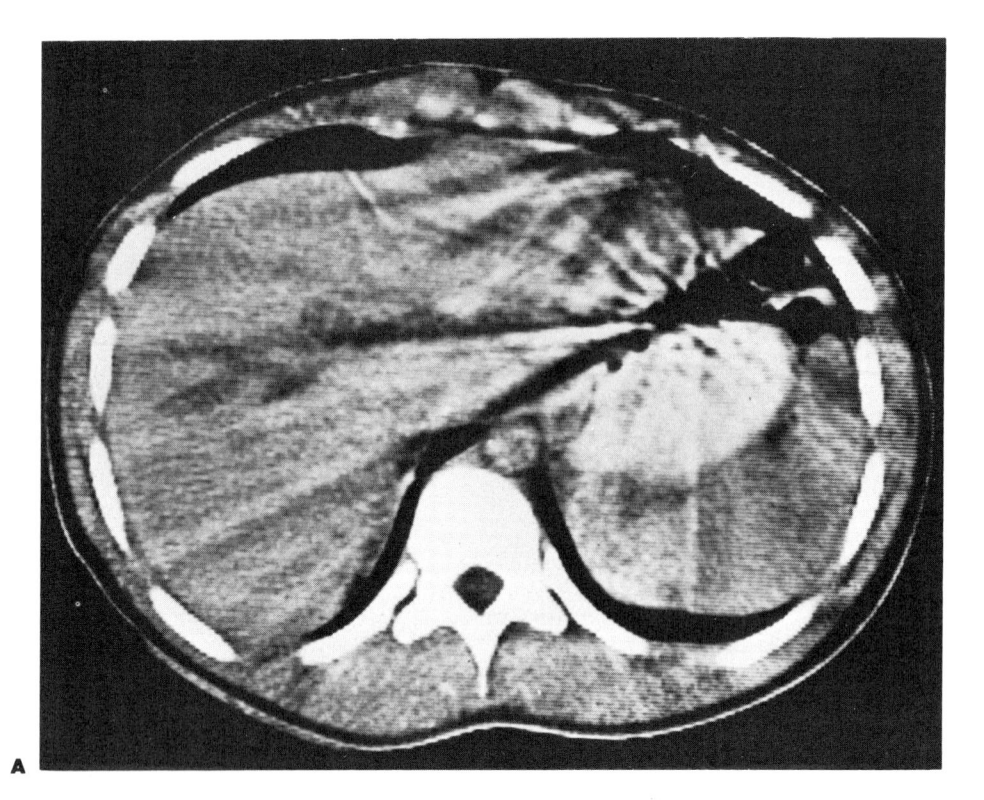

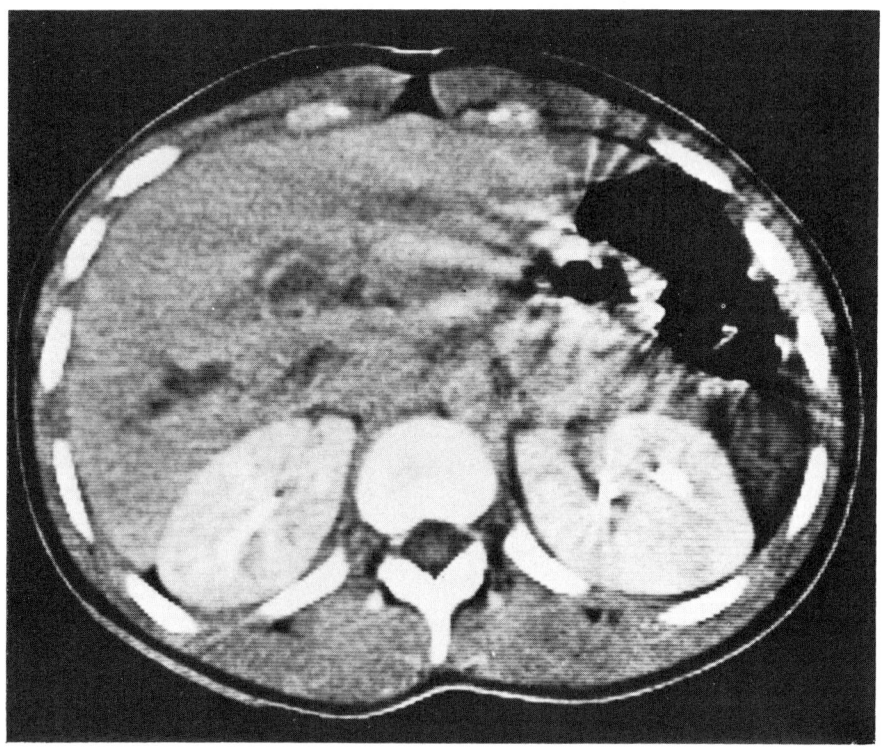

Figure 6–20. A and **B.** Multiple liver lacerations ("bear claw") simulate dilated bile ducts, but close examination of contiguous sections fails to show expected arborization pattern of dilated ducts. (From Moon KL, Federle MP: Computed tomography in hepatic trauma. AJR 141:309, 1983.)

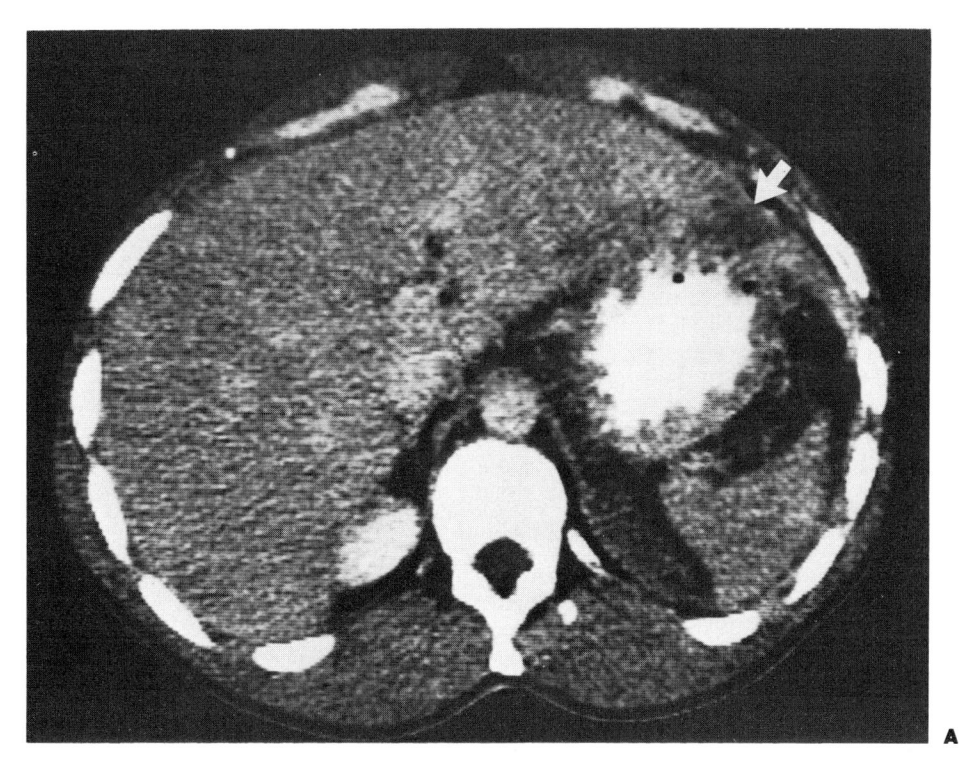

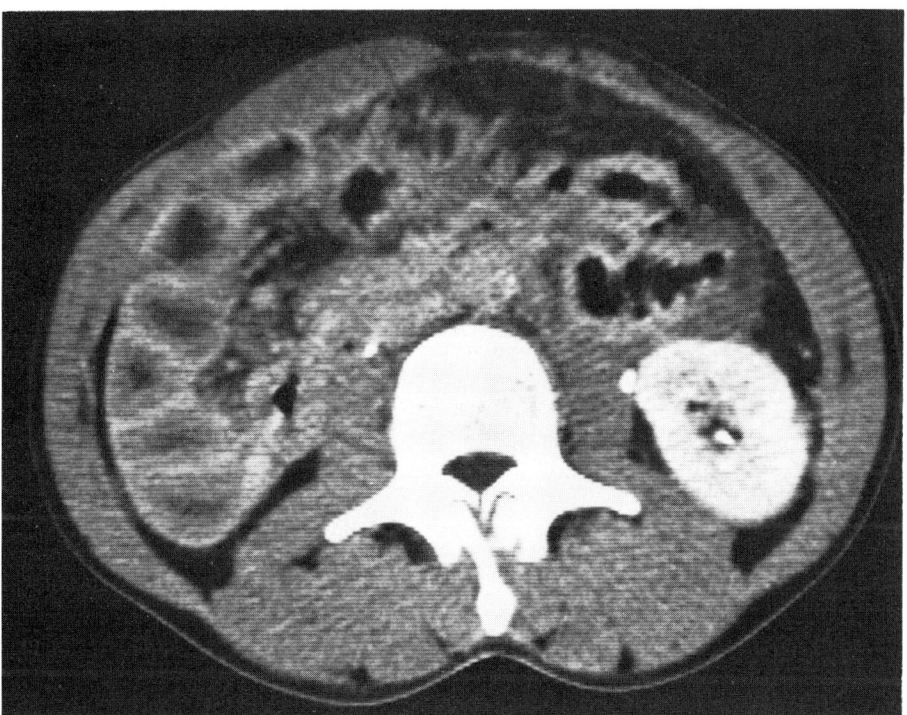

Figure 6–21. *A.* Traumatic laceration of left lobe. The fracture plane (arrow) separating the lateral segment of the left lobe from the rest of the liver might be overlooked without close attention to sequential axial sections. *B.* Relatively high-density blood surrounds multiple segments of small bowel, seen in cross-section, in the right flank. Findings confirmed at surgery.

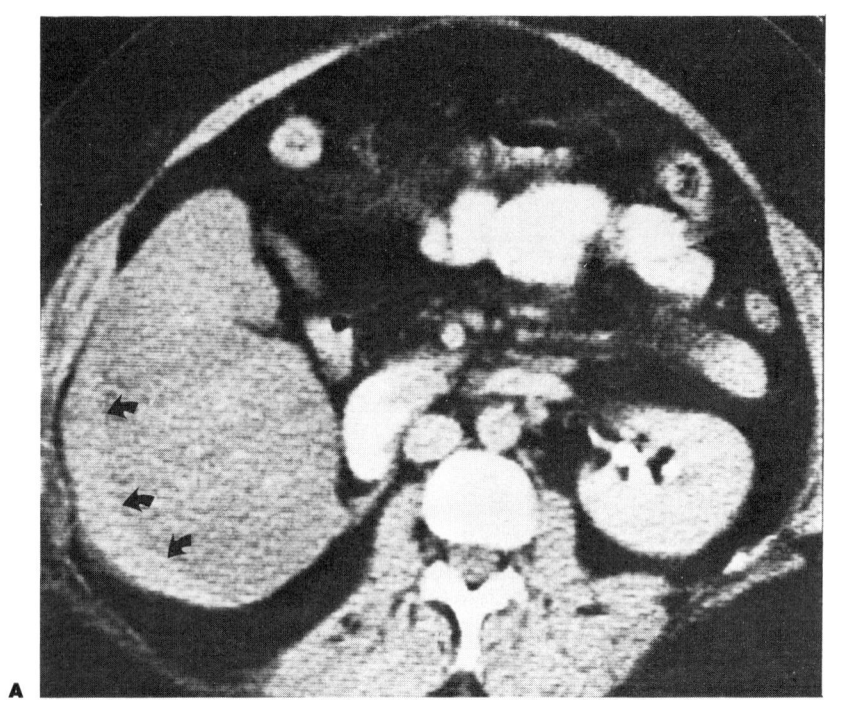

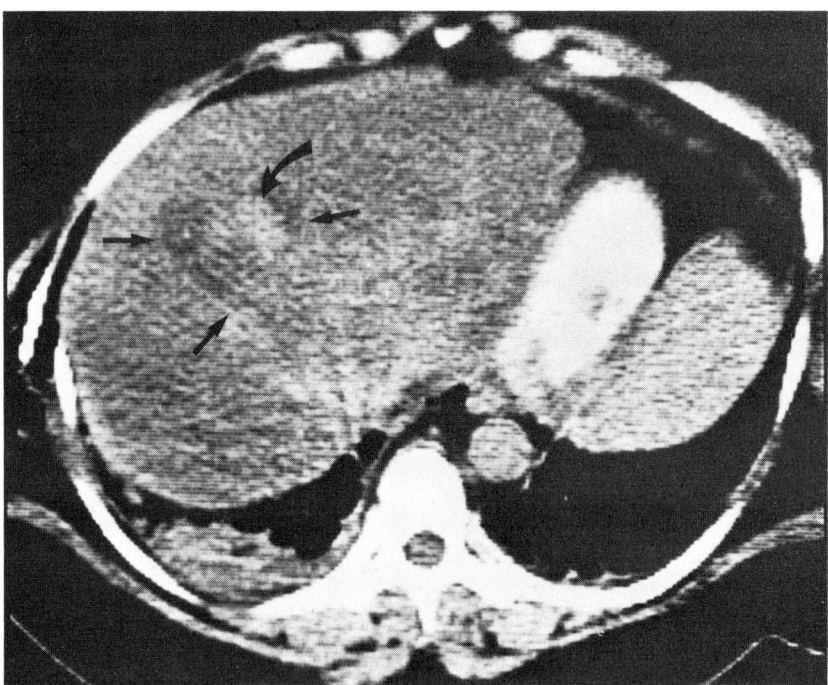

Figure 6–22. *A.* Acute subcapsular hematoma (arrows) is more dense (50 Hu) than underlying liver parenchyma (40 Hu) due to steatosis (fatty infiltration). *B.* Poorly defined region of mixed increased and decreased density (arrows) in right hepatic lobe; its appearance is less obvious than most intrahepatic hematomas. Area of increased density (curved arrow) probably represents formed clot. Hepatic parenchyma has abnormally low density compared to spleen.

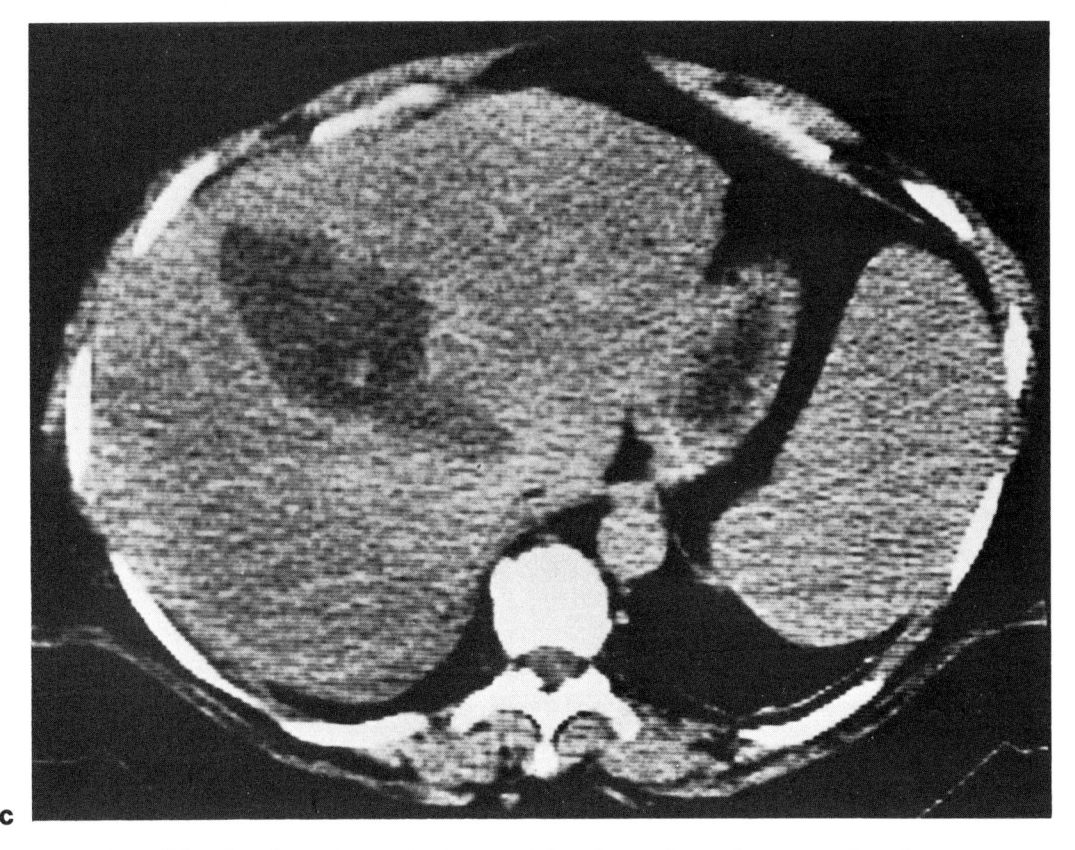

Figure 6-22. *C.* Nine days later. Laceration is now evident due to decreasing attenuation of intrahepatic hematoma and increasing attenuation of the surrounding liver. Patient was discharged from hospital same day without surgery. (Figs. 6-22 *A, B,* and *C* from Moon KL, Federle MP: Computed tomography in hepatic trauma. AJR 141:309, 1983.)

drainage. Aside from infection, delayed bleeding is a frequent problem, the source of which may be obscure.

CT is of value in evaluation of such patients. CT can exclude abscesses and continued bleeding (other than gastrointestinal) reliably. Conversely, the appearance of high attenuation fluid or dense clot within the liver or peritoneal cavity is evidence of continued blood loss. Many patients have nonspecific hepatic or peritoneal fluid collections postsurgically, with CT attenuation values near that of water. Such findings are nonspecific and are consistent with ascites, seroma, abscess, or biloma. CT may be of value in such cases in directing needle aspiration of these fluid collections for definitive analysis (38).

Advantages and Limitations Since we have reviewed all of the generally available imaging modalities for hepatic trauma, the role of CT may be discussed in this context. Following initial clinical and conventional radiographic evaluation, CT is the next imaging procedure of choice in virtually all cases of acute blunt trauma, should further radiographic evaluation be required by the surgeon. Other radiographic modalities are almost always reserved for specific indications in the subacute or postoperative evaluation of these patients. Angiography is employed for suspected persistent arteriovenous fistula. Radionuclide biliary scintigraphy and/or direct cholangiography give useful information in cases of hematobilia or traumatic bile leakage and biloma formation.

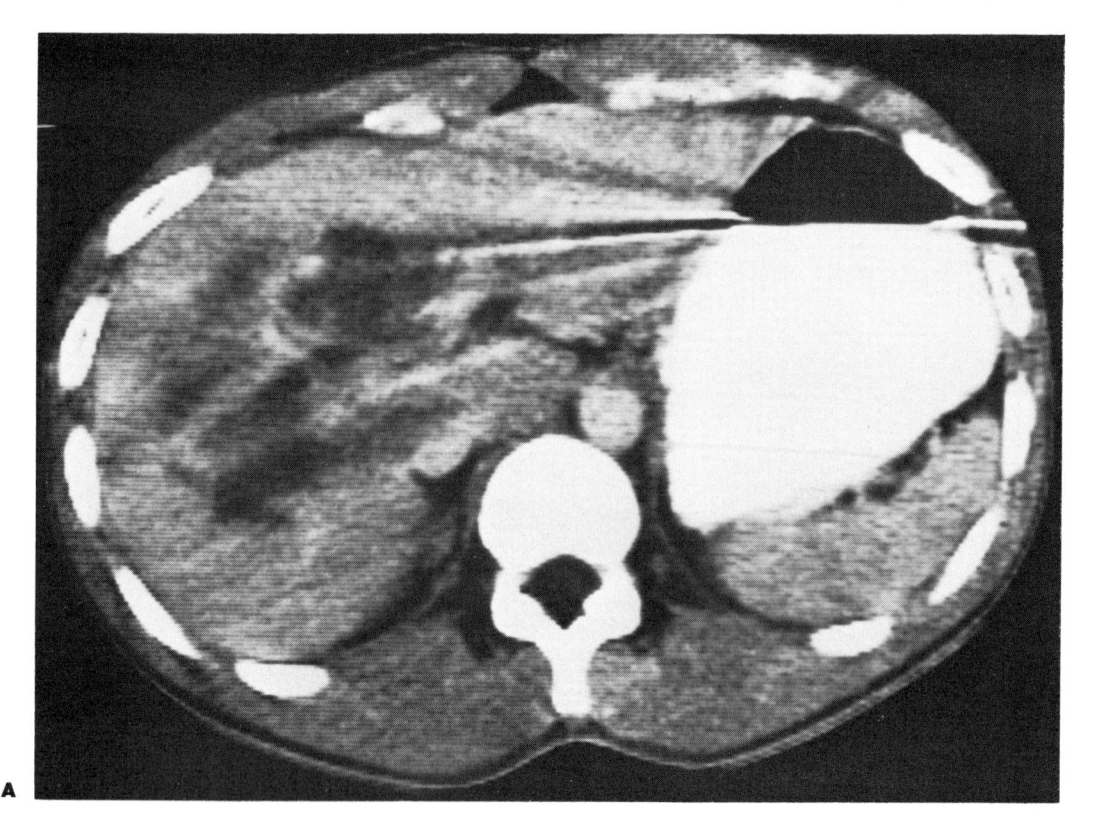

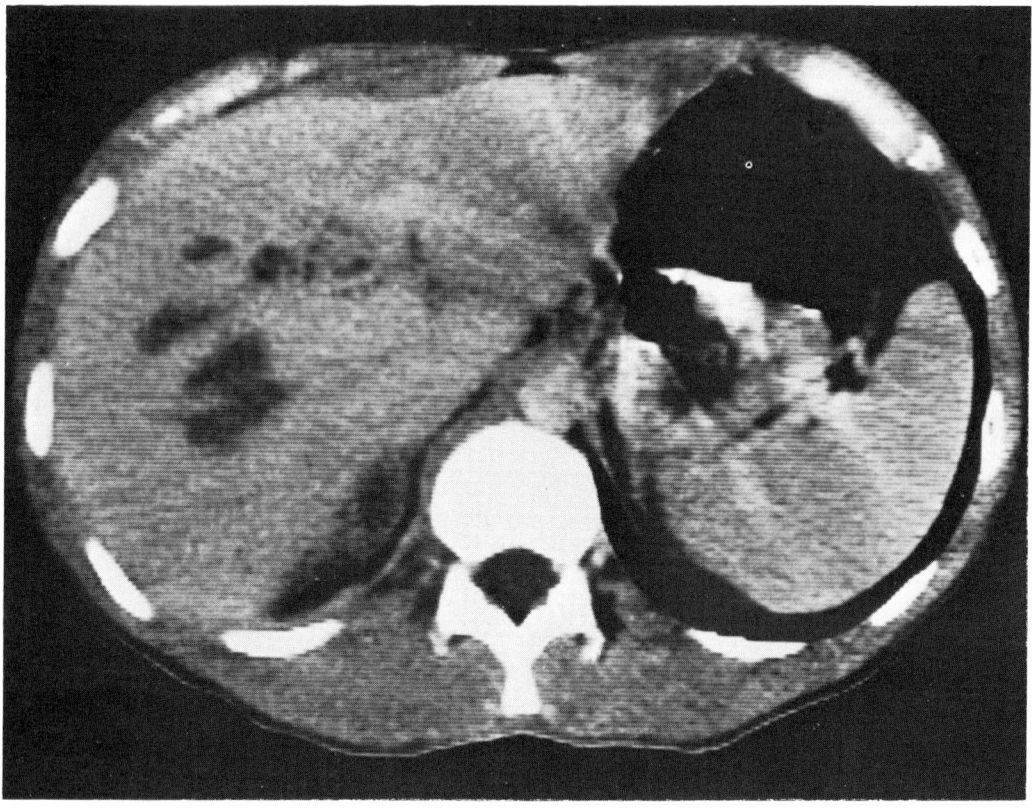

Figure 6–23. *A.* Large laceration (hematoma) in right lobe of liver. Despite this extensive lesion, there was very little blood in peritoneal cavity and patient was clinically stable. *B.* After 8 days of bed rest, substantial resolution of hematoma. (From Moon KL, Federle MP: Computed tomography in hepatic trauma. AJR 141:309, 1983.)

Ultrasonography is useful in detecting and sequentially following posttraumatic fluid collections and can guide diagnostic and therapeutic aspiration and drainage procedures.

In the acute setting, however, CT is the primary diagnostic modality. In a rapid and noninvasive fashion, it accurately defines the extent of hepatic injury, determines the presence of other abdominal injuries, and quantifies the size of associate hemoperitoneum. In addition to modifying the use of other imaging modalities, CT has decreased the use of diagnostic peritoneal lavage in blunt abdominal trauma. Peritoneal lavage is very sensitive in detecting peritoneal hemorrhage from hepatic (or other) injuries, being "positive" with as little as 25 mL of intraperitoneal blood. Lavage is limited by its inability to detect the source of bleeding, failure to detect retroperitoneal injuries, and its relative "invasiveness." Its sensitivity in detecting hemorrhage constitutes another problem in that patients with "positive" peritoneal lavage are frequently operated upon only to find insignificant amounts of blood from superficial hepatic or mesenteric lacerations that have already stopped bleeding (36). In our experience, such patients have little or no blood detected by CT and the source of the bleeding is usually evident. The policy of our surgeons is to avoid surgery on hepatic lacerations with small hemoperitoneum and stable vital signs.

REFERENCES

1. Lim RL: Injuries to the liver and extrahepatic ducts. In FW Blasidell, DD Trunkey (eds), Trauma Management. New York: Thieme-Stratton, 1982, vol. 1, pp. 123–147.
2. Lucas CE, Walt AJ: Critical decisions in liver trauma. Arch Surg 1970;101:277–282.
3. Morton JR, Roys GD, Bricker DL: The treatment of liver injuries. Surg Gynecol Obstet 1972;1343:298–302.
4. Richie JP, Fonkalsrud FW: Subcapsular hematoma of the liver: nonoperative management. Arch Surg 1972;104:781–784.
5. Federle MP, McCort JJ: Abdominal trauma. In AR Margulis, HJ Burhenne (eds), Alimentary Tract Radiology, 3rd ed. St. Louis: Mosby, 1983, pp. 455–480.
6. Frimann-Dahl J: Roentgen Examinations in Acute Abdominal Diseases, 3rd ed. Springfield, Ill.: Charles C Thomas, 1974.
7. Laurell A: A contribution to the differential diagnosis in the presence of free fluid in the abdomen. Acta Radiol 1935;16:424.
8. McCort JJ: Radiographic examination in blunt abdominal trauma. Philadelphia: Saunders, 1966.
9. Margulies M, Stoane L: Hepatic angle in roentgen evaluation of peritoneal fluid. Radiology 1967;88:51.
10. Keefe EJ, Gagliardi RA, Pfister RC: The roentgenographic evaluation of ascites. AJR 1967;101:388.
11. Redman HC, Reuter SR, Bookstein JJ: Angiography on abdominal trauma. Ann Surg 1969;169:57.
12. Berk RN, Wholey MH, Stockdale R: The angiographic diagnosis of splenic and hepatic trauma. J Can Assoc Radiol 1970;21:230.
13. Ben-Menachem Y: Angiography in Trauma: A Work Atlas. Philadelphia: Saunders, 1981.
14. Friedman GS: Radionuclide imaging of the injured patient. Radiol Clin of North Am 1973;11:461.
15. Evans GW, Antin FG, McCarthy HF, et al.: Scintigraphy in traumatic lesions of liver and spleen. JAMA 222:665,1972.
16. Froelich JW, Simeone JF, McKusick KA, et al.: Radionuclide imaging and ultrasound in liver/spleen trauma: a prospective comparison. Radiology 1982;145:457.

17. Mueller PR, Ferrucci JT, Simeone JF, et al.: Detection and drainage of bilomas. AJR 1983;140:715.
18. Esensten M, Ralls PW, Colletti P, Halls J: Posttraumatic intrahepatic biloma: sonographic diagnosis. AJR 1983;140:303.
19. Federle MP, Goldberg HI, Kaiser JA, et al.: Evaluation of abdominal trauma by computed tomography. Radiology 1981;138:637.
20. Gold L, Patel AA: Ultrasound detection of extrahepatic encapsulated bile: "biloma." AJR 1979;139:1014.
21. Zagel HB, Karty AB, Perlmutter GS, Goldberg BR: Ultrasonic characteristics of bilomas. JCU 9:21, 1981.
22. Weissman HS, Chun KJ, Frank M, et al.: Demonstration of traumatic bile leakage with cholescintigraphy and ultrasonography. AJR 1979;133:843.
23. Kuni CC, Klingensmith WC III, Koep W, Fritzberg AR: Communication of intrahepatic cavities with bile ducts: demonstration with Tc-99m-diethyl-IDA imaging. Clin Nucl Med 1980;5:349.
24. Van Sonnenberg E, Simeone JF, Mueller PR, et al.: Sonographic appearance of hematoma in liver, spleen, and kidney: a clinical, pathologic and animal study. Radiology 1983;147:507.
25. Wicks JD, Silver TM, Bree RL: Gray scale features of hematomas: an ultrasonic spectrum. AJR 1978;131:977.
26. Visconii GN, Gonzalez R, Taylor KJ, Crade M: Ultrasonic evaluation of hepatic and splenic trauma. Arch Surg 1980;115:320.
27. Corica A, Powers SR: Blunt liver trauma: an analysis of 75 treated patients. Trauma 1975;9:751.
28. Moon KL, Federle MP: Computed tomography in hepatic trauma. AJR 1983;141:309.
29. Toombs BD, Sandler CM, Rauschkolb EN, et al.: Assessment of hepatic injuries with computed tomography. J Comput Assist Tomogr 1982;6:72.
30. Iion S, Sawada T, Kusonobi T: Computed tomography in neonatal subcapsular hemorrhage of the liver. J Comput Assist Tomogr 1981;5:416.
31. Tylen U, Hoevds J, Nilsson U: Computed tomography of iatrogenic hepatic lesions following percutaneous transhepatic cholangiography and portography. J Comput Assist Tomogr 1981;5:15.
32. Berger PE, Kuhn JP: CT of blunt abdominal trauma in childhood. AJR 1981;136:105.
33. Federle MP: CT of abdominal trauma. In MP Federle, M Brant-Zawadzki (eds), Computed Tomography in the Evaluation of Trauma, Baltimore: Williams & Wilkins, 1982.
34. Federle MP, Jeffrey RB: Hemoperitoneum studied by computed tomography. Radiology 1983;148:187.
35. Axel L, Moss AA, Berninger W: Dynamic computed tomography demonstration of hepatic arteriovenous fistula. J Comput Assist Tomogr 1981;5:95.
36. Foley DW, Berland LL, Lawson TL, Maddison FE: Computed tomography in the demonstration of hepatic pseudoaneurysm with hemobilia. J Comput Assist Tomogr 1980;4:863.
37. Longmire WP, Cleveland RJ: Surgical anatomy and blunt trauma of the liver. Surg Clin North Am 1972;52:687.
38. Haney PJ, Whitley NO, Brotman S, et al.: Liver injury and complications in the postoperative trauma patient: CT evaluation. AJR 1982;139:271.

7

Hepatic Biopsies and Abscess Drainages

MICHAEL E. BERNARDINO

INTRODUCTION

Interventional radiology in the liver has added tremendously to patient care. This technique can obtain a tissue diagnosis or avoid significant abdominal surgery. This chapter deals with focal liver biopsies and hepatic abscess drainages. Specific attention will be paid to technique, results, and possible complications.

HEPATIC GUIDED-BIOPSY TECHNIQUES

Indications

Guided hepatic biopsies are performed to answer a specific question (usually to determine the etiology of a specific focal hepatic mass) (Figure 7-1). Also, they may be obtained to determine the viability of hepatic tumors after therapy or in patients who have ascites and/or cholestasis. Standard biopsy techniques in such patients increase the incidence of bile peritonitis. The small-needle biopsy rarely supplements the standard liver biopsy. The latter is performed to obtain information about the liver parenchyma rather than to determine whether or not malignant cells are present.

Technique

Needle Various types of needles can be used in obtaining a tissue specimen from the liver. Many have advocated fine needles (22–23 gauge) for obtaining specimens (1–5). The majority of these smaller-needle specimens are for cytologic diagnosis. This type of needle is used mainly in patients who have a known malignancy to determine whether the focal hepatic mass is metastatic. However, not every hospital has an expert cytolo-

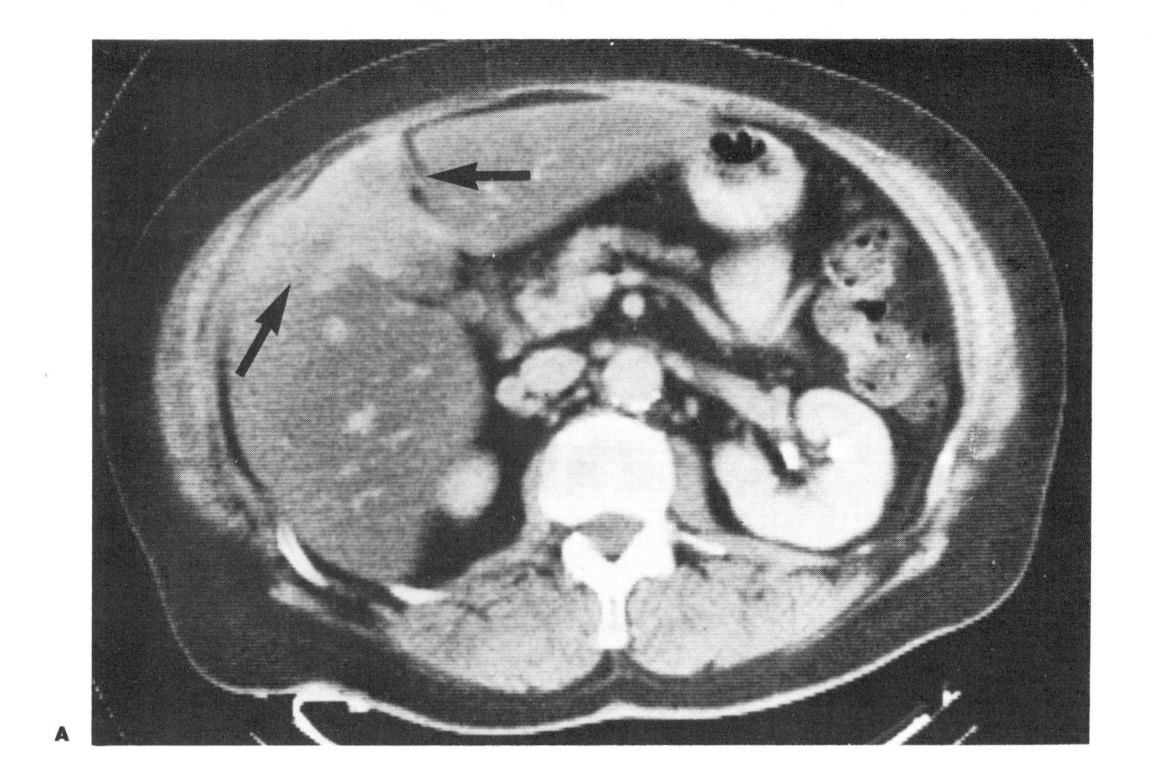

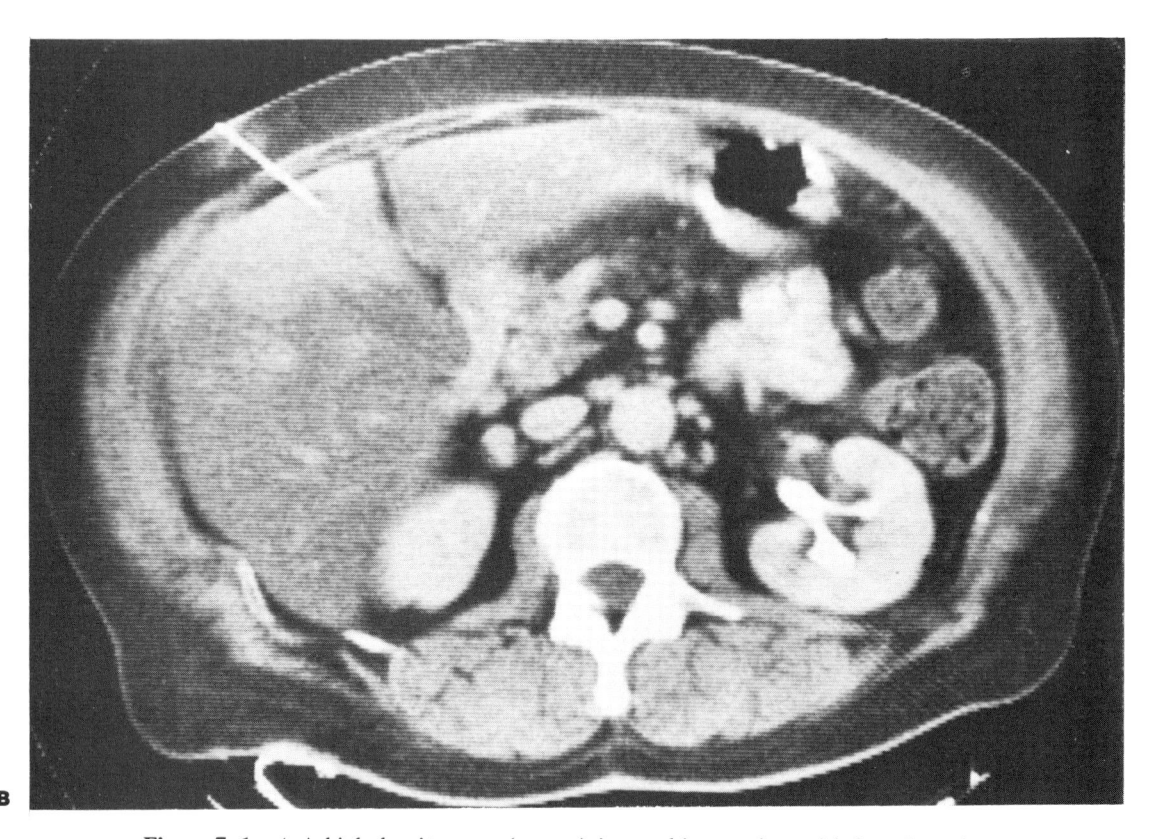

Figure 7-1. *A.* A high-density mass (arrows) is noted in a patient with fatty hepatic metamorphosis. Is this area malignant tissue, a hemangioma, normal tissue, or something else? *B.* A guided biopsy was performed to determine the lesion's etiology. It demonstrated adenocarcinoma.

gist. Thus, at many institutions, more tissue may be needed for a diagnosis. The use of smaller needles is more prudent in vascular lesion because they decrease the chance of hemorrhage. Also, smaller needles may be more applicable when lesions are in critical anatomic areas. However, small needles have a tendency to bend when entering the body, which may make them difficult to guide and may increase the procedure's length.

Larger needles up to 14 gauge in size, such as "True Cuts" and/or "Menghinis," obtain not only a cytologic diagnosis but a histologic diagnosis (6,7). Recent reports have shown that although the accuracy of both cytologic and histologic samples was roughly equal for making a diagnosis of carcinoma, the larger needles gave much more information about the focal mass in 54 percent of the cases (8). Another report demonstrated a definite increase in accuracy with larger needles (9). This was due to more consistent retrieval of adequate tissue for diagnosis. Also, there was no increase in complications using the larger needles (assuming that vascular lesions were excluded from the large-needle catagory).

Medium-sized needles, those between 20 and 19 gauge, also obtain adequate specimens. In one report an accuracy of greater than 94 percent was noted using these needle sizes (10). Most of these needles were aspiration needles, although cutting needles may be used in this size range. Basically, the choice of needle size should depend on the information needed, vascularity of the mass, and the pathologist.

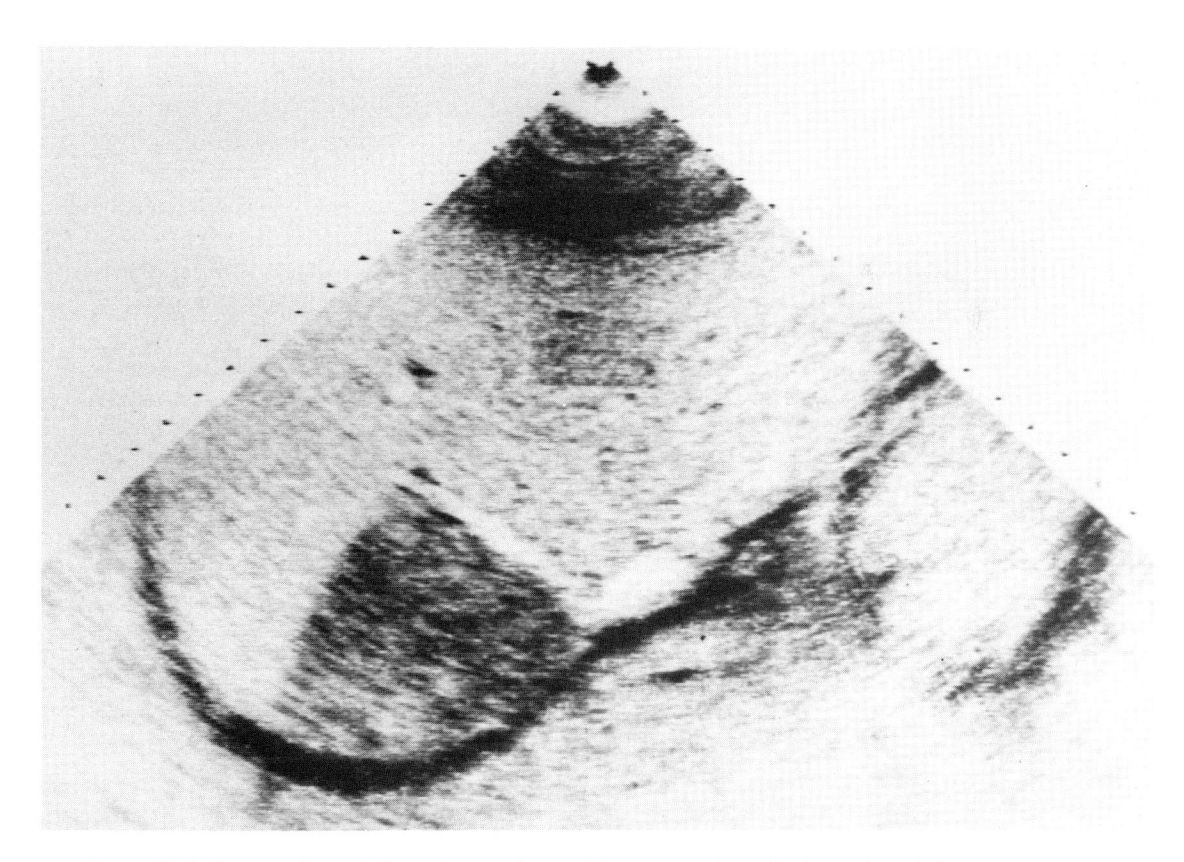

Figure 7-2. Large echogenic hepatic mass is noted by sonography. The large size of the mass makes sonography an excellent biopsy-guidance mechanism.

Choice of Imaging Modality The imaging modality used to guide the needle, whether into an abscess or neoplasm, is dependent upon the size, location, and depth of the lesion. Large lesions could conceivably be biopsied under fluoroscopy (11), although we routinely biopsy large, peripherally located hepatic masses under sonography. Deep lesions, small masses, or lesions located in difficult anatomical areas, such as the porta hepatis, are best biopsied under CT guidance. CT allows a much more accurate placement of the needle within the lesion. CT-guided biopsies may take more time than other forms of guidance. However, their accuracy rates are extremely high. If CT has been used as the guidance system, we routinely scan the biopsied area about 5 to 10 minutes after the procedure to determine if there is any significant hemorrhage present. Also, the patient's clinical condition is monitored closely in the x-ray department for 1 hour after the procedure.

Ultrasound A single-sector scan over the large (> 3 cm) or peripherally located lesion is obtained (Figure 7–2). The lesion can then be biopsied using a specially fitted ultrasound transducer for guidance, or by marking the scan directly below the midportion of the sonographic beam (12–16). The depth from skin surface to the mass's periphery is noted. This measurement will determine the final distance of needle placement. Again, it is important that the hepatic mass be large and peripherally located to obtain accurate placement. Most biopsy specimens should be obtained from the periphery of the mass. The periphery has more viable tissue, while the tumor's central area has more necrosis.

CT Guidance Using CT for guidance, a reference catheter is placed along the right midaxillary line or over the right side of the abdomen. Localization scans are then obtained to identify the lesion. The safest and shortest access route is determined. Distance measurements are made from the reference catheter to a point on the patient's skin directly anterior or lateral to the lesion (Figure 7–3). A measurement is made from this point by the CT computer to the mass. The patient is then marked while still in the scanner, using a laser beam at the proper scan level. The patient is removed from the scanner. Measurements are made on the skin from the marking catheter to the skin biopsy entry point (6,9). At this site, the skin is washed with antiseptic and local anesthesia is applied. Anesthesia is not only applied subcutaneously, but also along the proposed biopsy track to the liver capsule. The skin is then "nicked" with a scalpel blade and is widened using curved hemostats. The needle is placed into the liver the required distance. At this point, using a scanner with long reconstruction times, a "scout view" is obtained (Figure 7–4). The needle tip is localized and the scan is taken at the needle-tip level. It is important that the needle tip be localized since scanning at the skin entry site may not yield the needle tip. This is due to respiratory movement and the fact that the needle does not always traverse a straight course to the target (a significant problem with 22–23 gauge needles). Using faster reconstruction time scanners, multiple scans can be obtained in and around the needle entry site to localize the needle tip very quickly.

Once the needle has been placed properly within the lesion, a 10 ml syringe is attached to the aspiration needle and suction is applied. As the suction is applied, two to three rotary "in and out" movements are made into the lesion to obtain the specimen. This process is repeated three times to decrease sampling error. The specimen is then sent to the laboratory for analysis. If cores are obtained, a histologic as well as cytologic diagnosis can be ascertained. Each of the two to three needle placements should be in a different portion of the target lesion. This also decreases the chance of sampling error. After the procedure, repeat scans are made to check for acute hemorrhage.

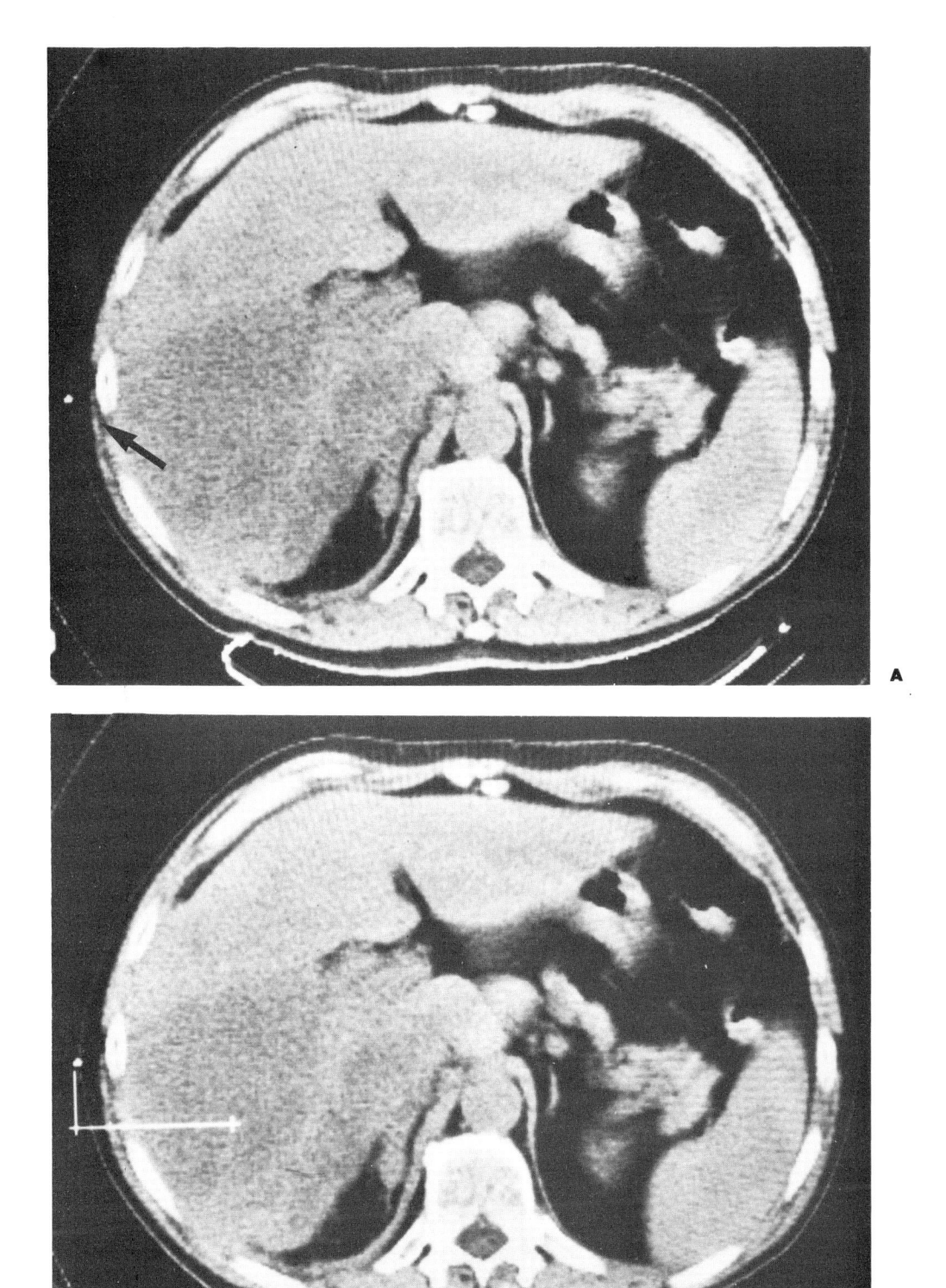

Figure 7-3. *A*. A reference-mark angiographic catheter (arrow) is placed on the patient's skin. *B*. Distances are determined by the CT computer for the optimum access route. These distances are then translated to the patient's skin and used to determine the needle excursion distance.

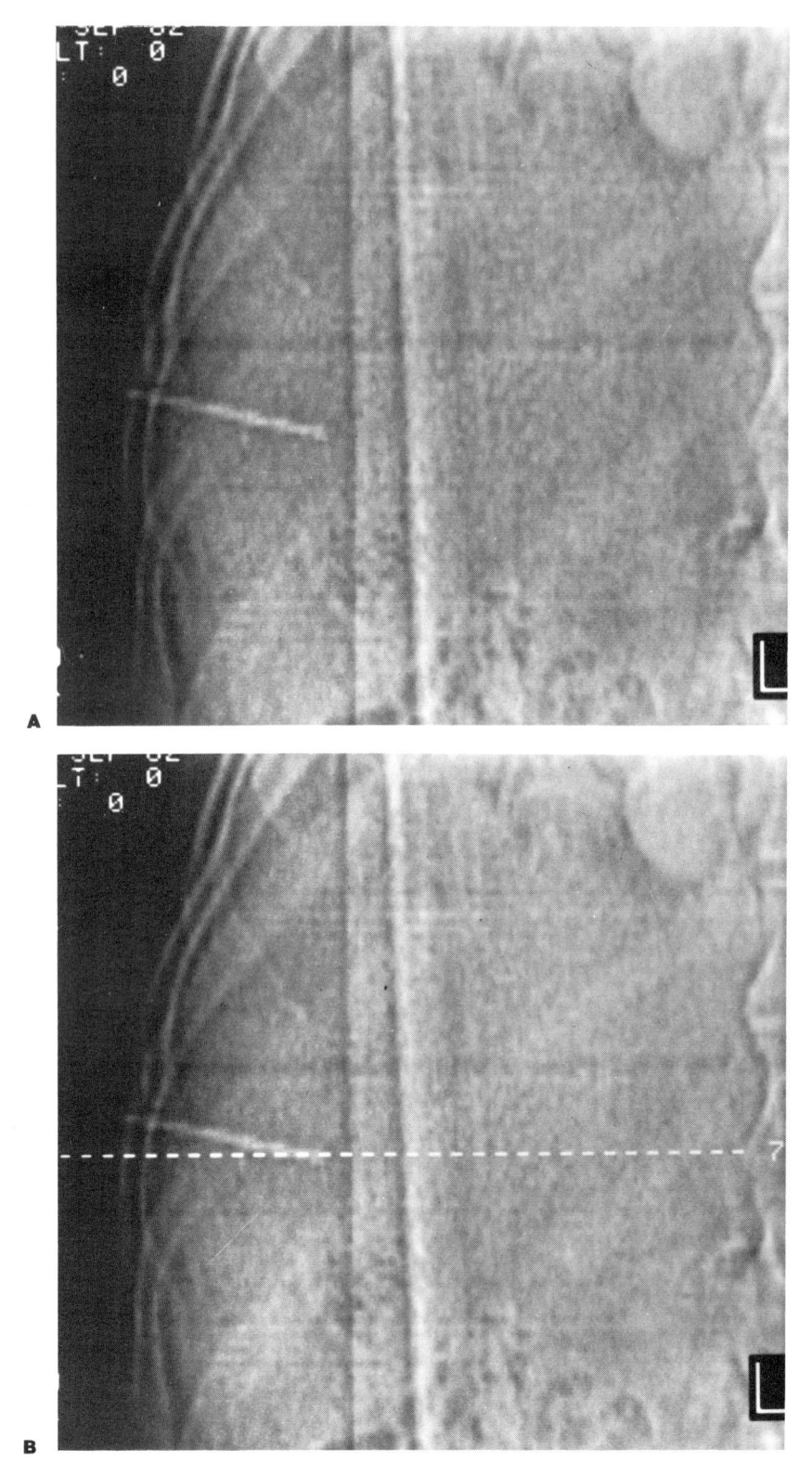

Figure 7-4. *A.* A digital radiograph is obtained to locate the needle tip. *B.* The exact location of the tip is noted and a scan obtained to determine the tip location. Note the tip is not where the needle entered the skin.

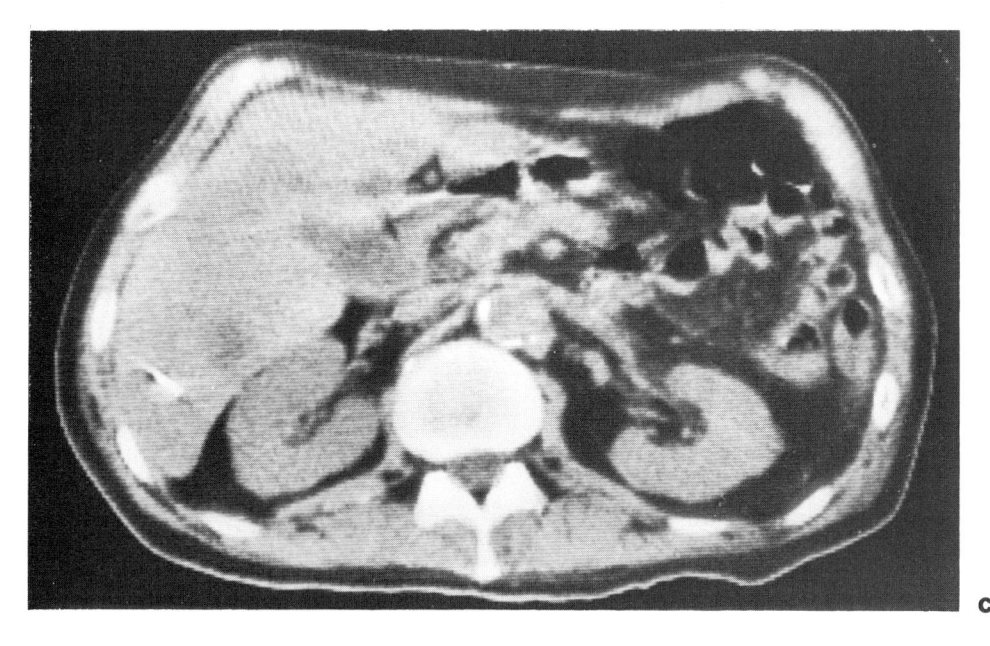

Figure 7-4. *C.* Biopsy of the hepatic mass shows the needle tip in the lesion. Note the needle tip and the needle skin-entrance point are not the same.

Accuracy

The accuracy of guided biopsies is between 83 and 94 percent (4,8–10,17–21) (Figure 7-5). Again, accuracy figures depend upon the size of the needle, type of specimens being obtained, expertise of the individual performing the biopsy, and the careful cooperation of the pathologist. Without proper pathologic support, high accuracy rates cannot be achieved (22).

Complications

Very few complications should occur if care is taken during a biopsy (23–25). Subcapsular hemorrhage may be seen in far more patients than has been expected previously, although it is usually asymptomatic. Also, vascular fistulas are noted angiographically in postbiopsy patients. These are asymptomatic and the angiographic abnormalities decrease with time. Vascular lesions should not be biopsied with large-bore needles because of the increased incidence of hemorrhage. The majority of reported deaths from percutaneous hepatic biopsies have been with large-bore needles ($\geq$ 18 gauge). In these cases, the lesions were hypervascular, such as a hypervascular metastasis and/or hemangioma. A CT flow study is recommended before the biopsy in such suspected cases. Another complication is septic shock. If an abscess is biopsied and not drained immediately, or if the patient is not covered with appropriate antibiotic before the procedure, septic shock is always a concern. Proper premedication and drainage of the abscess at the time of the biopsy decreases the possibility of sepsis. Bile peritonitis is another complication that may occur. Usually this is noted in the jaundiced patient after a large-needle ($\geq$ 18 gauge) biopsy.

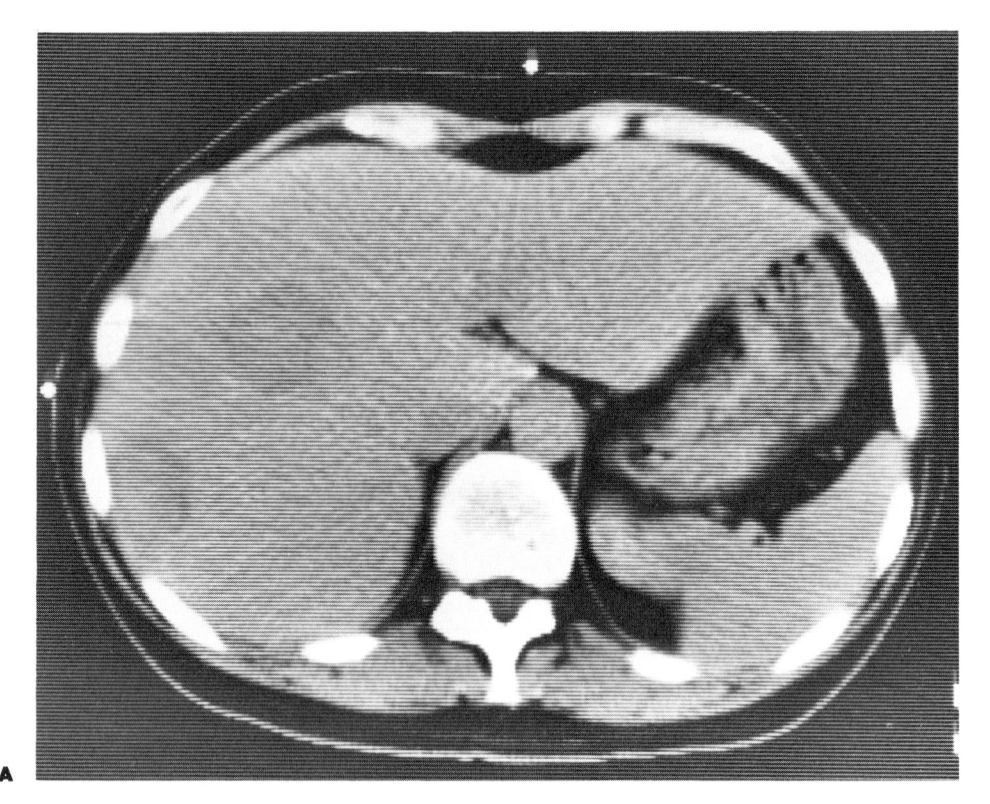

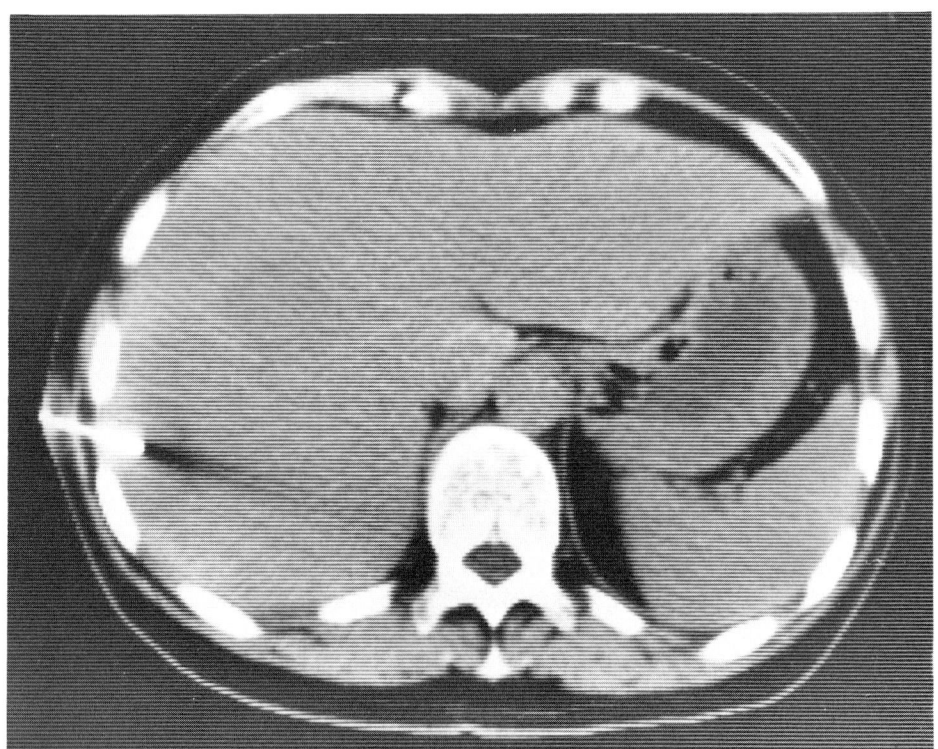

Figure 7-5. *A* and *B*. The accuracy of focal hepatic biopsies is quite high. One reason is knowledge that the specimen is obtained from the "targeted" hepatic mass.

ABSCESS DRAINAGE

Indications

Hepatic abscesses that are well-formed and offer a safe access route are excellent drainage candidates. Patients with multiple microabscesses, (Figure 7–6), who have coagulopathy problems, or who require more than two drainage tubes are poor candidates. However, greater than 95 percent of hepatic abscesses fulfill the acceptable criteria. Even well-circumscribed amebic abscesses are drainage candidates. They have not been candidates for percutaneous drainage in the past because they contain thick, tenacious material. Thus, amebic abscesses have been treated medically with metronidazole. However, we feel that percutaneous drainage is quite possible in these cases and that it decreases the patient's hospitalization (Figure 7–7).

Technique

Once an abscess has been diagnosed, drainage of the lesion can be performed under ultrasound or CT guidance (26–33). Again, larger, superficially located lesions can be drained with ultrasound. Deeper lesions in critical anatomical areas or smaller lesions are drained under CT guidance. The guidance system is similar to that used for biopsies. However, after the initial diagnostic study, one has to decide whether to use a Seldinger

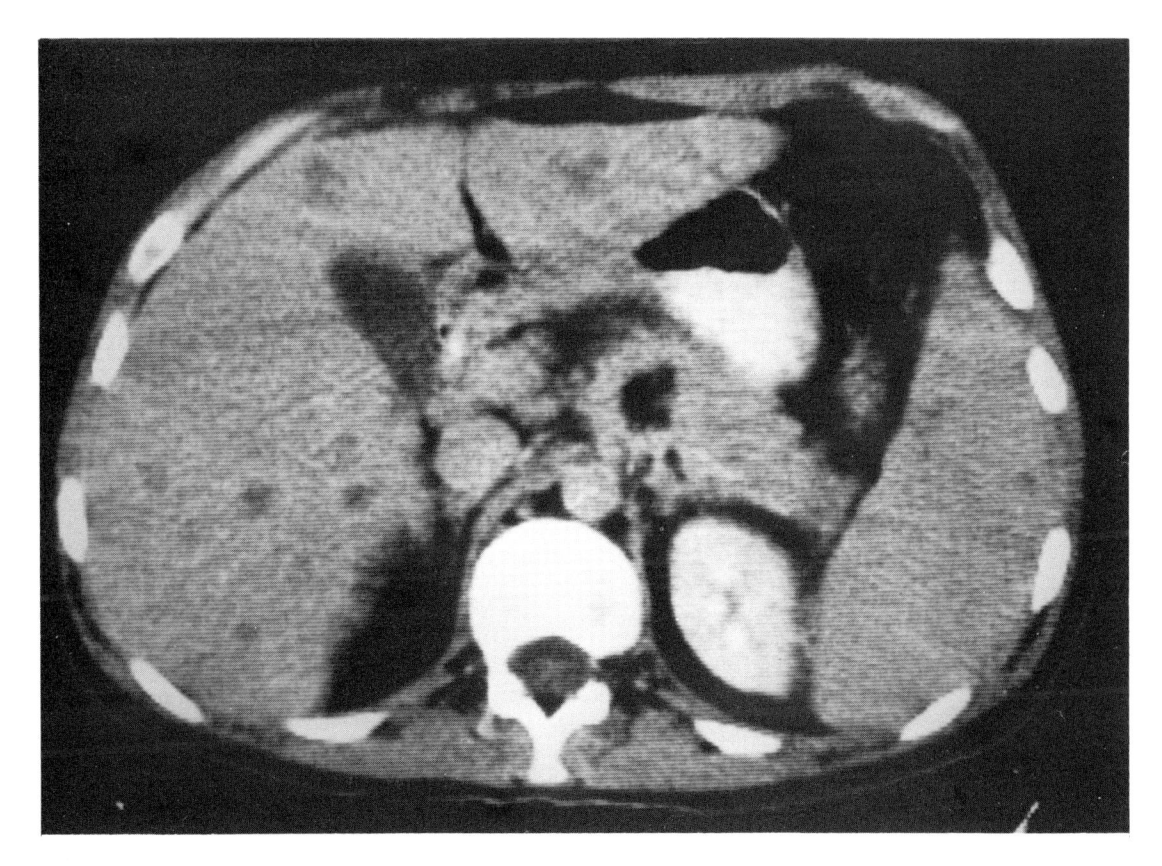

Figure 7–6. This patient with multiple hepatic and splenic abscesses is not a percutaneous drainage candidate.

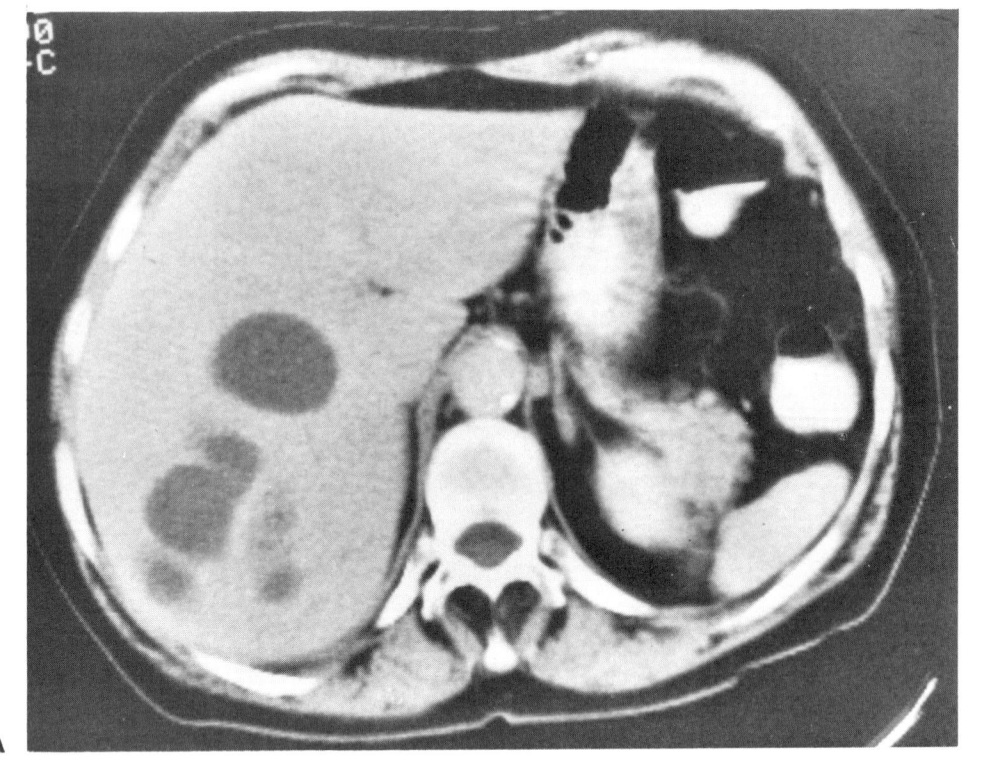

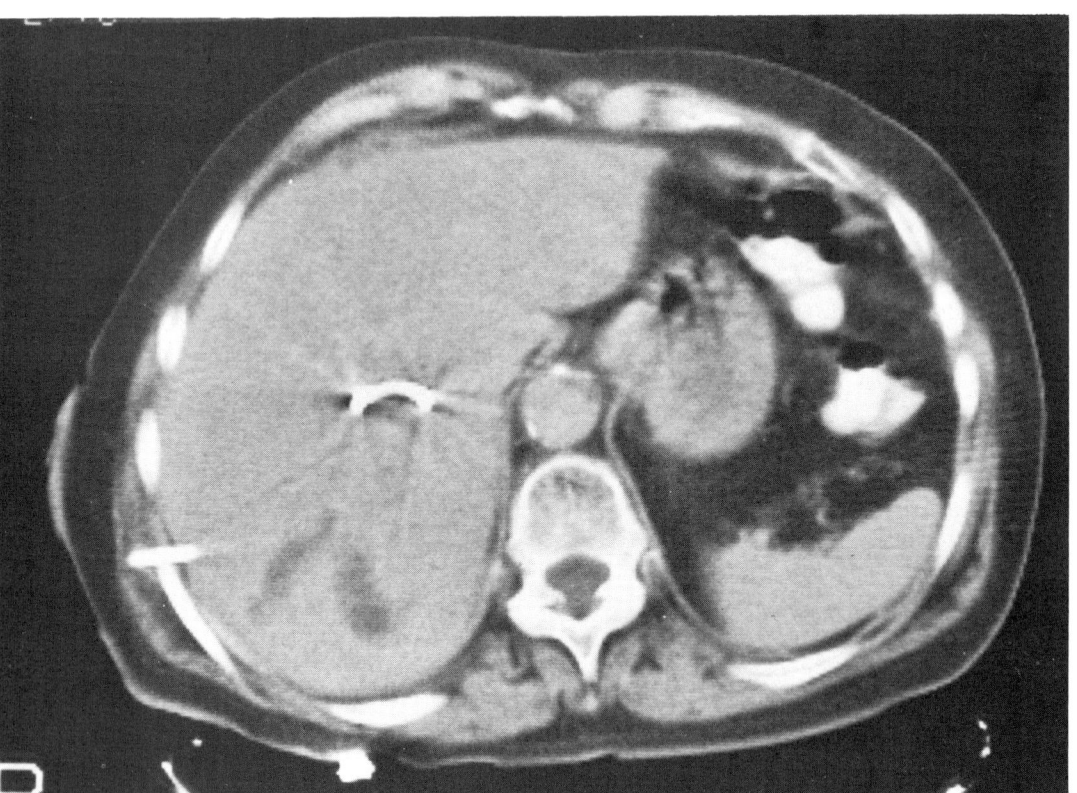

Figure 7-7. *A.* CT scan demonstrates multiple hepatic cystic pockets due to amebiasis. *B* and *C.* Using the Seldinger exchange technique, two 10 French nephrostomy catheters with mild saline irrigation were used for drainage. The patient was discharged from the hospital 4 days later.

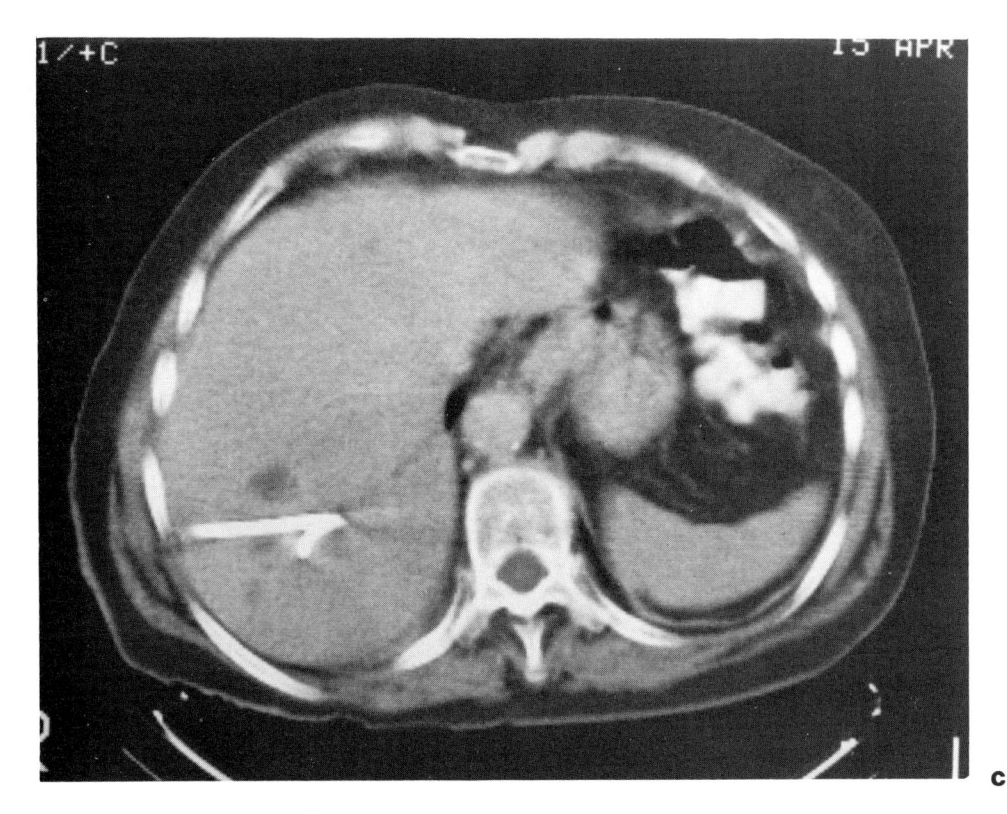

Figure 7-7. C. (*Continued*)

technique with a guide-wire exchange or the trocar method. This is usually dependent on the location and vicscosity of the lesion (Figure 7-8). If the guide-wire technique is used, dilating the track up to the proper sized catheter is mandatory. It is painful and time-consuming. Also, the size of the pigtail catheter is dependent upon the viscosity of the abscess (34). Usually a 7, 8, or 10 French pigtail nephrostomy catheter will suffice (35).

If the trocar technique is used, guidance of the trocar toward the lesion is performed as with a biopsy. A larger catheter, usually 12 or 14 French, is introduced by the trocar and slid gently into the abscess. The trocar is removed and the abscess is drained.

In abscesses that have a very high viscosity, utilization of either saline or acetylcysteine to decrease the viscosity has been advocated (36). This may mean multiple injections of the "wetting agent" into the abscesses and withdrawing the fluid and particulate matter. However, care should be taken since these injections may induce a septicemia. In most instances, gentle continuous suction is sufficient (37).

In all cases, surgical back-up should be available because of the possibility of sepsis, failure, and hemorrhage. Any specimens obtained from the abscess drainage should be sent for both aerobic and anaerobic bacterial culture. Anaerobes have been found in over 50 percent of the hepatic abscesses.

Length of Drainage

The length of drainage is dependent upon the type of abscess and the positioning of the catheter. It may be possible to remove a catheter within 48 hours; however, some

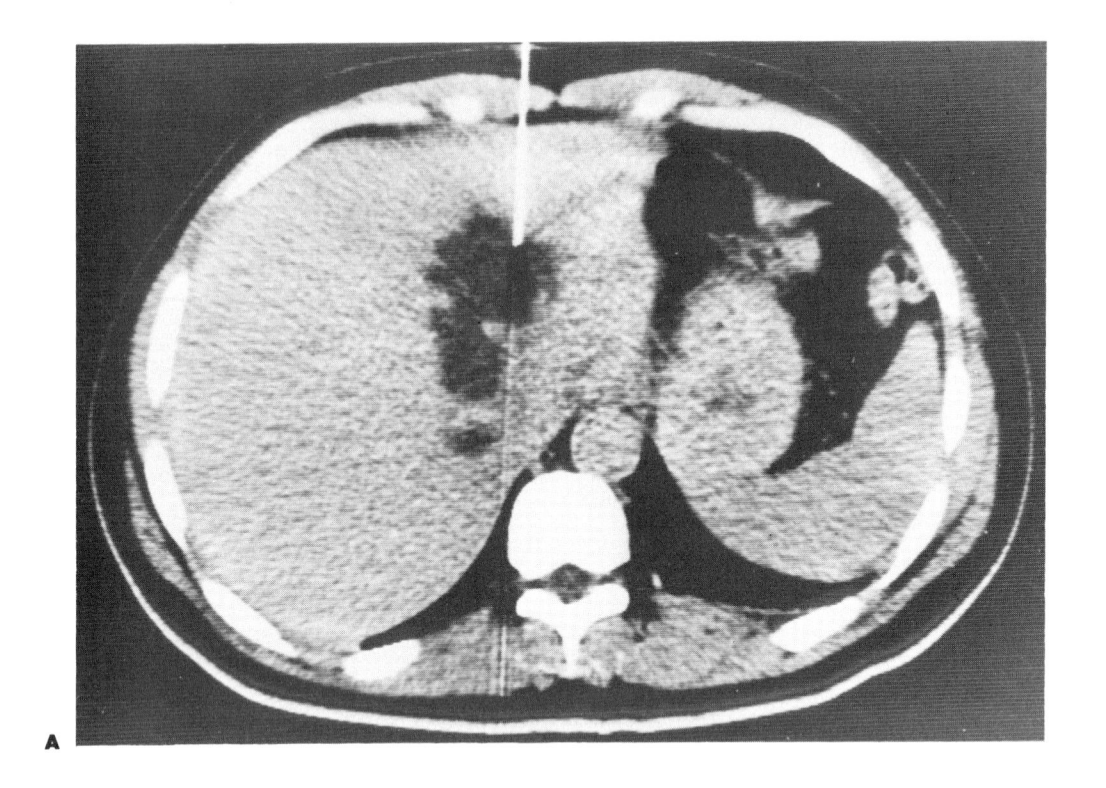

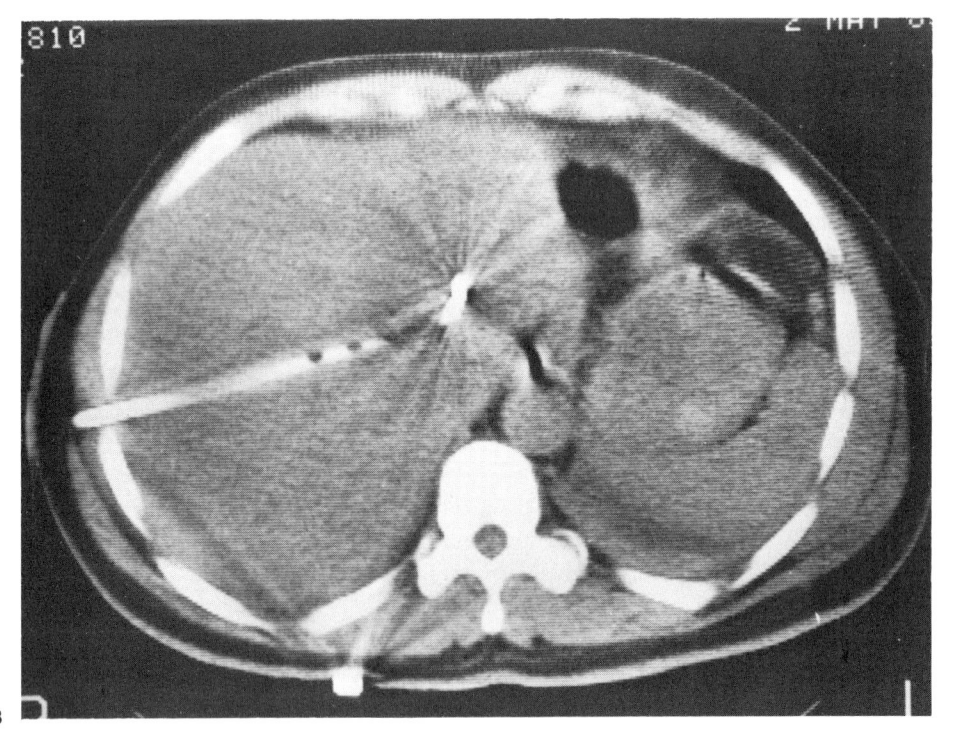

Figure 7-8. *A.* CT-guided biopsy shows a viscous abscess. *B.* The trocar method is chosen because of the thickness of the material. A 12F drainage tube is placed in the lesion. The patient was discharged from the hospital 5 days after the procedure.

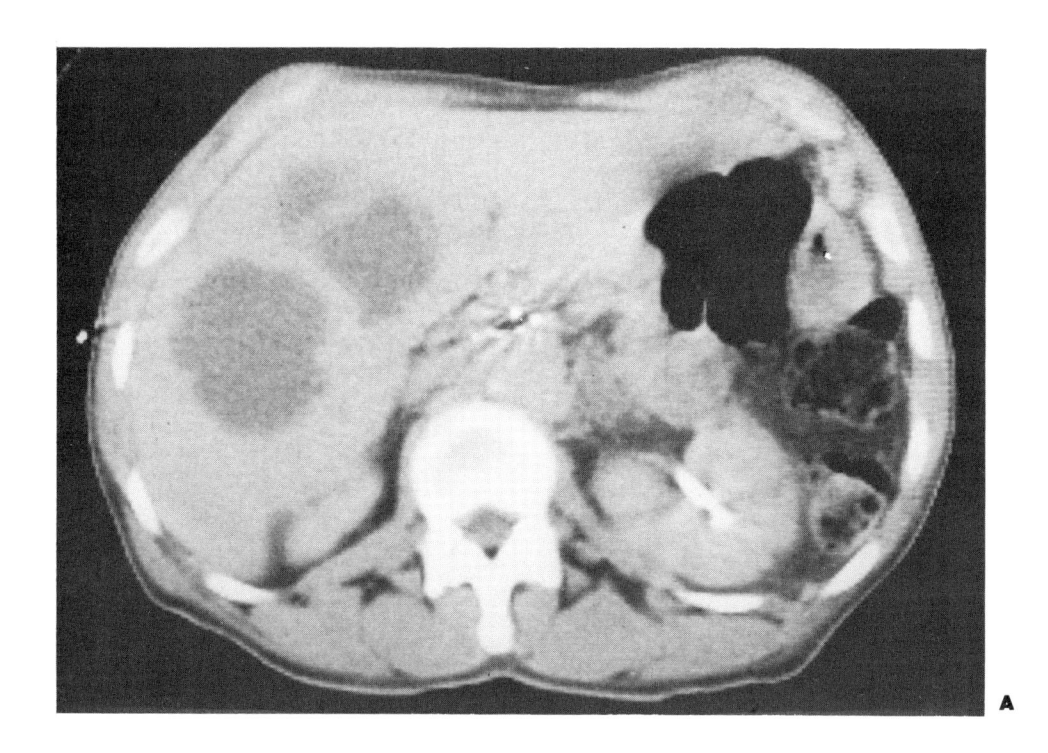

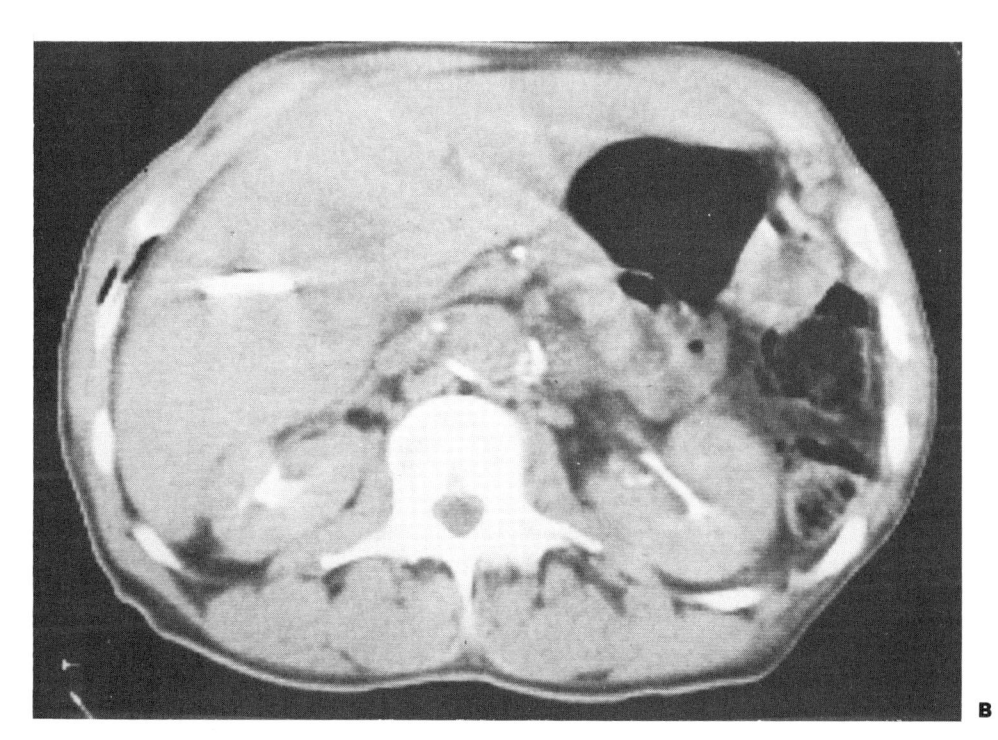

Figure 7-9. *A.* CT section demonstrates a multiseptated hepatic abscess. *B.* The abscess is drained with a single catheter.

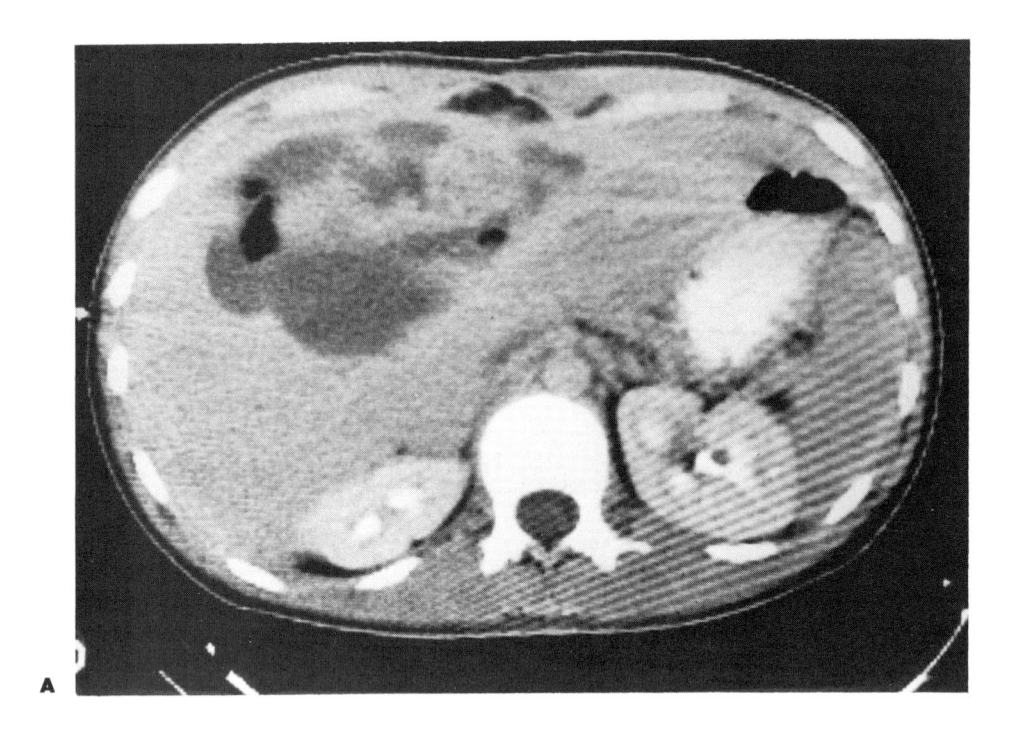

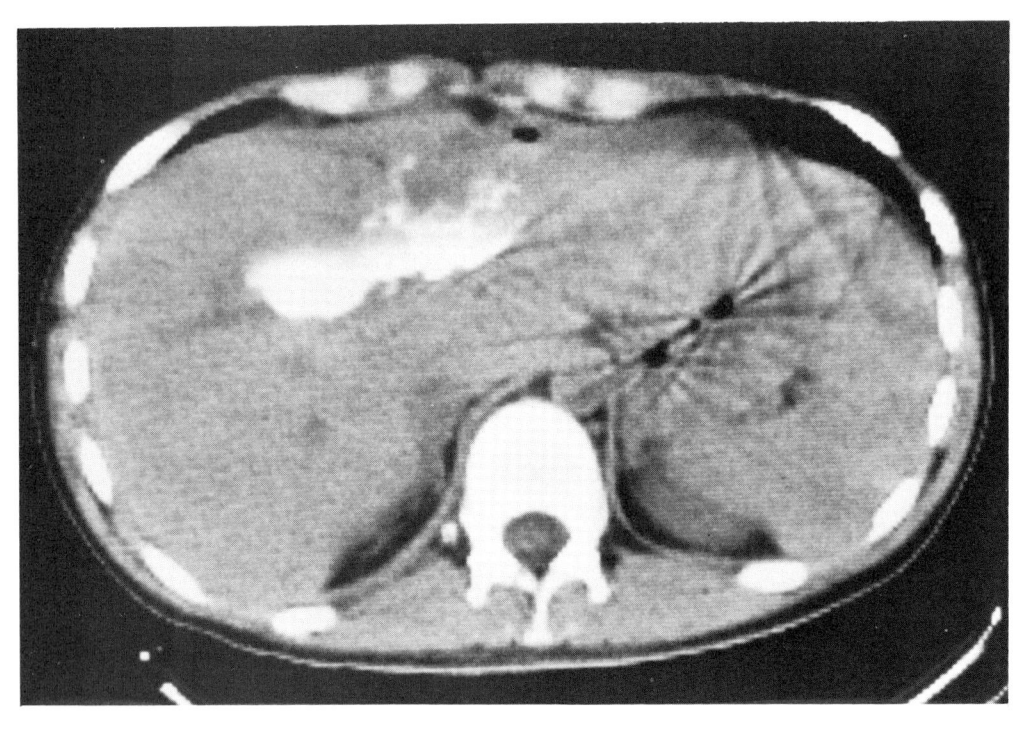

Figure 7-10. *A.* A multiseptated hepatic abscess is detected. Gas pockets are noted within the abscess. *B.* Contrast is injected within the abscess to determine if communication exists between the loculations.

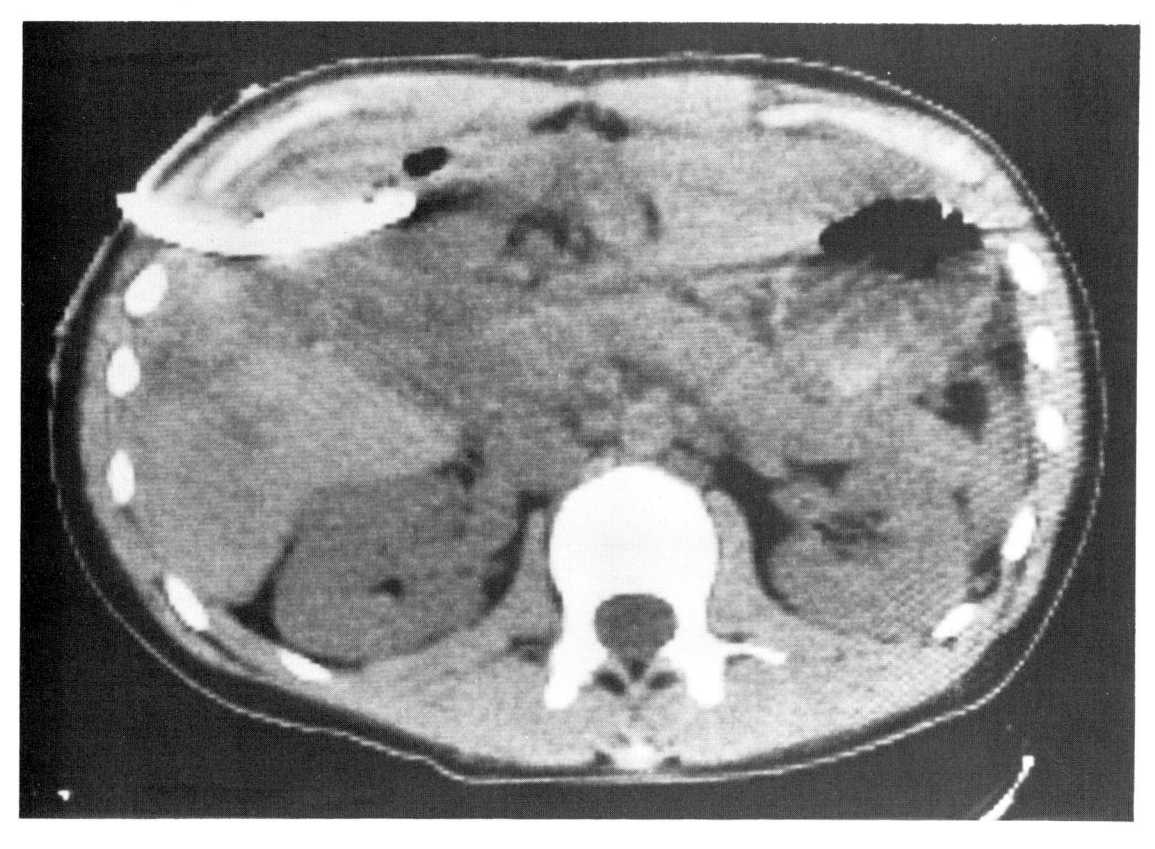

Figure 7–10. *C.* After multiple communications have been established between the abscess loculations, it is drained by a single catheter.

drainages may be longer than 20 days. As long as material is still draining, the catheter should remain in place. Periodic limited CT scans over the area of the abscess are suggested to insure proper positioning of the catheter within the abscess and adequate drainage. Injection of contrast into the cavity under fluoroscopy can be used as an alternative. However, the possibility of not visualizing other pockets or other hepatic abnormalities has caused us to use this method of follow-up sparingly. Once the drainage has stopped, and no lesion is noted on the follow-up CT scan, the catheter can be removed.

Results

The success of hepatic abscess drainage should be quite high. In reported studies it has been 33 to 93 percent (31,36,38). The success rate is dependent on the patient population and the experience of the reporter. The failures have been those due to infected necrotic tumors or those that have been complicated by a previous operation. Multiseptated or loculated abscesses are not a contraindication for drainage (9,39). (Figure 7–9, 7–10) In one series, 12 of 13 multiseptated lesions were drained successfully (38). The majority of these were drained with a single catheter. The one failure was due to an abscess with thick tenacious fluid whose viscosity could not be decreased with saline. Only one recurrence in twelve was noted. This was drained with repeat percutaneous catheter placement.

Complications

Major complications of hepatic abscess drainage are hemorrhage and sepsis. The incidence of bleeding increases with the use of larger catheters, the number of catheters used, the number of needle placements, and the location of the abscess. The incidence of sepsis decreases with proper premedication. Thus, we advocate the use of two broad-spectrum antibiotics for 24 hours before the procedure. After the offending organism(s) is identified, antibiotic therapy can be altered.

REFERENCES

1. Zornoza J: Abdomen. In J Zornoza (ed), Percutaneous Needle Biopsy. Baltimore: Williams & Wilkins, 1981, pp. 102–140.
2. Zornoza J, Wallace S, Ordenez N, Lukeman JM: Fine needle aspiration of the liver. AJR 1980;134:331–334.
3. Schultz TB: Fine needle biopsy of the liver complicated with bile peritonitis. Acta Med Scand 1976;199:141–142.
4. Isler RJ, Ferrucci JT Jr, Wittenberg J: Tissue core biopsy of abdominal tumors with a 22 gauge cutting needle. AJR 1981;136:725.
5. Wittenberg J, Mueller PR, et al.: Percutaneous core biopsy of abdominal tumors using 22 gauge needles: further observations. AJR 1982;139:75–80.
6. Haaga JR: New techniques for CT-guided biopsies. AJR 1979;133:633–641.
7. Haaga JR, Vanek J: Computed tomographic guided liver biopsy using the Menghini needle. Radiology 1979;133:405–508.
8. Haaga JR: Clinical comparison of small- and large-caliber cutting needles for biopsy. Radiology 1983;146:665–667.
9. Pagani, JJ: Biopsy of focal hepatic lesions: comparison of 18 and 22 gauge needles. Radiology 1983;147:673–675.
10. Alspaugh JP, Bernardino ME, Sewell CW, et al.: CT directed hepatic biopsies; increased diagnostic accuracy with low patient risk. J Comput Assist Tomogr 1983;7:1012–1017.
11. Pereira RV, Meiers W, Kunhardt B, et al.: Fluoroscopically guided thin needle aspiration biopsy of the abdomen and retroperitoneum. AJR 1978;131:197–202.
12. Reid MH: Real-time sonography biopsy guide. AJR 1982;140:162–163.
13. Buonocore E, Skipper GJ: Steerable real-time sonographically guide needle biopsy. AJR 1981;136:387–392.
14. Yeh E, Kronewetter C, Meade RC, Ruetz PP: Technical considerations in B-mode scanning with an aspiration transducer. Radiology 1978;129:527–530.
15. Rasmussen SN, Holm HH, Kristensen JK, et al.: Ultrasonically guided liver biopsy. Br Med J 1972;2:500–502.
16. Goldberg BB, Pollack HM: Ultrasonic aspiration biopsy techniques. J Clin Ultrasound 1976;4:141–151.
17. Ferrucci JT, Wittenberg J: CT biopsy of abdominal tumors: aids for lesion localization. Radiology 1978;129:739–744.
18. Ferrucci JT, Wittenberg J, Mueller PR, et al.: Diagnosis of abdominal malignancy by radiologic fine-needle aspiration biopsy. AJR 1980;134:323–330.
19. Nosher JL, Plafker J: Fine needle aspiration of the liver with ultrasound guidance. Radiology 1980;136:177–180.
20. Lieberman RP, Hafez GR, Crummy AB: Histology form aspiration biopsy: Turner needle experience. AJR 1982;138:561–564.
21. Sundaram M, Wolverson MK, Heiberg E, et al.: Utility of CT-guided abdominal aspiration procedures. AJR 1982;139:1111–1115.
22. Harter LP, Moss AA, Goldberg HI, Gross BH: CT-guided fine-needle aspirations for diagnosis of benign and malignant disease. AJR 1983;140:363–367.

23. Hollstein H, Boklke E, Pochhammer KF: Sonographically guided percutaneous needle biopsy of the liver. Ultraschall 1981;2:151–152.
24. Cremniter D, Chatel A, Bigot JM, et al.: Angiographic abnormalities following needle biopsy of the liver. J Radiol Electrol Med Nucl 1978;59:33–38.
25. Bernardino ME, Lewis E: Imaging hepatic neoplasms. Cancer 1982;50:2666–2671.
26. Johnson WC, Gerzof SG, Robbins AH, et al.: Treatment of abdominal abscesses: comparative evaluation of operative drainage vs percutaneous catheter drainage guided by computed tomography or ultrasound. Ann Surg 1981;194:510–520.
27. Gronvall S, Gammelgaard J, Haubek A, et al.: Drainage of abdominal abscesses guided by sonography. AJR 1982;138:527–529.
28. VanSonnenberg E, Ferrucci JT, Mueller PR, et al.: Percutaneous drainage of abscesses and fluid collections: techniques, results and applications. Radiology 1982;142:1–10.
29. Maklad NF, Doust BD, Baum JK: Ultrasonic diagnosis of postoperative intra-abdominal abscess. Radiology 1974;133:417–422.
30. Gerzof SG, Robbins AH, Johnson WC, et al.: Percutaneous catheter drainage of abdominal abscesses. A five-year experience. N Engl J Med 1981;305:653–657.
31. Martin EC, Karlson KB, Fankuchen EI, et al.: Percutaneous drainage of postoperative intraabdominal abscesses. AJR 1982;138:13–15.
32. Haaga JR, Weinstein AJ: CT guided percutaneous aspiration and drainage of abscesses. AJR 1980;135:1187–1194.
33. Gronvall S, Gammelgaard J, Haubek A, Holm HH: Drainage of abdominal abscesses guided by sonography. AJR 1982;138:527–529.
34. Kleinhaus U, Rosenberger A: Computed tomography-guided percutaneous drainage of right upper abdominal abscesses. Cardiovasc Intervent Radiol 1982;5:8–13.
35. Aeder MI, Wellman JL, Haaga JR, Hau T: Role of surgical and percutaneous drainage in the treatment of abdominal abscesses. Arch Surg 1982;118:273–280.
36. vanWaes PFGM, Feldberg MAM, Mali WPThM, et al.: Management of loculated abscesses that are difficult to drain: a new approach. Radiology 1983;147:57–63.
37. Edwards KC, Katzen BT, Woods C: Continuous, gentle suction apparatus for abscess drainage. Radiology 1982;145:537.
38. Bernardino ME, Berkman WA, Plemmons M, et al.: Percutaneous drainage of multiseptated hepatic abscess. J Comp Assist Tomogr 1984;87:38–41.
39. Greenwood LH, Collins TL, Yrizarry JM: Percutaneous management of multiple liver abscess. AJR 1982;139:390–392.

8

Diagnostic Hepatic Angiography: Mass and Diffuse Disease

ARINA VAN BREDA • ARTHUR WALTMAN

INTRODUCTION

The advent of angiography heralded a new era in the evaluation of a wide spectrum of hepatic abnormalities. Tentative diagnosis of the nature of hepatic lesions, as well as valuable vascular anatomy, was now available preoperatively. Increasing experience with angiography brought forth reports of "characteristic" or pathognomonic features of different entities, promising a high degree of accuracy of angiographic diagnosis. Further experience led to the realization that angiographic findings were often not completely specific, and overlap could and did occur (1). The development of newer, noninvasive imaging techniques complemented by fine-needle biopsy has reduced the indications for diagnostic hepatic angiography. However, angiography frequently can provide valuable diagnostic information not available with other modalities. Familiarity with angiographic appearance of diseases affecting the liver can allow the radiologist to contribute significantly to the evaluation of these patients.

TECHNIQUE

Prior to angiography, the radiologist should be familiar with the patient's history, clinical findings, pertinent prior radiologic examinations, and laboratory findings. Based on this data, the radiologist can entertain a list of possible diagnoses that may allow for more specific or focused angiographic examination and will ensure a satisfactory evaluation.

Frequently, hepatic angiography is performed on an elective basis for evaluation of an abnormality first noted on other studies. In this setting, proper patient preparation prior to the procedure is possible, including adequate hydration. When hepatic angiography is performed for the evaluation or treatment of trauma, adequate patient preparation may not be possible. Steps should be taken to ensure hemodynamic stabilization of the patient prior to and during the angiographic procedure. In all cases, there should be constant patient monitoring to prevent, recognize, and correct complications.

The technique of selective angiography has been well described elsewhere (2,3). The preferred approach is a femoral puncture using the Seldinger technique; where this is not possible, an axillary puncture may be necessary. The angiographer should be familiar with performance of selective catheterization of the visceral vessels from this approach. A rotating cradle top or C-arm fluoroscopy allows oblique visualization of the abdominal aorta, which facilitates catheterization of its branches and is particularly valuable in elderly patients with tortuous or calcified vessels.

Selective visceral angiography can generally be accomplished with preformed catheters (Cobra, Simmons, or side-winder shapes), but occasionally may require a catheter that is fashioned by steaming to conform to the patient's anatomy. A "headhunter," or multipurpose catheter can be used for selective catheterization from an axillary approach. The smallest catheter, 5F or 6F, that will allow sufficient torque control for selective catheterization should be used. Smaller catheters are necessary for pediatric angiography.

Seventy-six percent contrast is used in preference to lower density contrast agents because of its greater radiopacity. Extensive experience with the use of nonionic contrast in visceral angiography has not been reported. Injection rates for celiac angiography range from 6 to 10 ml/second with total contrast volume of 40 to 60 ml; similar rates and volumes are used for superior mesenteric angiography, although for satisfactory visualization of the portal venous system via superior mesenteric artery injection, total volume of contrast may be increased to 70 ml.

Rates and volumes used for subselective injections of the hepatic artery of its branches require assessment of the size of the artery being injected. Most commonly, 6 to 8 ml/second for a total contrast volume of 40 to 50 ml is used for the common hepatic artery. An infusion technique of hepatic arteriography has been described by a number of authors (4–6), consisting of a prolonged low rate of infusion of contrast into the hepatic artery (2 to 5 ml/second for 10 to 20 seconds) with delayed filming for better visualization of small primary liver tumors and metastatic lesions.

Hepatic vein visualization requires selective hepatic vein injection. This can be accomplished from the femoral, brachial, or transjugular venous approaches. Main hepatic vein injection is performed with an end and side hole catheter, injecting 25 to 30 ml at 10 to 12 ml/second. Wedged hepatic venography is performed with an endhole-only catheter, gently wedged into the hepatic parenchyma, or alternately, with a balloon occlusion catheter inflated in a main hepatic vein. Both techniques should be performed under fluoroscopic observation with small contrast volumes, generally 2 ml/second for 8 to 10 ml. Measurements of wedged and free hepatic vein pressures can be used to assess the portal vein pressure. The primary role of hepatic venography is in the assessment of cirrhosis or portal hypertension, although assessment of hepatic vein patency should be performed in the evaluation of hepatic tumors and of hepatic vein occlusion or Budd-Chiari syndrome (7–9).

Satisfactory visualization of the portal structures is generally possible with venous phase angiography after splenic or superior mesenteric arteriography, usually with concominant intraarterial vasodilators. Better delineation of portal structures can be obtained by splenoportography or transhepatic portography; the latter technique is more frequently performed. Portography is generally reserved for therapeutic applications, i.e., variceal embolization, and for the uncommon case of unsatisfactory portal vein visualization with standard arteriography (8,10,11).

The filming sequence for diagnostic hepatic arteriography must be tailored to the clinical problem but, in general, must include evaluation of the systemic arterial supply and the portal circulation. This necessitates a prolonged filming sequence, generally up to 30 seconds. Rapid early filming, 1 to 2/second × 6 seconds, is followed by a longer, slower sequence, 1 every 2 to 3 seconds for an additional 20 to 25 seconds. Hepatic angiography is generally performed in the AP position with oblique views added as indicated. Steep oblique views are sometimes necessary to distinguish extrahepatic mass lesions from intrahepatic processes (12). The right posterior oblique position is used in evaluating the main portal vein as it clears this structure from superimposition on the spine.

Pharmacoangiography

Vasodilators are frequently used to enhance the portal phase of splanchnic angiography, most commonly 25 to 40 mg of tolazoline injected directly into the superior mesenteric artery immediately before contrast injection. Other vasodilatory agents that have been utilized for the same purpose include papaverine and prostaglandins (14,15). Vasodilating agents are not used widely for purposes other than enhanced venous visualization.

Vasoconstrictive agents such as epinephrine, norepinephrine, vasopressin and angiotensin have not found widespread use in hepatic angiography. These agents may produce differential vasoconstriction of normal vessels relative to tumor vessels and thus may aid in identification of neoplasm, although they rarely uncover an abnormality not identifiable on standard arteriography (3,15). Additionally, the response of normal and abnormal vessels to these agents is variable and therefore the angiographic response is not specific (16).

Complications

Potential complications of diagnostic angiography are well-catalogued elsewhere (2,17). Specific complications of hepatic angiography include hepatic artery dissection, occlusion, and false aneurysm formation (18). Should occlusion occur as a complication of hepatic artery catheterization, the procedure should be halted if possible and resumed several days later when patency may be restored. The reversibility of these occlusions is probably due to the combined role of spasm and thrombosis as causative factors; both of these processes can be reversed endogenously. Occlusions of the common hepatic artery are generally well-tolerated and clinically inapparent because of the abundant potential collaterals that maintain hepatic arterial inflow, and to the dual blood supply via the portal system. Hepatic artery occlusions are of greater consequence in the face of decreased or reversed portal blood flow.

ANATOMY

Hepatic arterial anatomy is extremely variable, the "classic anatomy" being present in only 55 to 60 percent of the population. The common hepatic artery arises as one of the major branches of the celiac artery; it is termed the proper hepatic artery after the origin of the gastroduodenal artery. The proper hepatic artery divides into the right and left hepatic arteries; the middle hepatic artery arises as a separate branch of one of these arteries in most cases, or as a separate branch of the proper hepatic artery in approximately 10 percent. The right hepatic artery, after giving rise to the cystic artery, divides into branches to the anterior and posterior segments of the right lobe. These segmental branches subsequently divide to supply the superior and inferior divisions of these segments. The left hepatic artery divides into medial and lateral segmental arteries; the lateral segmental artery divides into superior and inferior branches. The middle hepatic artery supplies the medial segment of the left lobe, referred to in most anatomic texts as the quadrate lobe (8,19–21). Variations in hepatic arterial anatomy are common, with a replaced or accessory right hepatic artery present in approximately 25 percent of individuals, usually arising from the superior mesenteric artery, and a 25 percent incidence of replaced or accessory left hepatic artery (Figure 8–1), most frequently arising from the left gastric artery (Figure 8–1). Complete replacement of the hepatic artery from the superior mesenteric artery can occur, and rarely, one of the hepatic arteries can arise separately from the aorta. Awareness of the potential anatomic variations of hepatic arterial anatomy is important for complete angiographic assessment of the liver (22).

In normal individuals, the hepatic artery supplies 25 percent of inflow to the liver, the remainder being carried by the portal system. Therefore, complete angiographic evaluation of the liver must include visualization of the portal system. The pattern of involvement of the portal vein in evaluation of hepatic masses can help in differentiating the etiology of the mass (23). The main portal vein is formed by the junction of the superior mesenteric vein and the splenic vein after it receives its inflow from the inferior mesenteric vein. The portal vein enters the liver hilum in close relationship to the hepatic artery, lying dorsal to it and the common bile duct. The intrahepatic portal vein branching mirrors that of the hepatic artery and biliary ducts. The association of these three systems continues into the hepatic parenchyma to the microscopic level as portal triads.

The hepatic veins lie between the hepatic segments and drain into the inferior vena cava. The middle hepatic vein lies in the interlobar fissure; this is in distinction to the hepatic artery and portal vein branches, which do not cross lobar fissures. There are usually three major hepatic veins; the right drains into the inferior vena cava separately, whereas the middle and left hepatic vein often join before entering it. Several smaller veins may be present, draining the caudate lobe and entering the IVC directly. The hepatic veins are not usually visualized during arteriography of the liver unless venous catheterization and selective venous injection is performed. However, the hepatic vein may be visualized secondary to shunting in certain lesions, and differentiation of hepatic and portal veins may then be important. In addition, hepatic vein thrombosis or occlusions may lead to arterial or parenchymal abnormalities, and, therefore, visualization of this system should not be neglected in the evaluation of hepatic abnormalities (24,25).

Due to the greater contribution to total hepatic blood flow from the portal system, evaluation of the hepatic parenchyma is difficult by hepatic artery injection alone. Celiac or SMA injections, the latter enhanced by vasodilators, are most commonly used to evaluate the parenchyma. In the past, evaluation of the parenchymal phase was of particular value in the search for hypovascular mass lesions, although this is less important with improved sensitivity of noninvasive cross-sectional imaging techniques (26). However, a prolonged selective infusion of contrast into the hepatic artery, with careful attention to the early parenchymal phase and the pattern of contrast washout, has been described as a means of more specific differentiation of normal hepatic parenchyma from tumors (5,6).

The arterial parenchymal phase can have a mottled and inhomogeneous or finely nodular appearance, which can raise the possibility of a diffuse parenchymal abnor-

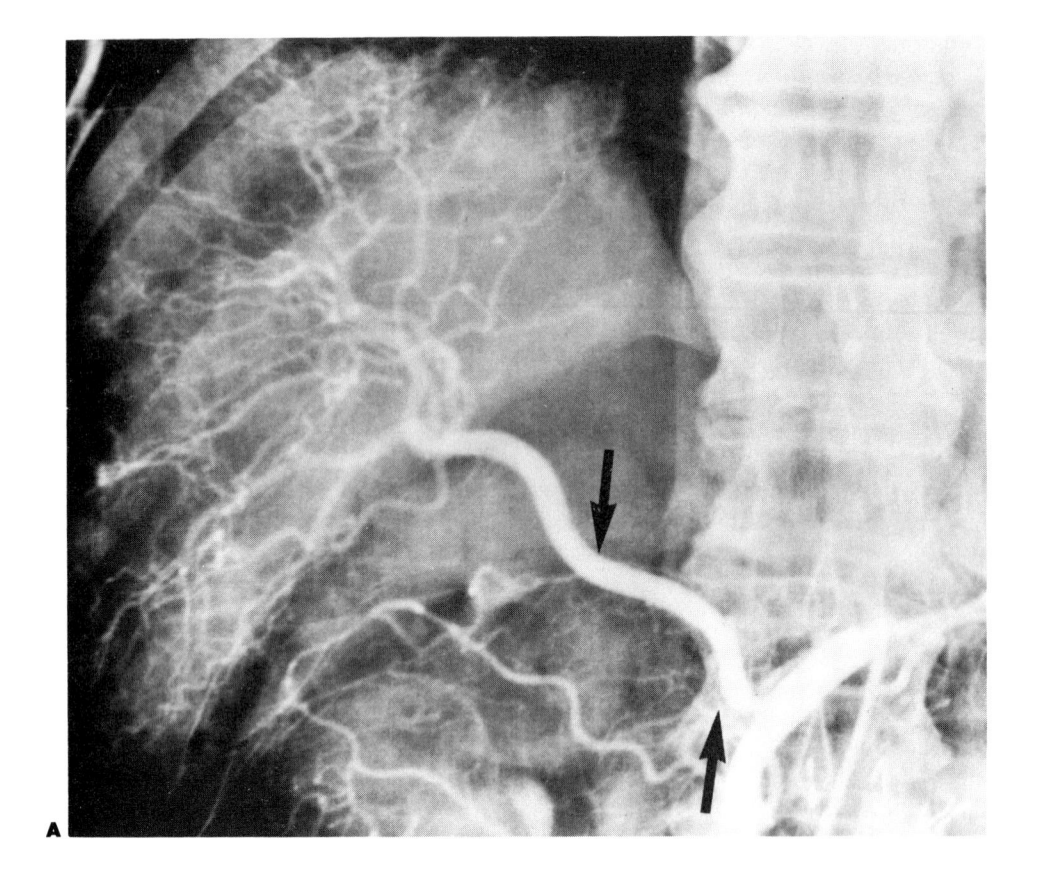

Figure 8-1. Usual hepatic arterial anatomic variants. *A.* Selective superior mesenteric arteriogram with right hepatic artery (arrows) arising from superior mesenteric artery.

mality. The wide range of appearance of normals must be borne in mind before making a pathologic diagnosis on the basis of this finding alone (8).

Pitfalls

The size of the left lobe of the liver is extremely variable, but is usually significantly smaller than the right; it is often very thin and partially overlies the spine. For these reasons, angiographic evaluation of the left lobe can be difficult. This may be somewhat overcome by subselective left hepatic artery injection. In addition, the left lobe lies in a relatively anterior position, making opacification of the left branch of the portal vein difficult due to posterior layering of contrast. Lack of awareness of these factors may lead to false-positive diagnosis of abnormalities of the left hepatic lobe.

The right lobe of the liver may have a relatively large Reidels lobe simulating a mass, but this should be readily recognized by a normal arterial, parenchymal, and venous appearance.

Differentiation of intrahepatic and extrahepatic masses can usually be made on the basis of noninvasive studies; however, the source of origin of large right upper quadrant masses, especially if hypovascular, can often present as a radiologic challenge. Careful attention to the hepatic vascular pattern can then provide a clue to the nature of the mass (12).

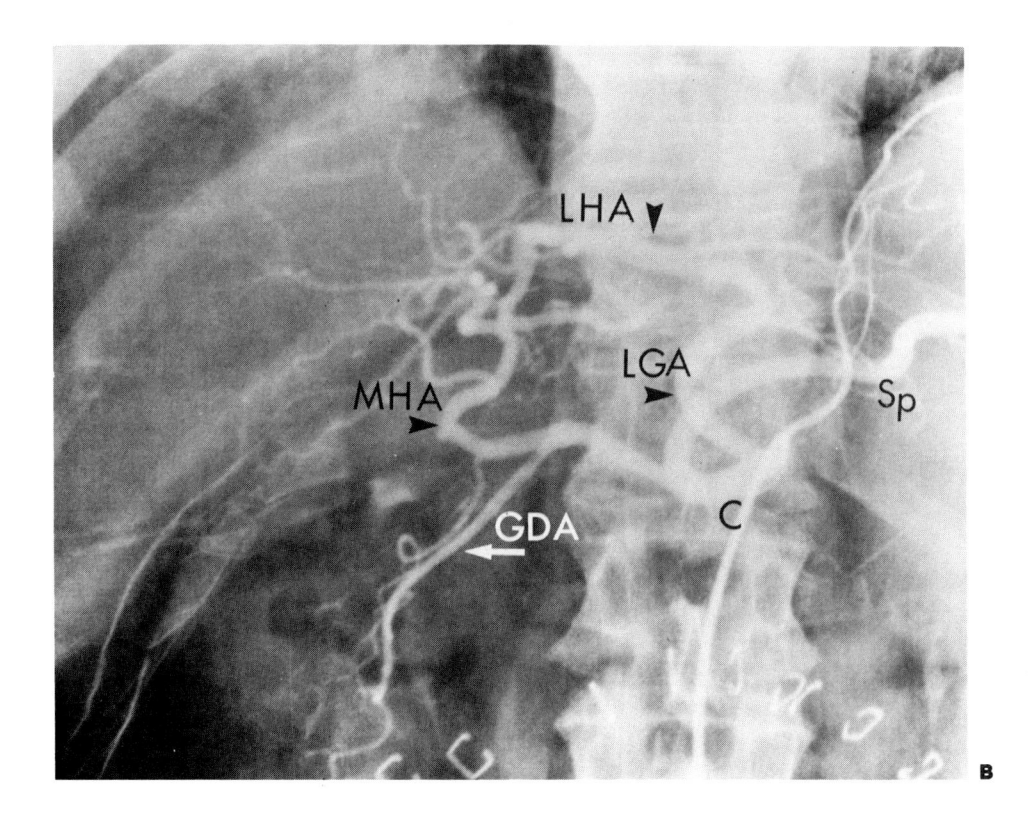

Figure 8-1. *B.* Selective celiac axis arteriogram demonstrating large left gastric artery (LGA) with left hepatic artery (LHA) (arrows). Common hepatic artery (CHA) supplies gastroduodenal (GDA) and middle hepatic arteries (MHA).

In the performance of selective angiography, the angiographer should always bear in mind the possibility of inducing spurious abnormalities by catheter or guidewire manipulation. Spasm of the hepatic artery or its branches can mimic vascular stenosis or occlusion due to atherosclerosis or tumor. If an abnormality is thought to be secondary to spasm, the administration of a vasodilating agent such as priscoline or nitroglycerin intraarterially may reverse the spasm. Often spasm will spontaneously subside after several minutes if no further manipulation of the affected artery is attempted.

VASCULAR DISORDERS

Peliosis Hepatis

Peliosis hepatis is a rare diffuse hepatic abnormality that produces a characteristic angiographic appearance (Figure 8-2). It is characterized by blood-filled cystic spaces of various sizes, which may or may not be lined by endothelium (27). Angiographically, multiple small areas of contrast accumulation are noted throughout the liver, ranging in size from minute pinpoints to 1 cm, which persist throughout the parenchymal and venous phase. This disorder has been associated with the ingestion of anabolic steroids, estrogens, oral contraceptives, and azothioprine. In addition, it has been noted in patients exposed to vinyl chloride. The pathogenesis may be cholestasis and vascular

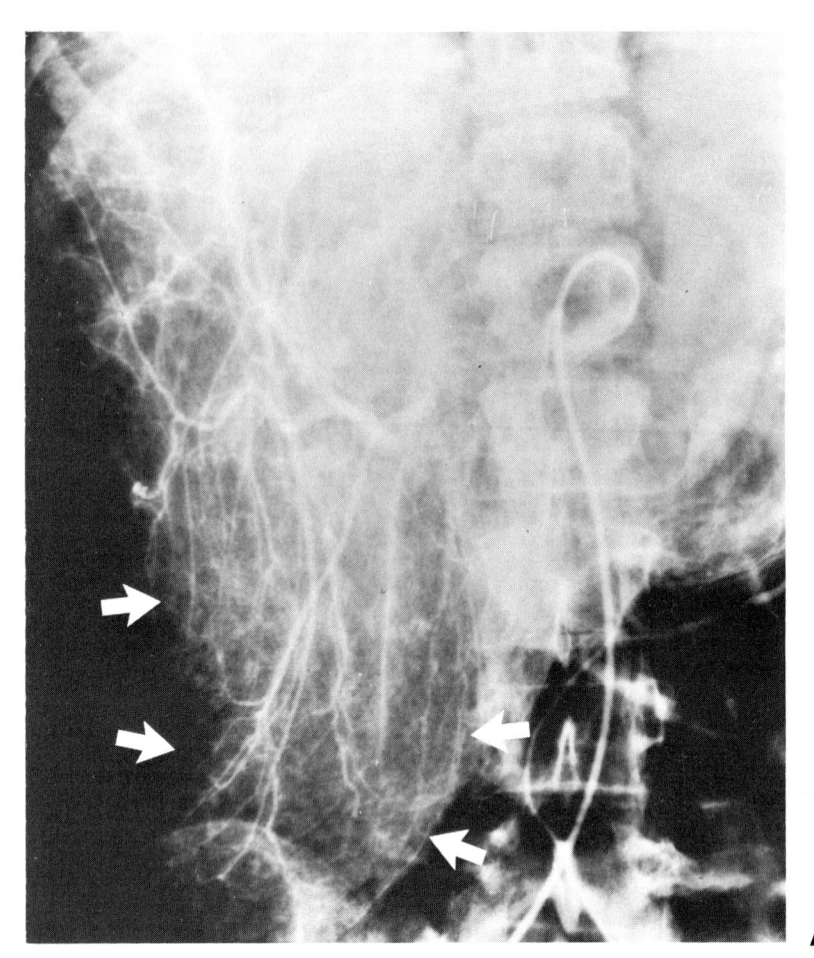

Figure 8–2. Twenty-nine-year-old female with acute right upper quadrant abdominal pain and palpable mass demonstrated on ultrasound and hepatic scan. *A.* Late arterial phase of selective hepatic arteriogram shows inhomogeneous staining of inferior aspect of right lobe (arrows). *B.* Capillary phase of magnification arteriogram shows abnormal and patchy hepatogram with small punctate collections.

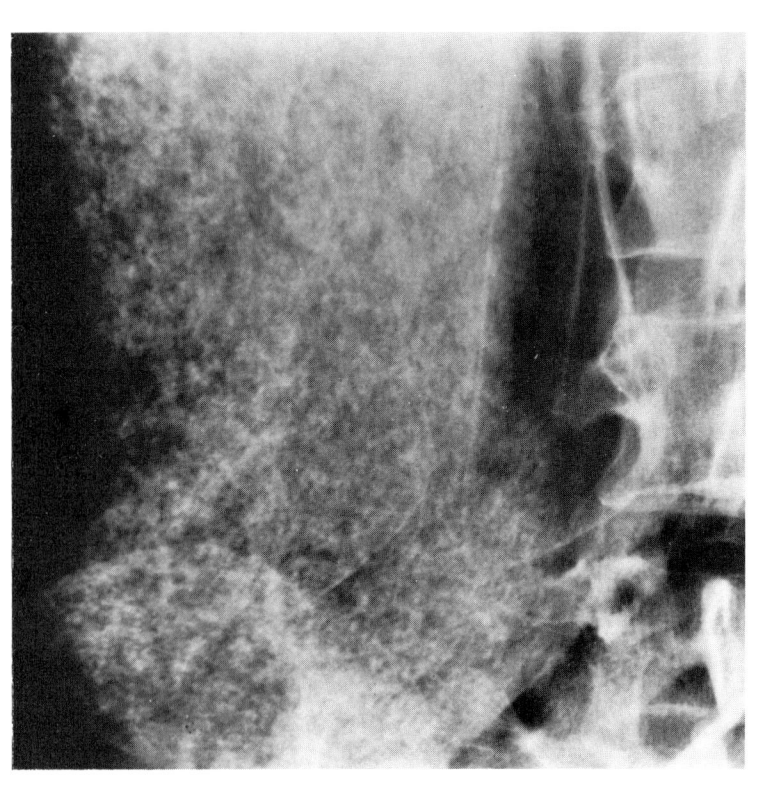

congestion leading to the development of venous lakes. Though generally considered a benign lesion that will resolve if the inducing agent is withdrawn, spontaneous rupture and intraperitoneal bleeding have been reported and can be life-threatening. In addition, peliosis has been reported in association with hepatic angiosarcoma, in patients with vinyl-chloride exposure and with hepatoma (28–30).

Polyarteritis Nodosa

Polyarteritis is a necrotizing vasculitis characterized by an inflammatory process that involves medium and small arteries. Multiple small fusiform or saccular aneurysms are the most prominent angiographic finding; these occur in the liver of approximately 40 to 60 percent of affected individuals, less frequently than renal involvement, which occurs in 80 to 100 percent. The aneurysms may rupture, producing intraperitoneal bleeding. Other angiographic findings include a decrease in the number of distal arteries in the involved organ and arterial irregularity and stenosis (3,8). Drug abuse produces a necrotizing angiitis with identical angiographic findings; as well, metastatic atrial myxoma and diffusely metastatic Wilms' tumor have been reported to produce a similar angiographic appearance due to transmural necrosis and direct tumor invasion of blood vessels (31).

Atherosclerosis

Atherosclerotic changes are seen frequently in arteriograms of older individuals; the importance of these changes is in the distinction of these lesions from other disease processes. The most common finding is plaque formation and stenosis, which must be differentiated from arterial changes of tumor encasement. The diffuse nature of atherosclerosis, with involvement of other celiac branches (most commonly the splenic artery), the occasional presence of vascular calcification, and the lack of associated parenchymal mass usually makes this differentiation quite straightforward, although occasionally, difficulties may arise. Similarly, atherosclerotic occlusions are readily recognized, but may create difficulties by precluding selective angiography. Most commonly, these occlusions involve the origins of major vessels such as the celiac or superior mesenteric artery, although isolated occlusions of the common hepatic artery can occur. These occlusions are usually accompanied by a well-developed collateral network. Atherosclerotic stenoses and occlusions must also be differentiated from spasm induced by catheter and guidewire manipulation.

Aneurysms

Aneurysms of the visceral arteries can be atherosclerotic, mycotic, or traumatic in origin, or may be due to a primary degeneration of the arterial walls (Figure 8-3). Differentiation as to etiology is often based on clinical grounds, rather than angiographic appearance (8).

Aneurysms that develop after trauma are generally pseudoaneurysms that may occur days or months after injury (32). Hepatic artery false-aneurysm formation has been described after subintimal dissection at angiography (18) and after liver biopsy (33). Another iatrogenic cause of hepatic artery aneurysms is intraarterial chemotherapy; aneurysms have been noted in up to 20 percent of individuals treated with hepatic artery infusions of 5-fluorouracil. These aneurysms appear to be related to direct toxicity of chemotherapeutic agents on the arterial wall (34).

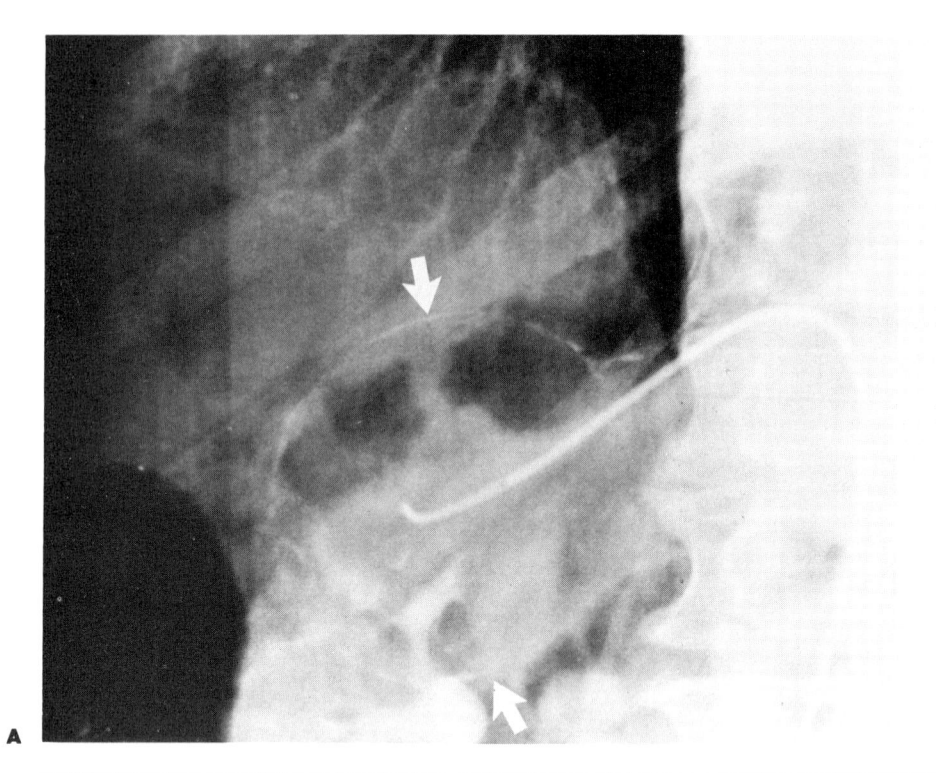

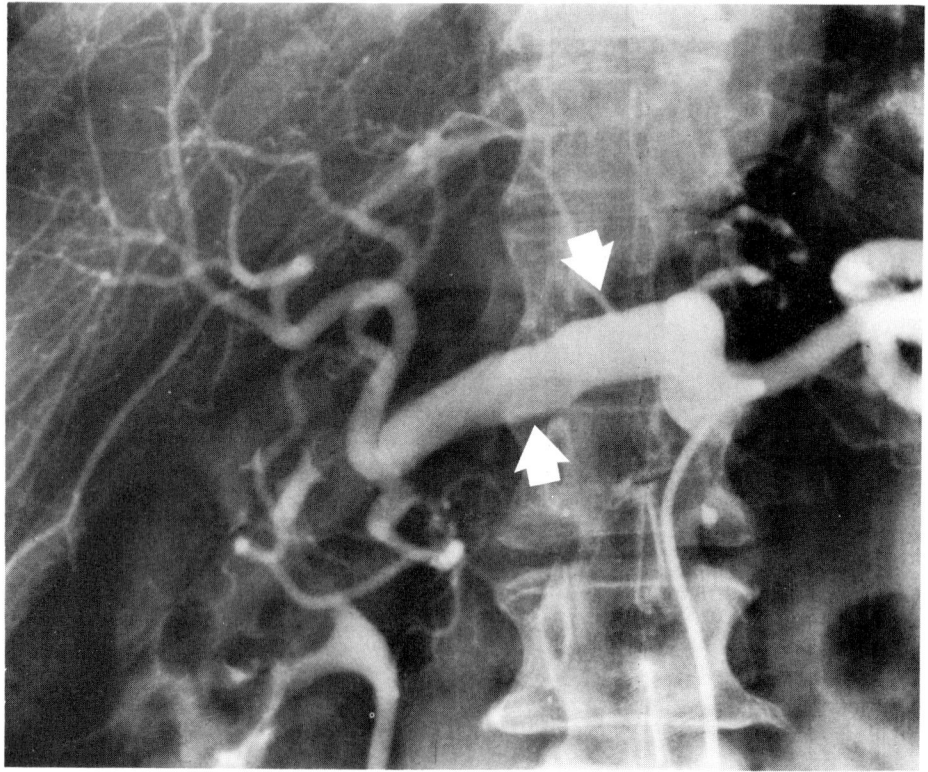

Figure 8-3. Patient with transient episodes of nausea and upper abdominal discomfort. Ultrasound demonstrated mass in right upper quadrant containing a tubular, central, sonolucent region. *A.* Plain film of right upper quadrant shows calcific rim of an 8-cm mass (arrows). *B.* Selective celiac axis arteriogram showing enlarged hepatic artery (arrows).

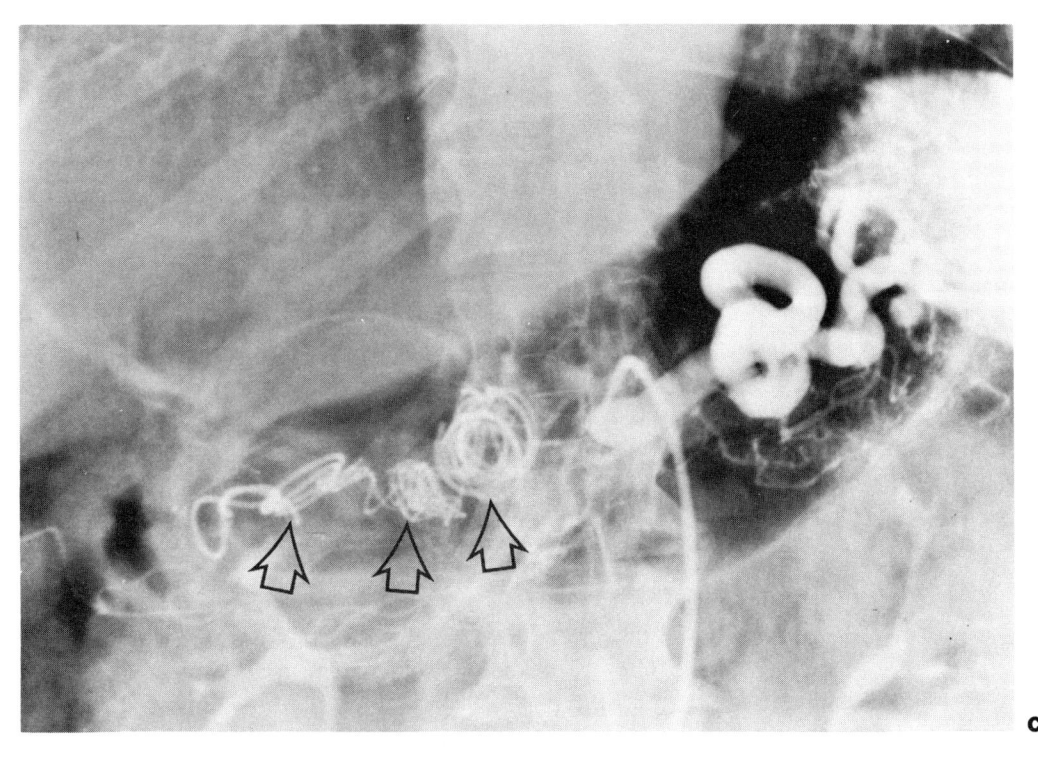

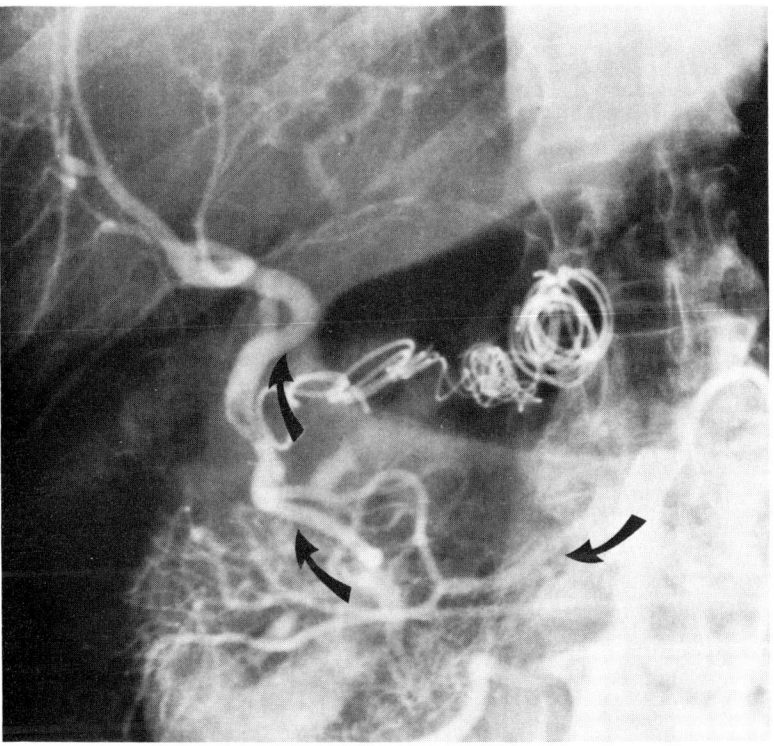

Figure 8–3. *C.* Selective splenic arteriogram, after multiple metallic coils (open arrow) placed in hepatic artery, demonstrates occlusion of hepatic artery. *D.* Superior mesenteric arteriogram with inferior pancreaticoduodenal artery reconstitution of gastroduodenal artery and intrahepatic arteries (curved arrows) after mechanical-coil occlusion of hepatic artery aneurysm.

Seventy-five percent of the reported cases of hepatic artery aneurysms have involved the extrahepatic course of the hepatic artery (35). There is a hazard of life-threatening rupture of the extrahepatic aneurysms (36); intrahepatic aneurysms can enlarge or develop communications with the biliary system, leading to hematobilia, or with the portal or systemic veins, producing AV fistulae (37). Jaundice can occur due to compression of the biliary system by the enlarging mass of the aneurysm. Aneurysms may be minute or quite large and present as an epigastric mass (38). Careful angiographic evaluation of the exact location of the aneurysm, its relationship to major hepatic artery branches and potential collaterals is important in planning the need for and method of therapy of these aneurysms (35). Although angiography is indispensable for accurate definition of the location of the aneurysm, occasionally patients can undergo serial evaluation by less invasive means, especially digital venous angiography, to determine the stability of the lesions and the need for treatment. The role of therapeutic embolization of aneurysms will be discussed elsewhere.

Amyloidosis

Widespread changes in the appearance of the hepatic and renal arteries have been described in amyloidosis. The changes consist of luminal irregularities with abrupt changes in caliber of the branches. An absence of changes in the more proximal portion of the vessels may help in differentiating the process from atherosclerosis. Similarly, lack of mass effect or tumor blush should help distinguish amyloidosis from encasement by tumor. The arteriographic changes are due to the deposit of abnormal mucopolysaccharide in and around the blood vessels (39).

INFLAMMATORY DISEASE

Diffuse inflammatory disease of the liver, hepatitis, can be due to infection, usually viral but occasionally bacterial, or to chemical toxins such as alcohol. Angiography does not play a role in the diagnosis of these processes, but familiarity with the arteriographic findings may be useful in distinguishing these abnormalities from other disease processes. Arteriographic findings in hepatitis are a spectrum ranging from an essentially normal arteriogram to fairly discrete abnormalities. Alcoholic hepatitis has been described as producing marked dilatation of the common and intrahepatic arteries; there may be significant hypervascularity of portions or of all the liver. There can be stretching of the intrahepatic branches and a mottled, irregular parenchymal phase; these findings represent the most severe changes produced. Since patients with prior inflammatory disease of the liver have an increased risk of hepatoma development, this must always be considered in the differential. The arteries in hepatitis should not have the irregular, widely varying caliber of neoplastic vessels, but nonetheless, differentiation from diffuse hepatoma can be difficult (8,40).

Increasing sophistication of diagnostic modalities, especially ultrasound and nuclear medicine, has allowed earlier diagnosis of pyogenic liver disease, enabling detection before the development of abscesses. Acute pyogenic hepatitis has been described as showing hypervascularity with a mottled, inhomogeneous parenchymal phase. In one case, arterial portal shunting was noted (41).

Once abscesses develop, the diagnosis is usually apparent by the clinical presentation and noninvasive diagnostic techniques. Prior to the development of these techniques, angiography was frequently required. The angiographic pattern of abscess in its early stages is similar to that of pyogenic hepatitis. As the abscess becomes better orga-

A

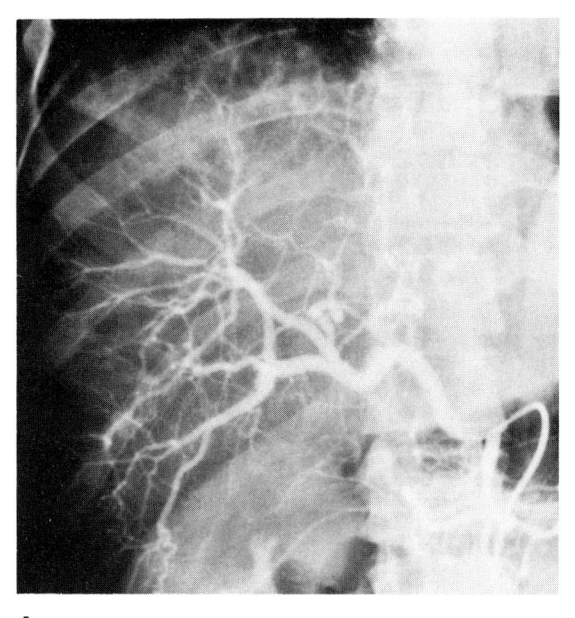

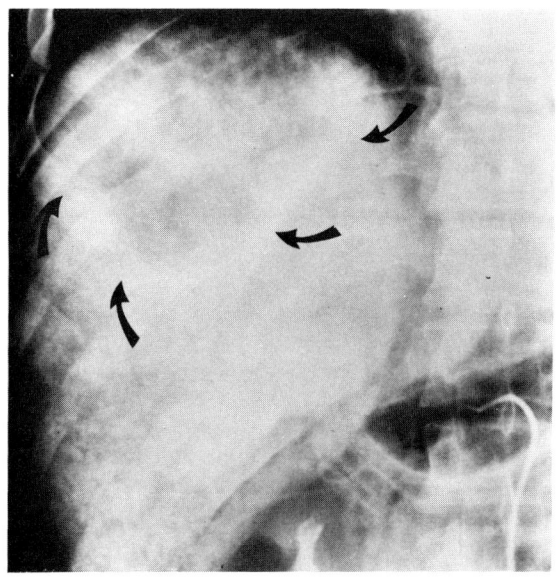

B

Figure 8-4. Middle-aged male with sudden onset of myalgia, diarrhea, fever, and chills with pleuritic and abdominal pain. Ultrasound evaluation identified diffuse inflammatory changes of right lobe. *A.* Selective hepatic arteriogram demonstrates no abnormal hepatic arterial branches. *B.* Capillary phase of hepatic arteriogram shows multilocular hypovascular mass of right lobe with thick hypervascular rind (curved arrows). Surgical resection and drainage of hepatic abscess was performed.

nized, mass effect with displacement of vascular structures is most frequently seen with a hypervascular rim or hypervascularity in surrounding parenchyma (Figure 8-4) (42). Arterial venous shunting has been reported (43). Multiple abscesses can be indistinguishable from metastatic disease.

Diffuse involvement of the liver with tuberculosis can occur and present clinically and radiographically as malignancy. The arteriographic pattern is one of diffuse hypervascularity with an irregular parenchymal phase and nodular irregularities of the distal arteries (44).

More indolent infections can produce a primarily hypovascular mass. In this instance, the angiographic appearance of pyogenic liver abscess can be difficult to distinguish from hematoma or parasitic abscesses. Amebic infestation is not an infrequent cause of hepatic abscess in the United States, accounting for up to 10 percent of cases (45). The arteriographic changes are similar to those described for pyogenic abscesses, with the more chronic abscess demonstrating less hypervascularity, leaving a thin rim around the cavity.

The liver is the most frequent site of involvement by echinococcal cyst formation. In the past, angiography has been employed to help define the location, number, and size of hydatid cysts, which are frequently multiple, but this indication no longer pertains. Angiography may be necessary for surgical planning. The angiographic appearance of hydatid cyst is not specific, but is fairly characteristic. The cyst itself is avascular with a sharply defined margin that is usually hypervascular. This hypervascularity is attributed to newly formed scar tissue in the ectocyst, which forms as a result of the

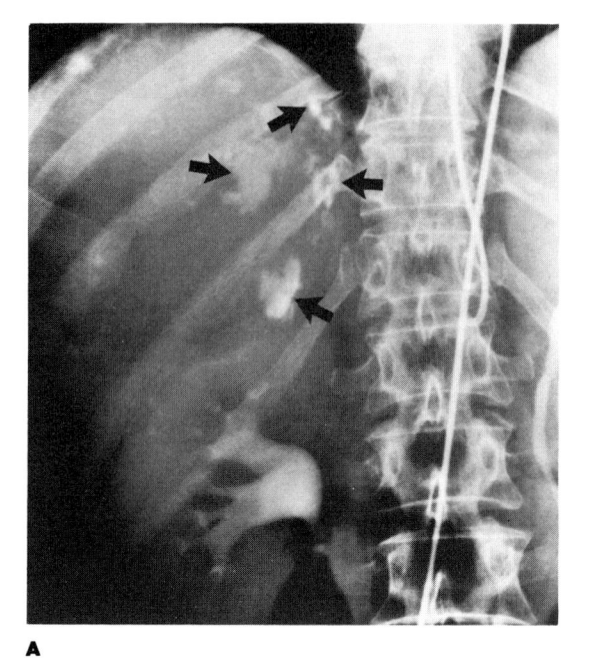

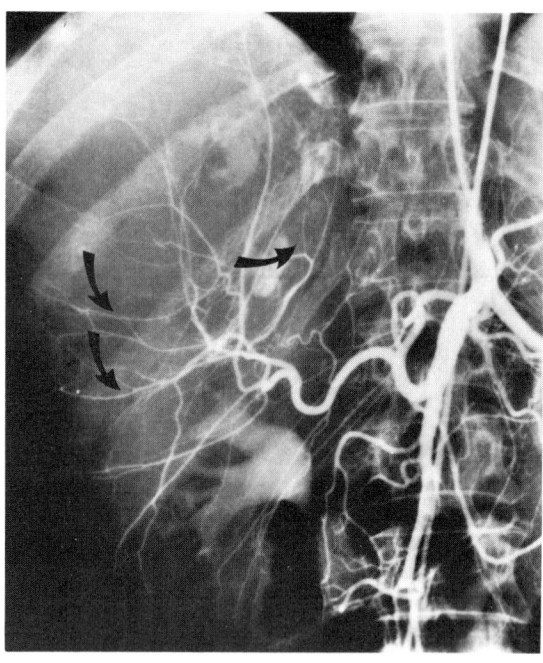

Figure 8–5. Forty-year-old female with enlarged liver. *A.* Plain film of right upper quadrant shows plaque-like calcifications (arrows). *B.* Celiac axis arteriogram shows bowing of intrahepatic arterial branches (curved arrows) in the right lobe with hypervascular rim.

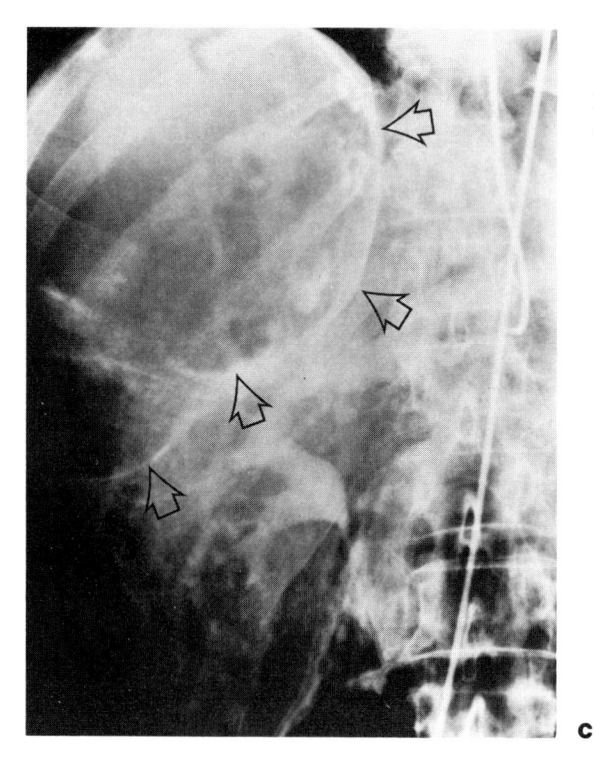

Figure 8–5. *C.* The lesion (open arrows) has a thin wall. An echinococcal cyst was resected.

continued growth and expansion of the hypovascular endocyst (46). The rim is usually only several millimeters thick, and the thickness of the rim has been used to differentiate echinococcal cyst disease from other focal hepatic masses (Figure 8–5) (45). However, this finding has been described in other lesions, as well (47).

CYSTS

Nonparasitic cysts of the liver are diagnosed with increasing frequency since the advent of ultrasound and CT. These cysts may be solitary or multiple; multiple cysts frequently are associated with polycystic disease of the kidneys, with cysts also noted in other organs. Cysts are usually an incidental finding in patients being evaluated for other problems, but if these cysts attain a large size, they may be the source of abdominal pain. The confidence of diagnosis by noninvasive technique should preclude the need for angiography in most instances, as ultrasound and CT are more accurate in defining the nature of these lesions (48). Although the angiographic appearance is usually described as that of an avascular mass, with perhaps a surrounding thin rim of compressed parenchyma, selective magnification arteriography can demonstrate hypervascularity in the rim of a benign cyst, suggesting tumor or abscess (47).

TUMORS

Benign Hepatic Tumors

Benign hepatic tumors of the liver are being discovered more frequently due to increased sensitivity of noninvasive techniques; previously, the discovery of these lesions was less common because of their asymptomatic nature. Unfortunately, these techniques often do not have the specificity to allow an unequivocal diagnosis of a benign process, and angiography still plays a key role in further defining these lesions.

Cavernous Hemangioma. Cavernous hemangiomas are the most common benign tumor of the liver and are found in up to 7 percent of individuals at autopsy (49). There is a female predominance, and their incidence increases with age. Pathologically, cavernous hemangiomas consist of blood-filled spaces, separated by fibrous septa and lined with endothelium (50). Central fibrosis occurs frequently and may replace the entire lesion (51). Calcification of these lesions may occur occasionally within a radiating pattern (52). Most are 1 to 3 cm in size, but they may become huge and present as an abdominal mass; they are not infrequently multiple. The great majority of these lesions are asymptomatic; however, they may cause abdominal pain due to spontaneous hemorrhage or mass effect on surrounding structures. Catastrophic bleeding has been reported after trauma or biopsy (53). Angiographically, their appearance is characteristic; the arteries supplying the liver are normal in size and demonstrate normal peripheral tapering. Multiple small vascular spaces are opacified late in the arterial phase and, unlike other vascular tumors, remain opacified during and past the venous phase up to 30 seconds after injection (Figure 8–6). Enlarged, irregular "neovascular" feeding vessels should not be present. The vascular spaces often have a ring or "C" shape, due to central fibrosis of the tumor or to central thrombosis or hemorrhage. Although arteriovenous shunting is generally considered pathognomonic of malignancy, it has been described in cavernous hemangioma (43,54). Dynamic imaging with CT may obviate the need for angiography in some instances, especially if a solitary large hemangioma with characteristic pattern of contrast enhancement is noted (55). However, angiography will still be required for definitive diagnosis in others. Occasionally, it can be diffi-

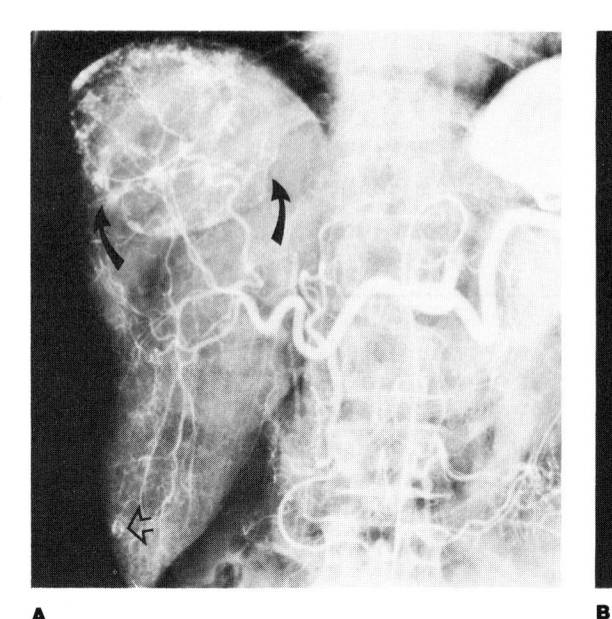

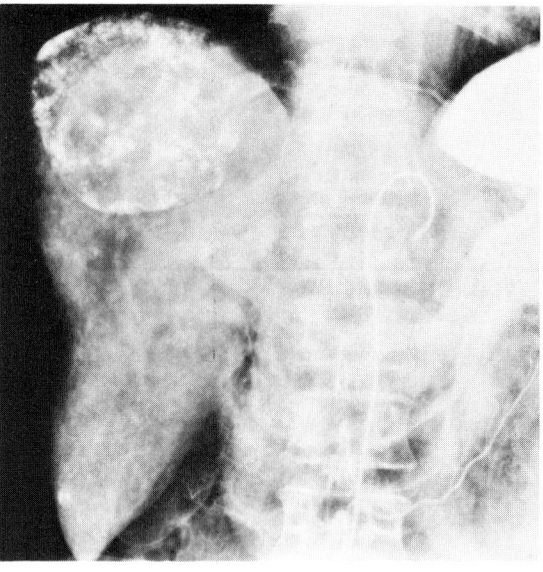

Figure 8-6. Forty-year-old female with recurrent right upper quadrant discomfort and ultrasound demonstration of mass lesion in the superior aspect of liver. *A.* Selective celiac axis arteriogram demonstrates large hypervascular mass lesion of dome of right lobe (curved arrows). Second small vascular mass (open arrow) is seen in the lower portion of right lobe. *B.* Venous phase of selective hepatic arteriogram with persistent peripheral contrast opacification ("puddling") of both lesions. Subsequent partial lobectomy of right lobe confirmed cavernous hemangioma and relieved patient's symptoms.

cult to differentiate small hemangiomas from hypervascular metastases, especially in patients with known hypervascular primary tumors such as renal cell carcinoma. Small vascular lesions in these patients are most likely hemangiomas; unfortunately, pharmacoangiography has not proven to be of value in these instances (56).

Hemangioendothelioma. Hemangioendothelioma is a less common benign vascular tumor of the liver. This tumor occurs primarily in infants and young children. It may be part of a clinical syndrome of multinodular hemangiomatosis of the liver (MHL), which consists of hepatomegaly, congestive heart failure, and cutaneous hemangiomas (57). These patients may also have thrombocytopenia, consumption coagulopathy, and abnormal liver-function tests. These lesions consist of enlarged sinusoidal channels that are lined by proliferating endothelial cells. Angiographically, these tumors are quite different from cavernous hemangiomas (Figure 8-7); marked enlargement of the feeding arteries, tortuous neovascularity, loss of normal arterial tapering, large vascular lakes, and arteriovenous shunting into the hepatic veins explain the clinical presentation of high output failure in these patients. The extent of venous shunting and the clinical presentation of congestive failure, as well as the prolonged opacification of large vascular lakes, can help differentiate this tumor from primary hepatocellular carcinoma or hepatoblastoma (58,59). Since these tumors may resolve spontaneously, initial management should be nonsurgical and directed toward controlling congestive failure and suppression of the tumor by corticosteroids or radiation therapy. Transcatheter embolization has been successful in the management of some of these lesions (60).

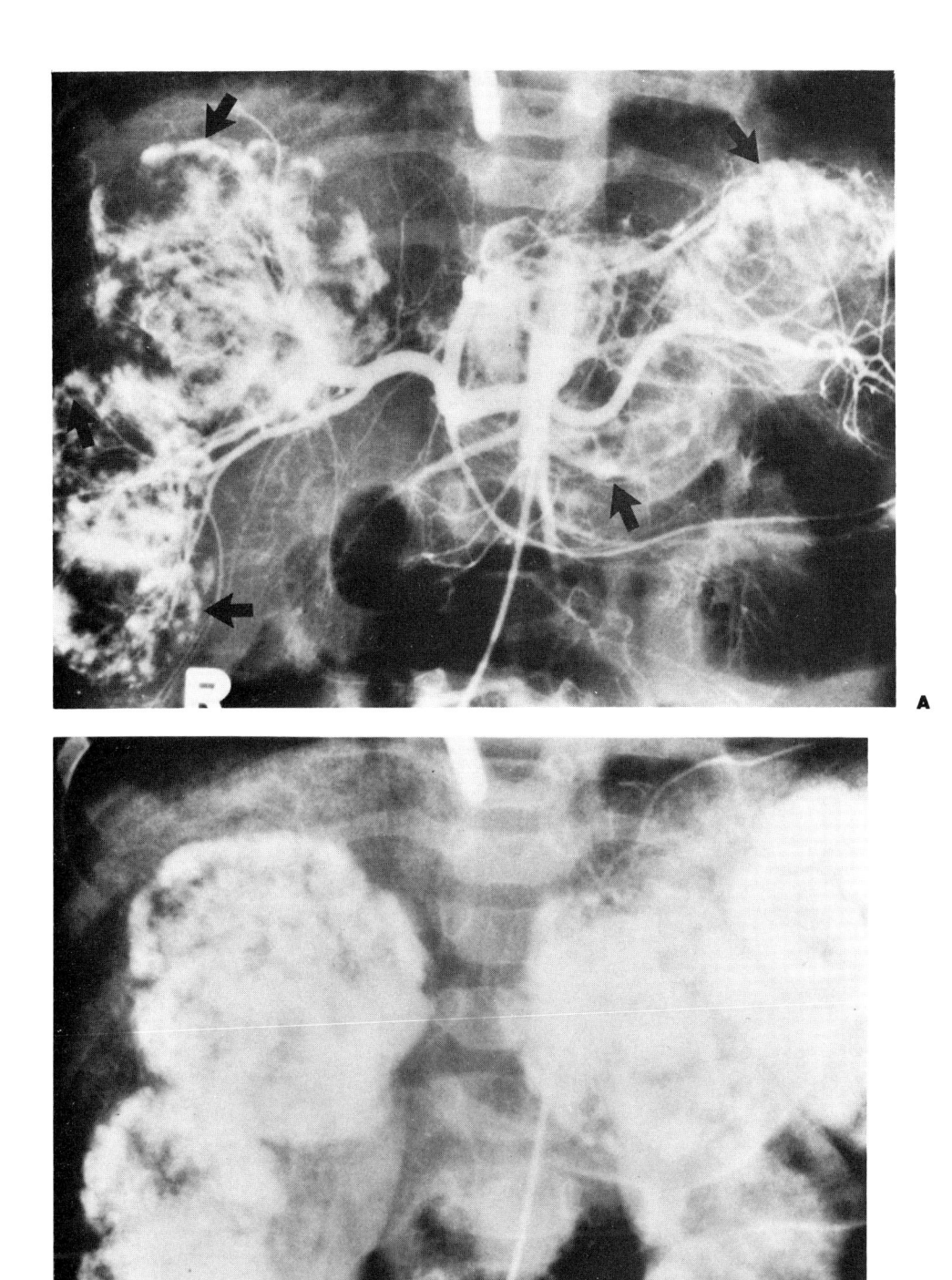

Figure 8-7. Five-month-old male with marked hepatomegaly and abnormal liver scan. *A.* Selective celiac axis arteriogram demonstrates five large vascular mass lesions with peripheral contrast puddling (arrows). *B.* Delayed film shows dense opacification of these mass lesions consistent with multiple cavernous hemangiomatosis of the infant.

Hepatic Adenoma. Hepatic adenomas are benign tumors consisting of hepatocytes without reticuloendothelial or biliary elements. There is a strong female predominance and an increased incidence associated with oral contraceptive use. This lesion appears to occur in men only if there is an associated use of androgens or other anabolic steroids. Though benign, these tumors have a propensity for spontaneous hemorrhage that can be life-threatening; additionally, there may be as slight chance of malignant degeneration. These characteristics indicate surgical removal. Adenomas have been described to resolve after cessation of oral contraceptives (61).

The angiographic appearance of hepatic adenomas is extremely variable, ranging from hypovascular to hypervascular (Figure 8–8). Neovascularity may be present, but there are generally no lakes or sinusoidal collections. Arteriovenous shunting does not occur. Feeding vessels have been described as starting from the periphery of the lesion, penetrating toward the center (62), though not all authors have found this point to be of use (63). Adenomas are generally well-circumscribed with a homogeneous capillary phase, though there may be associated hemorrhage or necrosis.

In the appropriate clinical setting and with a hypovascular mass on angiography, the diagnosis can be strongly suspected and surgical resection performed to prevent complications. However, in hypervascular masses, differentiation between adenomas and focal nodular hyperplasia may be difficult.

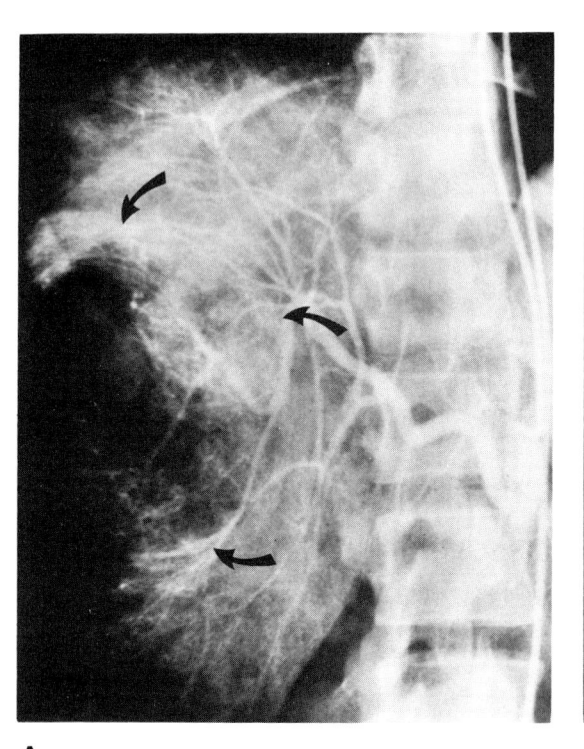

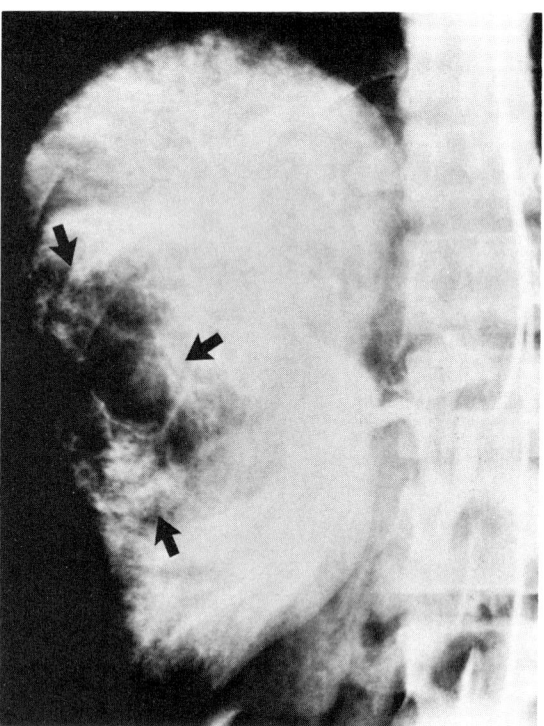

Figure 8–8. Thirty-year-old female with right upper quadrant discomfort and large mass demonstrated by ultrasound. *A.* Selective hepatic arteriogram demonstrates poorly vascularized mass (curved arrows), right lobe. *B.* Late capillary phase demonstrates some increased vascular staining (arrows). Subsequent surgical pathology revealed hepatic adenoma.

Focal Nodular Hyperplasia. Focal nodular hyperplasia (FNH) is a benign tumor or hamartoma composed of hepatocytes, biliary ducts, and Kupffer cells. The presence of reticuloendothelial cells enables uptake by Tc sulfacolloid in 40 percent of these lesions, as opposed to adenomas that are always "cold" on radionuclide scans. There is a female predominance in focal nodular hyperplasia, but not to the degree seen in adenoma; FNH can occur at any age (64), whereas adenoma occurs predominantly from the second to sixth decades.

There is no clear-cut relationship of FNH to steroid ingestion, although some association with oral contraceptives has been suggested. This lesion is clinically much more benign, with no malignant potential and without the risks of hemorrhage that accompany adenoma. The vast majority are asymptomatic. Lesions of focal nodular hyperplasia may be multiple in 20 percent of cases. These tumors are generally found in a subcapsular location (Figure 8–9) or may be pedunculated (Figure 8–10). On gross inspection, there is a stellate organization with a central fibrous core and septa radiating from center to periphery. The angiographic appearance is that of a well-defined, circumscribed, markedly hypervascular lesion with tortuous neovascularity. However, lack of encasement distinguishes this vascularity from hepatoma. The feeding vessel may

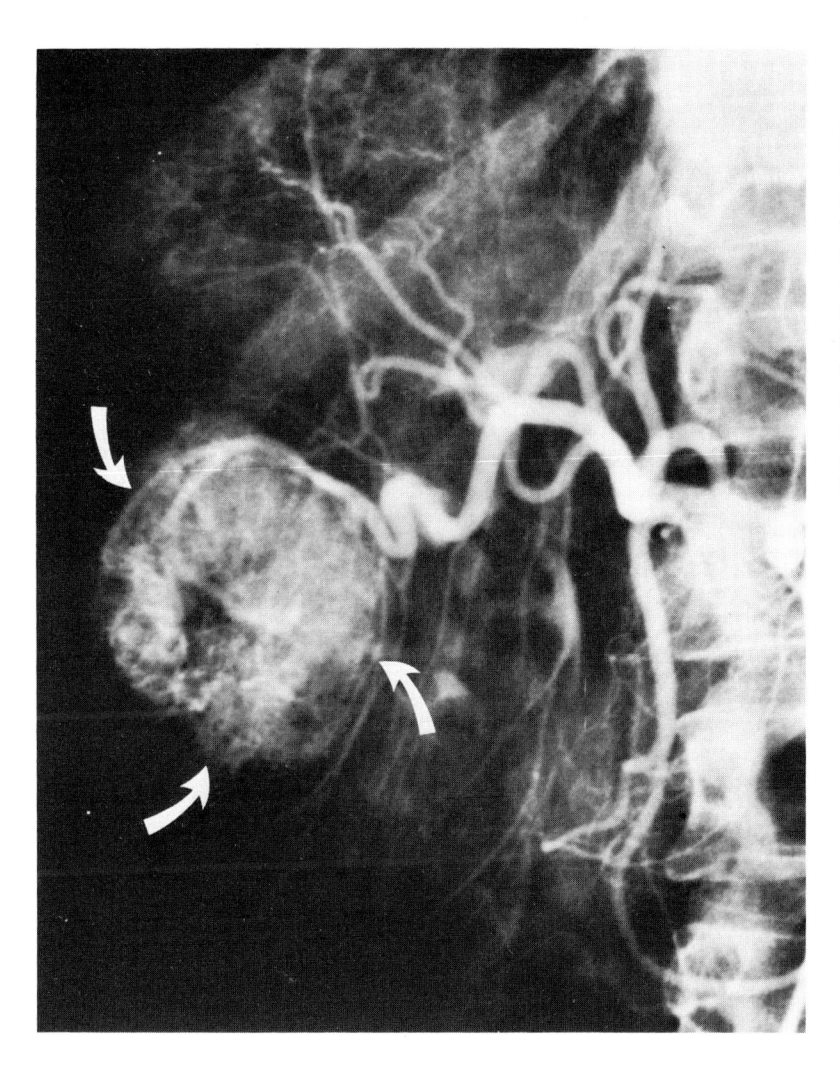

Figure 8–9. Incidental liver mass found at the time of pelvic surgery in a middle-aged woman. Selective hepatic arteriogram shows a well-circumscribed vascular tumor (curved arrows) of the right lobe of the liver with an arterial blood supply that appears to radiate from the center. Surgical biopsy confirmed focal nodular hyperplasia.

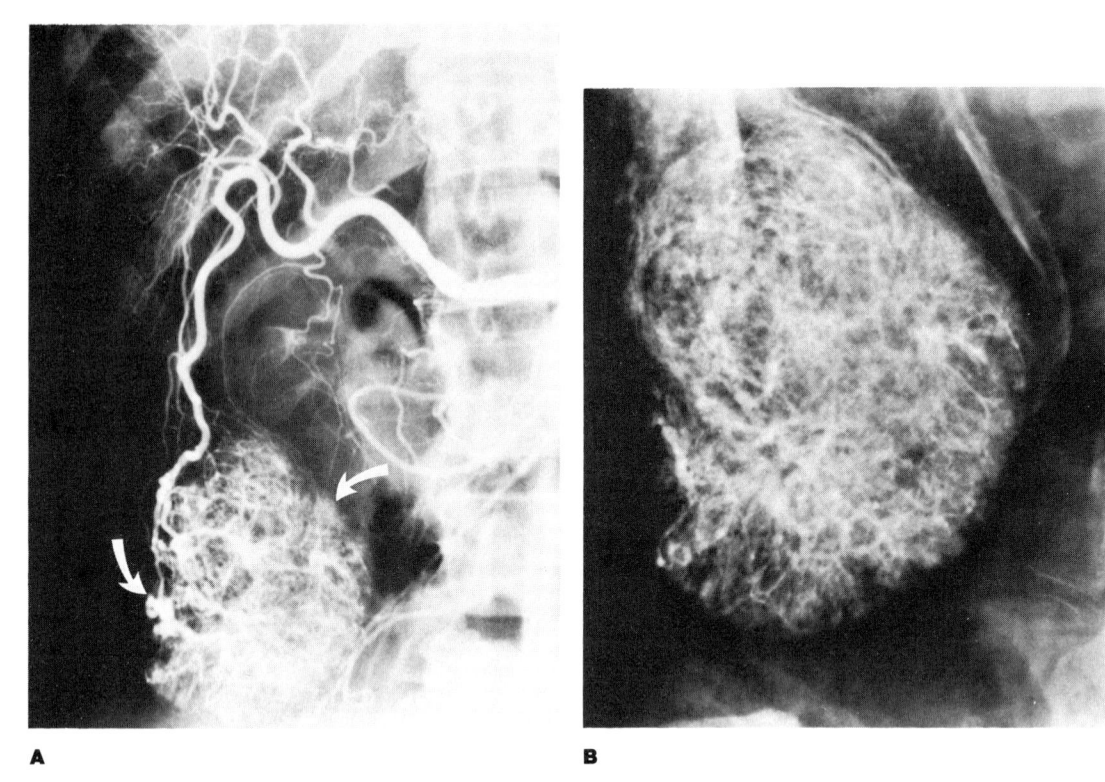

Figure 8-10. Middle-aged female with 10-year history of birth control medication and palpable right upper quadrant mass. *A.* Selective hepatic arteriogram demonstrates vascular mass of inferior margin of right lobe (curved arrows). *B.* Magnification arteriogram demonstrates orderly vascularity and septation. Surgical pathology revealed focal nodular hyperplasia.

appear to arise in the center of the lesion and radiate out to the periphery. Septation of the tumor may be noted during the capillary phase, which is usually quite dense. Arteriovenous shunting has been noted rarely. There is no portal or hepatic vein extension of the tumor. Though cases of avascular focal nodular hyperplasia have been reported (65), these probably represent adenomas; the confusion may be due to the variability of pathologic diagnoses accorded these lesions (63). Despite the use of radionuclide and angiographic criteria, the distinction between hepatic adenomas and focal nodular hyperplasia can be difficult (Figure 8-11). Hepatoma may present an angiographically similar appearance. If the diagnosis is not certain by imaging techniques, pathological confirmation should be obtained.

Malignant Hepatic Tumors

Hepatoma. The most common primary malignant tumor of the liver is hepatoma, or hepatocellular carcinoma. This tumor is often superimposed on an already diseased or abnormal liver, with cirrhosis present in 60 to 80 percent of patients with hepatoma (66,67). In diagnosing and planning treatment for hepatoma, angiography plays an important role, as it allows a detailed evaluation of vascular structures not possible by noninvasive means.

A   **B**

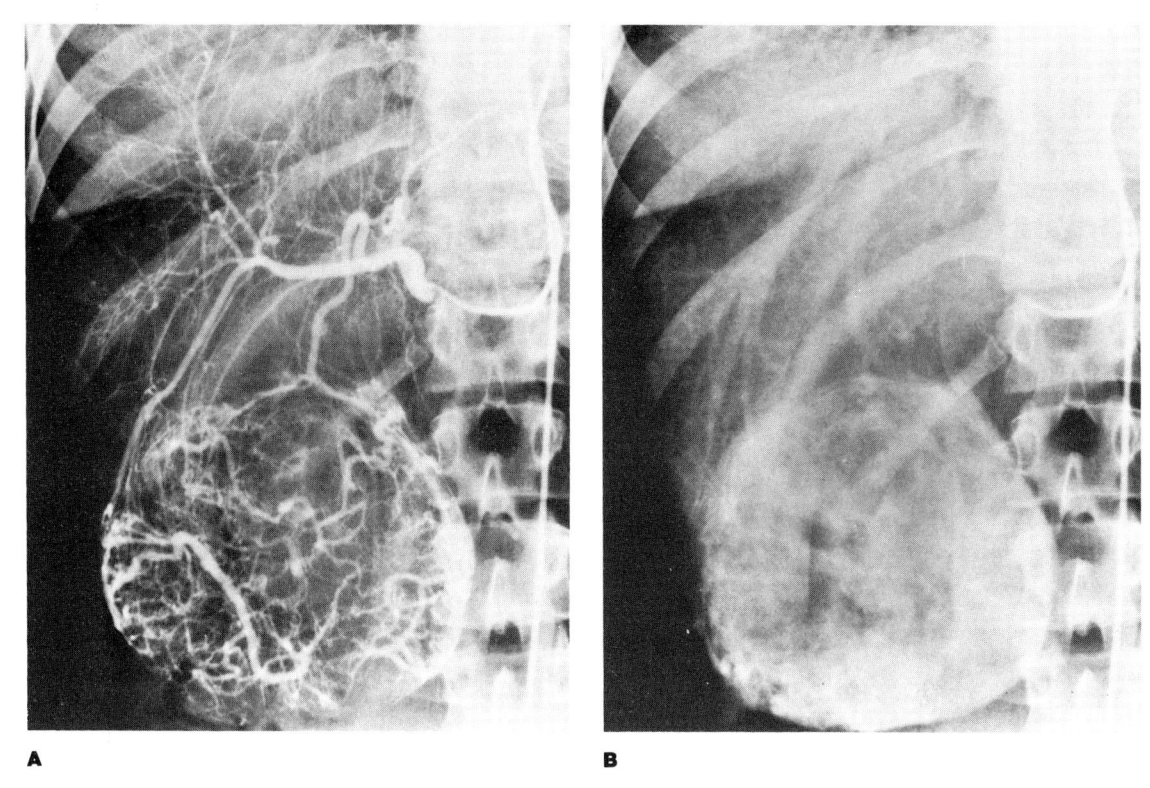

Figure 8-11. Twenty-one-year-old female with Stein-Leventhal syndrome and liver mass. *A.* Selective hepatic arteriogram demonstrates hypervascular mass of inferior margin of right lobe. *B.* Capillary phase demonstrates homogeneous opacification of lesion. Clinical and angiographic impression favored focal nodular hyperplasia, but surgical pathology revealed hepatocellular carcinoma. The vascularity is more disordered and purposeless than seen in focal nodular hyperplasia.

The angiographic appearance of hepatoma is most commonly that of a very hypervascular, solitary mass with enlargement of the feeding arteries, bizarre and irregular tumor neovascularity, and contrast accumulation in irregular vascular lakes (Figure 8-11). In addition to the solitary form, hepatoma can be multinodular (Figure 8-12), also usually hypervascular, or may present in a diffuse infiltrative form that may be hypovascular or hypervascular (3,66,68). Arterioportal shunting is highly suggestive of this diagnosis, especially in association with the other angiographic findings, although it has been reported in other entities, such as regenerating nodules and cavernous hemangiomas (43,54). In these latter cases, however, the portal vein should appear intrinsically normal, whereas careful evaluation in cases of hepatoma will show irregularity of the portal vein branches due to direct tumor invasion or compression (69). Hepatocellular carcinoma has a propensity for growth into the portal system, and the vascularity of the tumor thrombus can be identified angiographically (Figure 8-13) (67,69). The "threads and streaks" sign that this produces is highly specific for hepatoma, although similar findings have been described in hypervascular metastases (70). Differentiation of metastases is usually made relatively easy by the presence of a primary tumor and by the multiplicity of most metastases. Hepatic vein involvement and tumor extension into the inferior vena cava can also occur with hepatoma (71).

A small percentage of hepatomas has been described as hypovascular, frequently

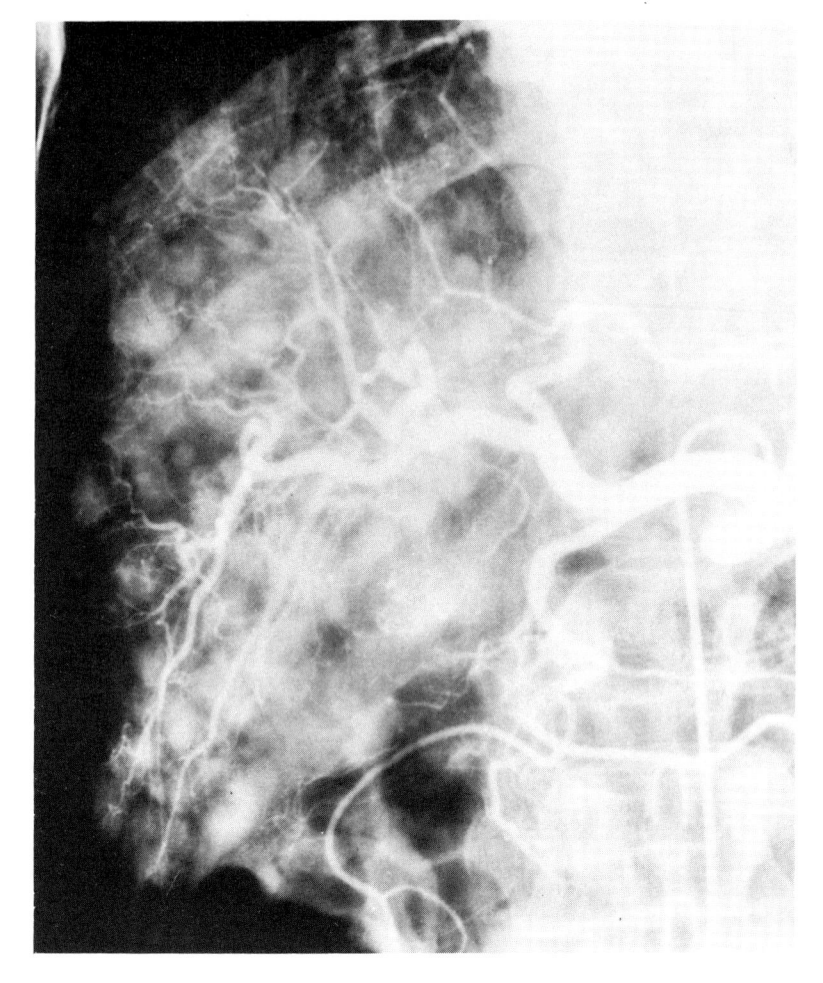

Figure 8-12. Sixty-seven-year-old man with anemia and abnormal hepatic ultrasound. Selective hepatic arteriogram demonstrates multiple hypervascular nodules. Two random hepatic biopsies were reported as normal hepatic architecture, and a third biopsy was consistent with benign hyperplasia. Surgical biopsy after 1 year revealed well-differentiated multifocal hepatocellular carcinoma.

those of the diffuse infiltrative type (66,67,72,73). These tumors in the setting of cirrhosis can be difficult to identify. Selective high-dose infusion techniques may better demonstrate hypervascularity in these tumors and increase diagnostic accuracy (4,5,74).

Attempts at surgical excision are reserved generally for the solitary form of hepatocellular carcinoma or tumor that has spared at least one hepatic segment (75). Computed tomography is well-suited to categorization of hepatocellular carcinoma based on gross anatomic appearance and extent. However, further evidence of resectability does depend on angiographic assessment of no major vessel involvement or direct vascular extension of tumor into hepatic or portal veins (76).

Cholangiocarcinoma. The diagnosis of cholangiocarcinoma does not generally require angiography, as these patients often present with jaundice and undergo evaluation by cholangiography and biopsy. These tumors are primarily adenocarcinomas that have an infiltrating scirrhous nature, producing an angiographic appearance of arterial encasement and invasion. These changes in the arterial phase are often the only abnormality and are characteristically serrated or serpiginous, with abrupt angulation of involved vessels. Fine, tortuous neovascularity may be present, but vascular lakes or pools and arteriovenous shunting are not noted. Encasement of portal venous structures

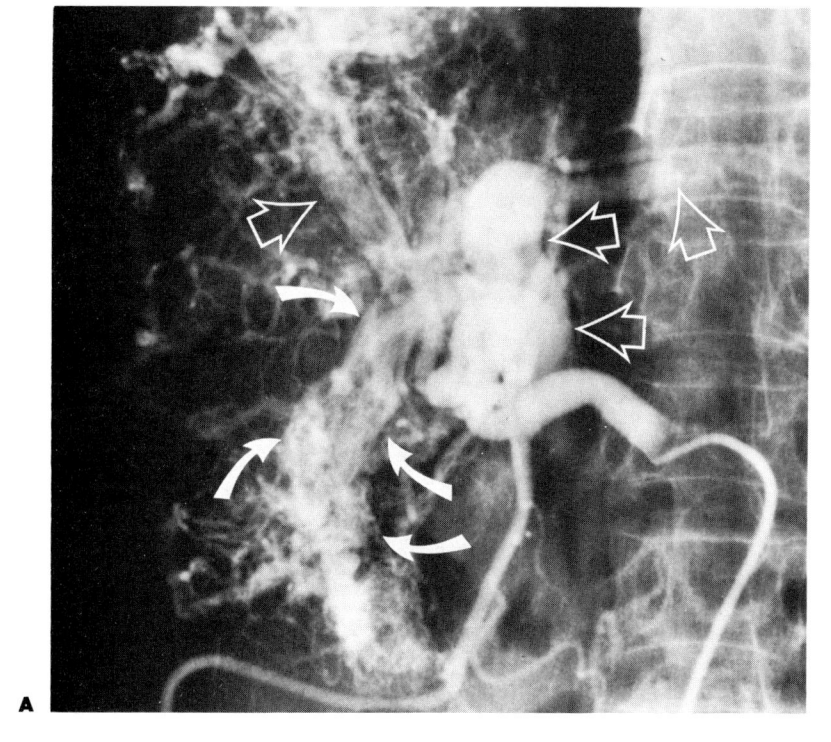

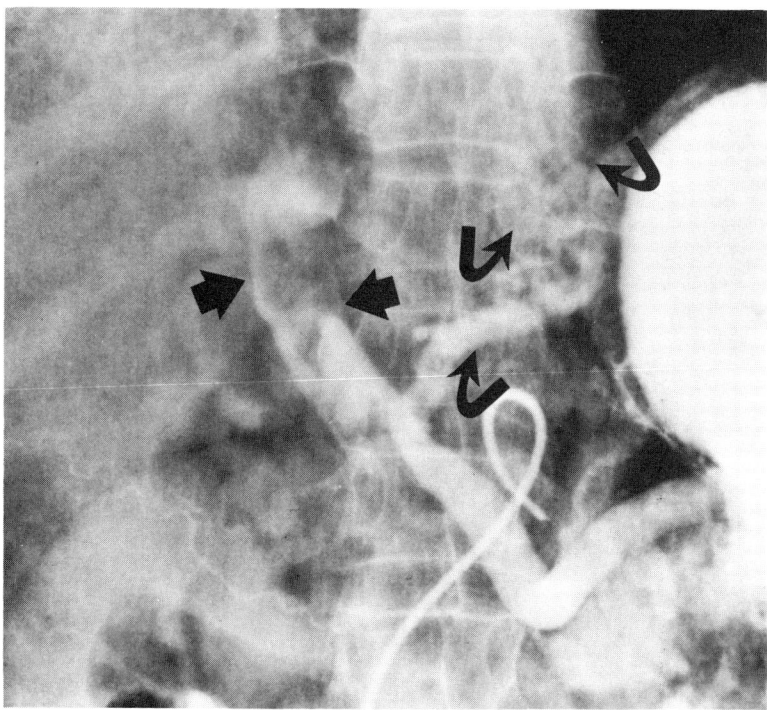

Figure 8–13. Elderly Oriental female with bloody ascites and hepatomegaly. *A.* Selective hepatic arteriogram demonstrates vascular mass of the right lobe of the liver, and small coiled vasculature in a tubular configuration (curved arrows) in right lobe extends into porta hepatis and is consistent with tumor thrombus of portal veins. Arteriovenous shunting opacifies portal vein (open arrows). *B.* Venous phase of a selective splenic arteriogram demonstrates thrombus within the portal vein (arrows). Curved arrows demonstrate coronary vein and gastroesophageal varices. Autopsy confirmed hepatocellular carcinoma with portal vein tumor thrombus.

and portal vein invasion can occur, though less frequently than with hepatoma. The tumor may spread along biliary ducts and be quite extensive before mass effect is noted (3,8,77).

Hepatoblastoma. Primary tumors of the liver in children are rare and are usually hepatoblastomas or hepatomas, though sarcomas can also occur. Hepatoblastomas are poorly differentiated tumors of hepatocellular origin. Hepatomas are somewhat better differentiated. These two entities are not distinguishable angiographically. Both are hypervascular, and the angiographic features are similar to those of hepatocellular carcinomas in adults. Diagnosis of these tumors is often suggested by noninvasive means, and angiography is reserved for cases in which the diagnosis is uncertain or prior to surgical resection (42,59,78,79).

Angiosarcoma. Angiosarcoma is a rare malignancy of the liver that has been linked epidemiologically in approximately 40% of cases with exposure to several substances including vinyl chloride, THOROTRAST, arsenicals, and radium (28). The arteriographic

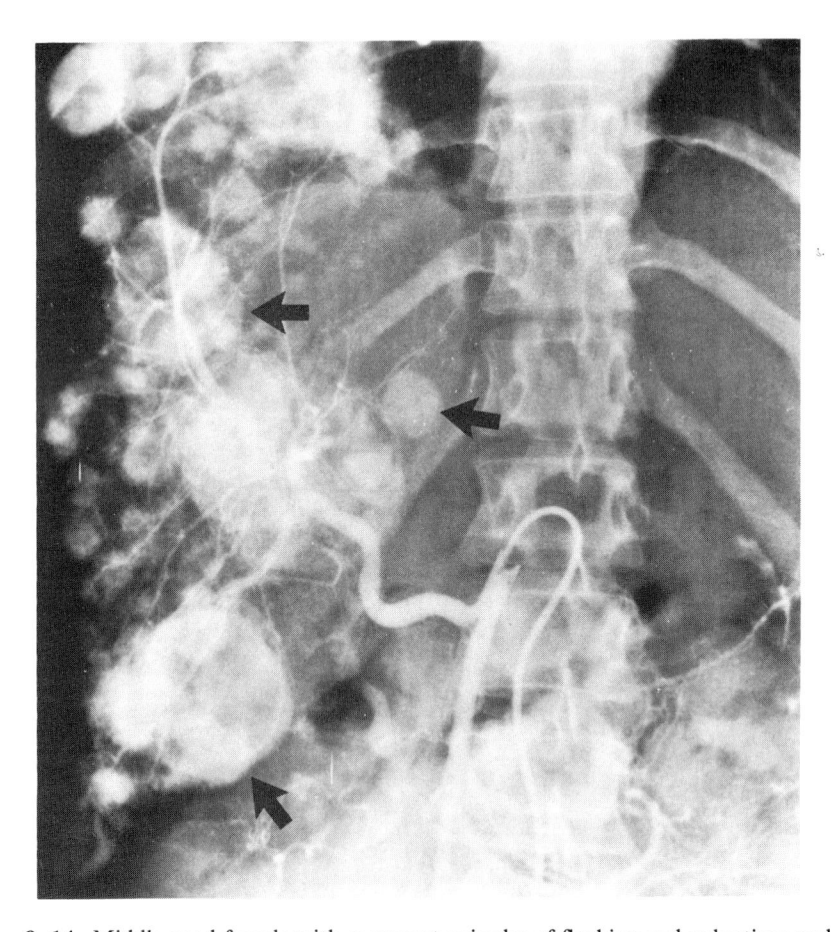

Figure 8-14. Middle-aged female with recurrent episodes of flushing and palpations and elevated 5-hydroxyindoleacetic acid levels. Selective superior mesenteric arteriogram with right hepatic artery arising from superior mesenteric artery shows multiple hypervascular mass lesions (arrows) of right lobe consistent with hypervascular metastases from carcinoid tumor. Subsequent embolization of hepatic arterial blood supply provided 9-month symptomatic relief.

findings include normal-sized hepatic arteries, peripheral tumor staining and puddling that lasts long beyond the arterial phase, and a central area of hypovascularity (30).

Other hepatic tumors that have been associated with THOROTRAST include sarcomas, hepatomas, cholangiocarcinomas and endotheliomas. Development of these tumors is due to concentration of radioactive thorium in the reticuloendothial elements of the liver (80).

Metastatic Disease. The liver is one of the organs most frequently affected by metastases. Indeed, they represent the most common hepatic malignancy. The most common site of origin of metastases to the liver is the gastrointestinal tract, followed by breast and the genitourinary tract. Angiography is rarely required for the diagnosis of metastatic disease; however, it may play an important role in the treatment planning if surgical resection or direct hepatic artery chemotherapy infusion is considered. The vascular pattern of metastases generally mirrors that of the primary lesion and is categorized by its vascularity relative to that of the liver, i.e., hypervascular, hypovascular, and those with vascularity similar to the liver (Figure 8–14). The hypervascular metastases include those arising from choriocarcinoma, hypernephroma, endocrine tumors, carcinoid tumors, and leiomyosarcomas. These metastases can be diagnosed while still quite small, and angiography is a quite sensitive tool for discovering these lesions. They are usually multiple and have increased contrast density in the capillary phase, which disappears promptly. There are no abnormal lakes or sinusoids, though neovascularity

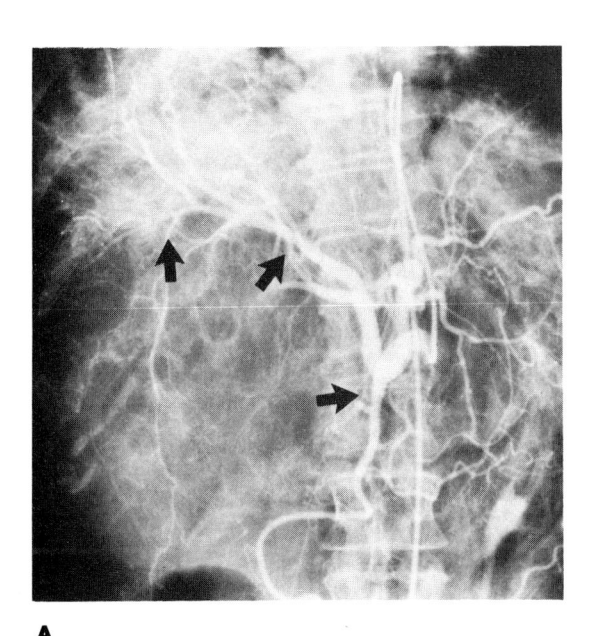

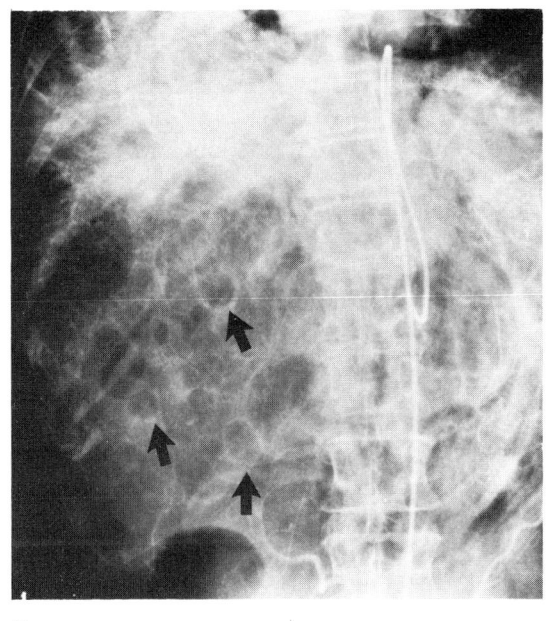

Figure 8–15. Middle-aged male with increasing hepatomegaly following resection of descending colon carcinoma. *A.* Selective hepatic arteriogram demonstrates enlargement of the right lobe with displacement of arterial structures medially and superiorly (arrows). *B.* Capillary phase of hepatic arteriogram using 60 ml of contrast at 5 ml per second demonstrates multiple small lucent mass lesions with rings of compressed hepatic tissue (arrows). Hypovascular metastases are typical for gastrointestinal adenocarcinomas. Following gastroduodenal artery occlusion, long-term (14 months) transaxillary intraarterial chemotherapy was administered with an implantable pump.

is not infrequently identified. Their peripheral location, multiplicity, and well-defined margins distinguish them from hepatoma and other vascular liver lesions. Solitary hypervascular lesions can occasionally be a diagnostic dilemma, as these often represent hemangiomas, even in patients with known vascular primaries (56). Surgical therapy of the primary should probably not be withheld from these patients if this is the only finding indicating metastases.

The hypovascular metastases (Figure 8–15) are less readily identified and must achieve a larger size before angiographic diagnosis is possible. Noninvasive techniques are more sensitive in diagnosing these lesions in their early stage. These tumors include breast, most gastrointestinal tract tumors, lung, and pancreas. Their angiographic recognition is based on defects in the parenchymal phase, often with little arterial changes other than displacement. Lymphoma, which not infrequently involves the liver, shares this angiographic appearance, as it is usually poorly vascularized. There may be focal filling defects or, if the liver is diffusely involved, stretching and displacement of the arteries is noted. Rarely, lymphoma may present as hypervascular mass (81).

Pharmacoangiography has been reported to improve visualization of both hypovascular and hypervascular metastases; vasoconstrictors such as epinephrine being most useful in hypervascular lesions, and vasodilators most useful when looking for hypovascular metastases. However, the variable response to these agents limits their use as a routine procedure, and they are best reserved for use in cases where initial angiography is not diagnostic, and there is strong clinical suspicion that a lesion is present.

Another approach to improving identification of liver metastases is infusion hepatic angiography. The classification of hepatic tumors into hypervascular and hypovascular is based on their appearance during celiac angiography, which combines both arterial parenchymal opacification via hepatic artery flow and portal parenchymal opacification that occurs later via contrast delivered into the splenic artery. Several authors have reported an improved diagnostic accuracy with selective infusion hepatic arteriography versus standard celiac arteriography. This technique exploits the exclusive hepatic-artery supply of primary and secondary liver tumors to increase contrast delivery to the tumor. The subsequent "washout" of the normal hepatic parenchyma by unopacified portal blood renders these tumors even more apparent (5,82). This technique produces a hypervascular appearance in nearly all tumors and metastases previously considered hypovascular by conventional angiography. In addition to improving the diagnostic accuracy of angiography in discovering liver metastases, this technique may allow for an assessment of tumor response to therapy by documenting, on serial angiograms, the conversion of a vascular lesion to a hypovascular or avascular one, as this change may reflect decreased tumor viability (5).

CIRRHOSIS

Angiography in patients with cirrhosis is limited generally to preoperative evaluation in patients with portal hypertension prior to portal systemic shunting, and to evaluation and treatment of patients with gastrointestinal bleeding from esophageal varices, issues that will be dealt with elsewhere in this volume. However, patients with cirrhosis are predisposed to development of hepatomas and regenerating nodules that may require angiography.

The cirrhotic liver in its early stages undergoes fatty replacement, with angiographic findings of hepatomegaly and diffuse stretching of the hepatic arteries. There is progressive scarring as fibrosis of the parenchyma develops with a decrease in the liver volume. This produces a tortuous and corkscrew pattern of the hepatic arteries. With

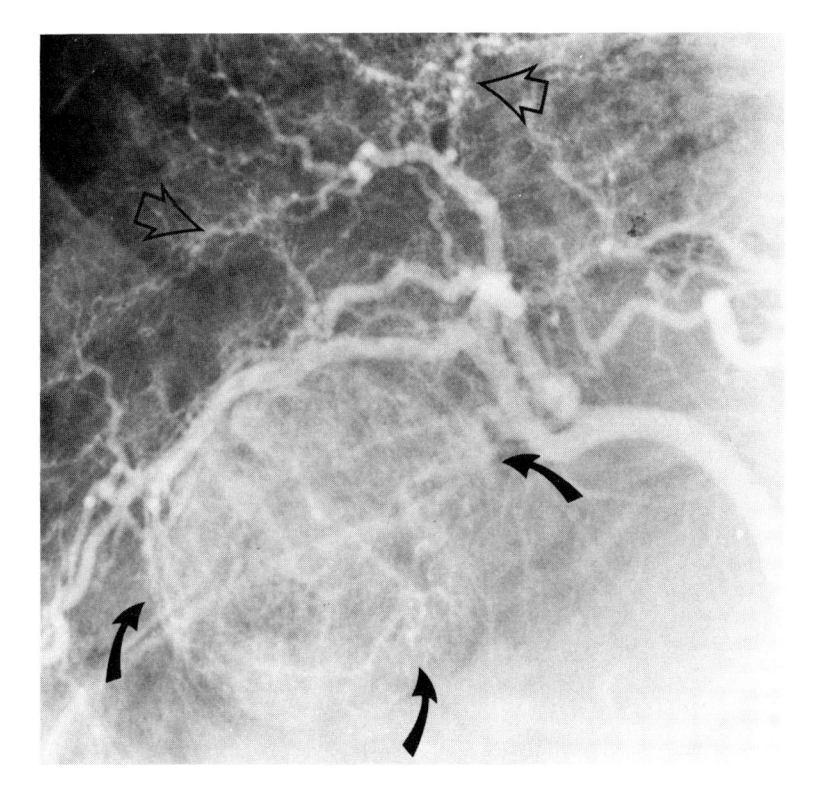

Figure 8-16. Ultrasound demonstrated a mass in patient with known postnecrotic cirrhosis. Open arrows point to increased tortuosity of arterial structures, so-called "corkscrew" changes of cirrhosis. Arrows point to a vascular mass of the right curved lobe of the liver containing regular arteries within and at the margins of the tumor. Angiographic differential diagnosis included hepatoma and regenerating nodule. Surgical biopsy confirmed regenerating nodule.

increasing fibrosis, there is increased resistance to portal blood flow, with resultant portal hypertension and in severe cirrhosis, reversal of portal blood flow. As resistance to portal flow increases, its contribution to total hepatic inflow decreases, and there is compensatory increase of hepatic inflow. This results in dilatation of the hepatic artery. The hepatic parenchyma appears inhomogeneous and dense. Opacification of the portal vein during hepatic artery injection, due to reversal of portal blood flow, can be seen (8,83).

Regeneration of the hepatic parenchyma is an integral part of the process of cirrhosis (50). Large regenerating nodules can develop and must be differentiated from hepatomas, which also occur with increased frequency in cirrhotic livers (Figure 8-16). Regenerating nodules are focal masses with stretched arteries penetrating toward the center of the mass. The supplying arteries may have fewer side branches than the surrounding parenchyma. The parenchymal phase is homogeneous, and often an enlarged, stretched portal vein branch is found extending through the nodule. Diffuse hypervascularity can occur, but without the wild neovascularity of most hepatomas. Arterial venous shunting is rare (3,8,83,84).

REFERENCES

1. Gutierrez OH, Rosch J: Limitations of angiographic differential diagnosis in major hepatic processes. Fortschr Geb Roentgenstr Nuklearmed Erganzungsband 1977;127:1-8.
2. Abrams H (ed): Angiography, 3rd ed. Boston: Little, Brown, 1983.
3. Johnsrude IS, Jackson DC: A Practical Approach to Angiography. Boston: Little, Brown, 1979.
4. Takashima T, Matsui O: Infusion hepatic angiography in the detection of small hepatocellular carcinomas. Radiology 1980;136:321-325.

5. Chuang VP: Hepatic tumor angiography: a subject review. Radiology 1983;148:633–639.
6. Roche J, Freeny P, Antonovich R, Gutierrez OH: Infusion hepatic angeography in diagnosis of liver metastasis. Cancer 1976;38:2278–2286.
7. Novak D, Butzow GD, Becker K: Hepatic occlusion venography with a balloon catheter in portal hypertension. Radiology 1977;122:623–628.
8. Reuter SR, Redman HC: Gastrointestinal Angiography, 2nd ed. Vol. 1 in Monographs in Clinical Radiology. Philadelphia: Saunders, 1977.
9. Cavaluzzi JA, Sheff R, Harrington DP, et al.: Hepatic venography and wedge hepatic vein pressure measurements in diffuse liver disease. AJR 1977;129:441–446.
10. Burcharth F: Percutaneous transhepatic portography: technique and application. AJR 1979;132:177–182.
11. Burcharth F, Nielbo M, Anderson B: Percutaneous transhepatic portography: comparison with splenoportography in portal hypertension. AJR 1979;132:183–185.
12. Shanser JD, Glickman MG, Palubinskas AJ: Pitfalls in the arteriographic differentiation of intrahepatic and extrahepatic masses. AJR 1974;121:420–429.
13. Legge D: The use of prostaglandin F_2 in selective hepatic angiography. Radiology 1977;124:331–335.
14. Widrich W, Nordahl D, Robbins A: Contrast enhancement of the mesenteric and portal veins using intra-arterial papaverine. AJR 1974;121:374.
15. Mills S, Doppman JL, Kahn ER: Metastatic islet cell carcinoma to the liver visualized after intraarterial epinephrine. AJR 1979;132:664–665.
16. Young SW, Hollenberg NK, Kazam E, et al.: Resting host and tumor perfusion as determinants of tumor vascular response to norepinephrine. Cancer Res 1979;39:1898–1903.
17. Hessel SJ, Adams DF, Abrams HL: Complications of angiography. Radiology 1981;138:273–281.
18. Long JA, Krudy A, Dunnick NR, et al.: False aneurysm formation following arteriographic intimal dissection. Radiology 1980;135:323–326.
19. Goss CM (ed): Gray's Anatomy. Philadelphia: Lea & Febiger, 1972.
20. Michaels NA: Newer anatomy of the liver and its variant blood supply and collateral circulation. Am J Surg 1966;112:337–347.
21. Gelfand DW: Anatomy of the liver. Radiol Clin North Am 1980;18:187–194.
22. Konstam MA, Novelline RA, Athanasoulis CA: Aberrant hepatic artery: a potential cause for error in the angiographic diagnosis of traumatic liver hematoma. Gastrointest Radiol 1979;4:43–45.
23. Roche A, Schmit P, Medina F, et al: The value of a portal study in determining the etiology of hepatic masses in the adult. Radiology 1982;143:387–393.
24. Nakamura S. Tsuzuki T: Surgical anatomy of the hepatic veins and the inferior vena cava. SGO 1981;152:43–50.
25. Gupta SC, Gupta CD, Gupta SB: Hepatovenous segments in the human liver. J Anat 1981;133:1–6.
26. Bernardino ME, Thomas JL, Barnes PA, Lewis E: Diagnostic approaches to liver and spleen metastases. Radiol Clin North Am 1982;20:469–485.
27. Pliskin M: Peliosis hepatis. Radiology 1975;114:29–30.
28. Locker GY, Doroshaw JH, Zwelling LA, Chabner BA: The clinical features of hepatic angiosarcoma: a report of four cases and review of the English literature. Medicine 1979;58:48–64.
29. Whelan JG, Greech JL, Tamburro CH: Angiographic and radionuclide characteristics of hepatic angiosarcoma found in vinyl chloride workers. Radiology 1976;118:549–557.
30. Herrera LO, Glassman CI, Teikido RA et al.: Peliosis hepatis associated with cavernous hemangioma and hepato carcinoma. Am Surg 1981;47:502–506.
31. Esterbrook JS: Renal and hepatic microaneurysms: report of a new entity simulating polyarteritis nodosa. Radiology 1980;137:629–630.
32. Levin DC, Watson RC, Sos TA, Baltaxe HA: Angiography in blunt hepatic trauma. AJR 1973;119:95–101.

33. Dunnick NR, Doppman JL, Berenton HD: Balloon occlusion of segmental hepatic arteries: control of biopsy-induced hemobilia. JAMA 1977;238:2524–2526.
34. Forsberg L, Hafstrom L, Lunderquist A, Sundquist K: Arterial changes during treatment with intrahepatic arterial infusion of 5 fluorouracil. Radiology 1978;126:49–52.
35. Mathisen DJ, Athanasoulis CA, Malt RA: Preservation of arterial flow to the liver. Ann Surg 1982;196:400–410.
36. Petrin P, Costantino V, Feltrin GP, et al.: Hepatic artery aneurysms. Am J Gastroenterol 1982;77:934–935.
37. Chen MF, Chou FF, Wang CH, Jang YI: Hematobilia from rupture hepatic artery aneurysms. Arch Surg 1983;118:759–761.
38. Countryman D, Norwood S, Register D, et al.: Hepatic artery aneurysm. Am Surg1983;49:51–54.
39. Yaghoobian J, Pinck RL, Naidich J, Hyman R: Angiographic findings in liver amyloidosis. Radiology 1980;136:332.
40. Rourke JA, Bosnick MA, Ferris EJ: Hepatic angiography in "alcoholic hepatitis." Radiology 1968;91:290–296.
41. Freeny PC: Acute pyogenic hepatitis: sonographic and angiographic finding. AJR 1980;135:239–252.
42. Novy SB, Wallace S, Goldman AM, Ben-Menachem Y: Pyogenic liver abscess. AJR 1974;121:388–395.
43. Adler J, Goodgold M, Mity H, et al.: Arteriovenous shunts involving the liver. Radiology 1978;129:315–322.
44. Dwek JH, Schechter LS, Grinberg ME: Hepatic angiography in a patient with tuberculosis of the liver. Am J Gastroenterol 1981;75:307–308.
45. Reeder MM: Tropical diseases of the liver and bile ducts. Semin Roentgenol 1975;10:229–243.
46. Rizk, GK, Tayyarah KA, Ghandur-Mnaymneh L: Angiographic changes in hydatid cysts of the liver and spleen. Radiology 1971;99:303–309.
47. Rosch J, Mayer BS, Campbell JR, Campbell TJ: "Vascular" benign liver cyst in children: report of two cases. Radiology 1978;126:2278–2286.
48. Hyde GL, Bertram RL, Schwartz RW: Solitary nonparasitic hepatic cysts. South Med J 1981;74:1357–1360.
49. Ishak KG, Rabin L: Benign tumors of the liver. Med Clin North Am 1975;59:995–1013.
50. Robbins SL: The Pathologic Basis of Disease. Philadelphia: Saunders, 1974.
51. McLoughlin MJ: Angiography in cavernous hemangioma of the liver. AJR 1971;113:50–55.
52. Pantoja E: Angiography in liver hemangioma. AJR 1968;104:874–879.
53. Taitelbaum G, Hinckley EJ, Herba MJ, Lough J: Giant hemangioma of the liver. Can J Surg 1982;25:652–654.
54. Winograd J, Palubinskas AJ: arterial-portal venous shunting in cavernous hemangioma of the liver. Radiology 1977;122:331–332.
55. Johnson CM, Sheedy PF, Stanson AW, et al.: Computed tomography and angiography of cavernous hemangiomas of the liver. Radiology 1981;138:115–121.
56. Madayag MA, Bosniak MA, Kinkhabwala M, Becker JA: Hemangiomas of the liver in patients with renal cell carcinoma. Radiology 1978;126:391–394.
57. Pereyra R, Andrassy RJ, Mahour GH: Management of massive hepatic hemangiomas in infants and children: a review of 13 cases. Pediatrics 1982;70:254–258.
58. Slovis TL, Berdon WE, Haller JO, et al.: Hemangiomas of the liver in infants. AJR 1975;123:791–801.
59. Moss AA, Clark RE, Palubinskas AJ, deLorimer AA: Angiographic appearance of benign and malignant hepatic tumors in infants and children. AJR 1971;113:61–69.
60. Stanley P, Grinell VS, Stanton RE, et al.: Therapeutic embolization of infantile hepatic hemangiomas with polyvinyl alcohol. AJR 1983;141:1047–1051.

61. Benedict KT, Chen PS, Janower ML, et al.: Contraceptive-associated hepatic tumor. AJR 1979;132:452–454.
62. Neiman HL, Goldstein HM: Angiography of benign and malignant hepatic masses. Semin Roentgenol 1975;10:197–205.
63. Casarella WJ, Knowles DM, Wolff M, Johnson P: Focal nodular hyperplasia and liver cell adenoma: radiologic and pathologic differentiation. AJR 1978;131:393–402.
64. Atkinson GO, Kodruff M, Sones PJ, Gay BB: Focal nodular hyperplasia of the liver in children: a report of three new cases. Radiology 1980;137:171–174.
65. Whitley NO, Cunningham JJ: Angiographic and echographic findings in avascular focal nodular hyperplasia of the liver. AJR 1978;130:777–779.
66. Okuda K, Sinnouchi S, Nagasaki Y, et al.: Angiographic demonstration of growth of hepatocellular carcinoma in the hepatic vein and inferior vena cava. Radiology 1977;124:33–36.
67. Marks WM, Jacobs RP, Goodman PC, Lin RC: Hepatocellular carcinoma clinical and angiographic findings and predictability for surgical resection. AJR 1979;132:7–11.
68. Gammill SL, Takahasi M, Kawanami M, et al.: Hepatic angiography in the selection of patients with hepatomas for hepatic lobectomy. Radiology 1971;101:549–554.
69. Okuda K, Musha H, Yanaski T, et al.: Angiographic demonstration of intrahepatic arterioportal anastomosis in hepatocellular carcinoma. Radiology 1977; 122:53–58.
70. Heaston DK, Chuang VP, Wallace S, deSantos LA: Metastatic hepatic neoplasms: angiographic features of portal vein involvement. AJR 1981;136:897–900.
71. Okuda K, Obata H, Jinnouichi S, et al.: Angiographic assessment of gross anatomy of HCC: comparison of celiac angiograms and liver pathology in 100 cases. Radiology 1977;123:21–29.
72. Reuter S, Redman HC, Siders DB: The spectrum of angiographic findings in hepatoma. Radiology 1970;94:89–94.
73. Watson RC, Baltaxe HA: The angiographic appearance of primary and secondary tumors of the liver. Radiology 1971;101:539–548.
74. Wirtanen GW: A new angiographic technique in the diagnosis of liver tumor. Radiology 1973;108:51–54.
75. Starzl TE, Bell RH, Beart RW, Putnam CW: Hepatic trisegmentectomy and other liver resections. SGO 1975;141:429–437.
76. Williamson BWA, Blumgart LH, Mekellar NJ: Management of tumors of the liver. Am J Surg 1980;139:210–215.
77. Walter JF, Bookstein JJ, Bouffard EV: Newer angiographic observations in cholangiocarcinoma. Radiology 1976;118:19–23.
78. Miller HH, Gates GF, Stanley P: The radiologic investigation of hepatic tumors in childhood. Radiology 1977;124:451–458.
79. Franken EA, Smith WL, Siddigui A: Liver disease in pediatrics. Radiol Clin North Am 1980;18:239–252.
80. Smoron GI, Battifora HA: Thorotrast induced hepatoma. Cancer 1973;31:1252–1257.
81. Castaneda-Zuniga WR, Amplatz K: Angiography of the liver in lymphoma. Radiology 1977;122:679–681.
82. Freeny PC, Antonovic R, Gutierrez OH, Rosch J: Diagnostic effectiveness of infusion hepatic angiography: a comparison with the conventional technique. Fortschr Geb Roentgenstr Nuklearmed Erganzungsband 1976;124:534–541.
83. Fullenwider JT, Nordlinger BM, Millikan WJ, et al.: Portal pseudoperfusion: an angiographic illusion. Ann Surg 1979;189:257–268.
84. Rabinowitz JG, Kinkabwala M, Ulreich S: Macroregenerating nodule in the cirrhotic liver. AJR 1974;121:401–411.

9

Hepatic Angiography: Portal Hypertension

THOMAS W. OLIVER, JR. • P. J. SONES, JR.

INTRODUCTION

Portal hypertension is usually a manifestation of underlying hepatic parenchymal disease, although it may be secondary to portal or hepatic venous thrombosis and rarely to hyperdynamic portal states. Portal hypertension may present as encephalopathy, ascites, jaundice, hepatic failure, or catastrophic upper gastrointestinal hemorrhage. Radiologic investigation should include indirect or direct measurements of portal pressure, assessment of portal venous perfusion, visualization of collaterals, and demonstration of arterial and venous anatomy for potential shunt procedure. Following survival of initial variceal bleeding, the most effective procedure to prevent recurrent hemorrhage is a shunt to decompress the varices. The decision whether to intervene medically or surgically during the acute hemorrhagic episode as well as the type of shunt used to prevent future hemorrhage is the subject of continuing controversy.

DEFINITION

Portal hypertension is defined as the persistent elevation of portal vein pressure above 10 mm Hg (15 cm saline). A normal portal venous pressure ranges from approximately 5 to 10 mm Hg (1). Portal venous pressure is dependent upon several factors: (1) rate of inflow from the splanchnic circulation, (2) resistance to outflow through the liver, and (3) resistance to outflow through portosystemic collaterals. Although the portal venous pressure is normally quite low, a small pressure head must be maintained in order to overcome the vascular resistance at the level of the sinusoids. Portal venous and hepatic arterial circulations provide a dual blood supply to the sinusoids, with approximately two thirds contributed by the portal system and one third by the hepatic artery. The normal arterial pressure is reduced greatly at the microcirculatory level and contributes little to sinusoidal pressure (2,3). Portal pressure may be measured by a variety of methods, including catheterization of the portal venous system directly at surgery, via the umbilical vein (4,5), by transhepatic route (6), by measurement of splenic pulp pressure at splenoportography, by hepatic wedge pressures, and by direct measurement of "hepatic tissue" pressure by a large-bore needle (7).

Although direct or indirect measurement of elevated portal pressure establishes the diagnosis of portal hypertension, the demonstration of portosystemic collaterals by barium swallow, endoscopy, computed tomography, sonography, or angiography is strong evidence of significant elevation of portal pressure. Occasionally, erroneous diagnosis of portal hypertension may be made if esophageal varices exist as "downhill" varices related to obstruction of the superior vena cava before the azygos vein enters. The development of collaterals is an expected evolution in any venous system with increased pressure and shunting into neighboring lower pressure veins. The major sites of portosystemic decompression via collaterals include gastroesophageal submucosa, parietal peritoneum, mesentery, umbilical vein (8), rectal submucosa, and splenic vein/left renal vein (spontaneous splenorenal shunt) (Figure 9-1).

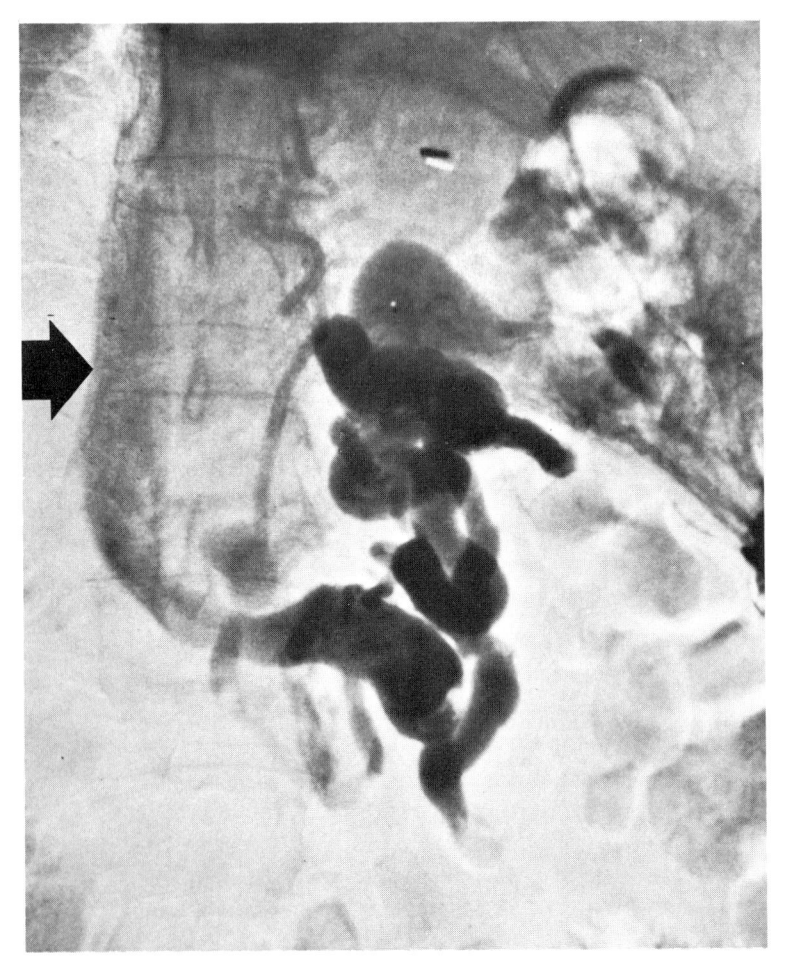

Figure 9-1. Splenoportogram demonstrating large serpiginous collaterals near the splenic hilus decompressing into the left renal vein and vena cava, forming a "spontaneous" splenorenal shunt. Arrow = IVC.

CLINICAL CONSIDERATIONS AND RISK OF GASTROINTESTINAL BLEEDING

The clinical manifestations of portal hypertension usually brings the patient for evaluation. Bleeding gastroesophageal varices are the most dramatic presentation of underlying portal hypertension, although ascites, hepatic encephalopathy, renal failure, and hypersplenism may be the presenting manifestation or may be present concomitantly. Significant hemorrhage from extraesophageal varices is rare. When it occurs, it may be difficult to diagnose and is often lethal (9–12). It is interesting to note that gastroesophageal varices have been shown to be the most common collateral in patients with portal hypertension. As might be expected, they are more frequently seen in patients who have bled than in those who have not experienced hemorrhage (13,14). It has been suggested that the presence of esophageal varices in approximately 95 percent of the hemorrhagic group (90 patients studied by splenoportography) is related to the esophagus's ability to discharge a greater amount of blood to the lower pressure systemic circulation compared to other collateral pathways (14). The suggested mechanism for the increased flow through the esophageal varices relates to the lower intrathoracic as compared with intraabdominal pressure, especially during inspiration. The precipitating mechanism in a varix hemorrhage has not been clearly elucidated. Factors suggested as causative or contributory include gastroesophageal reflux and esophagitis, variceal size, and portal pressure. Simpson and Conn (15) suggested that acid peptic erosion of the varix wall might precipitate hemorrhage. This has been disputed by other authors, however, who argue convincingly against the acid peptic hypothesis, presenting pathologic evidence obtained at the time of variceal hemorrhage and citing cases of varix hemorrhage recurring in patients with achlorhydria and those in whom gastrectomy has been performed (16,17). Although the presence or absence of varices correlates well with degree of elevation of portal pressure, the correlation between variceal size and risk of bleeding is mild at best (18). Varix hemorrhage is unlikely at low pressures (less than 10 mm Hg) but above this level, prediction of bleeding tendency from estimation of wedge pressures is unreliable (19,20).

The risk of portal hypertensive bleeding from esophageal varices without a history of prior hemorrhage is approximately one in four (21). If that one patient has experienced a previous variceal hemorrhage, the likelihood of another hemorrhage increases to two in three. Approximately 65 percent of patients will die from an acute variceal bleed. The impact of medical treatment, endoscopic sclerotherapy, or transhepatic varix embolization in controlling acute variceal bleeding is significant; however, these methods represent temporizing measures with little promise of preventing future hemorrhage (22). Surgical shunt is the only proven modality for controlling recurrent hemorrhage. Once a patient has undergone variceal bleeding, prognosis remains poor without shunt surgery. Five-year survival of patients randomized to medical therapy following variceal bleeding is approximately 35 percent in two separate prospective trials evaluating medical versus shunt therapy (23,24). The acute survival of the portal hypertensive patient with variceal bleeding can be predicted on the basis of (1) hepatic function (as measured by serum bilirubin, prothrombin time, and serum albumin), (2) presence or absence of ascites, and (3) amount of blood transfused (21). Long-term survival is associated intimately with degree of hepatic dysfunction. Patients with prehepatic portal hypertension have a more favorable prognosis than those with some form of cirrhosis. Unfortunately, in the United States the etiology of 90 percent of all cases of portal hypertension is alcoholic cirrhosis (25). Variceal bleed accounts for one third of cirrhotic deaths and is a contributory factor in cirrhotic deaths due to hepatic and renal failure, infection, and so on (26).

CAUSES OF PORTAL HYPERTENSION

The causes of portal hypertension have classically been divided into: (1) extrahepatic-presinusoidal, (2) extrahepatic-postsinusoidal, and (3) intrahepatic-presinusoidal, postsinusoidal.

Extrahepatic-presinusoidal

Prehepatic portal hypertension is usually secondary to mechanical occlusion by thrombus, tumor, or extrinsic compression of the portal vein. Rarely, the cause may be arteriovenous portal fistula or an increase in the portal venous flow without fistula—so-called "hyperkinetic portal hypertension" (28).

In a review of 97 patients with extrahepatic portal thrombosis, Webb and Sherlock (29) found that infection is the most common etiology for portal vein thrombosis, accounting for approximately 30 percent of the total. Umbilical neonatal sepsis, although not uncommon, rarely results in portal thrombosis. Umbilical-vein catheterization may result in acute portal thrombosis, but generally resolves and only rarely leads to chronic thrombosis. In over one half of cases, the cause of thrombosis remains obscure. Congenital portal venous anomalies have been suggested as a possible cause of occlusion (29). Upper gastrointestinal hemorrhage was the most common clinical manifestation of portal vein thrombosis.

Additional causes for portal vein thrombosis include hypercoagulable states such as polycythemia rubra vera, myeloproliferative diseases, and use of oral contraceptives. Trauma may initiate thrombosis. Hepatocellular carcinoma may extend into the portal system, resulting in occlusion. Splenic vein thrombosis is most commonly related to pancreatic disease; pancreatic carcinoma, pancreatitis, or pseudocyst formation may occlude the splenic vein. This results in formation of gastric fundal collaterals with drainage of blood via the coronary vein toward the liver. Splenomegaly and elevation of splenic pulp pressure is a constant feature in either portal or splenic thrombosis; ascites may or may not be present (20). Unless there is coexistent liver disease, liver biopsy and liver function studies are normal, as is the wedge pressure.

Rosch and Dotter (30) described the angiographic features of extrahepatic portal hypertension in 38 children. Splenoportography and/or selective superior mesenteric angiography is usually definitive and essential in patients with a suspected diagnosis of portal thrombosis. The technique of splenoportography is well-known and described later in this chapter. In utilizing selective splenic and superior mesenteric angiography, large volumes of contrast and long filming programs are essential to adequately visualize collaterals for potential shunt surgery. Both hepatopetal and hepatofugal collaterals develop. Hepatopetal collaterals often form a serpiginous web in the subhepatic region, tending to compensate for the partially or totally occluded portal vein. This complex has frequently been referred to as "cavernous transformation" of the portal vein (Figure 9-2). These collaterals represent dilated veins in the hepatoduodenal and hepatocolic ligaments, around the gallbladder and surface of the liver. In complete portal occlusion, these collaterals are often inadequate to carry the entire splanchnic and mesenteric blood supply, and hepatofugal flow also develops to decompress into the lower pressure systemic circulation. The hepatofugal collateral routes are similar to those seen in intrahepatic venous obstruction, with blood shunted through veins of the esophagus, stomach, retroperitoneum, and perisplenic and intestinal regions.

Hyperdynamic causes for extrahepatic presinusoidal hypertension are much less frequent than obstructive etiologies. Congenital arterial venous fistula occur in the splanch-

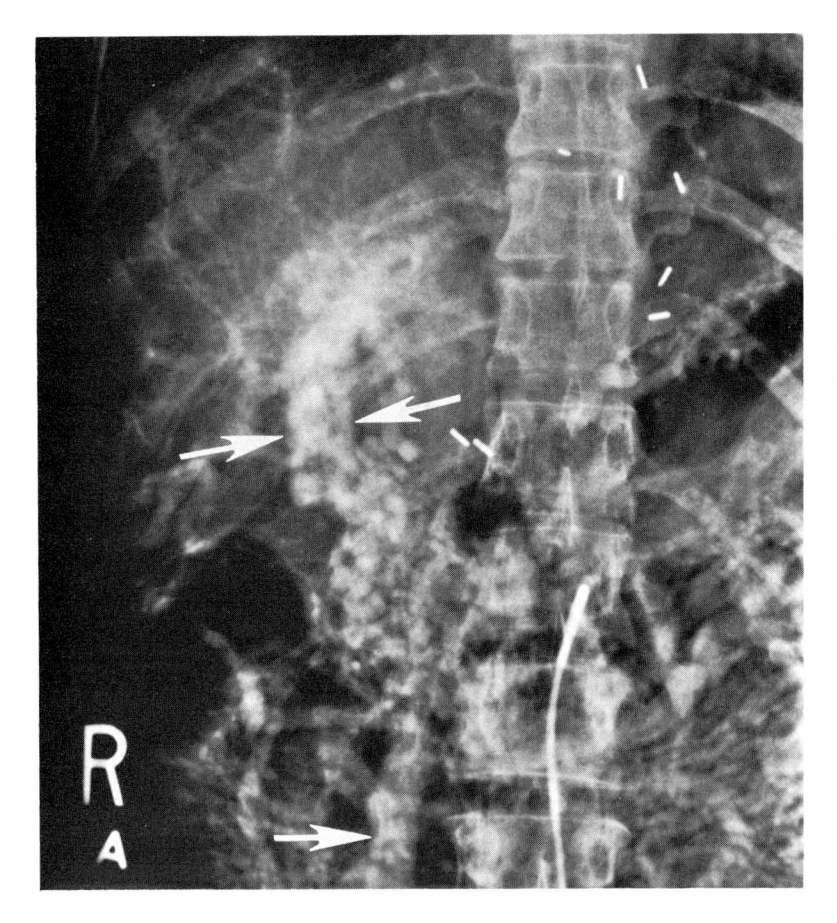

Figure 9-2. Distal superior mesenteric and portal vein thrombosis resulting in multiple collateral channels in the region of the porta hepatis (double arrow), termed "cavernous transformation" of the portal vein. Arrow defines patent proximal superior mesenteric vein.

nic circulation. Although rare, they may be associated with hereditary hemorrhagic telangiectasia. The most common causes for increased portal flow resulting in portal hypertension are rupture of aneurysm into the portal venous circulation and trauma—usually gunshot or knife wounds (31,32). In order for portal hypertension to develop in these individuals, the intrahepatic vascular resistance must increase in proportion to the portal flow to avoid the development of high-output heart failure. Whether this increased flow phenomenon eventually results in liver damage is unclear. Donovan *et al.* (33) report two patients with arteriovenous portal communications with thickened portal venous radicles and widened portal areas containing angiomatous structures, without pathologic findings suggestive of alcoholic cirrhosis. They employed the term "hepato-portal sclerosis" for these findings and proposed that they are secondary to chronic increased flow from the portal circulation. Their hypothesis is bolstered by similar pathologic findings in animals who have undergone arterialization of the portal system (34–36).

In the past, surgery was the therapy for arterioportal venous fistula. New advances in interventional radiologic techniques have allowed an alternative mode of therapy for these lesions. This mode will be discussed in detail in Chapter 10.

Extrahepatic-postsinusoidal

The occlusion of hepatic veins and/or the suprahepatic inferior vena cava is generally referred to as the Budd-Chiari syndrome (veno-occlusive disease). Acute occlusion of all hepatic veins results in a fulminant clinical course with congestive hepatomegaly, ascites, liver failure, and death. Occlusion of one or two hepatic veins may present a more insidious course, with the true diagnosis often unsuspected until autopsy. Budd-chiari may be divided into primary and secondary forms. Primary thrombosis is generally of unknown etiology, and the secondary type is usually the result of tumor from the kidney or liver (37). Other causes of hepatic venous thrombosis include recent trauma (37), hypercoagulable states, and use of oral contraceptives (38). A membranous obstruction or web involving the suprahepatic inferior vena cava is a common cause of Budd-Chiari in the Orient and Southern Africa.

The clinical diagnosis of this entity is difficult but important, since it is a potentially curable disease. Once Budd-Chiari is suspected, its definitive diagnosis rests on radiographic demonstration of the occluded hepatic veins or high vena cava. If there is total obstruction of the vena cava at the orifice of the hepatic veins, femoral vein catheterization and cavography reveal the occlusion and elevated pressures. Several methods are used to demonstrate intrahepatic vein thrombosis. Catheterization of the hepatic veins from the vena cava may provide the diagnosis in partially occluded veins or when a portion of the hepatic venous system remains patent. Kreel (39) used direct hepatic vein injection under high pressure and visualized a bizarre plexus of vessels for which he coined the term "spider web," which is considered pathognomonic for Budd-Chiari syndrome (Figure 9–3). He postulated that this network of interconnecting vessels represented hepatic vein-vein collaterals. This hypothesis was supported by work performed on monkeys in which serial venograms and subsequent cast studies of the liver were obtained following the induction of partial Budd-Chiari syndrome (40). Direct percutaneous intraparenchymal injection of contrast has also been advocated for demonstrating the occluded hepatic veins and pathognomonic spider-web appearance (41). Celiac or selective hepatic arterial injections into patients with partial Budd-Chiari reveal atrophy of the affected lobe and hypertrophy of the unaffected lobe. The arteries of the affected lobe are stretched, and there may be signs of portal hypertension. The affected lobe usually shows arterial stretching secondary to congestive hepatomegaly, although the appearance may mimic hepatoma (42). Hypertrophy of the caudate lobe is a frequent finding in Budd-Chiari due to unique venous drainage of two to four veins from this lobe directly into the infrahepatic vena cava. As the arterial evaluation of the liver in this syndrome is not definitive and may lead to diagnostic confusion, we feel that hepatic venography via percutaneous transhepatic injection or hepatic vein catheterization is the procedure of choice in the evaluation of this disease.

An interesting variant of Budd-Chiari has been termed veno-occlusive disease (a synonym for Budd-Chiari) and refers specifically to a common form of centrolobular fibrosis seen predominantly in children in Jamaica (43). The occlusion involves small and medium-sized hepatic venous radicles. The offending agents have been suggested to be alkaloids from crotalaria and senecio plants used to make "bush tea." The pathologic findings are similar to those seen in Indian childhood cirrhosis.

Intrahepatic

Cirrhosis is a chronic condition characterized by diffuse destruction and subsequent regeneration of hepatic parenchyma, with development of fibrous connective tissue dis-

A **B**

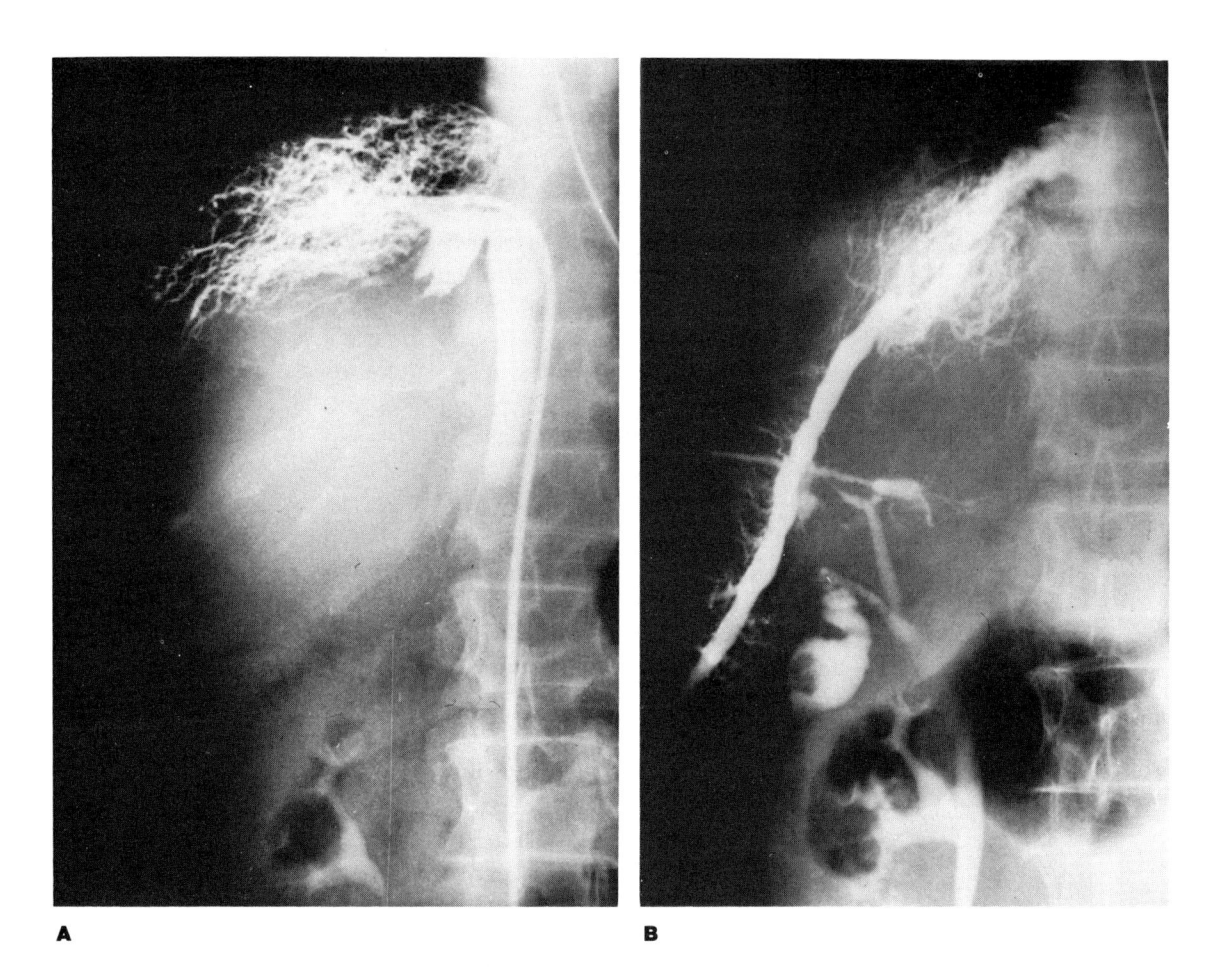

Figure 9-3. *A.* Hepatic vein injection demonstrates the multiple interconnecting collaterals referred to as "spider web" appearance, considered pathognomonic for Budd-Chiari syndrome. *B.* Percutaneous hepatic vein injection filling "spider web" collaterals in an antegrade fashion. Note filling of tributaries of the hepatic vein seen typically with hepatic vein obstruction.

torting the lobular and vascular architecture. The derangement occurs on both macroscopic and microscopic levels. It is the alteration in the microcirculatory unit that leads to portal hypertension and its potentially devastating sequelae. Cirrhosis is not a uniform disease throughout the liver; one lobe may be predominantly affected with inhomogeneity of the process within that lobe. The classification of cirrhosis has been and remains confusing, with an array of terms based on morphologic, clinical, or etiologic presentation. In the United States, alcohol is the most common cause of cirrhosis and portal hypertension, with the fibrotic process mostly involving the postsinusoidal hepatic venules. On a worldwide basis, schistosomiasis is the most prevalent cause. The ovae of the schistosomes are carried from mesenteric venules to small portal radicles within the liver. The subsequent granuloma formation in fibrosis destroys portal venules and leads to portal hypertension.

THE LIVER PACKAGE

At Emory University, the panangiographic evaluation of 612 patients (approximately 1,350 examinations) referred for examination and treatment of portal hypertension from 1972 to 1982 has led to a combination of arterial and venous studies collectively called "the liver package." Since most patients referred for workup have experienced at least one episode of variceal hemorrhage, the goals of the preoperative liver package are to stage the portal hypertension and determine if the patient is a candidate for shunt surgery. As the diagnosis of varices has usually been established by previous modalities (endoscopy, barium studies, CT, etc.), the angiographic assessment for surgery makes no special attempt to document the diagnosis of varices. As a result, 25 percent of patients with endoscopically proven varices have no demonstrable varices on routine liver package (44). Angiography following tolazoline (PRISCOLINE) injection and selective left gastric arterial injection would be expected to demonstrate varices in almost all of these patients.

The standard preoperative liver package consists of hepatic wedge pressure and injection; free hepatic vein, inferior vena cava, right atrium, and left renal vein pressures; left renal venography; and selective superior mesenteric and splenic arterial injections. In isolated cases, superior mesenteric arteriography following Priscoline injection, left gastric artery injection, or splenoportography are helpful.

Postoperatively, the liver package is modified with the following objectives: (1) evaluation of adequate shunt function, (2) assessment of hepatic portal flow, and (3) demonstration of varices. Postoperative shunt patients receive angiographic evaluation 1 week and 6 months following surgery and yearly thereafter according to protocol. Not all patients are studied as such, depending on complicating factors. Patients with suspected occluded shunt or development of encephalopathy undergo reevaluation at the development of symptoms. The postoperative liver package includes hepatic wedge, caval, left renal vein, and shunt pressures, shunt injection, and superior mesenteric arteriography, with special attention to portal flow and varices. Angiographic complications as a result of preshunt and postshunt evaluation are rare. In Nordlinger's review of 295 liver packages performed at Emory between 1971 and 1979, he discovered only three significant groin hematomas (44). In the last several years, the vast majority of patients at Emory University have received the selective distal splenorenal shunt, for reasons to be elaborated in the following sections.

HEPATIC WEDGE INJECTION

Technique

Following usual sterile preparation and local anesthesia of the groin, an 80 cm 6.7 French straight yellow catheter with single endhole is introduced into the inferior vena cava using standard Seldinger technique. The catheter is advanced to the approximate caval atrial junction, and a Cook deflector wire is used to deflect the catheter into a hepatic vein—usually the main right. The deflector wire is held in a 90° to 150° deflection, with the wire curve at the junction of the hepatic vein and vena cava, while advancing the catheter over the wire until the wedge position is achieved. Wedge position is confirmed by hand injection of a small amount of contrast demonstrating sinusoidal filling without reflux into the hepatic vein. Care is taken to avoid wedge positions along the extreme periphery of the liver, as power injection may rupture the liver and is irritating and painful in the subcapsular location. Injection is performed with a power

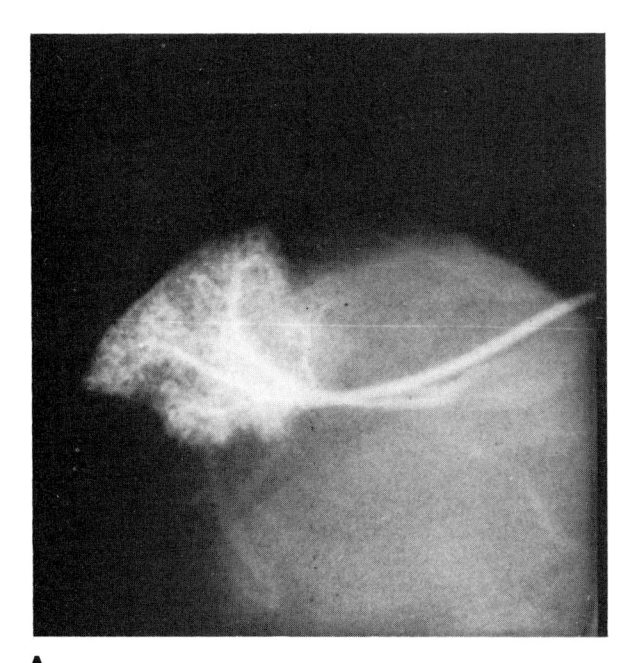

Figure 9-4. *A.* Hepatic wedge injection demonstrating Grade I portal venous flow (no portal reflux). Note the homogeneous, uniform parenchymagram.

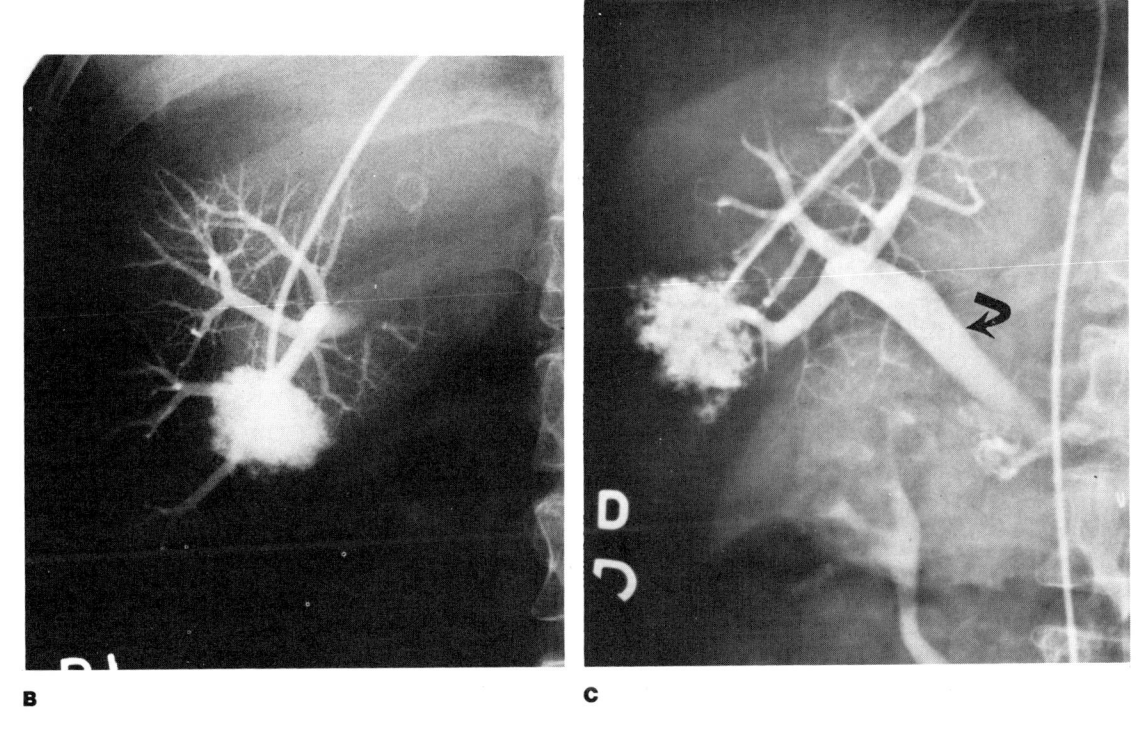

Figure 9-4. *B.* Hepatic wedge injection demonstrating significant reflux into the portal vein. This appearance may be seen with both Grade II and Grade III portal venous flow. The distinction between the grades rests on early flow into liver with Grade II and stagnation of flow with Grade III portal venous flow (see text). *C.* Hepatic wedge injection demonstrating retrograde flow into the portal vein (arrow), i.e., Grade IV portal flow.

injector at the rate of 2 ml per second for a total of 10 ml of contrast. Filming is one film per second for ten films.

Interpretation

The normal wedge venogram demonstrates a homogeneous, uniform parenchymogram (Figure 9-4A). Adjacent hepatic veins are frequently filled as the contrast under pressure seeks the lowest pressure system through sinusoidal communications. Flash filling of portal venous branches is often seen during the injection phase; however, rapid washout by unopacified blood occurs in normal (Grade I) flow. Persistence of portal venous opacification following the injection is abnormal. Portal veins can be distinguished from hepatic veins by their branching pattern. As reflux of contrast occurs in portal veins, the branches and tributaries will become opacified, giving a "branching tree" appearance. However, when the hepatic veins are filled, no branching pattern is observed, as unopacified blood is returning via tributaries into the main hepatic vein. Filling of hepatic vein branches is seen only in the case of hepatic vein obstruction, as in Budd-Chiari. The course of the vein is helpful in distinguishing hepatic from portal only in the middle and upper right lobes. In this region, the hepatic veins tend to follow an oblique course toward the caval atrial junction, whereas the portal vein follows a more horizontal path to the porta hepatis. In the inferior right lobe, the veins follow parallel paths, and therefore, course is not helpful in differentiating them.

Grade II portal flow by wedge injection is defined as the presence of significant reflux into the portal veins with rapid flow into the liver. Grade III flow is significant reflux into the portal veins, similar to Grade II, but present greater than 3 seconds following the end of injection (or the eighth film using filming program of one film per second for ten films) (Figure 9-4B). Grade IV is retrograde flow into the portal system (Figure 9-4C).

In patients with cirrhosis (postsinusoidal obstruction), the parenchymagram will demonstrate an inhomogeneous nodular pattern. The hepatic veins are truncated and stenosed, presumably secondary to fibrosis. Shunting from the hepatic to portal veins may be seen. The portal branches are normal but may be displaced by regenerating nodules. We have found the venous phase of the superior mesenteric artery (SMA) injection to be more accurate than estimation of portal flow by wedge injection (44). The greatest utility of the wedge injection in the preoperative liver package is to demonstrate reversal of portal flow in patients with Stage IV portal hypertension. In these patients, the venous SMA injection will fail to visualize the portal vein, and therefore, one cannot discriminate reversal of flow from portal thrombosis—an obviously critical distinction in shunt planning.

Bookstein *et al.*(45) correlated the wedged venographic appearance with various hepatic pathologies. Patients with periportal fibrosis (presinusoidal) demonstrated normal hepatic veins and nearly normal, slightly accentuated lobular parenchymagram. Patients with congenital hepatic fibrosis revealed a lobular parenchymagram and no visualization of portal veins. These findings in a recent study by Heeney *et al.*(46) serve to reiterate the concepts of presinusoidal and postsinusoidal obstruction and the information from hepatic venography that can be used to differentiate these two entities.

CORRECTED SINUSOIDAL PRESSURE

Technique

Corrected sinusoidal pressure (CSP) is obtained by subtracting the free hepatic vein (FHV) or inferior vena cava pressure from the wedged hepatic vein pressure (WHVP).

Wedged pressure determinations at multiple sites are needed to assess portal or CSP pressure accurately owing to the inhomogeneous nature of the cirrhotic process within the liver.

Interpretation

When a catheter is wedged in a hepatic vein, the portal pressure is transmitted through the sinusoids, giving an indirect measurement of portal pressure. Good correlation has been shown between indirect methods of obtaining portal pressure and measurements taken directly at the time of surgery (47,48). In cases of postsinusoidal obstruction (cirrhosis), the CSP should be elevated, while in presinusoidal obstruction (periportal fibrosis) or prehepatic obstruction, the CSP is normal. The normal WHVP is from 8 to 12 mm Hg (49) with a difference of approximately 5 mm Hg between the WHVP and the free hepatic vein or inferior vena cava. The gradient measurement allows differentiation between truly elevated sinusoidal pressure and that secondary to an elevated systemic venous pressure. A CSP of less than 5 mm Hg is normal, 5 to 15 mm Hg mildly elevated, 16 to 30 mm Hg moderately elevated, and greater than 30 mm Hg markedly elevated (50).

Studies by Lunderquist (51) have demonstrated how sinusoidal pressure is transmitted to a wedged hepatic-vein catheter despite postsinusoidal obstruction. By injecting cadaver livers with Microfil, he has demonstrated the irregular venous channels through fibrotic septi that serve to transmit the portal venous pressure to the hepatic veins. These irregular venous channels represent altered sinusoidal architecture.

CSP is helpful in distinguishing presinusoidal from postsinusoidal obstruction; however, no relationship between CSP and variceal size or risk of hemorrhage has been established (20).

LEFT RENAL VEIN

Technique

The distal splenorenal shunt is the predominant shunt performed at our institution; therefore, preoperative evaluation of the left renal vein is essential. Following the wedge injection and pressure in the right atrium and vena cava, the left renal vein is catheterized using the same 6.7 French straight endhole catheter and Cook deflector wire. Injection rate is 6 ml per second for a total of 18 ml and filming one film per second for a total of seven films. Following filming, the catheter is left in place and connected to a flush drip. This allows easy comparison of the left renal vein catheter position with the opacified splenic vein following selective splenic artery injection.

Interpretation

Preoperative knowledge of the left renal vein position and potential congenital anomalies is of great importance to the surgeon planning a distal splenorenal shunt (52). The variations in the left renal vein have been described by Chuang (53) as preaortic (80 to 90 percent), retroaortic (2 to 3 percent), circumaortic (6 to 17 percent) (Figure 9–5) and supernumerary (1 percent) (Figure 9–5). A left IVC occurs in approximately 0.5 percent of patients and may cause difficulty in left renal vein catheterization if unrecognized (54) (Figure 9–6). In 256 patients receiving a preoperative liver package, the left renal vein crossed the midline at L1 in 68 percent of patients (44). The position of the left renal vein in relation to the splenic vein is important in determining the

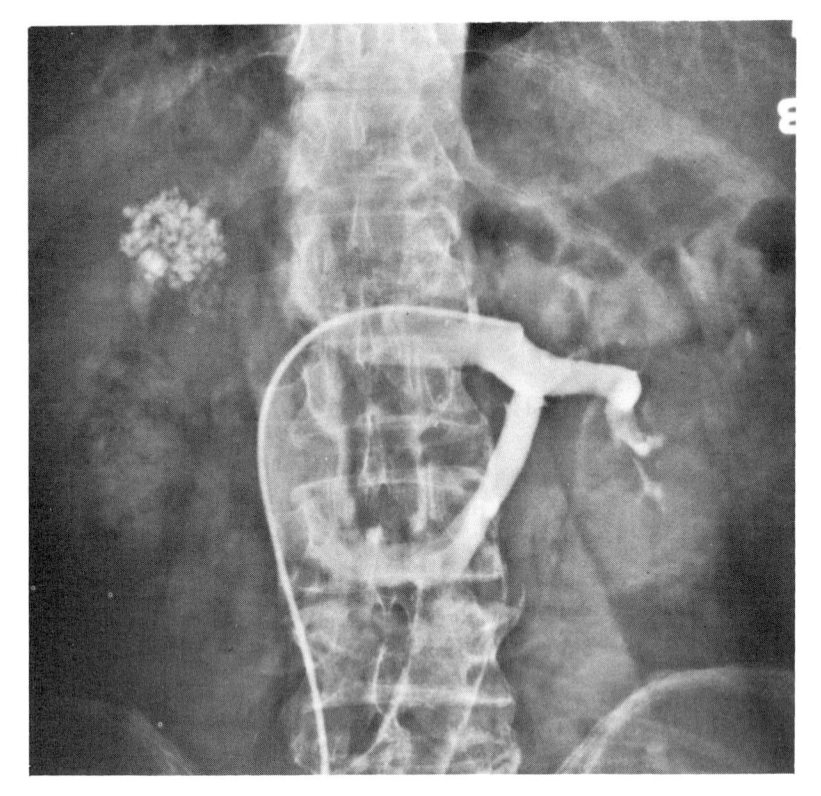

Figure 9-5. Left renal venography demonstrating circumaortic renal vein. The more cephalic limb is always ventral to the aorta, while the more caudal limb is dorsal to the aorta. Knowledge of this congenital anomaly is crucial for a surgeon planning a selective distal splenorenal shunt.

amount of splenic vein dissection and mobilization required for anastomosis with the left renal vein. Ideally, the splenic vein should be one vertebral body cephalad to the left renal vein.

Renal vein hypertension is not unusual in patients with portal hypertension and gastroesophageal varices (55). The normal left renal vein pressure should closely approximate that of the IVC. Greater than a 5 mm Hg gradient indicates significant renal vein compromise. Filling of collaterals from left renal venography is seen frequently (Figure 9-7) and seldom are these collaterals of any significance. The most frequently filled collaterals are left gonadal, left adrenal, and hemiazygos veins. These findings or the presence of renal vein anomalies do not preclude selective shunt surgery. However, significant collateral via the gonadal veins must be preserved at surgery in order to allow adequate postoperative decompression (Figure 9-8). Even in patients with normal renal vein anatomy, some degree of postoperative renal vein hypertension is not unusual and is caused by high flow through the shunt and edema from surgery. In time, this venous hypertension will clear as the renal vein and IVC enlarge and the postoperative edema resolves.

SUPERIOR MESENTERIC ARTERY INJECTION

Technique

Following selective SMA catheterization, an injection is made at 6 ml per second for a total of 60 ml. Filming program is variable, but should extend approximately 35

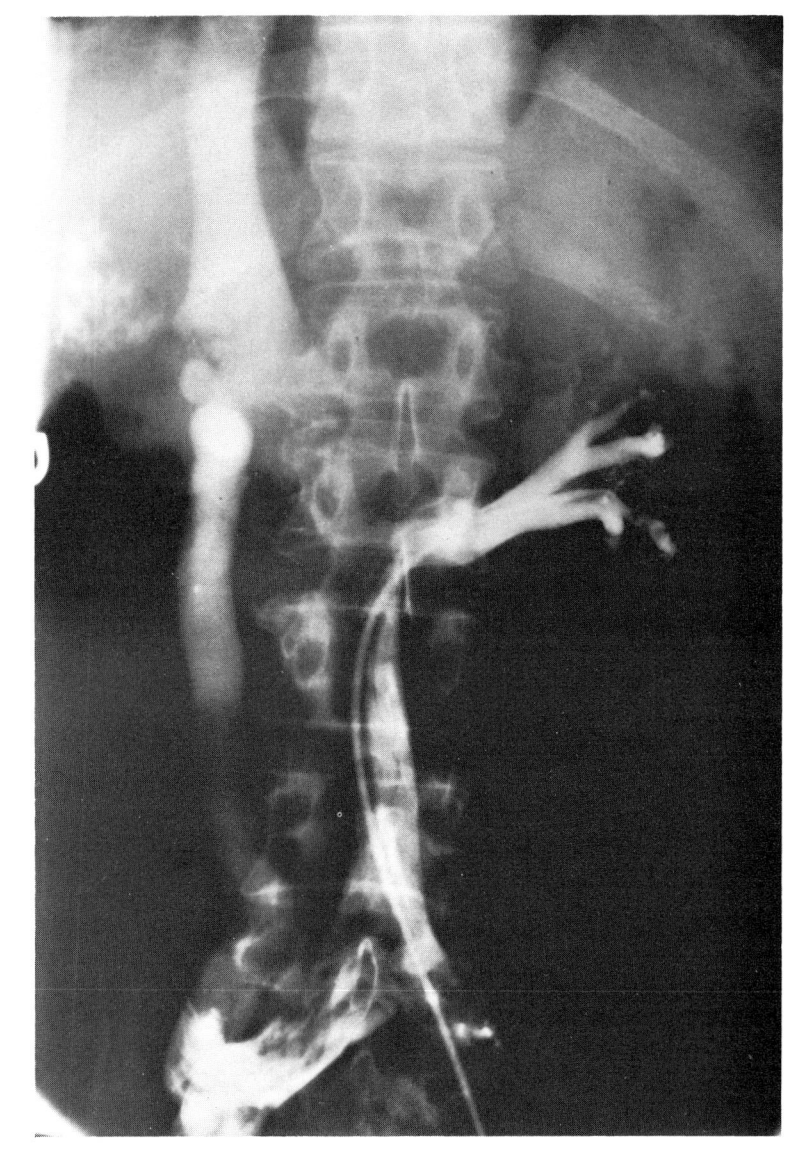

Figure 9-6. Left renal vein catheterization via a persistent left inferior vena cava. When difficulty is encountered catheterizing a left renal vein through a right femoral vein approach, this uncommon anomaly should be considered.

seconds for good visualization of the venous phase. Centering should be slightly to the right of midline with inclusion of the dome of the right lobe of the liver. If test injection reveals a replaced right hepatic artery, the catheter should be advanced past the orifice of the hepatic artery to avoid simultaneous arterial opacification of the liver.

Interpretation

The venous phase of the SMA injection (performed without drug augmentation) is used to grade the portal venous perfusion of the liver. The grading is assessed as follows (Figure 9-9): Grade I—normal hepatopetal flow with visualization of the branches of the portal vein to the periphery of the liver and staining of the hepatic parenchyma; Grade II—hepatopetal flow with visualization of tertiary portal venous branches not

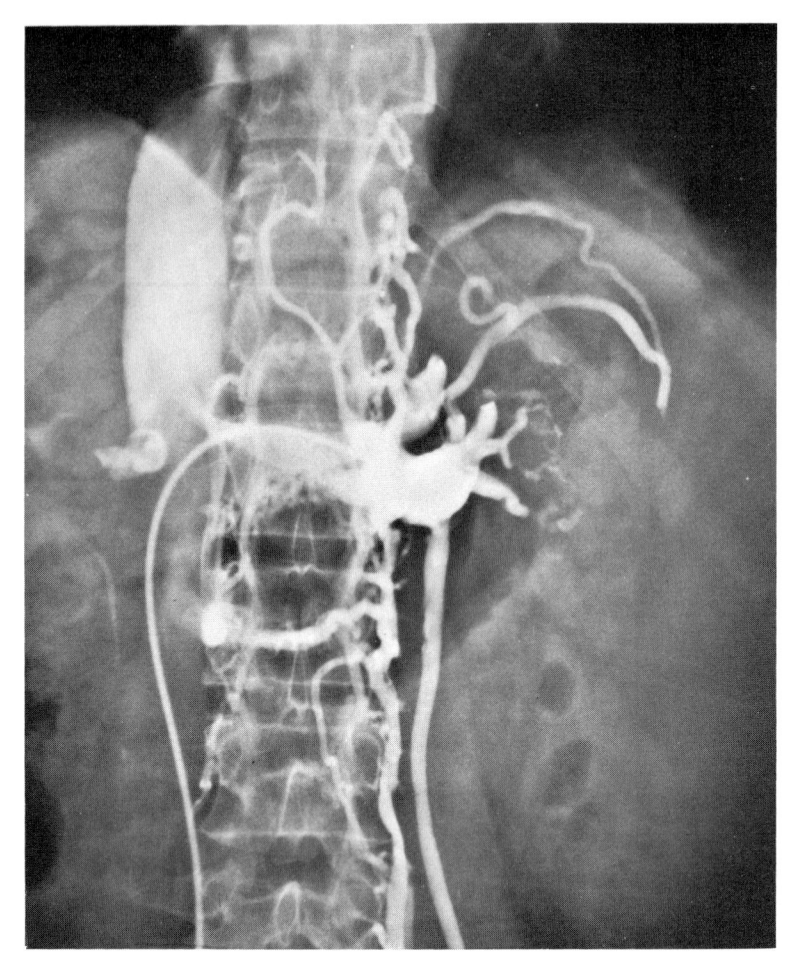

Figure 9-7. Left renal venography demonstrating multiple collaterals including the lumbar plexus, hemiazygous system, and gonadal vein. This patient demonstrated no pressure gradient from the left renal vein to the inferior vena cava, indicating that this collateral filling does not indicate compromise of renal venous drainage.

extending to the liver periphery, but with staining of the liver parenchyma; Grade III—poor hepatopetal flow with visualization of only first or second order portal branches and no liver stain; Grade IV—hepatofugal flow, i.e., reversal of portal flow and no visualization of portal vein. This grading of portal venous flow is a very important part of the preoperative liver package in determining the type of shunt to be performed. Patients with Grades I and II have good portal perfusion and are considered excellent candidates for the selective distal splenorenal shunt. Patients with Grade III flow are less than ideal, but benefit from the selective shunt. Patients with Grade IV flow have poor or absent portal perfusion and may be considered for the technically easier portocaval or mesocaval shunt. RPO projections of 15 to 20 degrees are often helpful in providing better visualization of the portal vein by projecting it off the vertebral column.

The continued postoperative portal perfusion of the liver is of great importance in preventing hepatic encephalopathy. This is the reason for performing the selective distal splenorenal shunt. (Figure 9-10). Claims have been made that portal perfusion is preserved following mesocaval shunt (56-59). However, it has been shown that this represents an angiographic illusion called "portal pseudoperfusion" and results from injection of the celiac axis, rather than selective SMA injection in the postoperative shunt patient (60). The apparent portal perfusion is the result of contrast injection into the

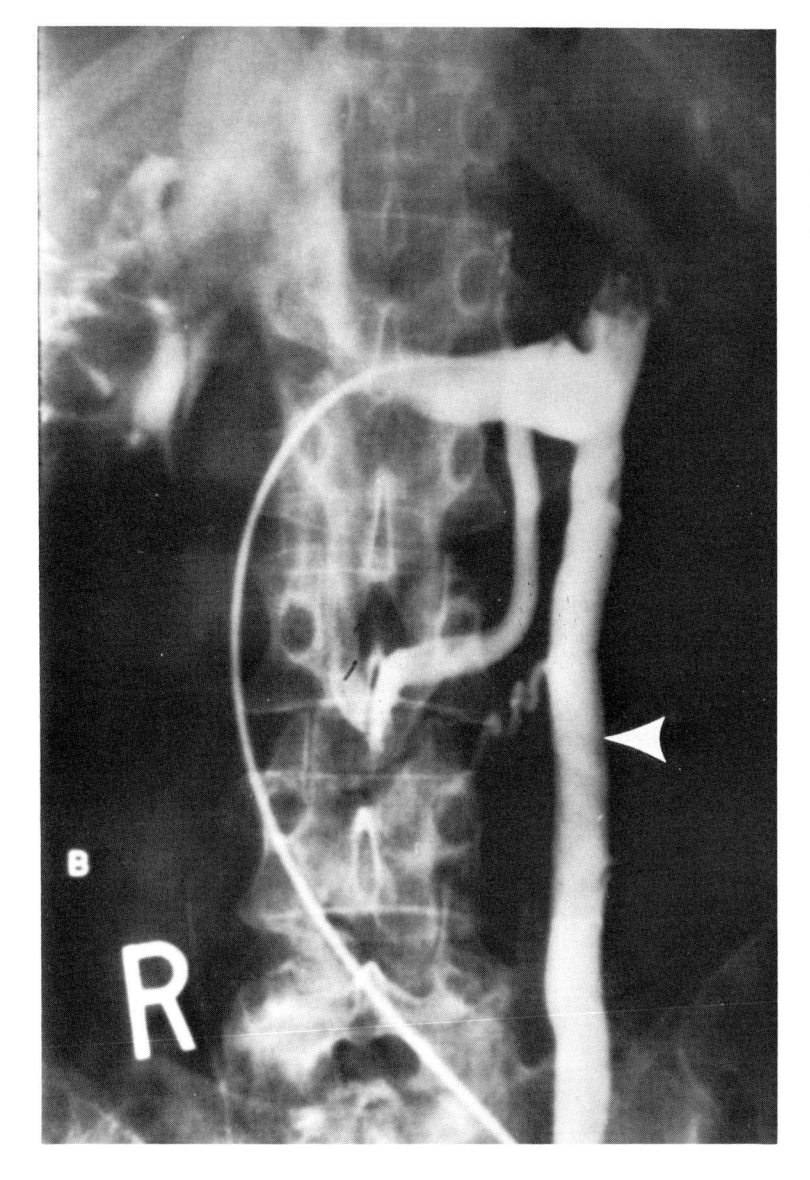

Figure 9-8. *A.* Preoperative left renal venogram demonstrating predominant drainage via the gonadal vein (arrow).

hepatic artery simultaneous to the splenic artery and resultant retrograde flow through the portal system. This simultaneous opacification of the splenic and portal veins has been interpreted incorrectly as portal perfusion. No patient with a functioning portosystemic shunt (mesocaval, portocaval, etc.) will demonstrate portal venous perfusion of the liver (Figure 9-11). Portal perfusion demonstrated by selective SMA injection following one of these systemic shunts is evidence of shunt thrombosis.

SPLENIC ARTERY INJECTION

Technique

Following selective splenic artery catheterization, 6 ml per second of contrast for a total of 60 mL is injected and filmed over approximately 35 seconds as previously dis-

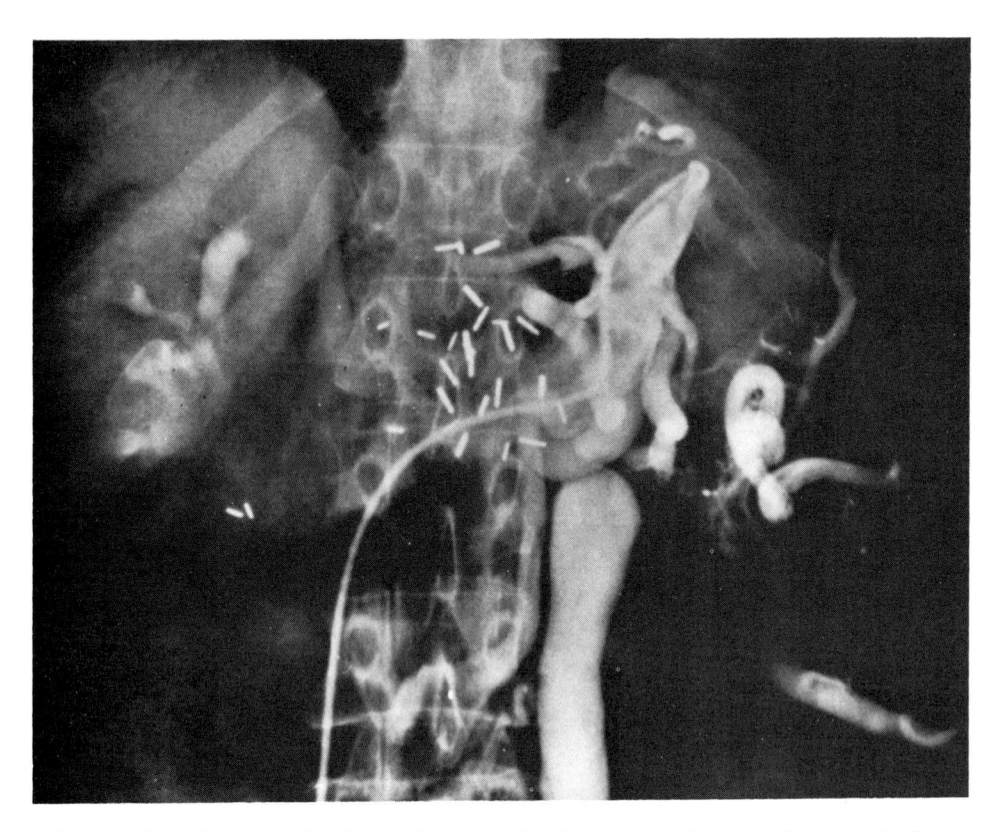

Figure 9-8. *B.* Postoperative distal splenorenal shunt catheterization revealing a markedly engorged gonadal vein. In cases of renal vein hypertension, the predominant collateral will usually enlarge to accommodate the increased flow from the splenic vein. This stresses the importance of preservation of this collateral at the time of surgery.

cussed with the SMA technique. If for technical reasons, the splenic artery cannot be catheterized, a celiac injection can be performed to show the position and patency of the splenic vein. Priscoline or other vasodilators may be necessary to demonstrate the splenic vein with a celiac artery injection.

Interpretation

Visualization of a patent splenic vein is essential in preparing for a distal splenorenal shunt (Figure 9-12). As previously discussed, the relative position of splenic to left renal vein is important in preoperative planning. Although specific efforts are not made, we have found that gastroesophageal varices are better visualized during the venous phase of the splenic injection than of the SMA injection (44).

ADDITIONS TO THE ROUTINE LIVER PACKAGE

Left Gastric Artery Injection

It is helpful occasionally to demonstrate the presence of esophageal varices in instances where splenic and superior mesenteric artery injections failed to detect these

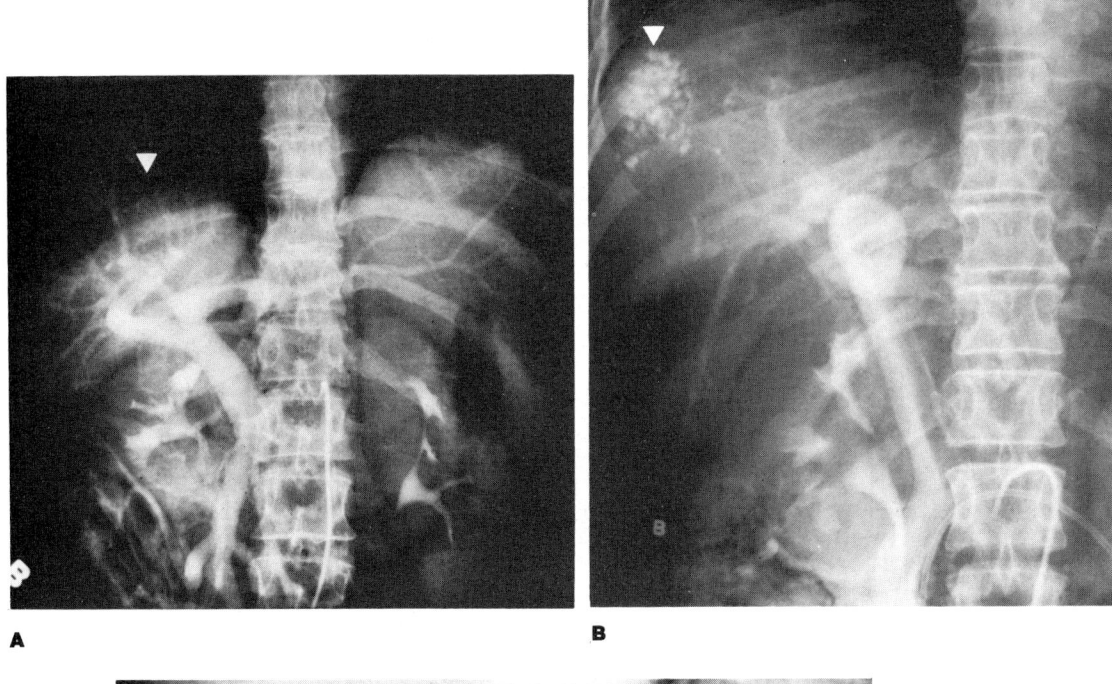

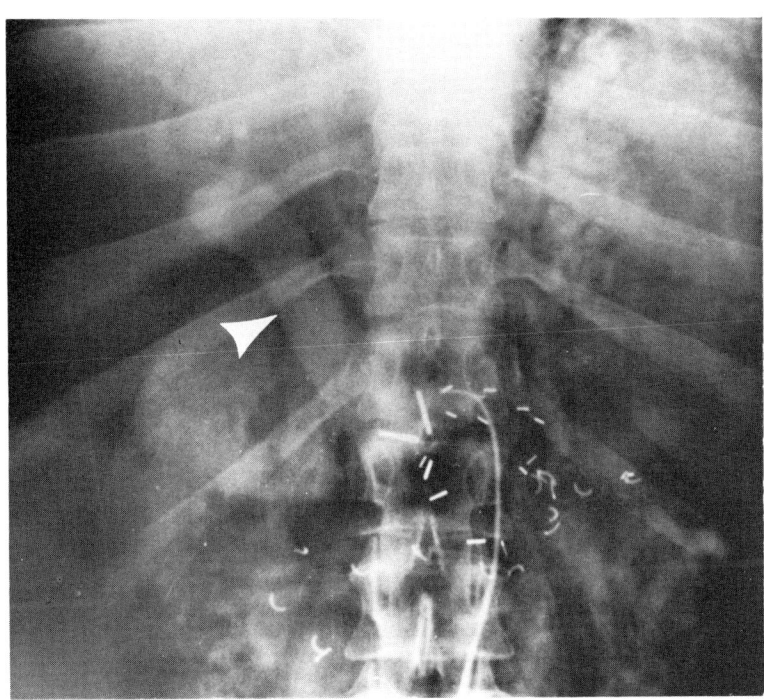

Figure 9-9. *A.* The venous phase of a superior mesenteric artery injection demonstrating Grade I portal flow. Note that the portal venous branches extend to the periphery of the liver (arrow). *B.* Grade II portal flow demonstrated by venous phase of superior mesenteric artery injection with visualization of portal venous branches, but not extending to the liver periphery. Residual stain from the hepatic wedge injection (arrow). *C.* Grade III portal flow revealing opacification of only the main portal vein without visualization of intrahepatic branches. This indicates virtual stasis of portal venous flow.

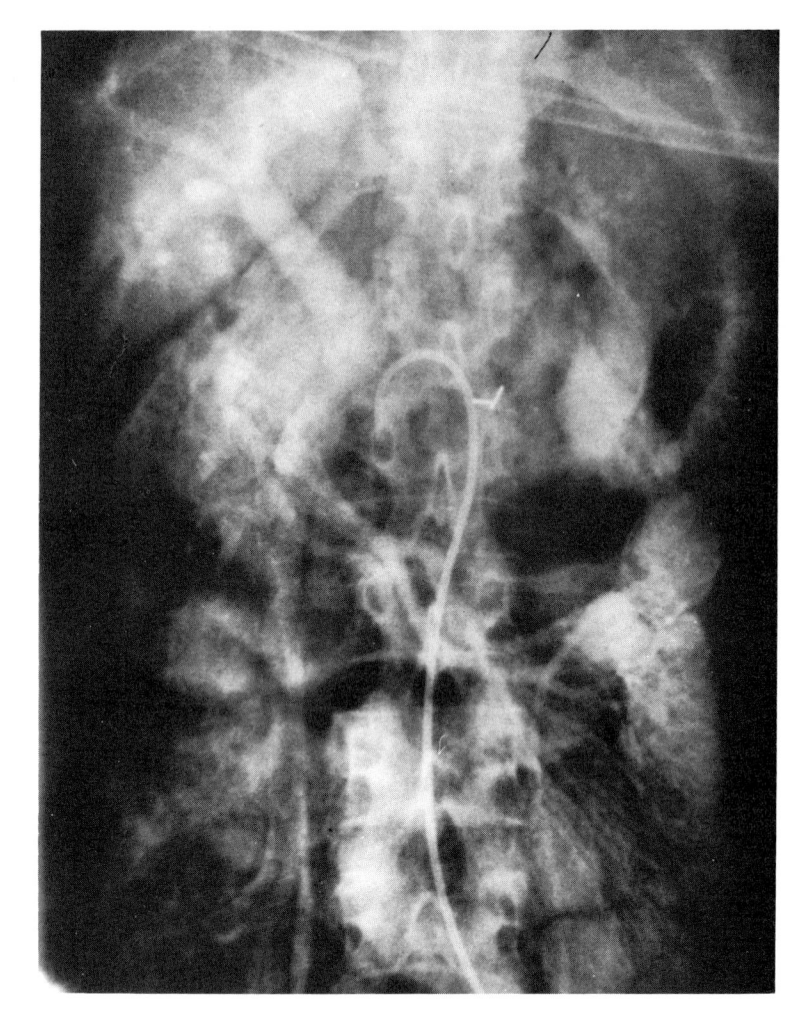

Figure 9-10. Well-preserved antegrade flow through portal vein demonstrated on venous phase of superior mesenteric artery injection following distal splenorenal shunt. No decrease in the corrected sinusoidal pressure was demonstrated postoperatively.

collaterals. High-dose left gastric artery injections (8 ml per second for a total of 50 to 70 ml) have given consistent demonstration of esophageal varices superior to that seen with splenoportography (61).

Priscoline

Priscoline (totazoline hydrochloride) is a vasodilator that may be given intraarterially approximately 30 seconds prior to contrast injection to increase flow and provide better visualization of the venous phase. The usual dosage ranges from 25 to 50 mg (25 mg per ml). Action is by direct effect on vascular smooth muscle. Care in administration tion is stressed, as this drug may cause tachycardia, cardiac arrhythmias, and anginal pain. Tolazoline (PRISCOLINE) has been implicated in contributing to myocardial infarction and severe hypotension(62).

Contraindications to Study

The liver package has been performed on a large number of patients with coagulopathies secondary to liver disease and acute hemorrhage with few significant compli-

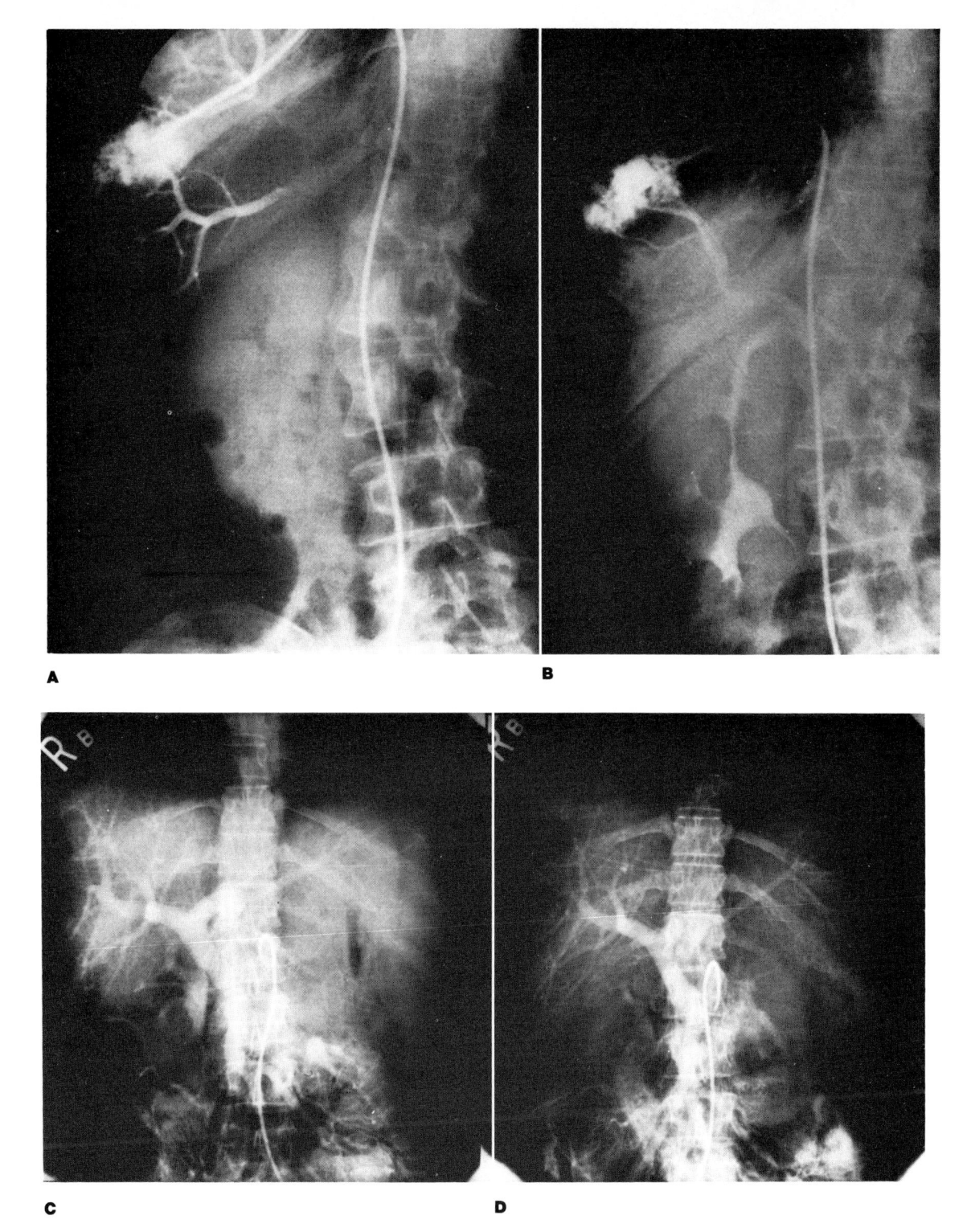

Figure 9-11. *A.* Preoperative hepatic wedge injection demonstrating Grade II portal flow. *B.* Following portocaval shunt, Grade II portal flow was converted to retrograde (Grade IV) flow. Although systemic shunts are effective in decompressing varices, they consistently result in loss of portal perfusion. *C.* Venous-phase superior mesenteric artery injection demonstrating Grade I portal perfusion. *D.* Left mesorenal shunt: demonstration of portal perfusion following nonselective shunt is evidence of shunt thrombosis, as occurred in this case. Portal perfusion will not be seen in a functioning nonselective shunt.

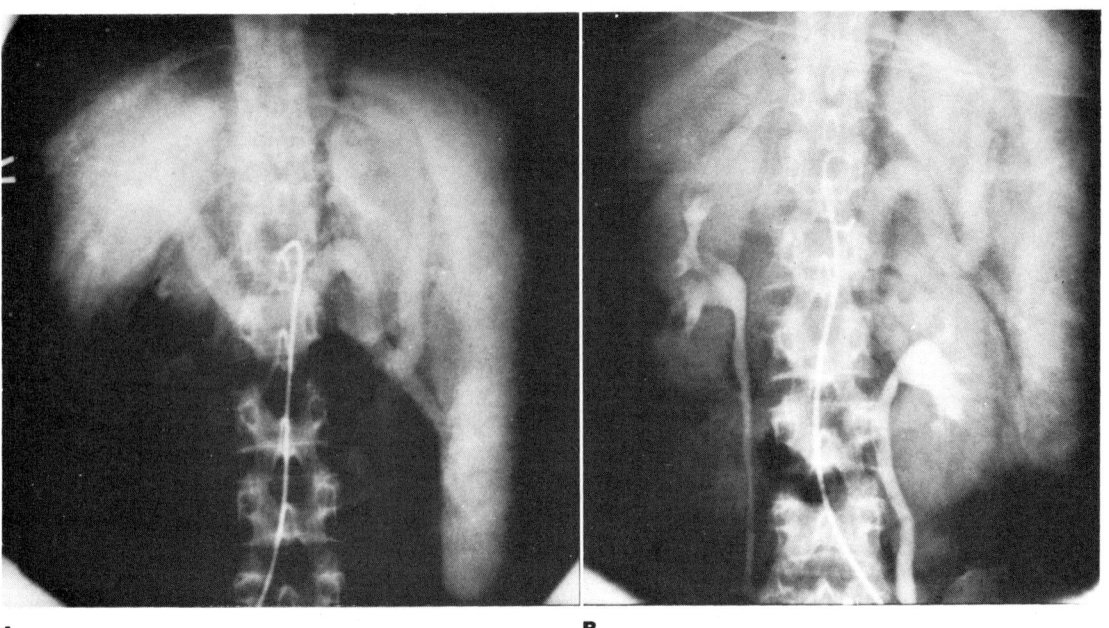

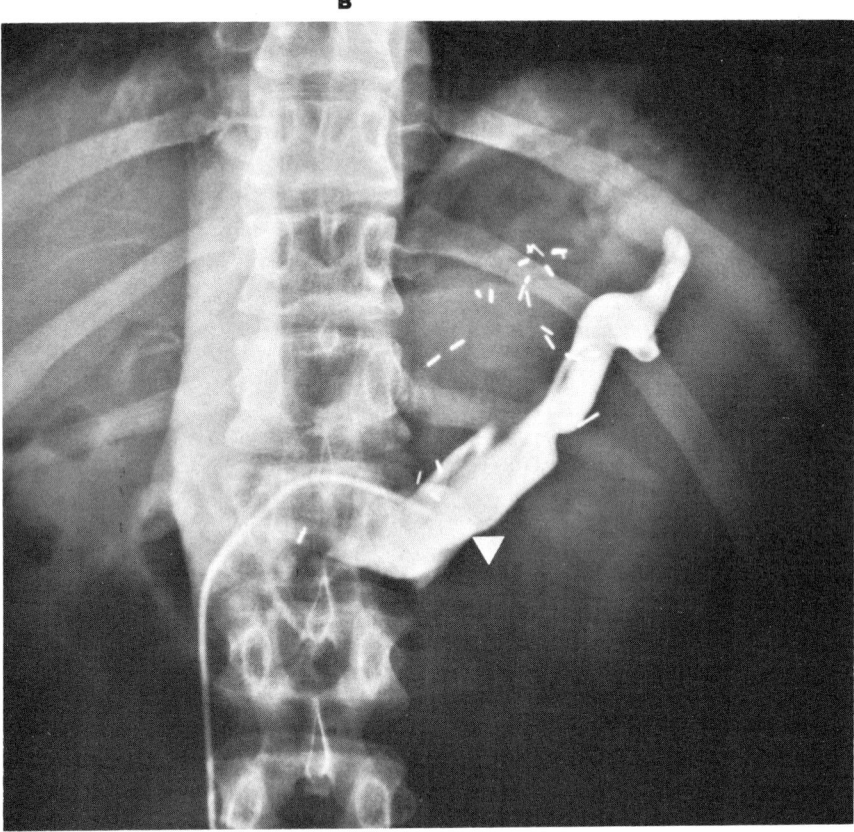

Figure 9-12. *A.* Venous phase of a selective splenic artery injection demonstrating good opacification of the splenic and portal veins. *B.* Same patient following distal splenorenal shunt demonstrates good visualization of the splenic vein, but poor visualization of the renal vein and inferior vena cava. This should not be misinterpreted as shunt thrombosis, but is secondary to dilution of the splenic venous contrast from the unopacified blood from the left renal vein and inferior vena cava. *C.* Good visualization of the distal splenorenal shunt can be achieved by direct venous catheterization. This method is preferable in that pressures across the anastomosis can be measured Arrow = anastomosis of splenic vein to left renal vein.

cations. Most patients will have low hematocrit and platelet counts, as well as abnormal clotting studies. We consider a platelet count of less than 30,000 or prothrombin time more than twice control as contraindications for angiography. Although a platelet count of 30,000 is less than the approximate 50,000 frequently cited in the literature, this is justifiable based on the risk associated with additional transfusion and the low incidence of bleeding complications encountered in this patient population.

Splenoportography

This technique is useful when there is suspected splenic or portal vein thrombosis (Figure 9-13) and when better visualization of these veins and variceal collaterals is desired (Figure 9-14). Ascites and coagulopathies are relative contraindications. With the patient in the supine position, the spleen is localized under fluoroscopy. Following sterile preparation and local anesthesia, an 18 French catheter-trocar set is directed in a cephalomedial direction from a point just dorsal to the midaxillary line. The puncture is performed during apnea, and the trocar is removed quickly to avoid splenic laceration. The tip of the catheter should lie within splenic pulp at the conclusion of the puncture.

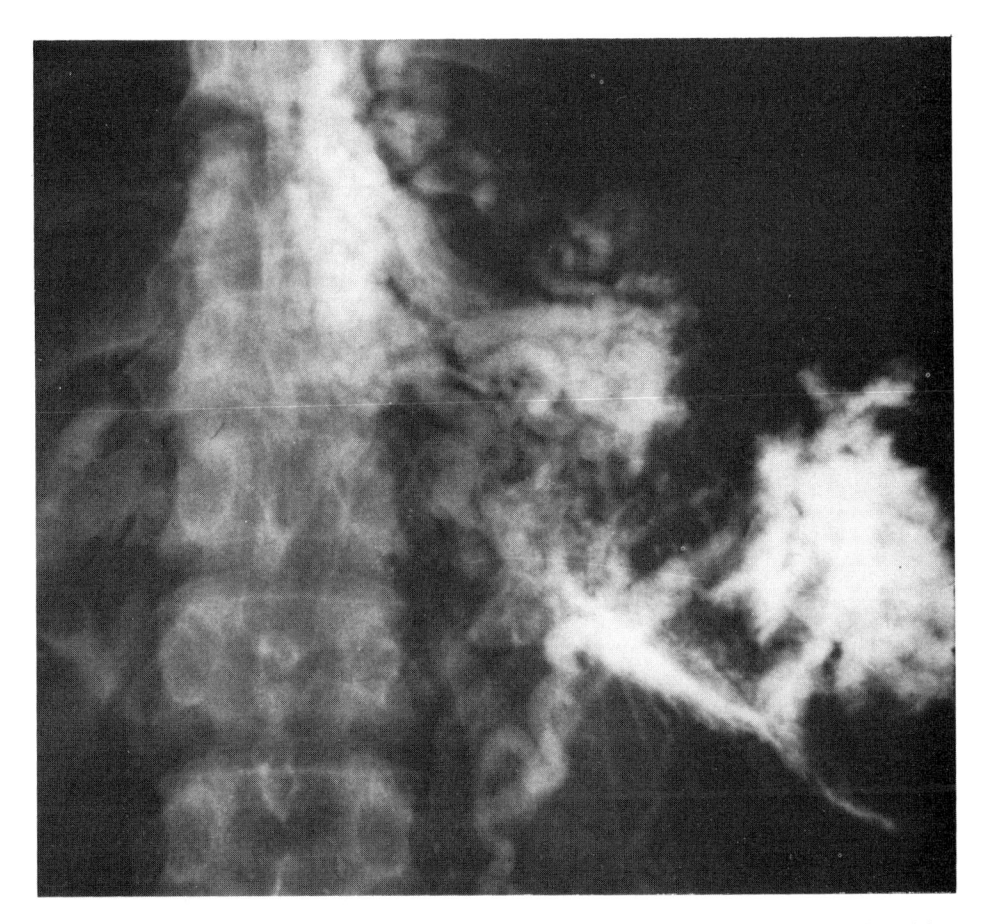

Figure 9-13. Splenoprotogram demonstrating nonfilling of the splenic and portal veins with opacification of multiple splenic hilum and gastroesophageal varices. This technique is especially useful in diagnosing splenic and portal vein thrombosis.

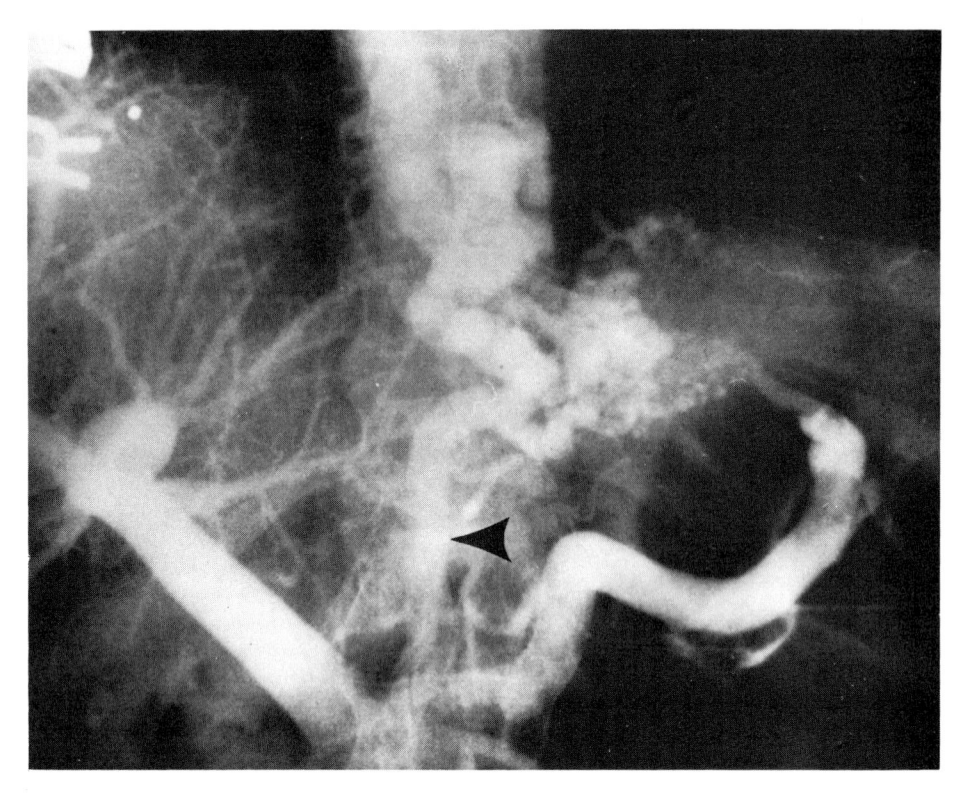

Figure 9-14. Splenoportogram demonstrating excellent opacification of the splenic and portal veins. Note the large coronary vein (arrow), as well as the gastroesophageal varices seen well with this technique.

A slow flow of blood from the catheter hub indicates the tip is within the spleen, though occasionally one must aspirate to obtain blood. A small test injection of contrast will confirm the correct position. Following splenic-pulp pressure measurement, a power injection is performed at approximately 6 ml per second for a total of 40 ml of contrast. On the normal examination, the splenic and portal veins are well-visualized. Gastroesophageal varices, splenic veins, and portal veins are well-demonstrated with this technique. Prone splenoportography is reported to result in better opacification of collaterals than supine positioning.

Complications following this procedure are uncommon. Hemorrhage is the major complication. Transfusion or splenectomy is very rare, and death secondary to the procedure was seen in 4 of 1,200 cases (63).

Transhepatic Portography

The use of transhepatic portography gives direct measurement of portal vein pressure, as well as superb visualization of the portal and splenic veins and collateral vessels. Routine use of this technique in the preoperative evaluation of patients for shunt procedures has been advocated (64,65). Although much information can be gained by its use, the potential risks have dissuaded most angiographers from using this technique for routine preoperative shunt evaluation. Transhepatic portography coupled with coronary vein embolization is a viable alternative in the patient with acute variceal bleeding and is discussed in Chapter 10. This approach simplifies the surgeon's task in performing a selective distal splenorenal shunt.

ADJUNCTIVE METHODS OF INVESTIGATION

The newer imaging modalities are capable of visualizing accurately the spectrum of pathologic changes associated with cirrhosis and portal hypertension. Computed tomography and ultrasound examinations are often used early in the evaluation of patients with diffuse liver disease, and findings suggestive of portal hypertension need to be recognized in order to further direct the diagnostic workup.

Real-time sonography has been particularly helpful in following the tortuous course of collateral veins presenting as serpiginous anechoic tubular structures located near the gastroesophageal junction, splenic hilum, and retroperitoneum. The anechoic recanalized umbilical vein within the echodense ligamentum terres and surrounding fat has been cited as a specific finding in portal hypertension (66,67) (Figure 9–15). Corroborative evidence of portal hypertension such as ascites, hepatic parenchymal disease, splenomegaly, and portal vein thrombosis may also be seen with sonography.

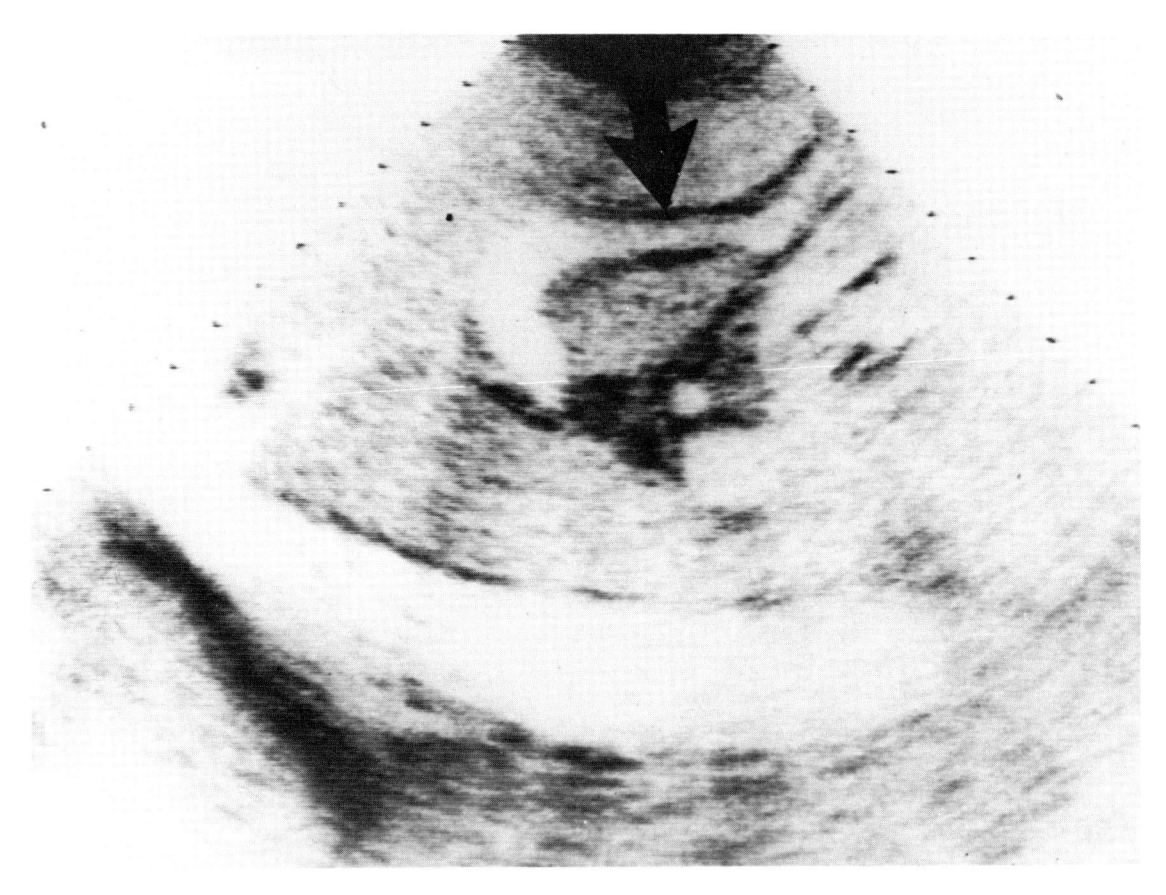

Figure 9–15. Longitudinal sonogram: visualization of the anechoic recanalized umbilical vein (arrow) within the echogenic ligamentum teres and surrounding fat is a specific finding in portal hypertension.

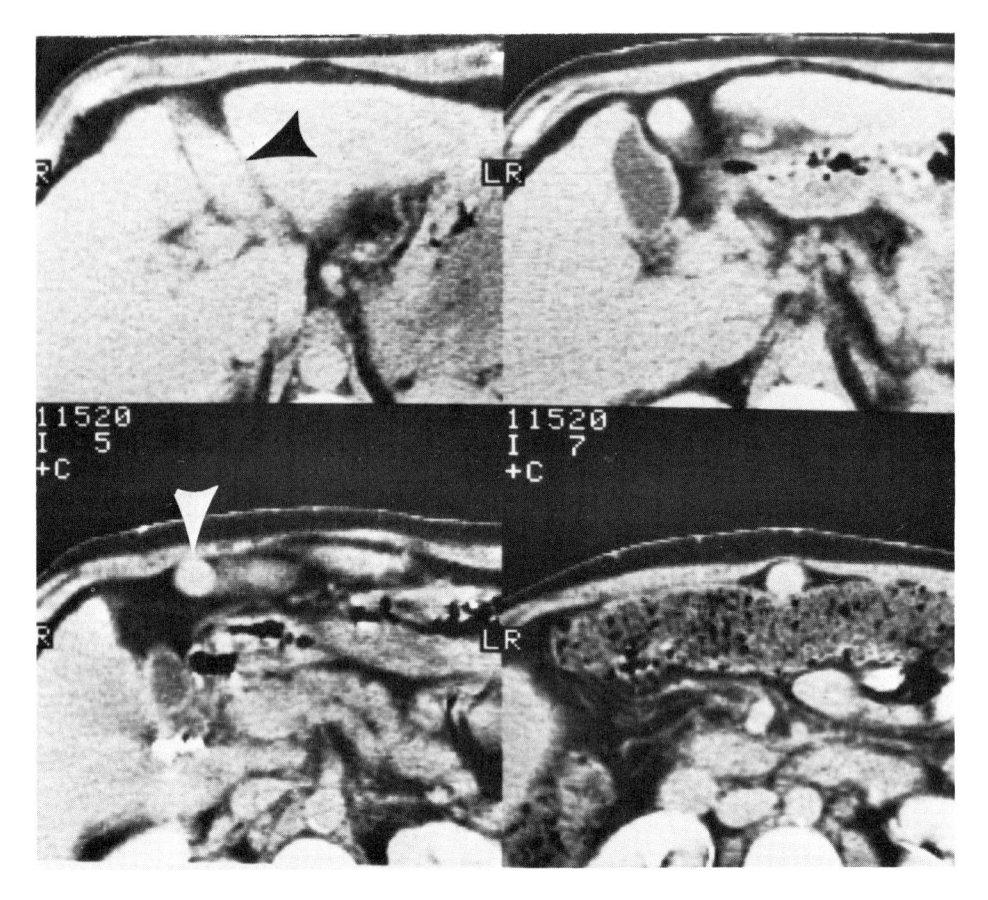

Figure 9–16. Sequential scans following intravenous contrast demonstrate the recanalized umbilical vein exiting the liver and coursing beneath the abdominal wall (arrow).

Computed tomography can effectively demonstrate collateral vessels and is most accurate when imaging is performed during contrast injection (68) (Figure 9–16). Varices are identified as lobulated or tubular structures occurring in the expected locations and demonstrating contrast enhancement. Correlation of CT and angiography (liver package) in the detection of varices has revealed that CT may image some varices not seen on angiography (69). However, it should be remembered that the liver package makes no routine attempt to visualize all varices, as this information is not essential in preoperative planning.

The use of digital subtraction angiography has been described for evaluation of patency and determination of flow direction in the portal vein (70). Although resulting in significant reduction of total contrast load compared with film-screen angiography, its practical application in the everyday evaluation of portal hypertension is yet to be determined.

The adjunctive methods described above are most helpful in the serendipitous detection of unsuspected portal hypertension. The comprehensive evaluation of portal hypertension requires the use of angiography to assess not only morphology, but more critically, the underlying hemodynamics.

Shunt Procedures

The primary goal of any portosystemic shunt is to prevent the recurrence of upper gastrointestinal hemorrhage. This is achieved by diverting the blood under high pressure within the portocollateral system into the low-pressure systemic circulation. Although a myriad of shunt procedures has been devised, they fall into two basic categories: (1) total or nonselective shunts, and (2) selective shunts (Figure 9-17).

Total or nonselective shunts are so called because they divert the entire blood supply from the portocollateral circulation into the low-pressure systemic venous circulation and, thus, effectively eliminate the chance of variceal bleeding. This type of shunt was first devised over 100 years ago when Eck performed the first portocaval anastomosis in dogs. Enthusiasm for this procedure in treatment of portal hypertension was rekindled by Whipple and Blakemore in the midtwentieth century. Over the next 20 years, many controlled studies were performed to assess the role of the shunt in the treatment of portal hypertension. One point became clear—the use of a "prophylactic shunt" (i.e., the operation on a patient with varices who has not yet hemorrhaged) was definitely not indicated. Three separate prospective trials revealed better survival among the medical (control) groups than the surgical (shunt) groups (71-73). Although the surgical group had a definitely decreased risk of hemorrhage, more patients died of hepatic failure and associated encephalopathy. Four prospective randomized trials were conducted to determine the effect portosystemic shunts would have on survival in patients with a prior variceal bleed ("therapeutic shunt") (74-77). In no case was there a statistically improved survival of the shunted patients as compared with the medical (controlled) groups. In addition, the quality of life was often impaired as a result of increasing hepatic encephalopathy. As was shown earlier, nonselective shunts result in total diversion of hepatic blood flow. The ensuing high incidence of encephalopathy and hepatic failure is based on two hypotheses: (1) portal blood appears to contain certain hepatotrophic factors necessary for maintaining hepatic integrity and regenerative ability (78,79), and (2) the shunting of portal blood from the liver prevents detoxification of nitrogenous wastes from the gut prior to entrance of the blood into the system circulation (80). In spite of the many variations on the portocaval shunt, none were effective in maintaining portal perfusion—an apparently crucial factor.

In 1967, Warren, Zeppa, and Foman (81) reported their findings of a new selective shunt procedure designed to prevent variceal hemorrhage while maintaining portal perfusion. This procedure, the distal splenorenal shunt, decompressed the gastroesophageal varices via the short gastrics with anastomosis of the distally ligated splenic to left renal vein. At the same time, the connections of the varices to the portal circulation were ligated and portal perfusion maintained via the superior mesenteric vein. This shunt is technically more difficult than a portocaval shunt, but carries no higher operative mortality in skilled hands.

In 1971, a prospective, randomized trial was begun comparing the efficacy of the distal splenorenal shunt to the nonselective shunt (total of 55 patients entered into the study). In 1979 (82), the results with a minimum followup of 3 years revealed a significant difference in the incidence of postshunt encephalopathy in the nonselective (52 percent) as compared with the selective (12 percent) shunt. No significant difference between the two groups was noted with respect to mortality, shunt occlusion, or recurrent variceal hemorrhage.

Even though the distal splenorenal shunt is superior to nonselective shunts in reducing postoperative encephalopathy, it is becoming clear that some patients continue to develop significant portosystemic collaterals and, therefore, may effectively convert the

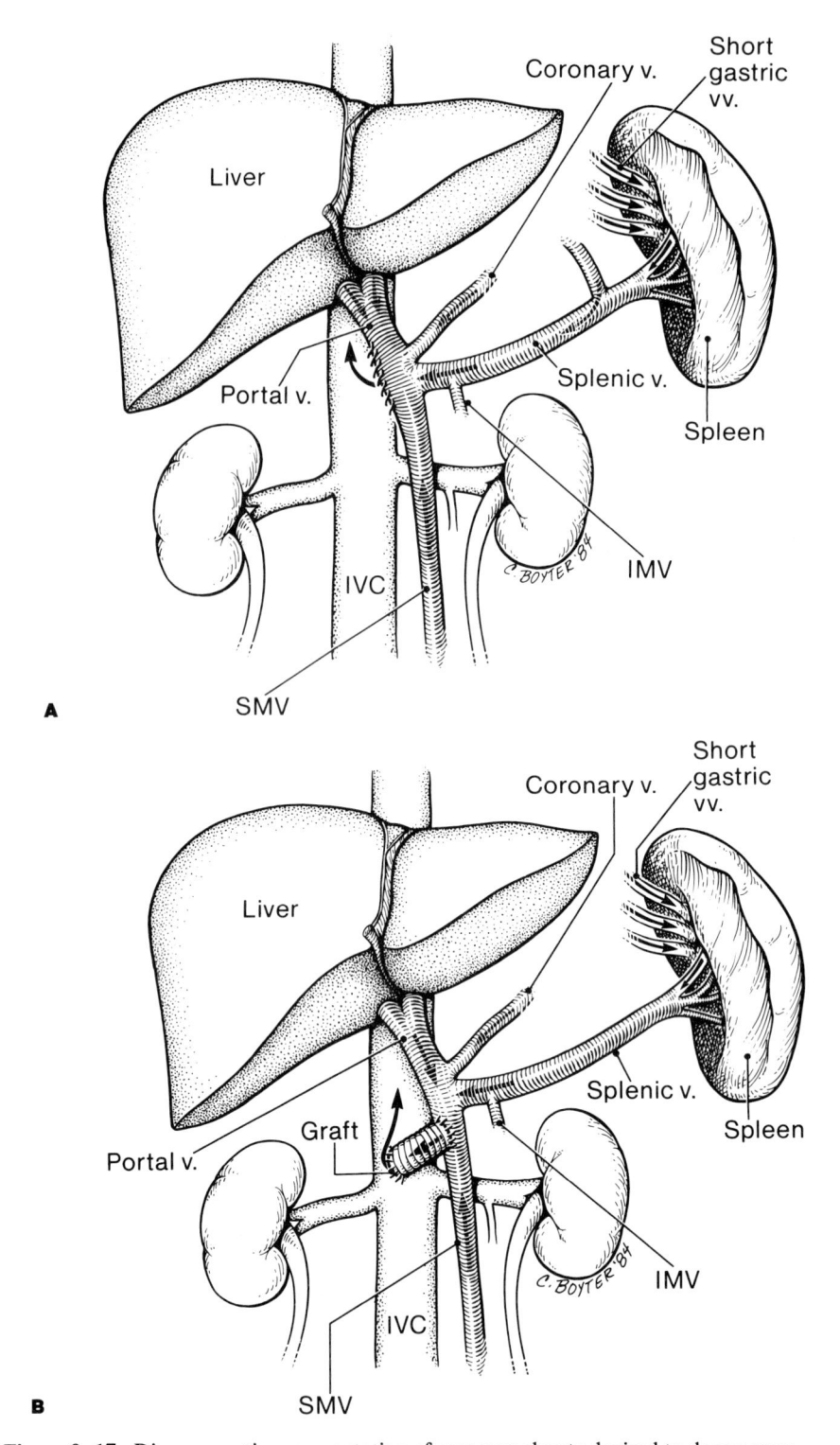

Figure 9-17. Diagrammatic representation of common shunts devised to decompress gastroesophageal varices. The arrows indicate the direction of blood flow. Note that the distal splenorenal shunt is a selective shunt and maintains portal perfusion while the others do not. *A.* Side-to-side portocaval shunt. *B.* H-type graft mesocaval shunt.

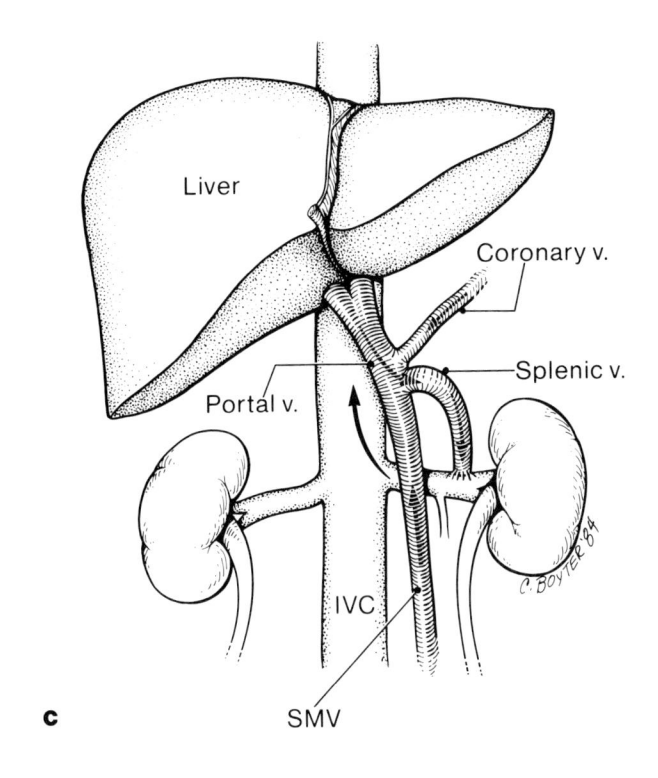

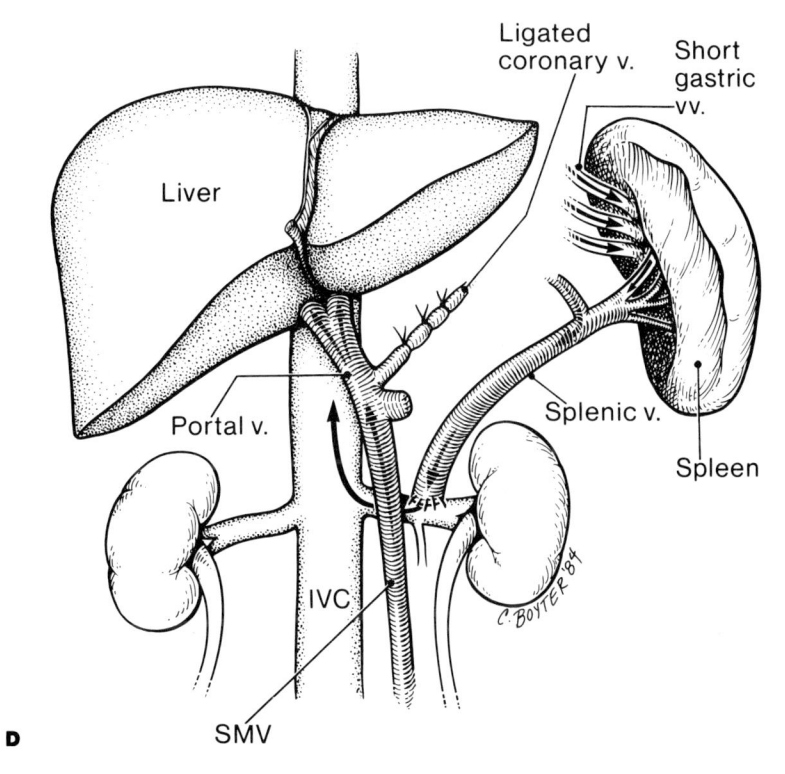

Figure 9–17. *C.* Conventional splenorenal shunt. *D.* Selective distal splenorenal shunt.

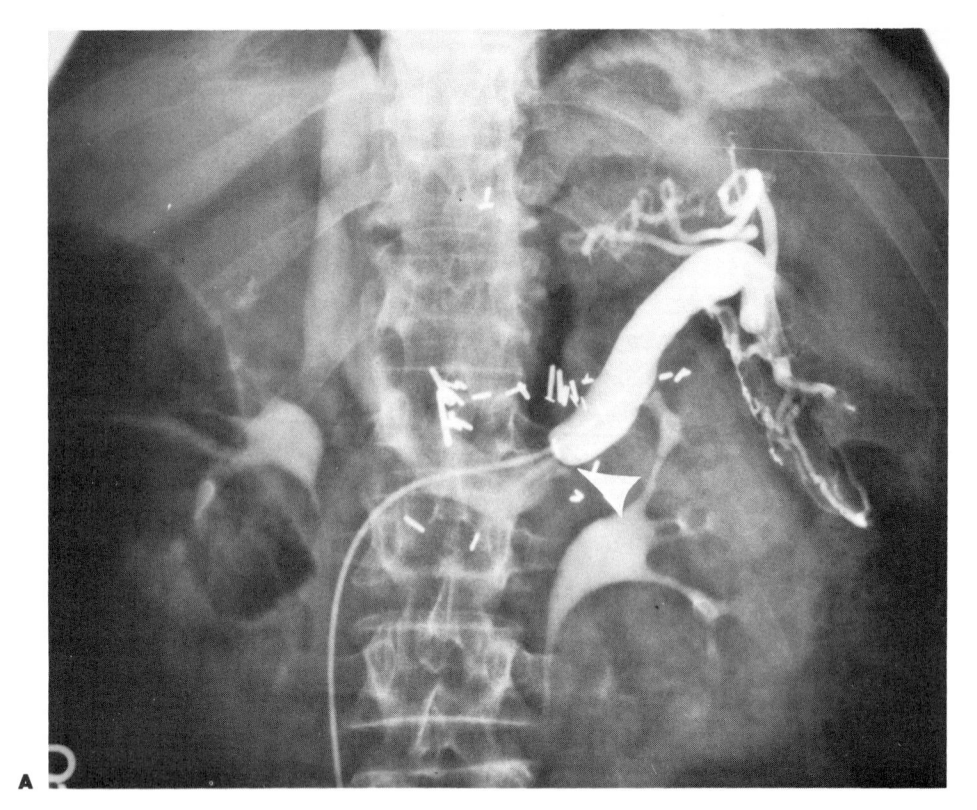

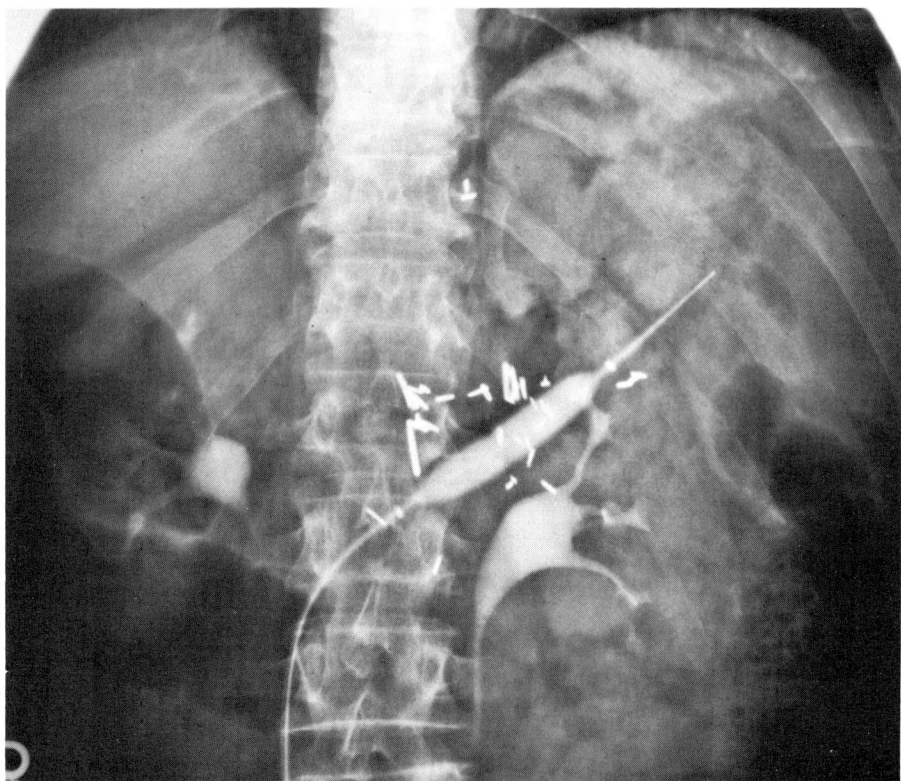

Figure 9-18. Successful dilatation of a stenosis occurring at the anastomotic site of the splenic to left renal vein in a distal splenorenal shunt. *A.* Predilatation study demonstrating stenosis (arrow) at the anastomotic site. The pressure within the splenic vein was 32 mm Hg with a left renal vein pressure of 14 mm Hg. *B.* Dilatation of the anastomosis was performed using a 12-mm balloon. (From Henderson JM, El Khishen MA, Millikan WJ, et al.: Management of stenosis of distal splenorenal shunt by balloon dilation. Surg Gynecol Obst 1983;157:43–48. By permission of *Surgery, Gynecology & Obstetrics.*)

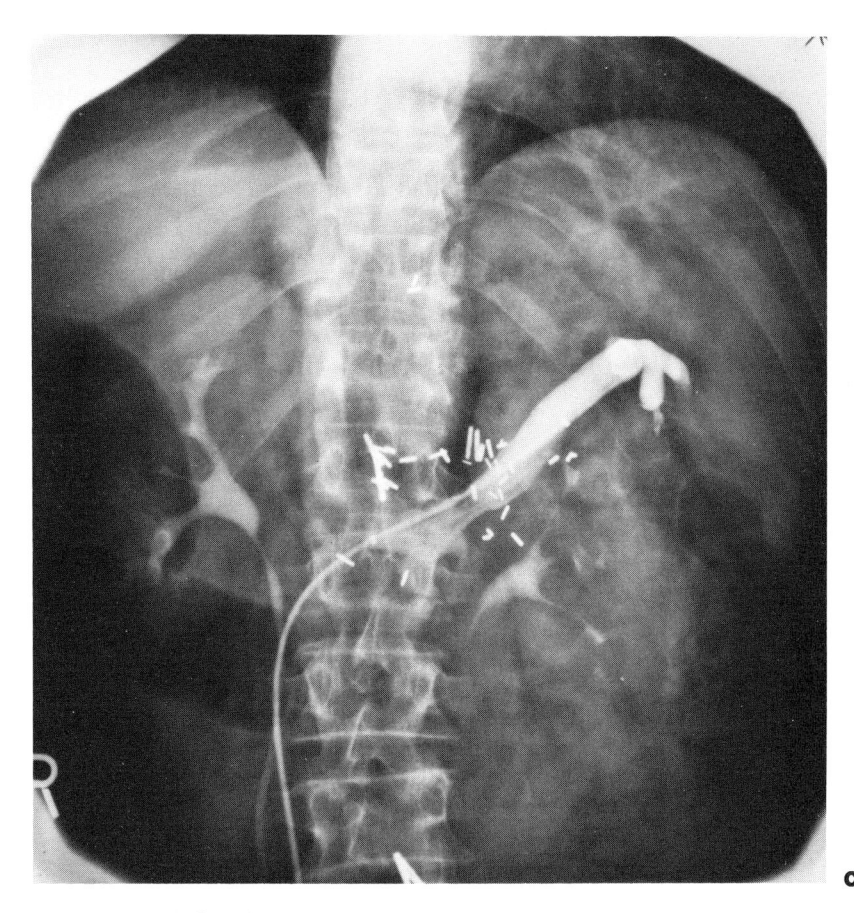

Figure 9-18. *C.* Significant improvement in the stenosis has been achieved postdilatation with the splenic vein pressure reduced to 22 mm Hg and a gradient of only 6 mm Hg. (From Henderson JM, El Khishen MA, Millikan WJ, et al.: Management of stenosis of distal splenorenal shunt by balloon dilation. Surg Gynecol Obst 1983;157:43–48. By permission of *Surgery, Gynecology & Obstetrics.*)

selective distal splenorenal shunt to a total shunt. Measurement of pressures across the shunt, as well as direct injection of the shunt, are a crucial part of the postoperative angiographic evaluation of patients following distal splenorenal shunt. A pressure gradient greater than 5 mm Hg from splenic vein to renal vein is an indication of stenosis at the anastomotic siste. Balloon dilation has been successfully employed to reduce pressure gradients across the shunt anastomosis in multiple cases (83) (Figure 9-18).

Although the selective distal splenorenal shunt appears to be a significant advance in the treatment of patients with portal hypertension, there are many unanswered questions in the medical and surgical management of these patients. There is a continuing search to provide variceal decompression while simultaneously maintaining portal perfusion and preventing hepatic encephalopathy. In some patients, hepatic deterioration will continue despite our best efforts.

REFERENCES

1. Schiff L, Schiff ER: Diseases of the Liver. Philadelphia: Lippincott, 1982.
2. Taylor FW, Rosenbaum D: The case against hepatic arterial ligation in portal hypertension. JAMA 1953;151:1066–1069.

3. Macleod JSR, Pearce RG: The outflow of blood from the liver as affected by variations in the condition of the portal vein and hepatic artery. Am J Physiol 1914;35:87–105.
4. Gonzales OC: Portography; a preliminary report of a new technique via the umbilical vein. Clin Proc Hosp DC 1959;15:120–124.
5. Spigos DG, Tauber JW, Tan WS, et al.: Work in progress: Umbilical venous cannulation: A new approach for embolization of esophageal varices. Radiology 1983;146:53–56.
6. Lunderquist A, Vang J: Transhepatic catheterization and obliteration of the coronary vein in patients with portal hypertension and esophageal varices. N Engl J Med 1974;291:646–649.
7. Vennes JA: Intrahepatic pressure: an accurate reflection of portal pressure. Medicine 1966;45:445–452.
8. Aagaard J, Jensen LI, Sorensen TIA, et al.: Recanalized umbilical vein in portal hypertension. AJR 1982;139:1107–1109.
9. Wilson SE, Stone RT, Christie JP, Passaro E: Massive lower GI bleeding from intestinal varices. Arch Surg 1979;114:1158–1161.
10. Perchik L, Max TC: Massive hemorrhage from varices of the duodenal loop in a cirrhotic patient. Radiology 1963;80:641–644.
11. Rosen H, Silen W, Simon M: Selective portal hypertension with isolated duodenojejunal varices. N Engl J Med 1967;277:1188–1190.
12. Hamlyn AN, Lunzer MR, Morris JS, et al.: Portal hypertension with varices in unusual sites. Lancet 1974;2:1531–1534.
13. Burcharth F: Percutaneous transhepatic portography I. Technique and application. AJR 1979;132:177–182.
14. Trenti A, Bracci F: Collateral circulations and bleeding oesophageal varices. In MJ Orloff, S Stipa, V Ziporo (eds), Medical and Surgical Problems of Portal Hypertension. New York: Academic Press, 1980.
15. Simpson JA, Conn HO: The role of ascites in gastroesophageal reflux with comments on the pathogenesis of bleeding esophageal varices. Gastroenterol 1968;55:17–25.
16. Liebowitz HR: Pathogenesis of esophageal varix rupture. JAMA 1961;175:874–879.
17. Orloff MJ, Thomas HS: Pathogenesis of esophageal varix rupture. Arch Surg 1963;87:301–307.
18. Baker LA, Smith C, Lieberman G: The natural history of esophageal varices. A study of 115 cirrhotic patients in whom varices were diagnosed prior to bleeding. Am J Med 1959;26:228–237.
19. Reynolds TB: The role of hemodynamic measurements in portosystemic shunt surgery. Arch Surg 1974;108:276–281.
20. McLeod MK, Eckhauser FE, Turcotte JG: Significance of corrected sinusoidal pressure (CSP) in patients with cirrhosis and portal hypertension. Ann Surg 1981;194:562–567.
21. Galambos JT (ed): Cirrhosis. Major Problems in Internal Medicine, Vol 17. Philadelphia: Saunders, 1979, pp. 253–287.
22. Conn H: The rational evaluation and management of portal hypertension. In F Schaffner, S Sherlock, CM Levy (eds), The Liver and Its Diseases. New York: Intercontinental Medical Book, 1974, pp. 289–306.
23. Jackson FC, Perrin EB, Felix WR, Smith AG: A clinical investigation of the portacaval shunt V. Survival analysis of the therapeutic operation. Ann Surg 1971;174:672–701.
24. Resnick RH, Iber FL, Ishihara AM, et al.: The Boston Inter-hospital Liver Group: a controlled study of the therapeutic portacaval shunt. Gastroenterol 1974;67:843–857.
25. Orloff MJ: Emergency diagnosis and medical management of bleeding esophageal varices. In MJ Orloff, S Stipa, V Ziparo (eds), Medical and Surgical Problems of Portal Hypertension. New York: Academic Press, 1980.
26. Garceau AJ, Chalmers TC: The Boston Inter-hospital Liver Group: the natural history of cirrhosis I. Survival with esophageal varices. N Engl J Med 1963;268:469–473.
27. Imanga H, Yamamoto S, Kuroyanagi Y: Surgical treatment of portal hypertension according to state of intrahepatic circulation. Ann Surg 1962;155:42–50.

28. Viamonte M, Danner P, Warren WD, Fomon J: A new technique for the assessment of hyperkinetic portal hypertension. Radiology 1970;96:539-542.
29. Webb LJ, Sherlock S: Extrahepatic portal venous obstruction. J Med 1979;48:627-639.
30. Rosch J, Dotter CT: Extrahepatic portal obstruction in childhood and its angiographic diagnosis. AJR 1971;112:143-148.
31. Stone HH, Jordan WD, Acker JJ, Martin JD: Portal arteriovenous fistulae. Am J Surg 1965;109:191-199.
32. Way CW, Crane JM, Riddell DH, Foster JH: Arteriovenous fistulae in portal circulation. Surgery 1971;70:876-890.
33. Donovan AJ, Reynolds TB, Mikkelsen WP, Peters RL: Systemic-portal arteriovenous fistulas: pathologic and hemodynamic observations in two patients. Surgery 1969;66:474-482.
34. Rather LJ, Cohn R: Some effects upon the liver of complete arterialization of its blood supply III. Acute vascular necrosis. Surgery 1953;34:207-210.
35. Schwartz SI, Morton JH, McGovern GR: Experimental arterialization of the liver. Surgery 1961;49:611-617.
36. Zuidema GO, Gaisford WD, Abell MR, et al.: Segmental portal arterialization of canine liver. Surgery 1963;53:689-698.
37. Deutsch V, Rosenthal T, Adar R, Mozes M: Budd-Chiari syndrome: study of angiographic findings and remarks on etiology. AJR 1972;116:430-439.
38. Hoyumpa AM Jr, Schiff L, Helfman EL: Budd-Chiari syndrome in women taking oral contraceptives. Am J Med 1971;50:137-140.
39. Kreel L, Freston JW, Clain D: Vascular radiology in the Budd Chiari syndrome. Br J Radiol 1967;40:755-759.
40. Maguire R, Doppman JL: Angiographic abnormalities in partial Budd Chiari syndrome. Radiology 1977;122:629-635.
41. Ramsay GC, Britton RC: Intraparenchymal angiography in the diagnosis of veno occlusive disease. Radiology 1968;90:716-726.
42. Galloway S, Cassarella WJ, Price JB: Unilobar veno occlusive disease of the liver: angiographic demonstration of interhepatic competition simulated hepatoma. AJR 1973;119:89-94.
43. Jelliffe DB, Bras G. Mukherjee KL: Veno occlusive disease of the liver and Indian childhood cirrhosis. Arch Dis Child 1957;32:369-385.
44. Nordlinger BM, Nordlinger DF, Fulenwider JT, et al.: Angiography in portal hypertension. Am J Surg 1980;139:132-141.
45. Bookstein JJ, Appleman HD, Walter JF, et al.: Histologic-venographic correlates in portal hypertension. Radiology 1975;116:565-573.
46. Heeney DJ, Bookstein JJ, Bell RH, et al.: Correlation of hepatic and portal wedged venography and manometry with histology in alcoholic cirrhosis and periportal fibrosis. Radiology 1982;142:591-597.
47. Vennes JA: Intrahepatic pressure: an accurate reflection of portal pressure. Medicine 1966;45:445-452.
48. Ruzicka FF, Carillo JF, D'Alessandro D, Rossi P: The hepatic wedge pressure and venogram vs. the intraparenchymal liver pressure and venogram. Radiology 1972;102:253-258.
49. Leery CM, Gliedman ML: Practical and research value of hepatic vein catheterization. N Engl J Med 1958;258:696-700.
50. Viamonte M Jr, Warren WD, Fomon JJ: Liver panangiography in the assessment of portal hypertension in liver cirrhosis. Radiol Clin North Am 1970;8:147-167.
51. Lunderquist A, Koolpe H, Mendez G Jr, Russell E: Wedged pressure recording and injection of contrast medium into the hepatic veins: a study performed on the livers of cadavers to explain clinical findings. Radiology 1980;136:619-622.
52. Warren WD, Salam AA, Hutson D, et al.: Selective distal splenorenal shunt. Arch Surg 1974;108:306-314.
53. Chuang VP, Mena CE, Hoskins PA: Congenital anomalies of the left renal vein: angiographic consideration Br J Radiol 1974;47:214-218.

54. Field S, Saxton H: Venous anomalies complicating left renal vein catheterization. Br J Radiol 1974;47:219–225.
55. Sones PJ Jr, Rude JC, Berg DJ, Warren D: Evaluation of the left renal vein in candidates for splenorenal shunts. Radiology 1978;127:357–361.
56. Bismuth H, Franco D, Hepp J: Portal-systemic shunt in hepatic cirrhosis: does the type of shunt decisively influence the clinical result? Ann Surg 1974;179:209–218.
57. Drapanas T, Lo Ciero J, Dowling J: Hemodynamics of the interposition mesocaval shunt. Ann Surg 1975;181:523–533.
58. Stipa S, Thau A, Schillaci A, et al.: Mesenterico-cava shunt with the internal jugular vein. Surg Gynecol Obst 1978;146:391–399.
59. Thompson B, Casali R. Read R, et al.: Results of interposition H grafts for portal hypertension. Ann Surg 1978;187:515–522.
60. Fulenweider TJ, Nordlinger BM, Millikan WJ, et al.: Portal pseudoperfusion. Ann Surg 1979;189:257–268.
61. Reuter SR, Atkin TW: High dose gastric angiography for demonstration of esophageal varices. Radiology 1972;105:573–578.
62. Nickerson M, Collier B: Drugs inhibiting adrenergic nerves and structures innervated by them. In LS Goodman, A Gilman (eds), The Pharmaceutical Basis of Therapeutics. New York: Macmillan, 1975.
63. Bergstrand I: Splenoportography. In HL Abrams (ed), Abrams' Angiography. Boston: Little, Brown, 1983, pp. 1573–1604.
64. Burcharth F, Nielbo N, Anderson B: Percutaneous transhepatic portography II. Comparison with splenography in portal hypertension. AJR 1979;132:183–185.
65. Widrich WC, Robbins AH, Johnson WC, Mabseth DC: Long term follow up of distal splenorenal shunts. Radiology 1980;134:341–345.
66. Schabel SI, Rittenberg GM, Jarid LH, et al.: The "bull's eye" falciform ligament: a sonographic finding of portal hypertension. Radiology 1980;136:157–159.
67. Kane RA, Katz SG: The spectrum of sonographic findings in portal hypertension: a subject review and new observations. Radiology 1982;142:453–458.
68. Waller RM III, Oliver TW Jr, McCain AH, Sones PJ Jr, Bernardino ME. Computed tomography and sonography of hepatic cirrhosis and portal hypertension. Radiographics 1984: (in press).
69. McCain AH, Bernardino ME, Sones PJ, et al.: Correlation of CT and Angiography in the detection of varices from portal hypertension. Radiology (in press).
70. Foley WD, Stewart ET, Milbrath JR, et al.: Digital subtraction angiography of the portal venous system. AJR 1983;140:497–499.
71. Conn HO, Lindenmuth WW, May CJ, et al.: Prophylactic portocaval anastamosis. Medicine 1972;51:27–40.
72. Jackson FC, Perrin EB, Smith AG, et al.: A clinical investigation of the portocaval shunt II. Survival analysis of the prophylactic operation. Am J Surg 1968;115:22–42.
73. Resnick RH, Chalmers TC, Ishihara AM, et al.: A controlled study of the prophylactic portocaval shunt. A final report. Ann Intern Med 1969;70:675–688.
74. Jackson FC, Perrin ED, Felix R, et al.: A clinical investigation of the portocaval shunt V. Survival analysis of the therapeutic operation. Ann Surg 1971;174:672–701.
75. Mikkelsen WP: Therapeutic protocaval Shunt. Preliminary data on controlled trial and morbid effects of acute alkaline necrosis. Arch Surg 1974;108:302–305.
76. Resnick RH, Iber FL, Ishihara AM, et al.: A controlled study of the therapeutic portocaval shunt in alcoholic cirrhosis. Gastroenterol 1974;67:843–856.
77. Rueff B, Degos F, Degos JD, et al.: A controlled study of the therapeutic portocaval shunt in alcoholic cirrhosis. Lancet 1976;1:655–659.
78. Starzl TE, Francavilla A, Halgrinson CG, et al.: The origin, hormonal nature and action of hepatotrophic substances in portal venous blood. Surg Gynecol Obstet 1973;137:179–199.

79. Marchioro TL, Porter ED, Brown BI, et al.: The effect of partial portocaval transposition on the canine liver. Surgery 1967;61:723–732.
80. Schenker S, Breen KJ, Hoyumpa AM: Hepatic encephalopathy: current status. Gastroenterol 1974;66:121–151.
81. Warren WD, Zeppa R, Fomon JJ: Selective transplenic decompression of gastroesophageal varices by distal splenorenal shunt. Ann Surg 1967;166:437–455.
82. Rikkers LF, Rudman D, Galambos JT, et al.: A randomized controlled trial of the distal splenorenal shunt. Ann Surg 1978;188:271–282.
83. Henderson JM, El Khishen MA, Millikan WJ, et al.: Management of stenosis of distal splenorenal shunt by balloon dilation. Surg Gynecol Obst 1983;157:43–48.

10

Vascular Interventional Techniques in Liver Disease

PETER J. SONES, JR. • THOMAS W. OLIVER, JR.

INTRODUCTION

Over the past 20 years, there has been a remarkable development in interventional radiologic techniques. This has been accompanied by a growing interest and body of knowledge relative to application of these techniques in liver disease. Only the vascular interventional techniques applicable to the liver will be discussed in this chapter.

EMBOLIC MATERIALS

Since many of the materials used in embolizing the hepatic artery are the same as those used in occluding varices, the properties of the various available embolizing agents will be discussed in this section. One of the first embolic agents employed was autologous clot. Autologous clot has the obvious virtue that it should be well-tolerated since it is constituted from the patient's own blood. One problem is that the blood of many cirrhotics will not clot spontaneously and that thrombin or some other agent must be used to accelerate clot formation. In addition, vessels occluded by autologous clot tend to recanalize in a relatively short period of time, making it a less desirable embolic agent (1). As a result of these problems, autologous clot is seldom used.

Gelfoam

Sterile surgical absorbable gelatin sponge (GELFOAM) can be cut into 2 mm to 5 mm cubes and injected through appropriately sized catheters. Multiple cubes can be loaded into a single tuberculin syringe which, because of its small bore, provides adequate pressure to force these particles through angiographic catheters. It is advantageous to wet the GELFOAM particles in radiographic contrast media, which greatly reduces the friction between these particles and the catheter. In addition, if the particles are loaded with contrast, they can be seen as negative defects under the fluoroscope while being injected. Once blood flow is visually slowed by the peripheral embolization of these particles, great care must be taken with additional embolization in order to avoid reflux of GELFOAM sponge from a static column of blood. Once the vessel in question is completely occluded, a very careful, low-volume contrast injection should be used to demonstrate the occlusion, since a forceful injection of contrast may produce turbulence and reflux of particles with embolization into vessels other than those desired. GELFOAM sponge is desirable because it is inexpensive, readily available, easy to work with, and well-tolerated. In addition, it is resorbed by the body over a period of several weeks. In some applications, this resorption can be used to advantage; however, in most embolization procedures where permanent occlusion is desired, this characteristic is a great disadvantage. Sclerosing agents, such as sodium tetradecyl sulfate, have been added to GELFOAM sponge in order to produce a more permanent occlusion. Widrich has indicated that the addition of this sclerosing agent produces better results in occlusion of esophageal varices (2). GELFOAM powder is available for embolization of precapillary vessels, but plays no role in the embolization of liver masses or varices.

Ivalon

IVALON, now called polyvinyl alcohol foam (Unipoint Industries, Highpoint, N.C.), is a compressible sponge material that expands considerably when immersed in fluid. Strips of IVALON sponge can be compressed and, following injection, will expand to 10 to 12 times their compressed length. This is an obvious advantage in attempting to occlude large vessels permanently. It is somewhat difficult to force compressed Ivalon through a catheter, presenting a limitation of its use.

IVALON particles are commercially available in prepared foam in three sizes: small (0.25–0.42 mm), medium (0.42–0.60 mm), and large (0.60–1.00 mm). The IVALON particles are stored in saline and can be heat-sterilized. IVALON particles tend to aggregate and settle at the bottom of the saline solution. In their aggregated form, they may be difficult or impossible to force through a diagnostic catheter. A double-syringe technique utilizing a Y connector has been described for flushing the particles rapidly from one syringe to another to suspend them in solution and break up the aggregates such that the Y connector could then be turned toward the patient and the particles rinsed through the catheter. We have found it much simpler to use a single syringe and flush the particles rapidly back and forth into a small basin. Once suitably suspended, one can move rapidly to the catheter for injection of the particles. IVALON has the distinct advantage that it is a permanent material and not reabsorbed over time. As a result, it produces a more permanent occlusion than GELFOAM. The smaller-sized IVALON particles tend to reach smaller vessels than GELFOAM, which, combined with permanence, is an advantage in embolizing hepatic tumors. Even in those hepatic tumors with the most impressive arteriovenous shunting, we have not seen the smallest particles traverse the tumor circulation. Gastroesophageal varices, on the other hand, may have sufficiently large communications for GELFOAM and IVALON particles to pass into the systemic circulation and thence into the lungs.

Coils

Initially, Gianturco coils were difficult to use in that they had to be threaded over an introducer fashioned from a guidewire mandrel and passed through a 7 French Teflon catheter with a nontapered tip. Subsequent developments have resulted in coils that are much easier to use. The present Gianturco coils can be introduced through a 5 French diagnostic catheter with a tip tapered to 0.035 inch. They no longer require mounting on a special introducer and can be pushed from their container through the catheter with an LLT guidewire (3). Coils can be obtained in multiple sizes ranging from 3 to 15 mm. Coils are effective in producing total occlusion of vessels up to approximately 5 mm. Vessels of high flow and larger size frequently require multiple coils for total occlusion. In some very large varices with high flow, even a large number of coils may not produce total occlusion. Additional particulate embolization into a "coil dam" may suffice to complete occlusion. Unfortunately, in very large vessels with high flow, even additional particulate embolization may not produce total occlusion. We have found that a "slurry" of AVITENE produced by mixing AVITENE powder with a small quantity of radiographic contrast media will be stopped by the coil baffle and produce total occlusion.

Cyanoacrylate

Isobutyl-2-Cyanoacrylate (Ethicon, Centerville, N.Y.) is a tissue adhesive that can be used to produce permanent vascular occlusion. It is not presently approved for clinical use, and an investigational new drug (IND) number is required for its use. The monomer is a liquid so it can be injected through small catheters. It undergoes polymerization within seconds of contact with an ionic solution such as saline or blood. It has the distinct advantage of forming an occlusive embolus larger than the catheter through which it is injected. One disadvantage of this material is that the rate of polymerization and formation of the adhesive embolus is difficult to control. If it polymerizes too quickly, it may occlude the catheter or potentially glue the catheter to the vessel being embolized. A coaxial system is recommended so that, if the injecting catheter becomes occluded, it can easily be exchanged (4). In addition, the tip of the injecting catheter should be coated with silicone in an effort to prevent adhesion of the catheter to the embolus. Five percent glucose solution should be used to rinse the injecting catheter promptly. If the cyanoacrylate polymerizes too slowly, it may pass well beyond the site of desired embolization. An occlusion balloon, to transiently obstruct the flow in the vessel to be embolized, can aid in preventing this migration. It is evident that this is a material that is difficult to control and should be used only by those who have obtained experience with its use in animals or as procedure assistants. Because fibrosarcoma was induced in cancer-prone rats following subcutaneous injection of Methyl-2-Cyanoacrylate, reservations have been raised about the possibility of carcinogenicity of Isobutyl-2-Cyanoacrylate (5). As yet, no cancer has been reported to be induced in humans by its use.

Absolute Alcohol

Alcohol has been used as a vascular occlusive agent in multiple sites. It appears to produce occlusion via two mechanisms. It has a direct irritant and sclerosing effect on the vascular wall. In addition, it crenates and destroys red blood cells leading to thrombus formation. It has been reported that alcohol is an equally effective occlusive agent when diluted with contrast (6). In our experience, dilution of the absolute alcohol has diminished its effectiveness. Alcohol is fairly rapidly diluted as it passes into major blood vessels, either arterial or venous, such that it seldom produces a problem by passing through the organ or lesion being embolized. It has been reported, however, as producing infarction of the left colon in several patients in whom renal occlusive procedures were being performed (7,8). Double-lumen occlusion balloon catheters can be used to prevent the reflux of alcohol from the vessel being injected. In addition, if alcohol passes very rapidly through high-flow arterial venous malformation, shunting tumor, or high-flow varix, it may have no significant effect because of its transient contact. The occlusion balloon can be very helpful in this situation by slowing the flow of blood so that alcohol can have the desired effect.

Avitene

AVITENE-microfibrillary collagen is a derivative of bovine collagen and was developed to produce hemostasis in surgical applications. The first use of this agent for transcatheter embolization was by Kaufman *et al.* (9) in swine. Use of AVITENE for human embolization was reported by Diamond *et al.* (10), who found it to be an excellent occlusive agent resulting in prompt thrombosis. It is readily available and easily passes through small bore catheters in the semiliquid state. Since it is highly thrombogenic, some concern has been expressed that inadvertent passage of AVITENE outside of the desired location may result in ischemia and tissue necrosis. Occlusion appears to be permanent, although some recanalization may occur.

VARICEAL EMBOLIZATION

Hemorrhage from gastroesophageal varices resulting from portal hypertension represents a clinical emergency of significant proportions. If uncontrolled, the mortality rate in this group of patients exceeds 40 percent. Many approaches are available to attempt to stop the hemorrhage in these patients. The usual first attempt is with intravenous infusion of vasopressin, since this route of infusion has proven to be just as effective as selective infusion of the superior mesenteric artery (11). Fortunately, a number of patients, especially those with lesser degrees of liver disease, will respond favorably to this method of treatment. At our institution, a Sengstaken-Blakemore tube is employed frequently as a second line of defense. While this tube, when properly positioned, will frequently control variceal hemorrhage, it is not universally successful. This is especially true in those patients bleeding from gastric varices. In addition, the use of this tube is attended by significant risk of esophageal or gastric erosion if it is employed for a prolonged period of time. Bleeding may recur when the tube is deflated.

If these methods of medical management fail, more invasive techniques must be employed. Endoscopic transesophageal sclerosis of varices represents a relatively atraumatic approach that may be effective in a large percentage of patients. Unfortunately, it may be difficult to identify and sclerose all of the offending varices in a blood-filled esophagus. The more massive the hemorrhage, the more difficult it is to effectively utilize this technique. Emergency surgery to construct a decompressive shunt represents the most definitive long-term treatment of bleeding in these patients, but is accompanied by a high mortality rate.

Transhepatic embolization of the coronary vein (Figure 10–1) and other venous collaterals perfusing gastroesophageal varices has proven to be an effective method for the acute control of variceal hemorrhage, with a relatively low rate of morbidity and

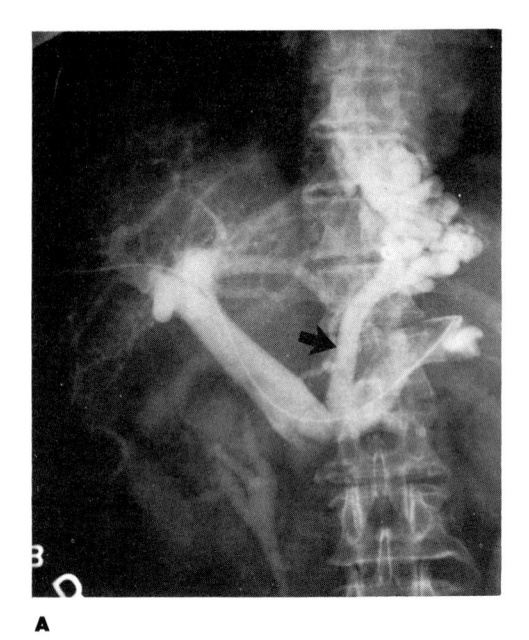

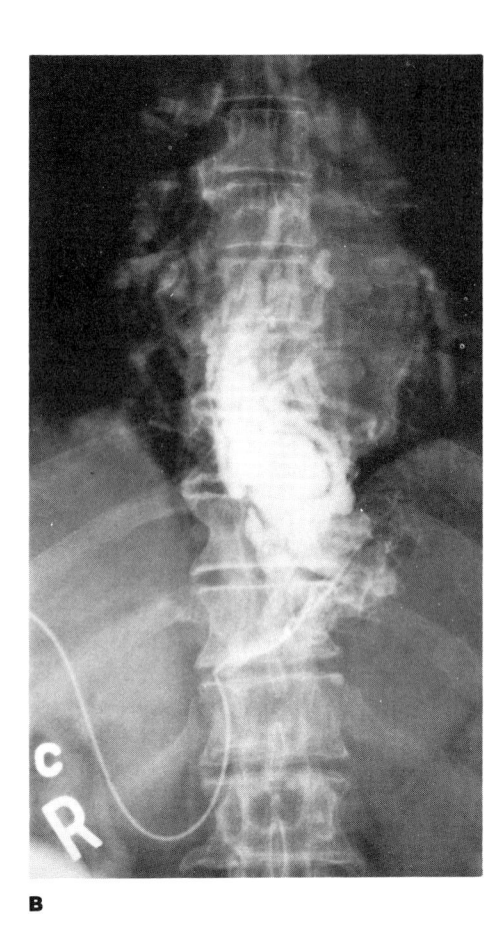

Figure 10-1. Transhepatic portography and coronary vein embolization. *A.* Transhepatic portogram with good visualization of large coronary vein (arrow) and gastroesophageal varices. *B.* Selective injection into the coronary vein with opacification of extensive esophageal varices.

mortality (2,11–13). Successful control of the acute variceal bleeding episode was reported in 83 percent of the patients attempted by Keller *et al.* (12), 90 percent of 150 patients attempted by Pereiras *et al.* (11), and 92 percent of 39 patients attempted at Emory University Hospital. In view of these results, it would appear that transhepatic embolization of varices is an effective means of controlling acute variceal hemorrhage and would appear to be employed reasonably if the less invasive methods of treatment, including endoscopic sclerosis, have been unsuccessful, and in preference to emergency surgery, which should be the last resort.

Technique

The procedure is best begun by placing a lead marker on the skin in the right midaxillary line two intercostal spaces below the costophrenic angle, as determined by anteroposterior fluoroscopy. This is followed by biplane transfemoral SMA angiography, which allows localization of the portal vein in relation to the skin marker. A site on the skin is then selected in relationship to the marker that allows entry into a large proximal

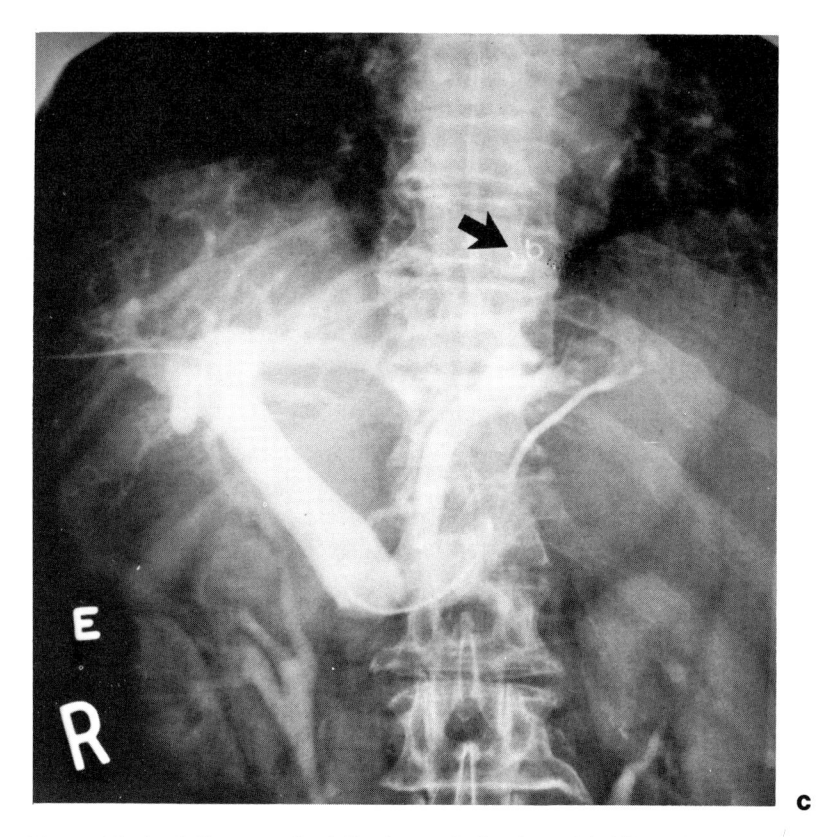

Figure 10-1. *C.* Portography following embolization with filling of only the proximal coronary vein and no visualization of the esophageal varices. In this patient, steel coils (arrow) were used to initially slow flow within the coronary vein, followed by absolute alcohol to sclerose the multiple serpiginous submucosal collaterals.

intrahepatic branch of the portal vein. The superior mesenteric arteriogram not only confirms patency and localization of the portal vein, but also excludes hypervascular lesions within the anticipated area of puncture. In cases where there is suspected reversal of portal flow, portal vein patency and localization can be achieved by hepatic wedge injection through a transfemoral venous approach. If biplane angiography is not available, a lateral radiograph is taken, and a point one vertebral body anterior to the spine is selected for site of puncture. After the puncture site has been localized, the area is sterilely prepped and draped, and the skin is anesthetized locally with 2 percent lidocaine. A small dermatotomy is made with a scalpel blade just above the rib in the selected intercostal space, and the skin is spread with a mosquito hemostat.

Following adequate sedation, in neutral suspended respiration, a 5 French radiopaque Teflon catheter 27 cm in length is introduced into the liver over a 19-gauge trocar (the tip of the catheter is bent into a gentle curve over steam to facilitate selective catheterization of the coronary and short gastric veins). The assembly is advanced under fluoroscopic guidance to within 3 cm of the right lateral aspect of the spine, directed toward the twelfth dorsal vertebral body, or otherwise as guided by AP films demonstrating the portal vein. The trocar is withdrawn, and the patient is allowed to breathe. The catheter is then withdrawn slowly with gentle aspiration until blood returns freely.

At this point, a small amount of contrast is injected to confirm location in the portal venous system. If the portal system has been catheterized, an 0.038 3-mm J guidewire is placed through the sheath, and the sheath and guidewire assembly advanced as a unit into the splenic vein. Frequently, only a few passes are required to cannulate the portal vein in patients with portal hypertension, but in some patients, as many as ten passes are required. In the event that a longer catheter is required, a 5 French radiopaque Teflon catheter is used. If the liver is exceptionally resistant, or if there is considerable ascites such that buckling of the catheter system is a problem, a Lunderquist exchange wire is used to exchange catheters. With the catheter in the splenic vein, a splenoportogram is performed initially for demonstration of coronary and short gastric veins. Tip-deflecting wires (Cook) designed to fit these catheters are used to facilitate selective catheterization of the coronary and short gastric veins. We have also found the Lunderquist torque control wire helpful in this regard.

The choice of embolic material historically involves all of the embolic materials previously discussed. Autologous clot and GELFOAM were used in the initial experiences with variceal embolization, but were abandoned because of rapid recanalization of the occluded varices (1). The use of Gianturco coils has been described by several authors (14,15); however, small particles or other sclerosing agents must be used in addition if the esophageal component of the varices is to be occluded. Lunderquist et al. (16) and Goldman et al. (17) have described the use of Isobutyl-2-Cyanoacrylate for variceal embolization. While this agent certainly is capable of producing long-term occlusion of varices, the difficulty in handling and requirement for IND limits its utility. Uflacker (18) described the use of alcohol for variceal sclerosis with no recurrent bleeding in 9 of 12 patients over 13 to 18 months. As described, the ability to inject this agent through small catheters and produce distal sclerosis along the length of the esophageal varices seems desirable. Unfortunately, there is a higher than usual incidence of portal vein thrombosis associated with its use. In addition, in our experience in large varices with very high flow, it may have no effect. This problem can be overcome by first using a large sized Gianturco coil and, once flow has slowed but not completely occluded, alcohol can be utilized to good effect. We have recently had the opportunity to occlude several large-caliber, high-flow vessels with a baffle formed by Gianturco coils followed by injection of AVITENE. This has produced rapid and total occlusion in these two incidences.

Mention should be made of the difficulty in obtaining clotting in many cirrhotics. These clotting factors are usually grossly deranged. A platelet count of less than 30,000, a prothrombin time (PTT) less than 50 percent control, or partial thromboplastin time greater than 50 percent control represent a relative contraindication to transhepatic puncture because of the potential for bleeding at the puncture site. This can be partially controlled by embolization of the catheter tract with GELFOAM at the completion of the procedure. It is highly desirable to correct the platelet deficiency to avoid transfusion with packed cells, since eight donors are utilized to produce one unit of packed cells. The potential for transfusion-transmitted diseases is thereby increased. Usually, the procedure can be adequately performed even with grossly disordered clotting mechanisms so long as some method other than the patient's clotting factors is relied on for occlusion.

We have reviewed 39 patients in whom variceal embolization was attempted for acute bleeding at Emory University. The portal vein was successfully cannulated and the coronary and/or short gastric vein selectively embolized with 37 (95 percent) of the 39 patients attempted. One failure occurred in a patient with massive ascites and a small cirrhotic liver who was unable to cooperate with breath-holding. The other failure occurred in a patient with thrombosis of the right portal vein.

Control of the acute bleeding episode was obtained in 36 (97 percent) of the 37 patients embolized. One patient continued to bleed despite an apparently successful occlusion of the gastroesophageal varices. Embolization in these patients was performed with a number of materials. These included GELFOAM, IVALON sponge, and Gianturco coils in combination with GELFOAM and IVALON.

Rebleeding occurred in 14 (39 percent) of the 36 patients initially controlled for embolization. The interval to rebleed varied from 10 days to 28 months with a mean of 2.8 months. There was no evidence of rebleeding in 22 (61 percent) of the 36 patients initially controlled. Of these 22, there were 13 patients surviving at the time of followup, which varied from 1 to 18 months. The remaining 9 patients had died during the followup period. One of the patients died at 5.5 months and the other 8 within 15 days of embolization. Six of these 8 patients had severe liver disease with highly compromised hepatic reserve and died of hepatorenal failure without rebleeding.

A total of six patients in this study were embolized with control of bleeding prior to distal splenorenal shunt. There was no recurrence of bleeding in any of these patients at followup, which varied from 6 to 18 months. Even though this represents a small group of patients, we feel that the results lend validity to our impression that patients who have bleeding controlled by embolization prior to surgery have a reduced surgical mortality when compared with those not controlled prior to surgery. These results with emergent transhepatic variceal embolization compare favorably with those of other investigators cited earlier.

Recently, Spigos *et al.* (19) reported successful embolization of esophageal varices with control of acute bleeding in seven consecutive patients utilizing an umbilical vein approach provided by a cutdown on the umbilical vein. All of these patients died during the relatively short followup.

We feel that our results, as well as those reported by others, indicate that transhepatic variceal sclerosis can clearly control acute variceal bleeding. It would, of course, be most reasonable to employ those less invasive methods of control, including transesophageal sclerosis, and utilize transhepatic embolization only when those methods fail.

Transhepatic variceal sclerosis has been suggested as a method to attempt to control bleeding in patients who are deemed to have too little hepatorenal reserve to be surgical candidates. It is our impression that this represents a poor indication. Most of our patients had very poor hepatorenal reserve, and many of them, as well as all of the seven patients reported by Spigos *et al.*, died within a few months of embolization.

Embolization Following Selective Distal Splenorenal Shunt

A critical element of the selective distal splenorenal shunt is the ligation of all varices communicating between the portal system on the right side of the abdomen and the splenic vein on the left. If any of these vessels are not ligated at the time of surgery, they tend to siphon blood away from the portal circulation into the shunt, such that the shunt functions essentially like a portosystemic shunt. Over a period of time, many patients who have had adequate ligation of these communications at the time of surgery develop additional communications that lead to decreased portal perfusion. As these events occur, the patients tend to develop hepatic encephalopathy. In addition, there is an increased rate of hepatic atrophy and a decrease in hepatic reserve when portal perfusion is not maintained. As a result, the transhepatic portal approach can be used to embolize these collateral channels and, to the extent that one is successful in occluding

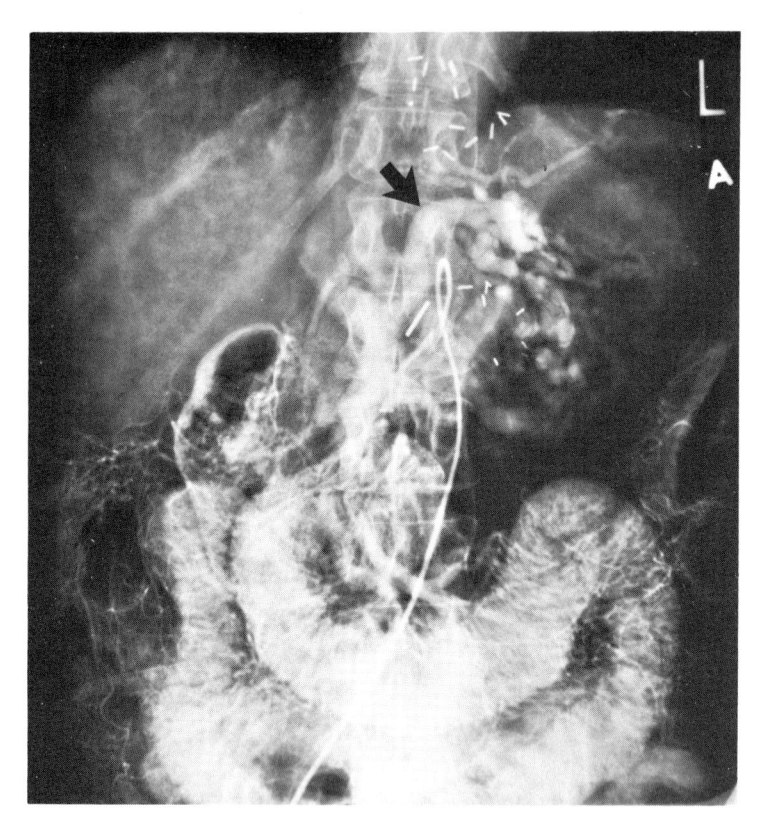

Figure 10–2. Following distal splenorenal shunt and recent onset of hepatic encephalopathy. *A.* Venous phase of SMA injection revealing lack of portal perfusion with shunting of portal blood through a large coronary vein (arrow) and multiple gastric varices.

Figure 10–2. *B.* Venous phase of SMA injection. Transhepatic embolization of several collateral channels including the large coronary vein (arrow = coils) has resulted in marked improvement in portal flow and resolution of encephalopathy.

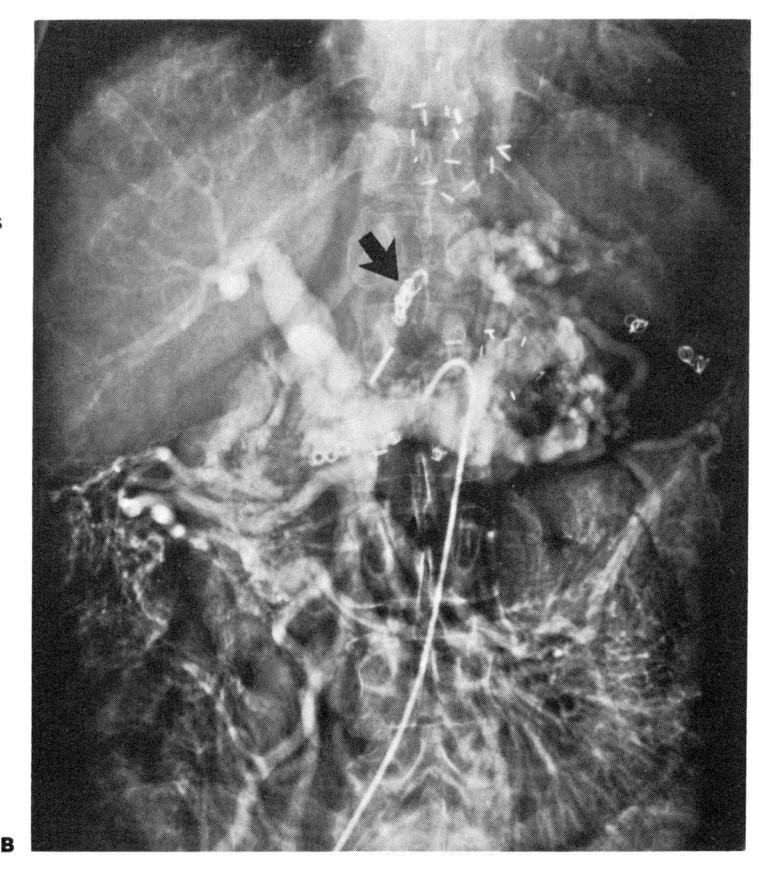

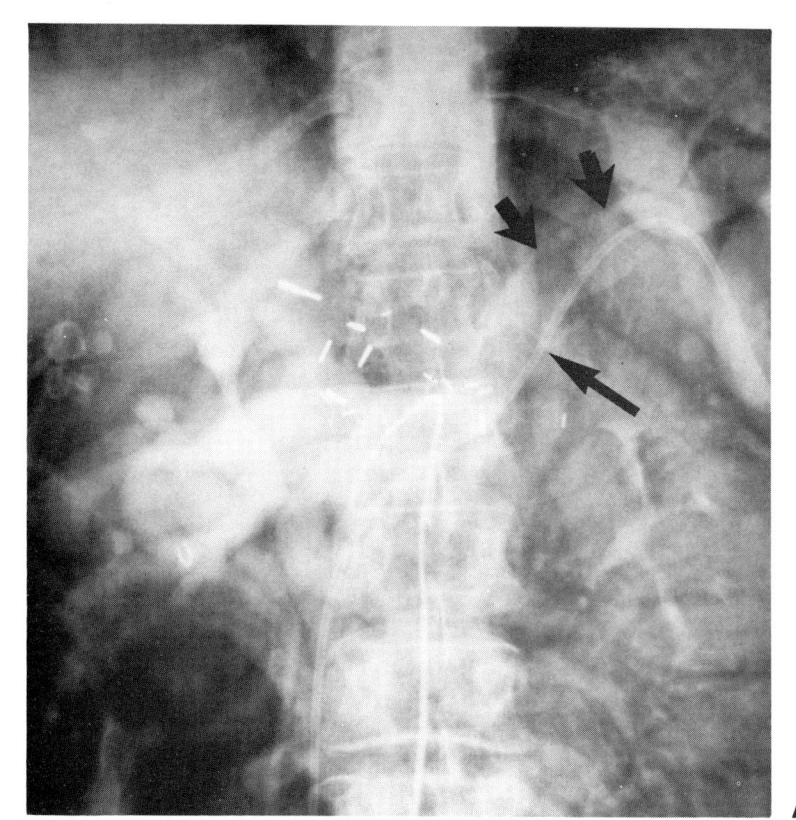

Figure 10–3. *A.* Following distal splenorenal shunt: venous phase of superior mesenteric artery injection revealing poor portal perfusion and siphoning of portal blood via a large colonic collateral (arrows) connecting the portal system with the lower pressure shunt. The venous catheter (arrow) is positioned within the splenic vein: left renal vein shunt.

Figure 10–3. *B.* Venous phase of repeat SMA injection following embolization of the large colonic collateral. Note improved portal and absence of filling of colonic collateral.

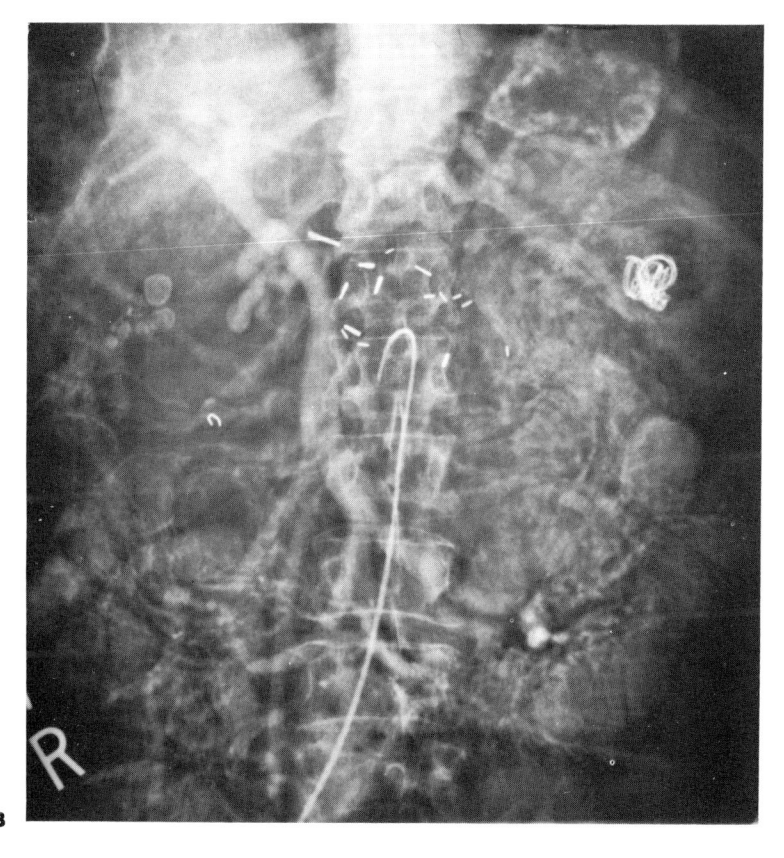

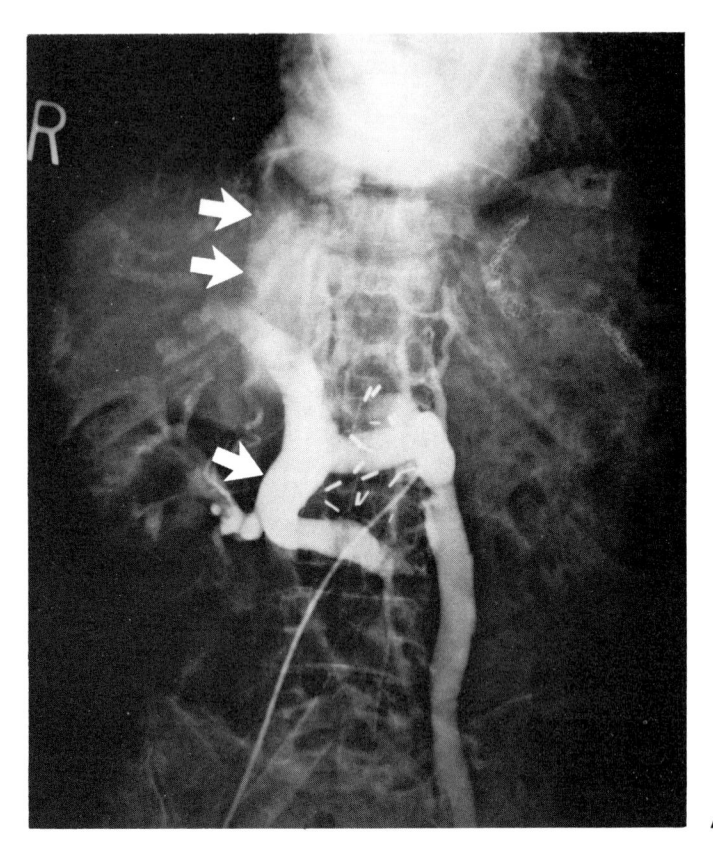

Figure 10-4. Radiologic conversion of nonselective to selective shunt. This middle-aged female had a history of multiple variceal bleeds and failed endoscopic variceal sclerosis. A recurrent variceal hemorrhage necessitated an emergency inferior mesenteric vein to left renal vein shunt (nonselective). Two weeks following the shunt, she became encephalopathic. *A.* Placement of catheter from IVC into renal vein and through inferior mesenteric vein shunt into portal system. There is simultaneous opacification of portal system (arrow) and IVC (double arrows).

Figure 10-4. *B.* Representation of shunt and position of catheter. Note circumaortic left renal vein. In order to convert the nonselective to a selective shunt, a Debrun balloon was placed to occlude the distal splenic vein and prevent retrograde portal flow through the shunt and into the lower pressure IVC.

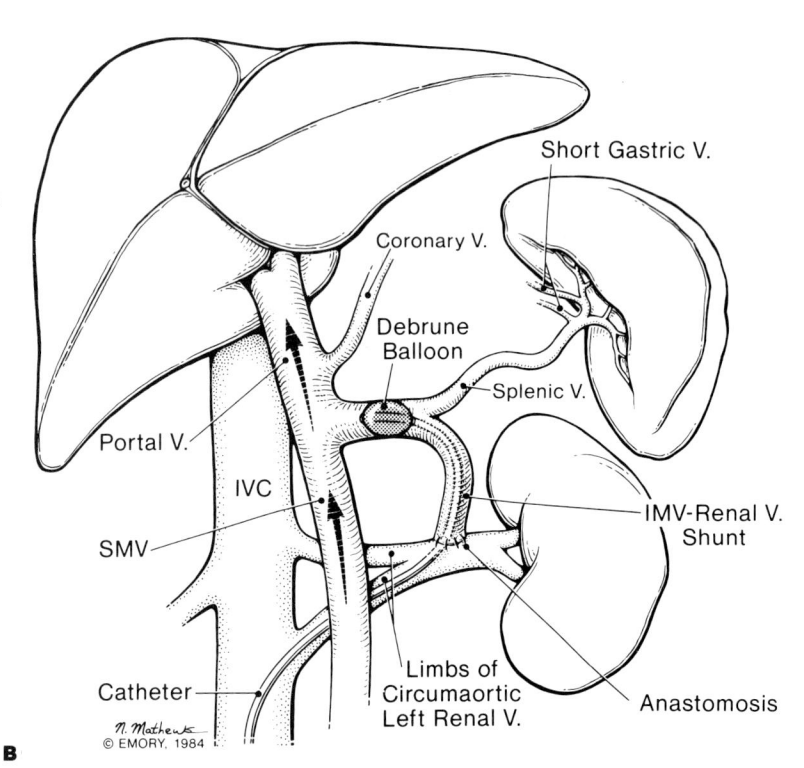

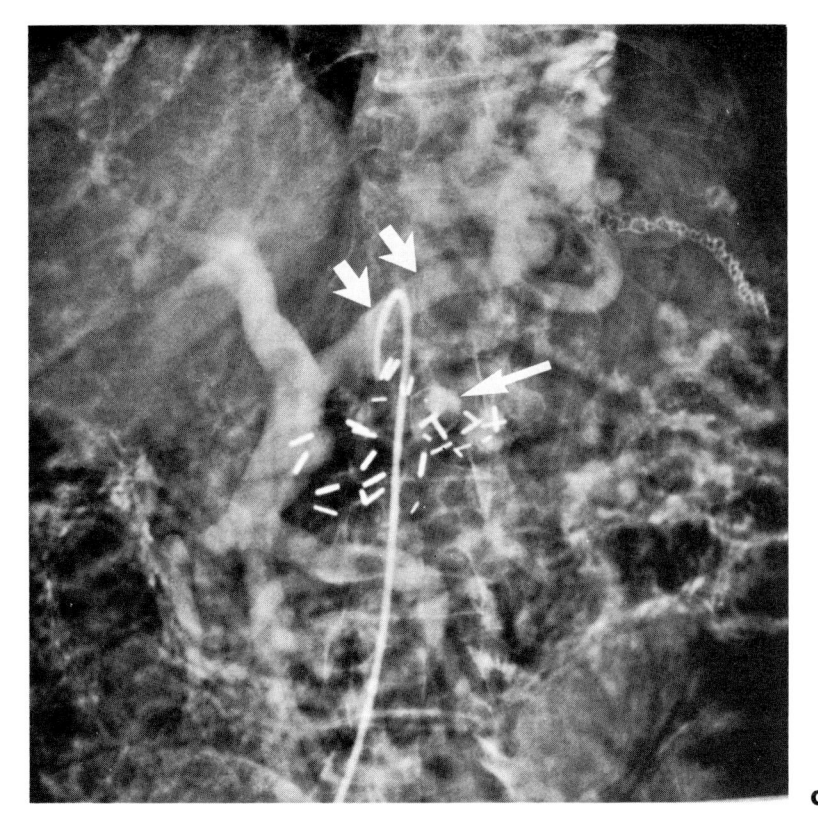

Figure 10-4. *C.* Venous phase of SMA injection. Following placement of balloon (arrow), the portal flow has been converted from retrograde to prograde, and the encephalopathy has cleared. However, there remains a large coronary vein (double arrows) with gastroesophageal varices. The increased portal pressure within these varices caused recurrence of upper gastrointestinal bleeding.

Figure 10-4. *D.* To convert to *selective* distal splenorenal shunt, transhepatic embolization of the coronary vein was performed using alcohol and steel coils. This venous phase of an SMA injection postembolization reveals good portal perfusion with no collateral filling (arrow = inflated Debrun balloon).

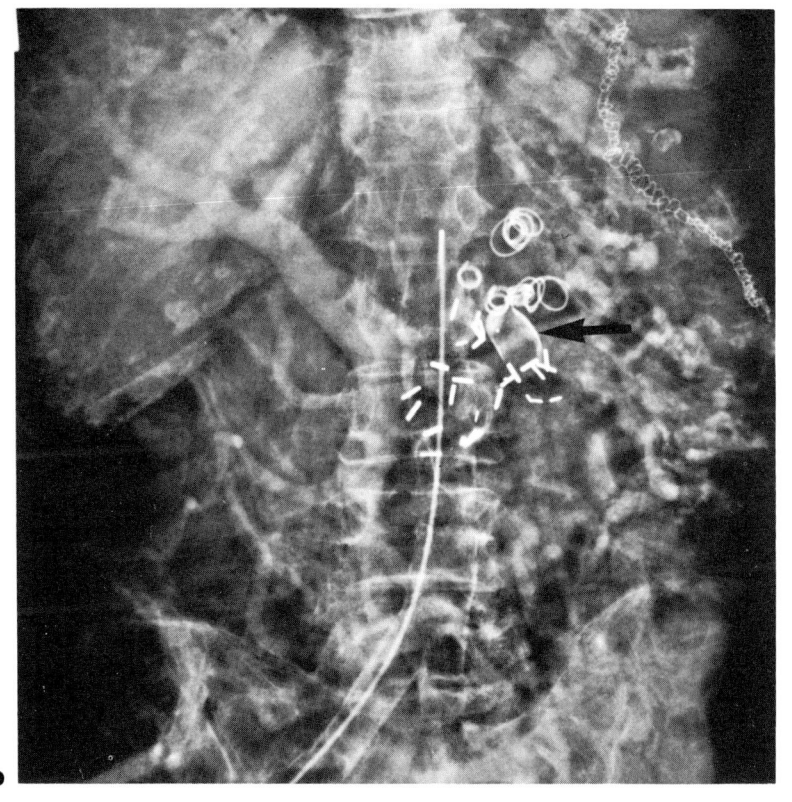

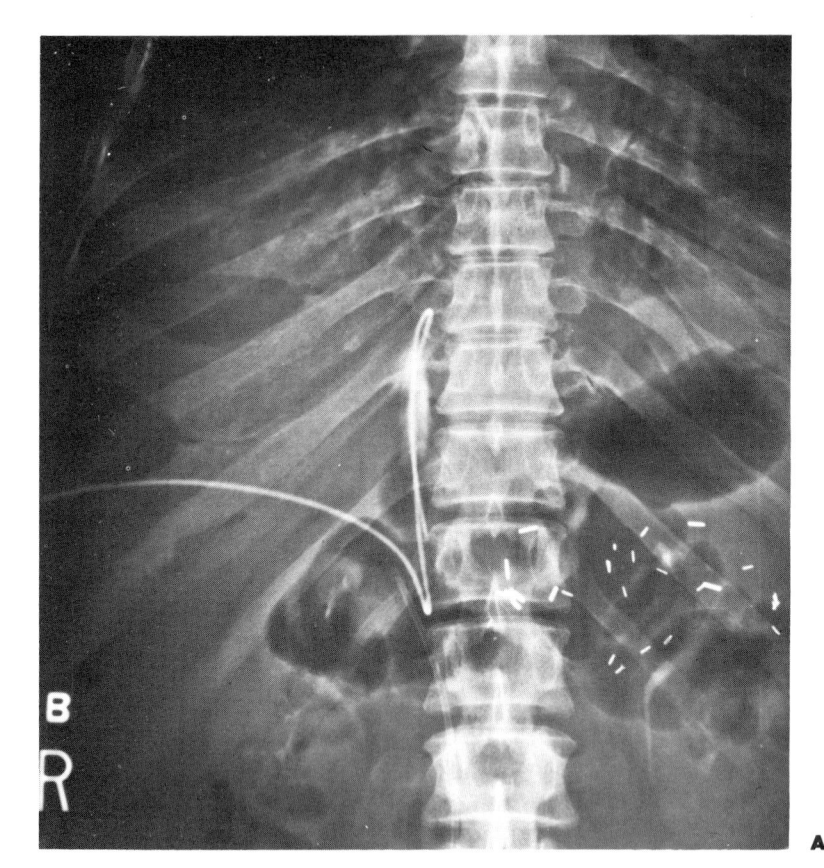

Figure 10-5. Several days postoperative distal splenorenal shunt. *A.* At surgery, a catheter was placed into umbilical vein for potential transcatheter embolization of collateral vessels missed at surgery or streptokinase infusion for postoperative portal vein thrombosis.

Figure 10-5. *B.* Injection through umbilical vein catheter opacifying portal system with visualization of single small collateral (arrow). No embolization was attempted in this case. Note retrograde inferior mesenteric vein drainage.

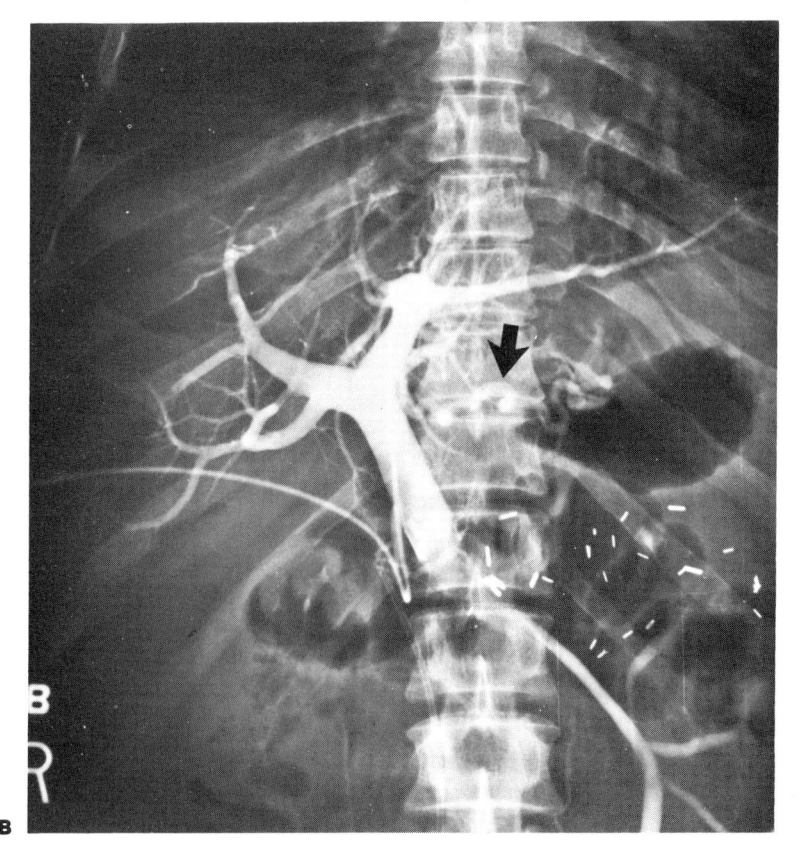

the siphon of blood into the shunt, the portal pressure is elevated and portal perfusion increased (Figure 10-2). It has become obvious that there are three major collateral pathways from the mesenteric portal circulation to the splenorenal shunt. These are (1) collaterals across the stomach via the short gastrics into the shunt, (2) transhepatic collaterals that originate from those veins draining the duodenum and communicating across the pancreatic bed to the splenorenal shunt, and (3) mesenteric collaterals which tend to course along the transverse colon through the splenocolic ligament to enter the splenic vein close to the splenic hilum (Figure 10-3). Occlusion of all of these various collateral pathways may be an arduous and time-consuming process. Since these tend to be large, high-flow channels, occlusion with large-size Gianturco coils alone may be difficult to accomplish. We have found a combination of coil baffle followed by AVITENE embolus to be an effective method of dealing with these collateral pathways.

Patients presenting with intractable variceal hemorrhage may be forced to undergo emergency portocaval shunt for variceal decompression. Many of these patients will subsequently develop hepatic encephalopathy. Interventional radiologic techniques may be employed to convert a nonselective to selective shunt to increase portal perfusion (Figure 10-4).

A useful technique to approach any collaterals that remain inadvertently unligated following selective distal splenorenal shunt has recently been utilized at our institution. This involves leaving an umbilical vein catheter positioned in the umbilical vein at the time of surgery. After a 5- to 10-day stabilization period, this catheter can be advanced into the splenorenal system to produce excellent opacification (Figure 10-5). Any collateral channels visualized at this time can be occluded.

HEPATIC ARTERY EMBOLIZATION (NONTUMOR CONSIDERATIONS)

The use of therapeutic hepatic artery ligation for hepatic trauma, arteriovenous portal fistula, and hepatic artery aneurysm has been the subject of controversy until the last few years. Some surgeons considered hepatic artery ligation to carry an unacceptably high mortality rate; this notion was based in part on review of the literature by Graham and Cannel indicating a 60 percent mortality rate associated with ligation of the hepatic artery [20]. Other authors [21-23] have demonstrated the efficacy of hepatic artery ligation primarily in the setting of traumatic hemorrhage. This technique was first suggested as a viable form of therapy by Madding [24]. Initial concern regarding this mode of treatment was based on fear of hepatic ischemia and resultant necrosis. However, several studies have shown the very rapid appearance of collateral vessels following hepatic artery ligation [25,26] with increase in size of the collateral vessels over the ensuing months. This rapid revascularization following ligation is made possible by the rich collateral supply within the liver and adjacent regions described by Michels [27,28] following over 200 cadaver dissections.

Although surgical ligation of the hepatic artery proved fruitful in the treatment of hepatic trauma and control of resultant hemorrhage, the risks of surgery and anesthesia remain high in this situation. As interventional techniques blossomed during the 1970s and early 1980s, transcatheter arterial embolization became an accepted mode of therapy to control hemorrhage, as well as occlude arterial venous portal fistulas and hepatic artery aneurysms. The early and mid-1970s found multiple reports attesting to the utility and safety of arterial catheter embolization and control of hemorrhage from gastrointestinal sources [29,30], and pelvic [31,32] and renal [33,34] trauma.

Traumatic Hemorrhage

In 1977, Jander et al. (35) reported one of the first uses of arterial embolization in the control of massive hepatic hemorrhage secondary to blunt trauma. Embolization was life-saving following failure to fully identify and control a bleeding site in the right hepatic lobe at surgery. A four-month followup arteriogram in this patient revealed revascularization of the right lobe through multiple collaterals including intrahepatic, left gastric and gastroduodenal arteries. Reuben and Katzen (36) simultaneously reported their experience with selective arterial embolization using GELFOAM to control hepatic bleeding following blunt trauma, obviating the need for surgery. Considering the frequent association (15 to 20 percent) of hepatic injury with abdominal trauma (37), angiography for localization of bleeding followed by selective embolization seems an attractive alternative to surgery in selected patients. Transcatheter embolization appears preferable to a surgical approach by allowing delineation of the bleeding site, more precise occlusion of the involved artery, and confirmation of cessation of hemorrhage by repeat arterial injection following embolization. The potential risks of anesthesia and surgery can thus be avoided.

Hepatic Artery Aneurysm

In addition to acute hemorrhage, the formation of an hepatic-artery pseudoaneurysm is a complication of blunt and penetrating abdominal injury. Trauma is the cause of hepatic artery aneurysms in approximately 10 percent of cases with infection, atherosclerosis, periarteritis nodosa, representing other etiologies (38–40). Infection is the most common etiology for hepatic artery aneurysms. Hepatic artery aneurysms may rupture into the peritoneal cavity (44 percent), biliary tract (41 percent), gastrointestinal tract (11 percent), and portal vein (5 percent) (41). The presence of the aneurysm is usually unsuspected prior to its rupture, often producing life-threatening hemorrhage. Arteriography readily detects these aneurysms, with 75 percent of the cases being extrahepatic and the majority involving the common hepatic artery (41). Surgical treatment for hepatic artery aneurysms has included extirpation of the aneurysm, endoaneurysmorrhaphy, and ligation of the feeding artery. Over the past several years, transcatheter embolization has proven a safe and effective method for treatment (42–44). The site of embolization, as well as choice of embolizing agent, is dependent on the location of the aneurysm. Proximal aneurysms may require the use of steel coils to effectively occlude the larger vessel. With more distal aneurysms, the choice of embolic agent may include GELFOAM, coils, IVALON, detachable balloons or Isobutyl-2-Cyanoacrylate. Rosen and Rothberg (45) reported the use of coils and GELFOAM in the occlusion of an hepatic artery pseudoaneurysm following biliary drainage, with the unique approach via the transhepatic tract.

Hemobilia

Hemobilia is defined as blood within the biliary tree and most commonly presents as severe colicky right upper quadrant pain and melena. Trauma is the most common cause for hemobilia, accounting for 55 perecent of the 355 detailed cases in Sandblom's extensive review of the literature prior to 1972 (46). Inflammatory and vascular disorders, gallstones and tumor are responsible for the remaining cases of hemobilia. Iatrogenic trauma contributed a not insignificant 30 percent of the total trauma cases. This figure has undoubtedly increased as the era of interventional radiology produced an increase in percutaneous transhepatic procedures, including cholangiography, biliary drainage, and biopsies. In an attempt to assess the frequency of hemobilia following percutaneous biliary drainage, Hoevels and Nilsson (47) performed hepatic angiography in 83 patients following drainage procedures. They discovered postprocedure vascular lesions (aneurysm, hematoma, arterial venous fistula) in 27 of the 83 patients. Only 5 of these patients had clinically significant hemobilia, with 2 resultant fatalities. The frequency of vascular injury following biliary drainage is not surprising, considering the close proximity of the bile ducts and vascular structures. It is probably true that the majority of cases of hemobilia following percutaneous drainage and biopsy are incidental and transient with spontaneous resolution, requiring no intervention.

The treatment of hemobilia has undergone radical change in the past decade. Sandblom (46) compiled the prognosis of surgical versus conservative treatment in the decade prior to 1972. Conservative measures yielded a mortality rate of 43 percent as compared with 21 percent of deaths following surgical treatment. Surgical methods include (1) local hepatic suture and control of bleeding, (2) hepatic artery ligation, and (3) partial hepatectomy. The advent of interventional vascular radiology has added a safer and, hopefully, more effective mode of therapy—that of transcatheter embolization. Walter *et al.* in 1976 (48) described the use of transcatheter arterial embolization for control of hemobilia secondary to liver biopsy. Subsequently, multiple case reports have attested to the efficacy of this approach in control of hemobilia (49–52). Angiographic embolization as an initial alternative to surgery is attractive for a number of reasons. Surgery carries a higher mortality and morbidity with a prolonged convalescence period compared with angiographic embolization. Transcatheter embolization can usually be performed safely in patients who are poor surgical risks. Selective angiography delineates precisely the bleeding site and vascular anatomy, allowing superselective embolization techniques so that only a portion of the hepatic arterial tree needs to be occluded. Lastly, transcatheter embolization may be repeated if necessary and does not preclude future surgery if unsuccessful. Recurrence of bleeding following surgical extrahepatic arterial ligation for hemobilia has been estimated to be approximately 20 percent (51) and may prevent the future use of transcatheter embolization. Although the number of cases of hemobilia treated by embolization to date is small, it has so far proven effective with relatively low risk. We believe it is the current procedure of choice and, in general, should precede surgery in the treatment of hemobilia.

Arteriovenous Portal Fistula

Discussion of arteriovenous portal fistulas and their treatment naturally follows the preceding descriptions of hepatic artery aneurysm and hemobilia. Hemobilia may accompany arteriovenous portal fistulas, as all three structures (portal vein, hepatic artery, and bile duct) lie in close proximity. Rupture of an hepatic or splenic artery aneurysm into the portal venous system is the most common cause of arteriovenous portal fistulas (53). Trauma is the second leading cause of this malady, with other etiologies including cirrhosis, tumor (especially hepatoma), and congenital malformation. Approximately onehalf of individuals with these fistulae will develop portal hypertension and the potential sequelae of bleeding varices. Congestive heart failure may develop, especially with large fistulas, although this is uncommon as the increased flow is dampened by the portal circulation and sinusoids (54). Treatment should be directed toward correction of the fistula, rather than creation of a shunt in patients with secondary portal hypertension, as the shunt will promote the onset of heart failure.

The diagnosis of arteriovenous portal fistula is usually first suspected clinically. The

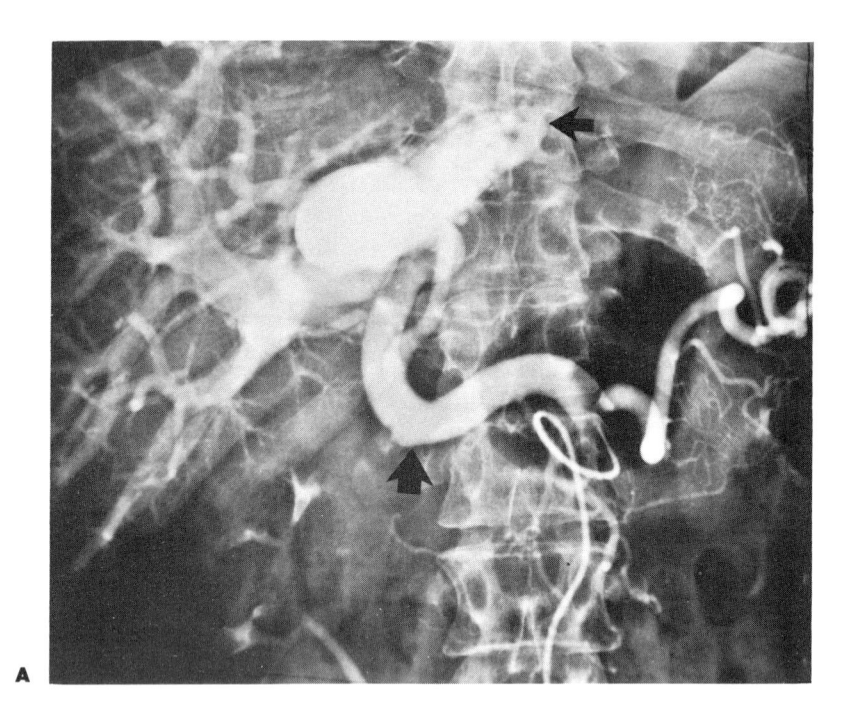

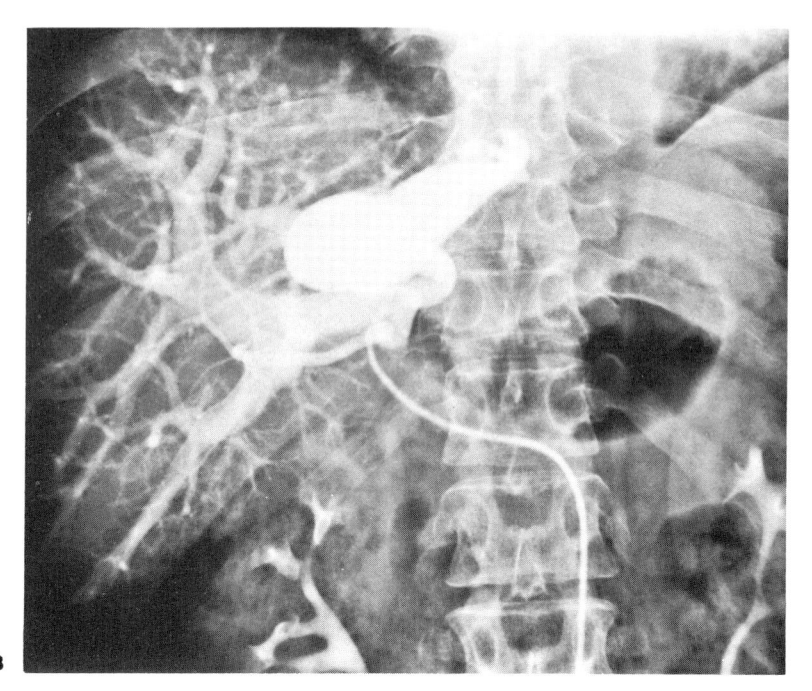

Figure 10-6. Traumatic arteriovenous portal fistula. Blunt abdominal trauma was sustained several years earlier with recent onset of high-output heart failure. *A.* Celiac arteriography demonstrating markedly with enlarged right hepatic artery (large arrow), immediate opacification of the portal venous system via arteriovenous communication with the left portal vein (small arrow). Two branches of the right hepatic artery contribute to the fistula. *B.* The catheter has been advanced into the larger right hepatic arterial branch and occlusion performed with a combination of steel coils and AVITENE.

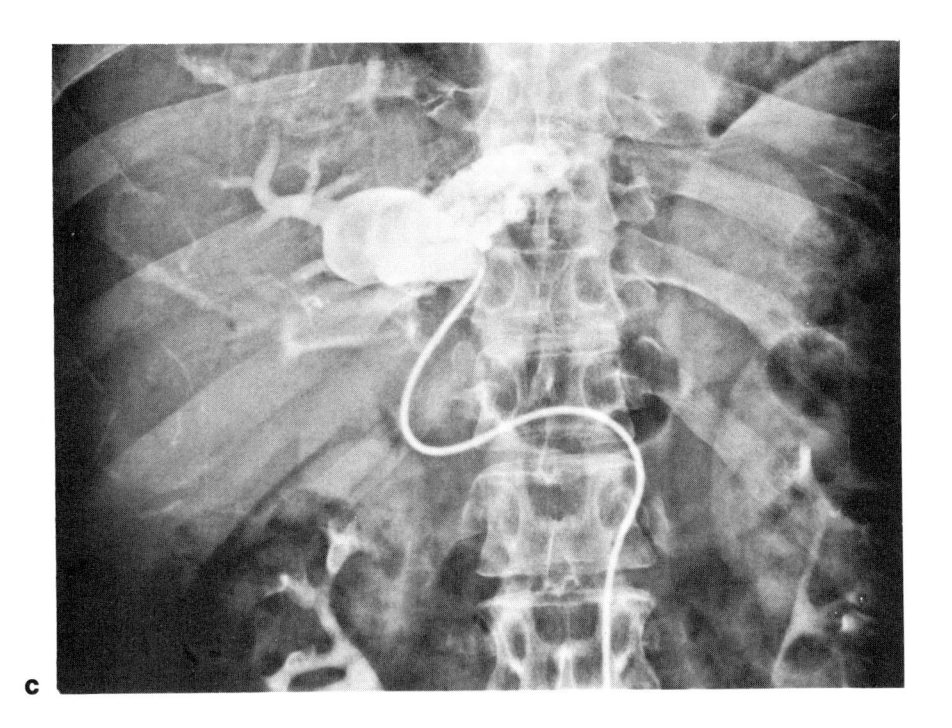

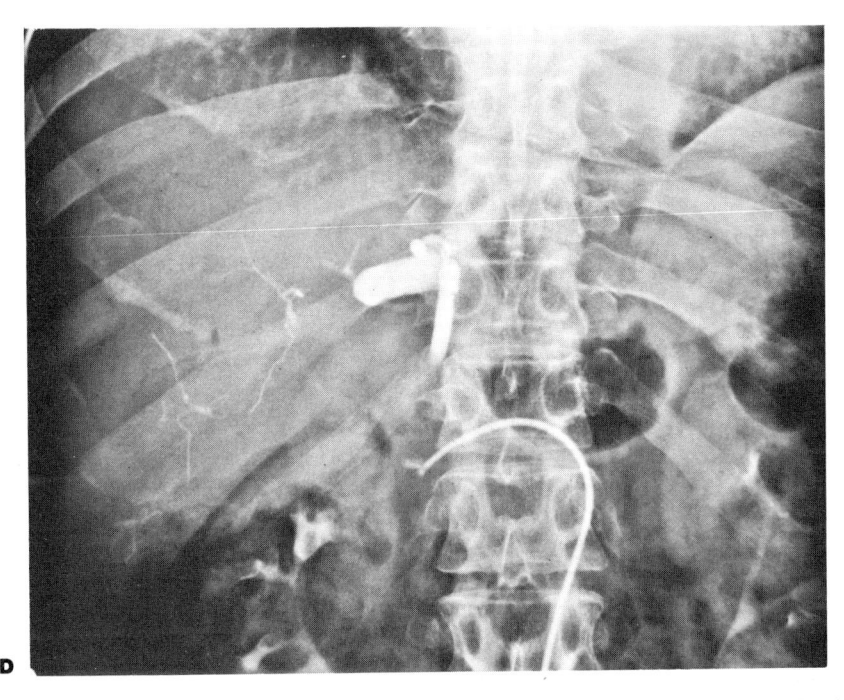

Figure 10-6. *C.* Selective catheterization of the smaller arterial vessel supplying the fistula with occlusion via coils and AVITENE. *D.* Appearance following embolization of both right hepatic arterial branches supplying the fistula with contrast embedded within the AVITENE embolus.

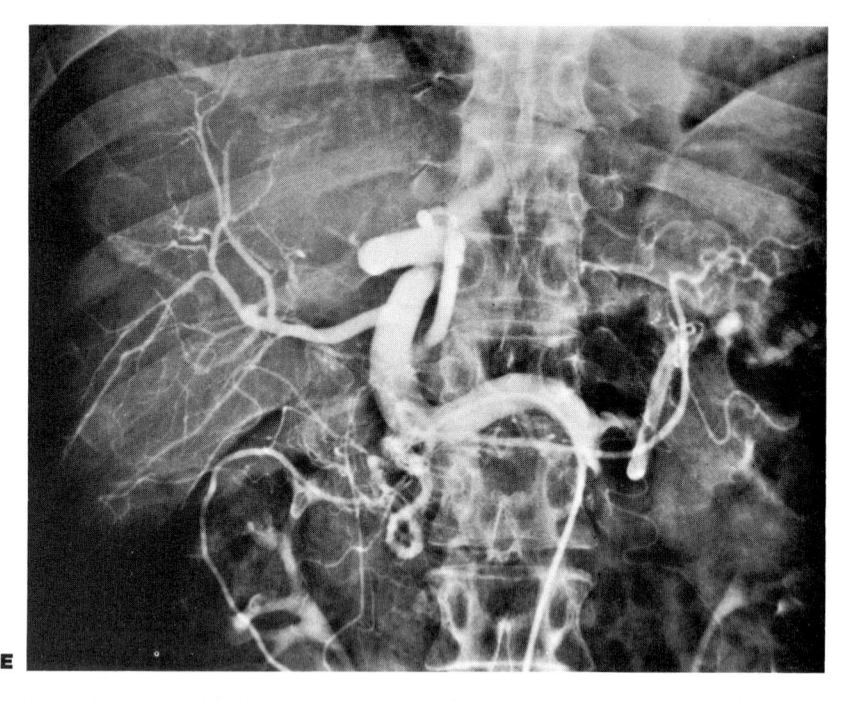

Figure 10-6. *E.* Repeat right hepatic arteriogram demonstrating preservation of right hepatic arterial flow with total occlusion of the arteriovenous portal fistula. Compare with *A,* above. The patient has remained asymptomatic.

vast majority of patients will have an abdominal bruit. Angiography is the definitive diagnostic modality, demonstrating an enlarged hepatic artery and a fistulous communication immediately opacifying the portal venous system. Moeller *et al.* (55) described the use of sonography in first proposing the diagnosis of arteriovenous portal fistula in a patient with a 6 year prior history of stab wounds to the upper abdomen.

Transcatheter embolization of arteriovenous portal fistulas is in an embryonic age, and many technical difficulties associated with the procedure have yet to be resolved (Figures 10-6, 10-7). Large fistulae may be very difficult to successfully occlude, as the torrential flow makes permanent placement of an embolic agent proximal to the fistula difficult. Small particulate embolic material such as Ivalon is not appropriate for occlusion. Autologous clot and GELFOAM have been shown to recanalize on two separate occasions after attempted embolization of arteriovenous portal fistula (56). Isobutyl-2-Cyanoacrylate was used successfully in occlusion of an hepatic arterial portal fistula (57); however, the long-term deleterious effects of this agent, if any, are unknown. Other investigators have reported success in transcatheter embolization of these fistulas (58,59). Stainless steel coils are available in multiple sizes and have been used frequently in embolization elsewhere in the body. Detachable balloons offer the unique advantage of controlled placement and the option to deflate and reposition. They have the disadvantage of being malleable and have the potential to dislodge and migrate. In addition, balloons require a nontapered catheter and sheath for introduction.

A more satisfactory method may be the use of a spider acting as a baffle, against which a variety of embolic agents may be "packed" to occlude the vessel (60,61). The spider is a stainless steel device with six prongs designed to embed into the vessel wall.

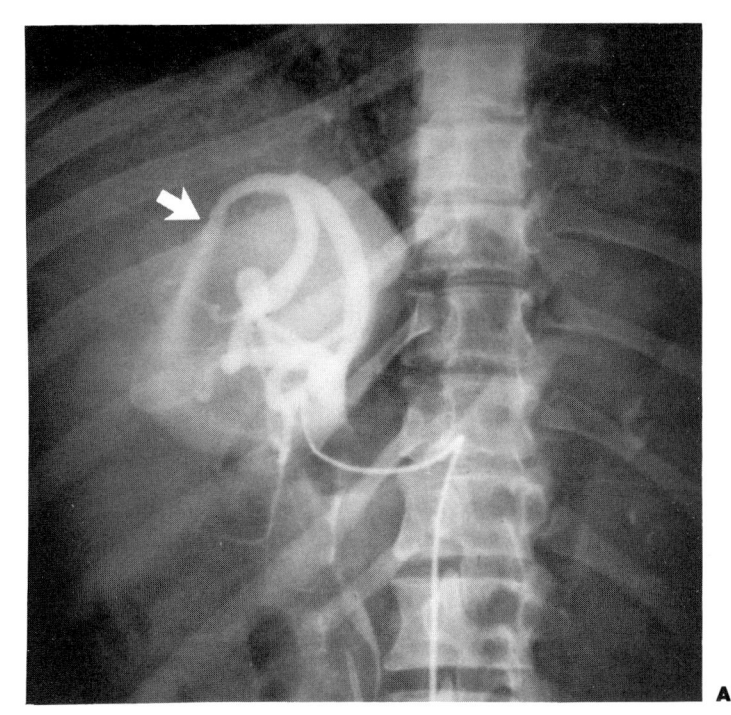

Figure 10-7. This young female presented with bleeding esophageal varices as a result of portal hypertension from a congenital arteriovenous portal fistula. *A.* Selective hepatic arteriogram demonstrating an enlarged hepatic artery with early filling of the portal system via a fistulous communication (arrow).

Figure 10-7. *B.* Later phase of same injection revealing massive arteriovenous portal fistula (arrow = portal vein).

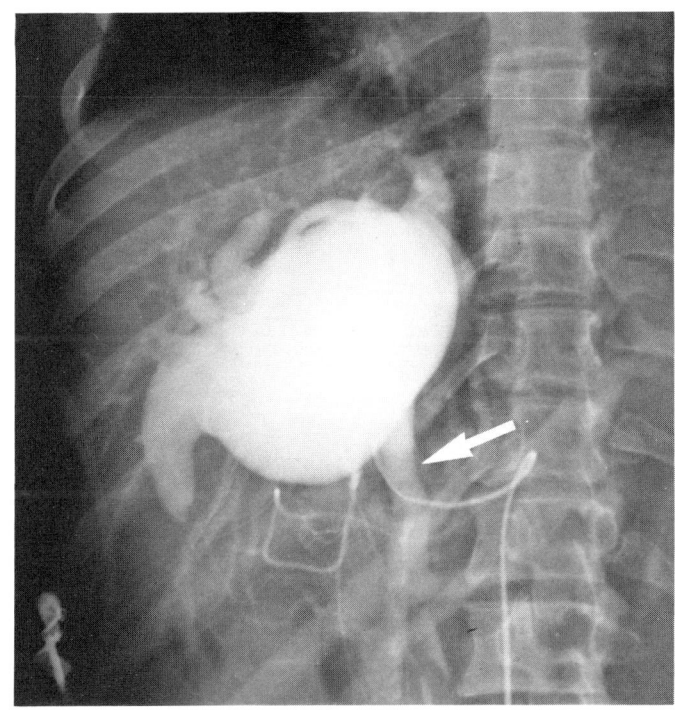

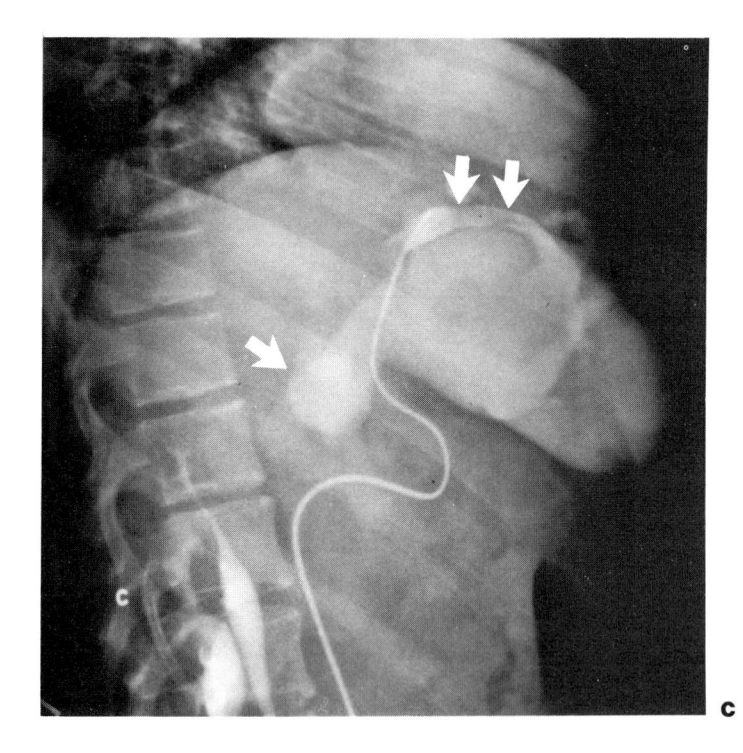

Figure 10-7. *C.* Lateral view demonstrating simultaneous opacification of hepatic artery (double arrows) and portal vein (arrow) by the fistula.

Figure 10-7. *D.* Following placement of detachable balloon (arrow) in hepatic artery proximal to fistulous communication, repeat hepatic arteriogram reveals filling of hepatic artery branches, but no opacification of fistula or portal system. Unfortunately, the balloon migrated through the fistula into the portal vein 1 week later, with recurrent upper gastrointestinal hemorrhage. Repeat arteriogram revealed a patent fistula, which was successfully reoccluded with coils and balloons. The patient followed a benign course and was later taken to surgery for excision of the fistula. At surgery, the fistula was markedly decreased in size and was removed without difficulty.

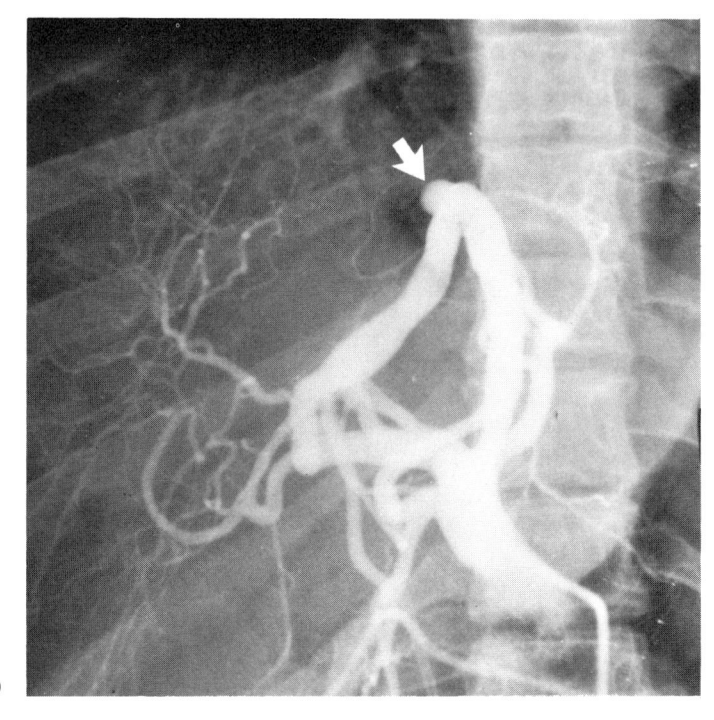

It is introduced in a collapsed state through a catheter. Balloons or coils may then be placed proximal to the spider to decrease flow. Once flow has been slowed significantly, AVITENE slurry may then be injected proximally to form an embolic plug to permanently occlude the vessel.

HEPATIC ARTERY EMBOLIZATION: TUMORS

Hepatic Neoplasms

The treatment of patients with hepatic neoplasms has included partial hepatectomy, systemic and intraarterial chemotherapy, radiation, and hepatic artery embolization. Partial hepatectomy remains the procedure of choice in hopes of obtaining a cure in patients, assuming (1) no distant metastases are present, and the operation is expected to be curative; (2) the overall medical condition is such that the patient can reasonably be expected to withstand the surgery and postoperative course; and (3) enough liver remains postoperatively to maintain adequate hepatic function. Most patients will not be candidates for resection for one or more of the above reasons. Partial hepatectomy carries a significant morbidity and mortality.

The indications for hepatic artery embolization of benign liver tumors are few. Hepatic adenomas may spontaneously hemorrhage, with catheter embolization an alternative to conservative management or surgical therapy. The most common benign liver tumor is the cavernous hemangioma, occurring in 0.4 to 7.3 percent of the population (62). Symptoms referable to the hemangioma have been reported to occur in from 13 to 50 percent of patients and may be secondary to hemorrhage or infection within hematoma (63,64). Pain may also be caused by mass effect if the hemangioma reaches a large size. Figure 10-8 illustrates a case in which hepatic artery embolization resulted in relief of pain caused by a large cavernous hemangioma in the right hepatic lobe.

Systemic chemotherapy for malignant liver disease has not proven to prolong median survival (65). As a result of these findings, researchers began experimenting with infusion of the chemotherapeutic agent directly into the hepatic artery in hopes that the higher concentration would prove more cytotoxic. In patients with metastatic colon carcinoma receiving intraarterial chemotherapy, the median survival did improve to 7 to 8 months (66,67). Median survival of patients with untreated metastatic liver disease of all types from the time of initial diagnosis ranges from 2.5 to 4.5 months (68,69). Because of the frequent presence of an aberrant hepatic artery in approximately half the population, either two simultaneous infusions would need to be performed or a portion of the liver would remain uninfused. To cope with this obstacle, embolization of the aberrant hepatic artery with steel coils and Gelfoam has been performed in an effort to redistribute blood flow and thereby allow infusion to the entire liver through a single artery (70).

The use of hepatic artery ligation as a treatment for metastatic liver disease was first suggested by Markowitz in 1952 (71). This concept of treatment is based on knowledge that the liver tumor receives virtually all of its blood supply from the hepatic artery, while normal hepatic parenchyma has a dual blood supply. Selective obliteration of the hepatic arterial bed would be expected to result in tumor necrosis. Surgical ligation of the hepatic artery may not permanently prevent arterial flow to the tumor because of the rapid formation of collateral circulation following hepatic artery ligation (72). For this reason, transcatheter hepatic artery embolization has gained popularity in hepatic tumor treatment (Figures 10-9, 10-10).

The indications for hepatic artery embolization in tumor treatment are (1) to

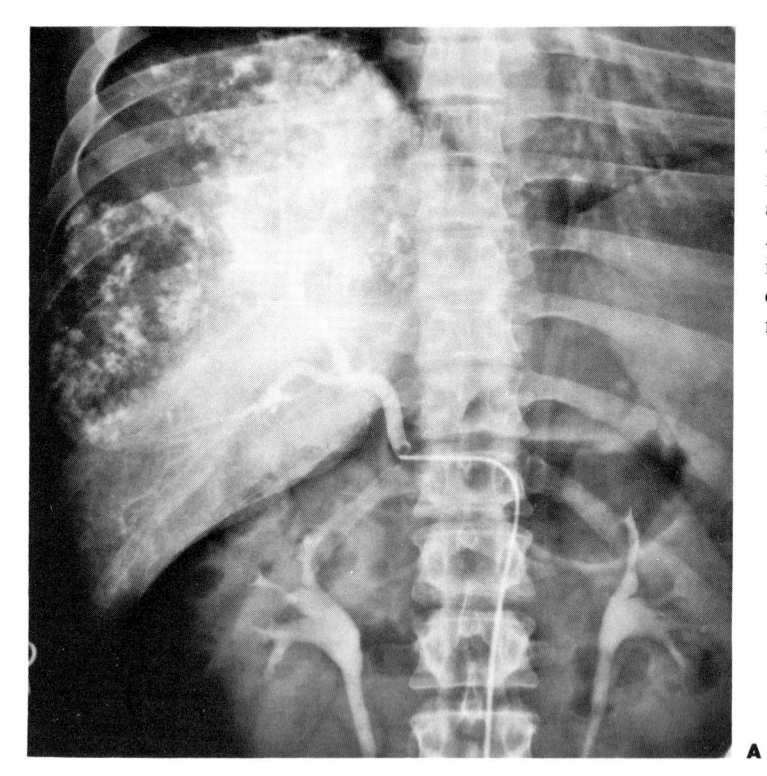

Figure 10-8. Embolization of cavernous hemangioma in a young male with a history of hepatomegaly and upper abdominal pain. *A.* Arterial phase of right hepatic artery injection reveals hypervascular mass occupying the major portion of the right hepatic lobe.

Figure 10-8. *B.* Venous phase from same injection demonstrating typical pooling of contrast within vascular lakes.

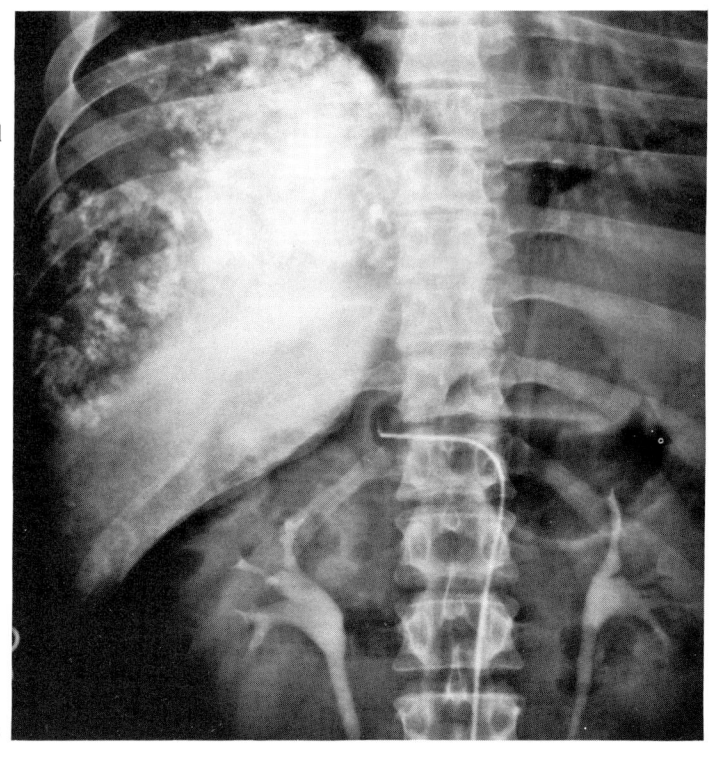

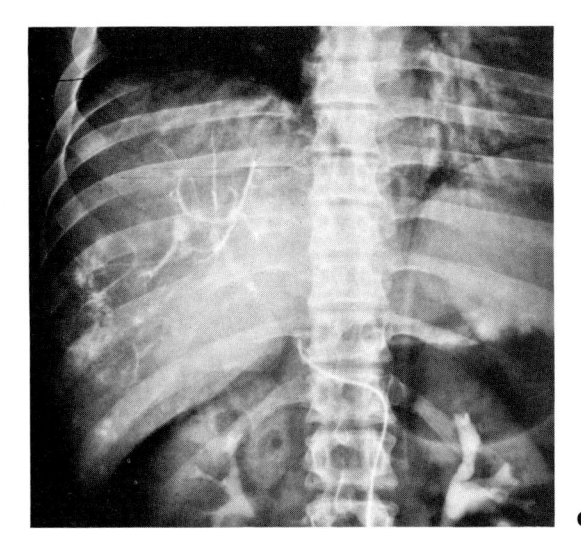

Figure 10-8. *C.* Following embolization with IVALON particles and GELFOAM, a late-phase arteriogram shows only minimal residual contrast puddling. The liver subsequently decreased in size with alleviation of pain.

decrease tumor size, (2) to alleviate pain, and (3) to reduce symptoms from metastatic endocrine tumor such as carcinoid. The ultimate goal in hepatic tumor embolization is to prolong survival. Chuang and Wallace (73) performed hepatic artery embolizations in 47 patients with median survival of 11.5 months from the time of embolization. Twenty of the patients had failed systemic or intraarterial chemotherapy prior to embolization. This makes the median survival data of 11.5 months more impressive in that time was lost from the initial diagnosis of liver metastasis until embolization. It appears that hepatic artery embolization is superior to either systemic or intraarterial chemotherapy, while avoiding the potential side-effects of the chemotherapeutic agent.

The technique of hepatic artery embolization involves initial diagnostic celiac, hepatic, and superior mesenteric arteriography. The celiac injection provides arterial mapping to document any aberrant blood supply to the liver. The selective hepatic angiogram defines tumor extent and which lobe should be embolized initially. The superior mesenteric injection gives information on aberrant hepatic arterial supply and patency of the portal vein. Portal vein occlusion is a contraindication to embolization of the entire liver, as no blood supply would remain to nourish the normal hepatic parenchyma. Unilobar embolization may be performed in the setting of portal vein thrombosis, although it is a relative contraindication, and each case should be judged on its own merit. Although prophylactic antibiotics are recommended by some to prevent the potential formation of abscess, Chuang (74) has experienced no abscess formation without the use of antibiotics in approximately 300 patients following hepatic embolization.

Once superselective catheterization of the right or left hepatic artery is achieved, particles of IVALON mixed with contrast are slowly injected. The amount of IVALON needed for complete embolization is determined by assessing the progressive reduction of blood flow under fluoroscopy. Once the flow approaches stasis, one or two GELFOAM cubes complete the embolization. A repeat angiogram at approximately 2 ml per second for 4 to 6 ml total contrast will reveal lack of arterial blood supply to the tumor. The patient can return in weeks or months for embolization of the remaining lobe if needed, or repeat embolization of the same lobe if progressive disease is discovered.

The postinfarction syndrome consists of a combination of upper abdominal pain, fever, nausea, vomiting, and transient elevation of liver function studies following hepatic embolization (75). This syndrome is expected to occur in approximately 90 per-

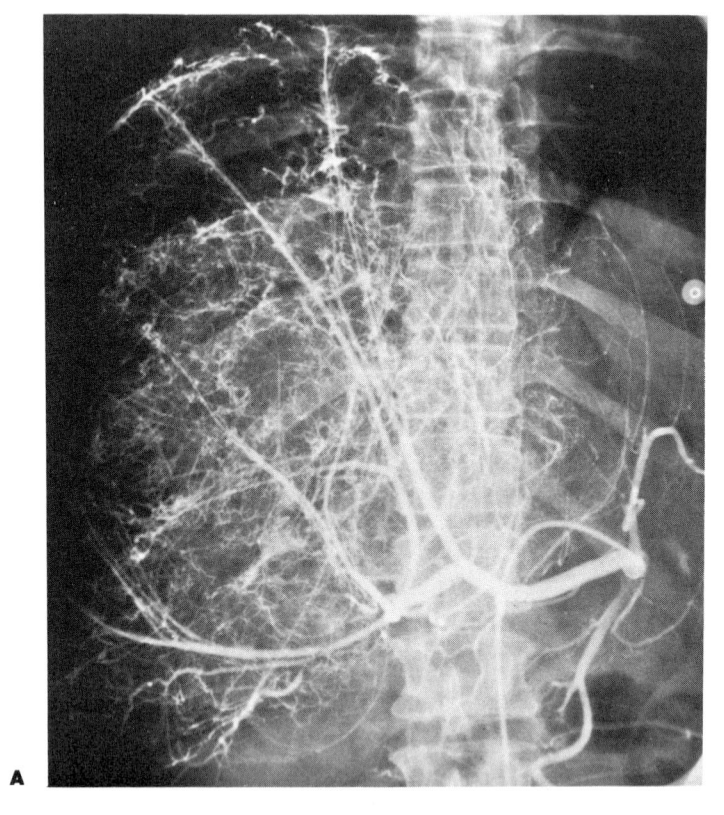

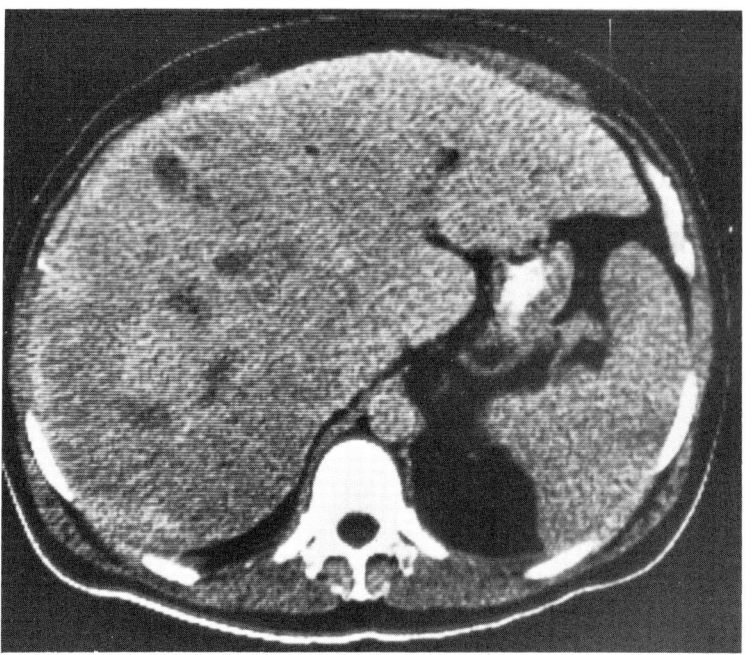

Figure 10-9. Hepatocellular carcinoma: embolization. *A.* Angiography demonstrating massive tumor involvement of right hepatic lobe with extensive neovascularity. No arterioportal shunting was seen. *B.* Corresponding computed tomographic scan prior to embolization with inhomogeneous density of right lobe, with small central areas of low density probably representing tumor necrosis.

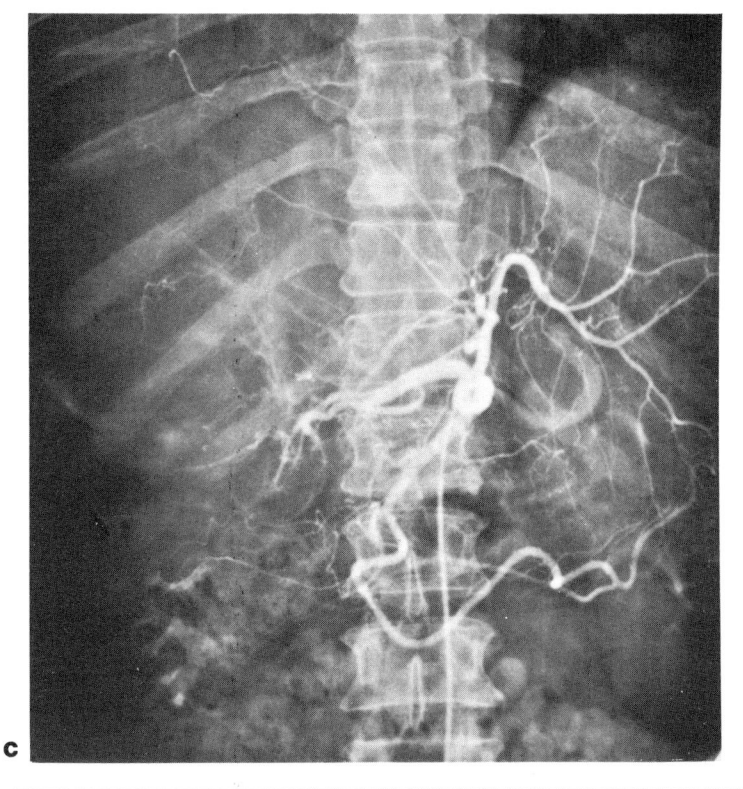

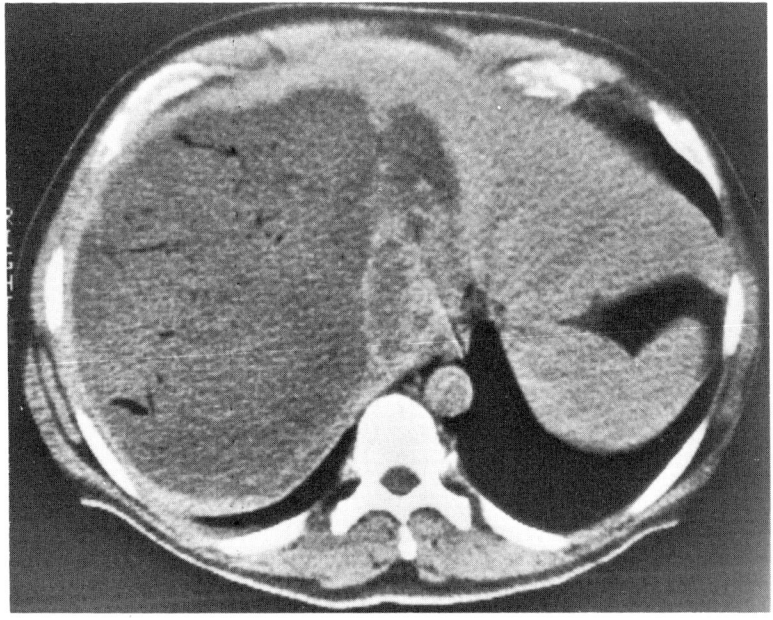

Figure 10-9. *C.* Following right hepatic artery embolization with IVALON and GELFOAM, there is a marked reduction in vascularity. *D.* CT several days following embolization revealing a more homogeneous low-density appearance likely representing diffuse tumor necrosis. The lateral segment of the left lobe is spared. Gas within necrotic tumor is frequently seen postembolization (Bernardino ME, Chuang VP, Wallace S, et al.: Therapeutically infarcted tumors: CT findings. AJR 1981;136:527–530) and has been suggested to represent a benign process rather than abscess, possibly due to air inadvertently injected at the time of embolization or the release of oxygen or carbon dioxide from infarcted tissues (Marks WM, Filly RA: Computed tomographic appearance of intraarterial air following hepatic artery ligation. Radiology 1979; 132:665–666).

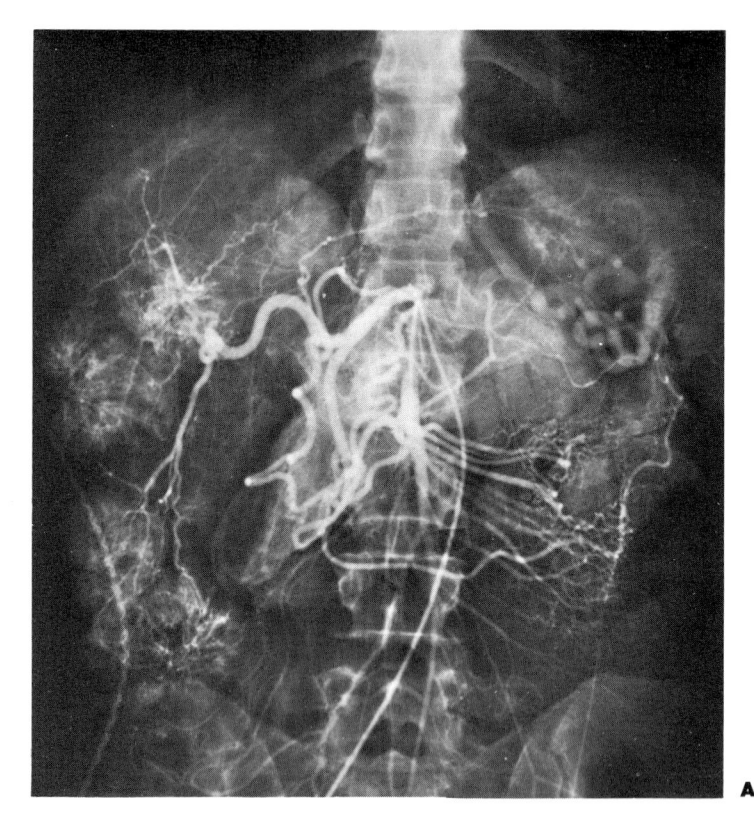

Figure 10-10. Metastatic melanoma. Forty-three-year-old female with recently resected primary melanoma from left shoulder. Hepatic metastases were unresponsive to chemotherapy. Progressive weight loss, hepatomegaly, abdominal pain, and malaise prompted referral to the Radiology Department for hepatic embolization. *A.* Arterial phase demonstrating multiple hypervascular metastatic deposits within both hepatic lobes.

Figure 10-10. *B.* Venous phase outlining the metastatic lesions.

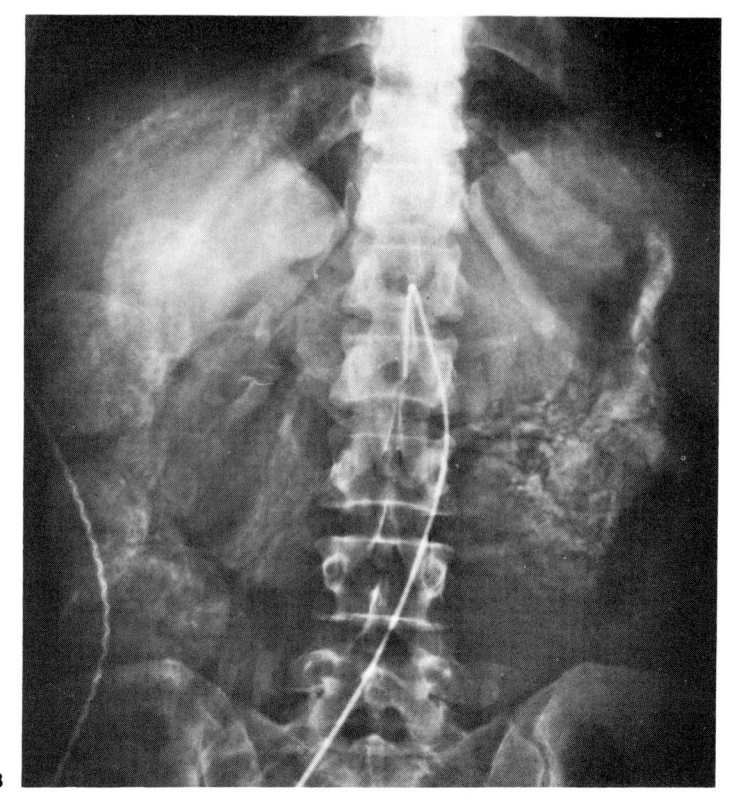

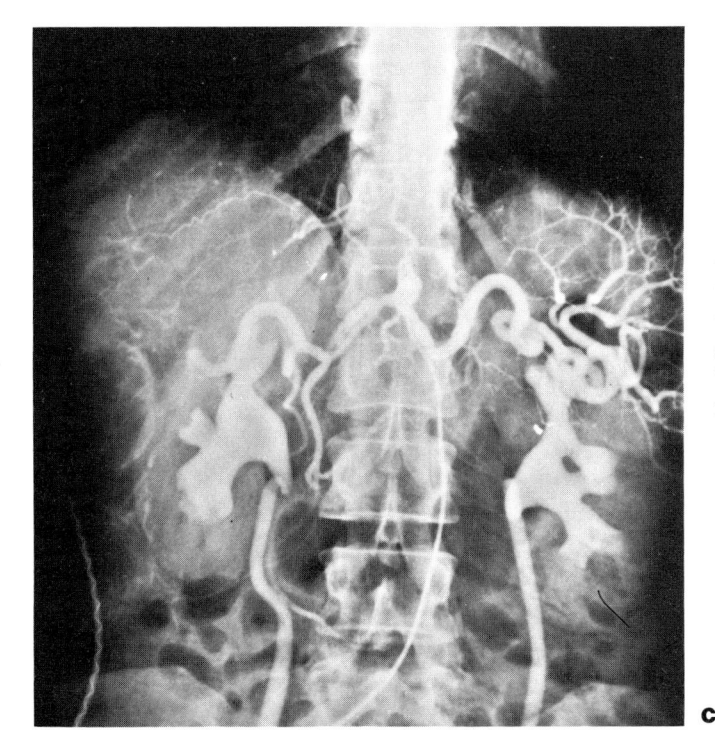

Figure 10-10. *C.* Following embolization of both lobes with Ivalon and Gelfoam, there is marked reduction in tumor vascularity. Over the ensuing months, the patient's condition improved considerably with weight gain and regained feeling of well-being such that she was able to return to playing tennis. At 6 months follow-up, she had no symptoms referable to her liver, but had unfortunately developed cerebral metastases.

cent of patients receiving hepatic embolization and should resolve within days to a week. The more extensive the embolization, in general, the more severe the symptoms. Symptoms of pain may begin immediately following embolization and usually require narcotics for control. Prior to embolization, patients should be forewarned to anticipate this side-effect. Wallace and Chuang (76) report their experience with 150 hepatic embolizations in 100 patients, with 7 fatalities occurring within a month of embolization. Their observations led to the assumption that 4 of the 7 patients probably died as a result of progression of their primary disease, and the embolization likely contributed to death in the remaining 3 patients as a result of hepatic failure. The deaths occurred for the most part in patients who were moribund, with the embolization performed to alleviate pain associated with rapid progression of hepatic metastasis.

REFERENCES

1. Lunderquist A, Simert G, Tylen U, Vang J: Follow-up of patients with portal hypertension and esophageal varices treated with percutaneous obliteration of gastric coronary vein. Radiology 1977;122:59–63.
2. Widrich W, Johnson WC, Robbins AH, Nasbeth DC: Esophagogastric variceal hemorrhage. Arch Surg 1978;113:1331–1338.
3. Chuang VP, Wallace S, Gianturco C: A new improved coil for tapered-tip catheter for arterial occlusion. Radiology 1980;135:507–510.
4. Gunther R, Schubert U, Bohl J, et al.: Transcatheter embolization of the kidney with Butyl-2-Cyanoacrylate: experimental and clinical results. Cardiovasc Rad 1978;1:101–108.
5. Page RC, Larson EJ, Siegmund E: Chronic toxicity studies of methyl-2-Cyanoacrylate in dogs and rats. In JE Healey, Jr (ed), Proceedings of the Symposium on Physiological Adhesives. University of Texas, Houston, Feb 3–4, 1966, pp. 11–23.

6. Ellman BA, Parkhill BJ, Curry TS III, et al.: Ablation of renal tumors with absolute ethanol: a new technique. Radiology 1981;141:619–626.
7. Cox GG, Lee KR, Price HI, et al.: Colonic infarction following ethanol embolization of renal cell carcinoma. Radiology 1982;145:343–345.
8. Mulligan BD, Espinosa GA: Bowel infarction: complication of ethanol ablation of renal tumor. Cardiovasc Intervent Radiol 1983;6:55–57.
9. Kaufman SL, Strandberg JD, Barth KH, et al.: Transcatheter embolization with microfibrillar collagen in swine. Invest Radiol 1978;13:200–204.
10. Diamond NG, Casarella WJ, Bachman DM, Wolff M: Microfibrillar collagen hemostat: a new transcatheter embolization agent. Radiology 1979;133:775–779.
11. Pereiras R, Schiff E, Barkin J, Hutson D: The role of interventional radiology in diseases of the hepatobiliary system and the pancreas. Radiol Clin North Am 1979;17:555–605.
12. Keller FS, Rosch J, Vaur GM, et al.: Percutaneous angiographic embolization: a procedure of increasing usefulness. Am J Surg 1981;142:5–11.
13. Passariello R, Rossi P, Simonetti G, et al.: Emergency transhepatic obliteration of bleeding varices. Cardiovasc Radiol 1979;2:97–106.
14. Funaro AH, Ring EJ, Freiman DB, et al.: Transhepatic obliteriation of esophageal varices using the stainless steel coil. AJR 1979;133:1123–1125.
15. Witt WS, Goncharenko V, O'Leary JP, et al.: Interruption of gastroesophageal varices: steel coil technique. AJR 1980;135:829–833.
16. Lunderquist A, Borjesson B, Bengmark S. Isobutyl-2-Cyanoacrylate (Bucrylate) in obliteration of gastric coronary vein and esophageal varices. AJR 1978;130:1–6.
17. Goldman ML, Freeny PC, Tallman JM, et al.: Transcatheter vascular occlusion therapy with Isobutyl-2-Cyanocacrylate (Bucrylate) for control of massive upper gastrointestinal bleeding. Radiology 1978;129:41–49.
18. Uflacker R: Percutaneous transhepatic obliteration of gastroesophageal varices using absolute alcohol. Radiology 1983;146:621–625.
19. Spigos DG, Tauber JW, Tan WS, et al.: Work in progress: Umbilical venous cannulation: a new approach for embolization of esophageal varices. Radiology 1983;146:53–56.
20. Graham RR, Cannell D: Accidental ligation of the hepatic artery. Br J Surg 1933;20:566–579.
21. Lewis FR, Lim RC, Blaidsell FW: Hepatic artery ligation: an adjunct in the management of massive hemorrhage from the liver. J Trauma 1974;14:743–755.
22. Mays ET: Lobar dearterialization for exsanguinating wounds of the liver. J Trauma 1972;12:397–407.
23. Aarons, Fulton RL, Mays ET: Surgical ligation of the hepatic artery for trauma of the liver. Surg Gynecol Obstet 1975;141:187–189.
24. Madding GF: Injuries of the liver. AMA Arch Surg 1955;70:748–756.
25. Koehler RE, Korobkin M, Lewis F: Arteriographic demonstration of collateral arterial supply to the liver after hepatic artery ligation. Radiology 1975;117:59–54.
26. Mays ET, Wheeler CS: Demonstration of collateral arterial flow after interruption of hepatic arteries in man. N Engl J Med 1974;290:993–996.
27. Michels NA: Newer anatomy of the liver and its variant blood supply and collateral circulation. Am J Surg 1966;112:337–347.
28. Michels NA: Collateral arterial pathways to the liver after ligation of the hepatic artery and removal of the celiac axis. Cancer 1953;6:708–724.
29. Rosch J, Dotter CT, Brown MJ: Selective arterial embolization: a new method for control of gastrointestinal bleeding. Radiology 1972;102:303–306.
30. Reuter SR, Chuang VP: Selective arterial embolization for control of massive upper intestinal bleeding. AJR 1975;125:119–126.
31. Ring EJ, Athanasoulis C, Waltman AC, et al.: Arteriographic management of hemorrhage following pelvic fracture. Radiology 1973;109:65–70.
32. Ring EJ, Waltman AC, Athanasoulis C: Angiography in pelvic trauma. Surg Gynecol Obstet 1974;139:375–380.

33. Kalish M, Greenbaum L, Silber S, Goldstein H: Traumatic renal hemorrhage treatment by arterial embolization. J Urol 1974;112:138–141.
34. Chuang VP, Reuter ST, Walter J, et al.: Control of renal hemorrhage by selective arterial embolization. AJR 1975;125:300–306.
35. Jander JP, Laws HL, Kogutt MS, Mihas AA: Emergency embolization in blunt hepatic trauma. AJR 1977;129:249–252.
36. Rubin BE, Katzen BT: Selective hepatic artery embolization to control massive hepatic hemorrhage after trauma. AJR 1977;129:253–256.
37. Steichen FM: Hepatic trauma in adults. Surg Clin North Am 1975;55:387–407.
38. Erskine JM: Hepatic artery aneurysms. Vasc Surg 1973;7:106–125.
39. McAlexander RA, Lawrence GH: Operative repair of hepatic artery aneurysm. Arch Surg 1966;93:409–414.
40. Mallory HR, Jason RS: Aneurysm of the hepatic artery. Am J Surg 1942;57:359–363.
41. Guida PM, Moore SW: Aneurysm of the hepatic artery: report of five cases with a brief review of the previously reported cases. Surgery 1966;60:229–310.
42. Johnson K, Bjernstad A, Erikson B: Treatment of hepatic artery aneurysm by coil occlusion of the hepatic artery. AJR 1980;134:1245–1247.
43. Kadir S, Athanasoulis CA, Ring EJ, Greenfield A: Transcatheter embolization of the intrahepatic arterial aneurysms. Radiology 1980;134:335–339.
44. Goldblatt M, Goldin AR, Shaff MI: Percutaneous embolization for the management of hepatic artery aneurysms. Gastroenterol 1977;73:1142–1146.
45. Rosen RJ, Rothberg M: Transhepatic embolization of hepatic artery pseudoaneurysm following biliary drainage. Radiology 1982;145:532–533.
46. Sandblom T: Hemobilia (Biliary Tract Hemorrhage). Springfield, Ill.: Thomas, 1972.
47. Hoevels J, Nilsson V: Intrahepatic lesions following nonsurgical percutaneous transhepatic bile duct intubation. Gastroentest Radiol 1980;5:127–135.
48. Walter JF, Paaso BT, Cannon WB: Successful transcatheter embolic control of massive hematobilia secondary to liver biopsy. AJR 1976;127:847–849.
49. Fagan EA, Allison DJ, Hodgson HJF: Treatment of haemobilia by selective arterial embolization. Gut 1980;21:541–544.
50. Hirsch M, Avinoach I, Keynan A, Khodadadi J: Angiographic diagnosis and treatment of hemobilia. Radiology 1982;144:771–772.
51. Heimbach A, Ferguson GS, Harley JD: Treatment of traumatic hemobilia with angiographic embolization. J Trauma 1978;18:221–224.
52. Perlberger RR. Control of hemobilia by angiographic embolization. AJR 1977;128:672–673.
53. Van Way CW, Crane JM, Riddell DH, Foster JH: Arteriovenous fistula in the portal circulation. Surgery 1971;70:876–890.
54. Mooney CS, Honaker AD, Griffin WO Jr: Influence of the liver on arteriovenous fistula. Arch Surg 1970;100:154–156.
55. Moeller DA, Rogers JV, Allan NK, Mack LA: Ultrasound appearance of a traumatic hepatic artery-portal vein fistula. J Clin Ultrasound 1983;11:237–239.
56. Vujic I, Meredith HC, Ameriks JA: Embolization for hepatoportal arteriovenous fistula. Am Surg 1980;46:366–370.
57. Ramchandani P. Goldenberg NJ, White RI: Isobutyl-2-Cyanoacrylate embolization of a hepatoportal fistula. AJR 1983;140:137–140.
58. Clark RA, Gallant TE, Alexander ES: Angiographic management of traumatic arteriovenous fistulas: clinical results. Radiology 1983;147:9–13.
59. Schafani SJA, Nauaranaswamy T, Mitchell WG: Radiologic management of traumatic hepatic artery-portal vein arteriovenous fistulae. J Trauma 1981;21:576–580.
60. Castaneda-Zuriga WR, Tadavarthy SM, Galliani CA, et al.: Experimental venous occlusion with stainless steel spiders. Radiology 1981;141:238–242.
61. Grimmell VS. Flanagan KG, Mehringer CM, Hieshima GB: Occlusion of large fistulas with detachable valved balloons and the spider. AJR 1983;140:1259–1261.

62. Ishak KG, Rabin L: Benign tumors of the liver. Med Clin North Am 1975;59:995–1015.
63. Park WC, Phillips R: The role of radiation therapy in the management of hemangiomas of the liver. JAMA 1970;212:1496–1498.
64. Johnson CM, Sheedy PF II, Stanson AW, et al.: Computed tomography and angiography of cavernous hemangiomas of the liver. Radiology 1981;138:115–121.
65. Zubrod CG: The limited usefulness of 5 fluorouracil (5-FU) and 5-fluorodeoxy-uridine (5-FUDR) in the management of patients with adenocarcinoma. In FJ Ingelfinger, AS Relman, M Finland (eds), Controversy in Internal Medicine. Philadelphia: Saunders, 1966, pp. 591–600.
66. Oberfill RA, McCaffrey JA, Polio J, et al.: Prolonged and continuous percutaneous intraarterial hepatic infusion chemotherapy in advanced metastatic liver adenocarcinoma from colorectal primary. Cancer 1979;44:414–423.
67. Ansfield FJ, Ramirez G, Davis HL, et al.: Further clinical studies with intrahepatic arterial infusion with 5-fluorouracil. Cancer 1975;36:2413–2417.
68. Jaffee BM, Donnegan WL, Watson F: Factors influencing survival in patients with untreated hepatic metastases. Surg Gynecol Obstet 1968;127:1–11.
69. Donnegan WL, Harris HS, Spratt JS: Prolonged continuous hepatic infusion. Arch Surg 1969;99:149–157.
70. Chuang VP, Wallace S: Hepatic arterial redistribution for intraarterial infusion of hepatic neoplasms. Radiology 1980;135:295–299.
71. Markowitz J: The hepatic artery. Surg Gynecol Obstet 1952;95:644–653.
72. Koehler RE, Korobkin M, Lewis F: Arteriographic demonstration of collateral flow of the liver after hepatic artery ligation. Radiology 1975;117:49–54.
73. Chuang VP, Wallace S: Hepatic artery embolization in the treatment of hepatic neoplasms. Radiology 1981;140:51–58.
74. Chuang VP. Personal communication.
75. Chuang VP, Wallace S, Soo CS, et al.: Therapeutic Ivalon embolization of hepatic tumors. AJR 1982;138:289–294.
76. Wallace S. Chuang VP: Liver tumors: Diagnosis and management. In H Herlinger, A Lunderquist, S Wallace (eds), Clinical Radiology of the Liver. New York: Dekker, 1983, pp. 715–865.

Index*

A

Abdomen, plain film of, 4
Abscess
  hepatic, 65–66
    amebic, 30, **31**
    calcified, 8, 9
    CT guided biopsy for, **208, 209, 210**
    CT of, 128, **129**
    differential diagnosis of, 101
    drainage of
      complications of, 212
      indications for, 205
      length of, 207, 211
      results of, 211
      technique of, 205, 207, **211**
    etiology of, 65
    plain film diagnosis of, 30, 32
    in pyogenic hepatitis, 224–225
    scintigraphy for, 65–66
  perihepatic, 31–32, **33, 34**

Adenocarcinoma, guided hepatic biopsy for, **198**
Adenoma
  CT of, 124, **125, 126**
  hepatic, angiography of, 230
  of liver cell. *See* Liver cell adenoma
Air, plain film manifestations of
  in gallbladder, 24–28, **25, 26**
  vs. gas, 24–34
Alcohol
  cirrhosis due to, 248–249
  as vascular occlusive agent, 278, 282
  use of, 279
Alcoholism, hepatitis due to, angiography in, 224–227
Amebiasis
  hepatic abscess due to, 30, **31**
  hepatic cysts due to, **206**
Amyloidosis, angiography in, 224
Amylopectinosis, plain film diagnosis of, 40, 40t

*Numbers in **boldface** type refer to pages on which illustrations appear; t indicates a table.

Anderson's disease, plain film diagnosis of, 40, 40t
Anechoic mass, in metastic hepatic malignancy, 87, **93**
Anemia, plain film diagnosis of, 39
Aneurysm
  angiography in, 221, **222, 223,** 224
  of hepatic artery, embolization for, 290
Angiography, hepatic
  of adenoma, **126**
  in amyloidosis, 224
  for aneurysms, 221, 224
  for angiosarcoma, 236–237
  of arteriovenous portal fistula, 294
  in artherosclerosis, 221
  for benign tumors, 227–232
  for cavernous hemangioma, 97, 227–228, **229**
  for cholangiocarcinoma, 234–236
  in cirrhosis, 238–239
  complications of, 216
  for cysts, 227
  in diffuse liver disease, **102**
  digital subtraction, 266
  for focal nodular hyperplasia, **62, 63, 127,** 231–232
  for hemangioendothelioma, 228, **229**
  for hemangioma, **64, 141**
  for hepatic adenoma, 230
  hepatic anatomy with, 216–218
  in hepatic trauma
    advantages of, 174
    of arteriovenous fistula, **176, 177**
    limitations of, 174–175
    of liver laceration, **173**
    and perihepatic fat, **174**
    signs in, 173–174
    technique of, 173
  for hepatoblastoma, 236
  in hepatocellular carcinoma, **300–301**
  for hepatoma, 232–234
  in inflammatory disease, 224–227
  infusion hepatic, 238
  for malignant tumors, 232–238
  for metastatic disease, 237–238
  in peliosis hepatitis, 219–221
  pitfalls in, 218–219
  in polyarteritis nodosa, 221
  radionuclide, of primary hepatic tumor, 60
  in Stein-Leventhal syndrome, **233**
  technique of, 213–216
  in vascular disorders, 219–224
  vasoconstrictors in, 216

vasodilators in, 216
  of vena cava obstruction, **68**
Angiosarcoma, angiography in, 236–237
Angiotensin, in angiography, 216
Antibody, radiolabeled, for metastatic hepatic malignancy, 59–60
Antigen, carcinoembryonic. *See* Carcinoembryonic antigen
Armillifer armillatus, hepatic calcification due to, 11
Arsenic, and angiosarcomas, 236–237
Arteriography, hepatic
  for aneurysms, **222, 223,** 224
  of arteriovenous portal fistula, **292–294, 295–296**
  for cavernous hemangioma, **228**
  in diffuse liver disease, **102**
  filming sequence for, 216
  in hepatitis, **225**
  infusion hepatic, 239
  of intrahepatic mass, **92**
  in peliosis hepatis, **220**
Arteriovenous portal fistula
  arteriography of, **292–294, 295–296**
  spider in, 294
  treatment for, 291
Artery, hepatic. *See* Hepatic artery
Ascaris lumbicoides, hepatic calcification due to, 12
Aseptic necrosis, **38**
  in liver disease, 38
Aspiration biopsy
  of hepatic cysts, 95
  of hepatic masses, 89
  with CT, **94**
Atherosclerosis, angiography in, 221
Au-198, in hepatic scintigraphy, 51
Autologous clot
  in arteriovenous fistulas, 294
  as embolic agent, 276, 282
Avitene, 278
  in arteriovenous portal fistula, **292–293**
  as embolic material, 279, 282, 289
Azothioprine, oral, and peliosis hepatis, 219

B

"Bear claw" lacerations, 185, **190**
Bibasilar interstitial infiltrate, precirrhotic, **39**
Bile, leakage of, cholescintigraphy for, 176
Bile duct, obstruction of, 73–74, **75**

Bile duct system, plain film manifestations of, gas in, 28–29
Bile pseudocyst
　cholangiography for, 175–176
　sonography of, **178**
Biliary atresia, vs. neonatal hepatitis, 74, 77
Biliary calculus disease, internal biliary fistulae and, 27
Biliary cirrhosis, CT in, 134
Biliary fistula
　enteric, 25–26
　internal, 27
　gallbladder gas due to, 25
Bilirubin, level of, in cholestasis, 74
Biloma
　CT of, **181, 185,** 186
　cholangiography for, 175–176
　cholangiography of, **181**
　sonography of, **178**
Biopsy, hepatic
　accuracy of, 203
　aspiration
　　of hepatic cysts, 95
　　of hepatic masses, 89
　　with CT, **94**
　complications of, 203
　digital radiography in, **202**
　focal, **204**
　imaging modalities for, 200
　indications for, 197, **198**
　technique of, 197, 199
Bleeding
　of GI varices
　　due to portal hypertension, 245
　　embolization for
　　　approaches to, 279–280
　　　following splenorenal shunt, 283, **284, 285, 286,** 289
　　　technique of, 280–283
　hepatic artery embolization for, following trauma, 290
Blood pressure, portal
　elevation of. *See* Portal hypertension
　measurement of, 244
Blood-pool scan, hepatic, in hemangioma, 64–65
Bone, abnormalities of, in hepatic disorders, **36, 37**
Bone marrow, colloid uptake by, in cirrhosis, 71, **72**
"Branching tree," of wedge venogram, 252
Bromsulphalein, retention of, 69
Brucella abortus, calcified granulomas and, 8

Brucella melitensis, calcified granulomas and, 8
Brucella suis, calcified granulomas and, 8
Budd-Chiari syndrome
　diagnosis of, 248
　radionuclide scan and, 66, 68–69

C

Calcification, hepatic. *See* Hepatic calcification
Carcinoembryonic antigen
　in radiolabeled antibodies, 59–60
　in serial testing, 59
Carcinoma. *See also specific type*
　hepatic calcification due to, 12–18
　hepatocellular. *See* Hepatocellular carcinoma
Caroli's disease, hepatic calcification in, 19
Catheter, in angiography, 215
Cavernous hemangioma
　angiography for, 97
　arteriography of, **228**
　calcified, **98**
　CT for, 98, **99**
　embolization of, **298–299**
　hepatic calcification in, 14
　incidence of, 227–228
　ultrasonography for, 98
Chilaiditi's syndrome, 33
Chlonorcis sinensis, hepatic calcification due to, 12
Cholangiocarcinoma
　angiography in, 234–236
　CT of, **157**
　hepatic calcification due to, 13
　NMR imaging of, **157**
Cholangiography, hepatic
　in hepatic trauma
　　advantages of, 176
　　for common duct obstruction, **180**
　　limitations of, 177
　　signs, 175
　　technique of, 175
　of intrahepatic biloma, **181, 185**
Cholangitis, plain film diagnosis of, 40, **41**
Cholecystitis
　emphysematous, 24
　　plain film diagnosis of, **25**
　hepatobiliary imaging for, 73, **74, 75**
Cholecystoenteric fistula, gallbladder gas due to, 25

Cholelithiasis, hepatobiliary imaging for, 73, **74, 75**
Cholescintigraphy, hepatic
　for bile leakage, 176
　in hepatic trauma, 175
Cholestasis, hepatobiliary imaging in, 74
Chondrocalcinosis, in Wilson's disease, 41, **42**
Chondromyxocarcinoma, of salivary gland, 18
Chronic granulomatous disease, hepatic calcification in, 8
Cirrhosis. *See also specific type*
　angiography in, 238–239
　biliary, CT in, 134
　causes of, 249
　in children, 37
　clotting in, 282
　CT in, 265, **266**
　description of, 248–249, 34
　hepatic
　　CT of, 135, **136**, 137
　　liver-spleen volume in, 137
　hepatic scintigraphy in, 70–71, **71**
　hepatocellular carcinoma and, 232–234, **235**
　plain film diagnosis of, 34–39, **35, 37–38**
　sonograpy in, 103–104, **265**
　syphilitic, hepatic calcification and, 8
Clonorchiasis, plain film manifestations of, **12**
Clot, autologous
　in arteriovenous fistulas, 294
　as embolic agent, 276, 282
Clotting, in cirrhosis, 282
Coccidiomycosis, hepatic calcification due to, 12
Coil
　in arteriovenous portal fistula, **292–293**, 294
　as embolic material, 278, 282, 283, 289, 290
"Cold" lesion, in radionuclide scanning, 53
Collateral pathways
　CT for, 266
　hepatopetal, 246
　portosystemic, development of, 244
　following splenorenal shunt, 289
Collimation, in CT, 110
Colloid(s)
　in hepatic scintigraphy, 51, 52
　sulfur, in hepatic trauma, 175
　uptake of
　　by bone marrow, 71, 72
　　in cirrhosis, 71
　　in focal nodular hyperplasia, 100–101
　　by hepatic cells, 70
　　by spleen, 71, **72**
Computed angiotomography, hepatic
　description of, 114
　of hepatic artery, **116**
　of multifocal hepatoma, **115**
　of superior mesenteric artery, 116
Computed tomography (CT), hepatic
　of abscess, 128
　of adenoma, 124, **125**
　anatomy of liver with, 116, **117, 118**, 119
　vs. angiography, 266
　in biliary cirrhosis, 134
　for biloma, **179**
　in biopsy guidance, 200, **201**
　for cavernous hemangioma, 98, **99**
　of cholangiocarcinoma, **157**
　in cirrhosis, 265
　collimation in, 110
　computed angiotomography and, 114, **115, 116**
　differential diagnosis by, of hepatic masses, 87–89, **93**
　in fatty liver, 103, 131–132, **133, 192**
　of focal nodular hyperplasia, 126, **127**
　future developments in, 137–138
　in glycogen storage disease, 134
　of hemangioma, 130, **141**
　of hematoma, **184, 185, 186**
　in hemosiderosis, 132, 134
　of hepatic artery, 114, 116
　in hepatic cirrhosis, 135
　of hepatic cyst, **21**, 67, **157, 206**
　of hepatic metastases, 121–124, **122, 151, 158, 160, 161, 162**
　vs. hepatic scintigraphy, 82
　in hepatic trauma
　　advantages of, 193
　　hemoperitoneum and, **188**, 189
　　limitations of, 195
　　postoperative evaluation of, 189–193
　　signs, 184–186
　　technique of, 180, 184
　in hepatocellular carcinoma, **300–301**
　of hepatomas, 120–121
　of intrahepatic biloma, **181, 185**
　iodinated contrast in, 111, 114
　liver-spleen volumes and, 137
　in lymphoma, 134
　of multiple lacerations, **190, 191**

vs. NMR imaging, 150, 152
radiation and, 134
sensitivity of, 135, 137
slice spacing in, 110–111
of superior mesenteric artery, 116
technique of, 109–110
vs. ultrasonography, 83–84, 106
in Wilson's disease, 134
window widths and levels in, 111, **112**
Contraceptive, oral
adenomas and, 124, **125, 126**
hepatoadenoma and, 62, **63**
and peliosis hepatis, 219
Contrast, intravenous
in CT, 111, **113, 114, 120**
of hemangioma, **131**
future developments in, 137–138
in hepatic cirrhosis, 135, **136**
Copper, hepatic deposits of, CT in, 134
Cori's disease, plain film diagnosis of, 40, 40t
Coronary vein
in distal splenorenal shunt, **284–288**
embolization of, 279, **280**
Corrected sinusoidal pressure (CSP), interpretation of, 253
Cyanoacrylate
in arteriovenous portal fistulas, 294
as embolic material, 278, 282, 283, 289, 290
Cyst, hepatic
aspiration of, **94**
benign, ultrasonography of, **92**
calcification in, 8–9
computed tomography of, **21**
congenital, 91, 95
CT of, **92**, 128–129, **130, 157**
differential diagnosis of
CT for, **93**
sonography for, 87–89
echinococcal, 225, **226**, 227
gray scale ultrasonography for, 66, **67**
hyatid, 9
NMR imaging of, **157**
nonparasitic, angiography for, 227
rim calcification in, **10**
types of, 95
ultrasonography for, 91, **92**
Cystic disease, plain film diagnosis of, 40, **41**

D

Debrun balloon, **286**
Decay curve, in NMR imaging, 152, 153

Diatrizoate meglumine, in CT technique, 184
Digital radiography, in hepatic biopsies, **202**
Diisopropyliminodiacetic acid, in hepatobiliary scanning, 73
Dimethyliminodiacetic acid, for scintigraphy, in hepatic trauma, 175
Distal splenorenal shunt
collateral pathways and, 289
embolization following, 283, **284–288**
"Dog ears," in hepatic trauma, 172
Dracunculus medinensis, hepatic calcification due to, 11

E

Echinococcus granulosus
hepatic calcification due to, 8–9
hepatic cyst due to, 9, **10**, 11
hyatid disease due to, 96–97
Echinococcus multilocularis, hepatic cyst due to, 9, 11
Echo time, in NMR imaging, 149t, 150
Echogenic mass, in metastic hepatic malignancy, 86
Echogenicity
of hemangioma, 98
of metastases, **102**
in metastatic hepatic malignancy, 86–87
Embolic material, 276–279
Embolization, 294
transcatheter, 290
in arteriovenous portal fistula, **295–296**
in hepatic neoplasms, 297
Emphysematous cholecystitis, 24
plain film diagnosis of, **25**
Entamoeba histolytica, hepatic abscess due to, 65
EOE-13, in CT, 137, **138–141**
Epinephrine, in angiography, 216
Escherichia coli, hepatic calcification and, 22
Estrogen, and peliosis hepatis, 219

F

18-F, in scintigraphy, 52
Fasciola gigantica, hepatic calcification due to, 11
Fatty liver
in children, 37
cirrhosis and, 37
CT of, 131–132, **132, 133, 163, 192**

Fatty liver (*cont.*)
  NMR imaging of, **163**
  plain film of, 23-24, **24**, 36-38
  sonography of, 103, **104**
Felty's syndrome, colloid uptake in, 72
"Flank stripe," in hepatic trauma, **170**, 171
Focal liver disease, scintigraphy for, 52-55
Focal nodular hyperplasia, 62-64
  angiography in, **62, 63,** 231-232
  CT of, 126, **127**
  vs. liver cell adenoma, 99-100
  scintigraphy for, 66
  sonography for, **100**
Forbes' disease, plain film diagnosis of, 40, 40t

G

Gallbladder
  gas in, plain film manifestations of, 24-28, **25, 26**
  in hepatic sonography, 84, **85**
  obstruction of, **75**
  scintigraphy of, 73-74
Gallium-67
  for hepatic abscess, 65, **66**
  in hepatocellular carcinoma, 61-62, **61**
Gallstone(s)
  diagnosis of, 24-28
    barium in, 27, **27**
    plain film in, 26-27
  noncalcified, **36**
Gallstone ileus, diagnosis of, 26-27, **28**
Gallstone obturation, diagnosis of, 26-27, **28**
Gas
  vs. air, 24-34
  plain film manifestations of
    in bile duct system, 28-29
    in gallbladder, 24-28, **25, 26**
    in gallstone fissures, **36**
    in hepatic abscess, 30, **31**
    in portal vein, 29-30, **29**
Gas gangrene, hepatic, 30
Gas-air, plain film manifestations of, 24-34
Gastric artery injection, left, 258, 260
Gastrografin, in CT technique, 184
Gaucher's disease, plain film diagnosis of, 40, **41**
Gelfoam, 299
  in arteriovenous portal fistulas, 294
  as embolic material, 276, 282, 283, 290
  in metastatic hepatic malignancy, 303
  use of, 277

Gianturco coil
  in arteriovenous portal fistulas, 294
  as embolic material, 278, 282, 283, 289, 290
Glycogen storage disease
  CT in, 134
  plain film diagnosis of, 40, 40t
  type I, sonography for, 104-105
Granuloma
  calcified brucella, 8
  calcified hepatic
    diagnosis of, 7, 8
    plain film of, 9
  calcified splenic, 8

H

Hemangioendothelioma
  angiography for, 228, **229**
  hepatic calcification due to, 13, 16
Hemangioma, 64-65
  angiography of, **141**
  cavernous
    angiography for, 97
    arteriography of, **228**
    calcified, **98**
    CT for, 98, **99**
    embolization of, **298-299**
    incidence of, 227-228
    ultrasonography for, 98
  CT of, 130, **131, 141**
Hemangiomatosis, multinodular, angiography for, 228
Hematoma
  CT of, **184, 185, 186, 187, 192, 194**
  plain film radiography of, **169**
  scintigraphy for, **178**
  sonography of, **182, 183**
Hemobilia
  hepatic artery embolization for, 290-291
  treatment of, 291
Hemoperitoneum, effect of, on CT, 189
Hemorrhage
  of GI varices
    due to portal hypertension, 245
    embolization for
      approaches to, 279-280
      following splenorenal shunt, 283, **284, 285, 286,** 289
      technique of, 280-283
  hepatic artery embolization for, following trauma, 290
Hemosiderosis, CT in, 132, **133**

Hepar lobatum, hepatic calcification and, 8
Hepatic abscess
  amebic, 30, **31**
  calcified, 8, 9
  CT guided biopsy for, **208, 209, 210**
  CT of, 128, **129**
  differential diagnosis of, 101
  drainage of
    complications of, 212
    indications for, 205
    length of, 207, 211
    results of, 211
    technique of, 205, 207, **211**
  etiology of, 65
  plain film diagnosis of, 30, 32
  in pyogenic hepatitis, 224–225
  scintigraphy for, 65–66
"Hepatic angle," in hepatic trauma, 170, **171**
Hepatic arterial perfusion scanning, 60
Hepatic artery
  aneurysm of, 290
    embolization for, 290
  CT of, 114, **116**
  embolization of, 289
    for arteriovenous portal fistula, 291–297
    following trauma, 290
    for hemobilia, 290–291
    for hepatic neoplasm, 297, **298–299, 302**
      technique of, 299
    in metastatic hepatic malignancy, **302–303**
    and pain, 303
  Hepatic calcification in, 18–19
  perfusion scanning of, 60
Hepatic-binding protein, in scintigraphy, 52
Hepatic calcification, 6–12
  capsular, 22
  in childhood, 8
  circumferential, **10**
  CT of, **123, 124**
  diffuse, **22**
  due to parasites, 8–12
  plain film diagnosis of, 40, **41**
    granulomatous, 7–12
    neoplastic, 12–18
    "popcorn-type," 7
    vascular, 18–19
  rim, 8–9, 21
Hepatic cyst
  aspiration of, **94**
  benign, ultrasonography of, **92**
  calcification in, 8–9
  computed tomography of, **21**
  congenital, 91, 95
  CT of, **92**, 128–129, **130**, 157
  differential diagnosis of
    CT for, **93**
    sonography for, 87–89
  echinococcal, 225, **226**, 227
  gray scale ultrasonography for, 66, **67**
  hyatid, 9
  NMR imaging of, **157**
  nonparasitic, angiography for, 227
  rim calcification in, **10**
  types of, 95
  ultrasonography for, 91, **92**
Hepatic cystic disease
  plain film diagnosis of, 42–43
  tomography of, **43**
Hepatic lymphoma, sonography for, 104, **105**
Hepatic osteoarthropathy, plain film diagnosis of, **36, 37**
Hepatic vein, angiography of, 215
Hepatic wedge injection
  interpretation of, 252
  preoperative, **261**
  technique of, 250, **251**
Hepatitis
  angiography in, 224–227
  neonatal, vs. biliary atresia, 74, 77
  pyogenic, 224–225
  sonography for, 103
  viral, **39**
Hepatoadenoma, 62–63, **63**
  incidence of, 62
Hepatobiliary scanning, 72–77
  in bile duct obstruction, **75**
  in biliary atresia, **76**
  in cholecystitis, 73, **74**
  in heptocellular disease, **76**
  in metastatic carcinoma, **77**
Hepatoblastoma, angiography in, 236
Hepatocellular carcinoma
  angiography in, 232–234, **235**
  embolication, **300–301**
  hepatic calcifization due to, 13
  hepatic sonography in, 86, **86**
  radionuclide scanning for, 60–62, **60, 61**
Hepatocellular disease, hepatobiliary imaging in, 74, **76**
Hepatocyte
  function of, 72
  in scintigraphy, 72–73

313

Hepatoma
  angiography in, 232–234, **235**
  computed angiotomography of, **115**
  CT of, 120–121, **120**
  plain film diagnosis of, **15**
Hepatomegaly, plain film diagnosis of, 5
Hepato-portal sclerosis, 247
Her's disease, plain film diagnosis of, 40, 40t
Histoplasmosis, and calcified liver granulomas, 7
Hormones
  adenomas and, 124, **125, 126**
  hepatoadenoma and, 62, **63**
"Hot" background, in radionuclide scanning, 53
"Hot spot"
  definition of, 66
  in focal nodular hyperplasia, 62
  in superior vena cava obstruction, 68, **69**
Hyatid cyst, angiography for, 225, **226,** 227
Hyatid disease
  hepatic, 96–97
  hepatic calcifications and, 8–9
Hyperechoic mass, in metastatic hepatic malignancy, **87**
Hypertension, portal. *See* Portal hypertension
Hypoechoic mass, in metastatic hepatic malignancy, 86, **87, 89, 95, 96**

I

I-131
  in hepatic scintigraphy, 51
  in hepatobiliary scanning, 73
  in radiolabeled antibodies, 59–60
Iminodiacetic acids
  in hepatic scintigraphy, 51
  in hepatobiliary scanning, 73, **75**
Indium-111
  for hepatic abscess, 65, **66**
  WBC technique, 66
Indium-113, in hepatic scintigraphy, 51
Inferior vena cava
  calcification in, 18–19
  in hepatic sonography, 84, **85**
Inflammatory disease, angiography in, 224–227
Intestinal pneumatosis, plain film diagnosis of, 30
Intravenous contrast
  in CT, 111, **113, 114, 120**

future developments in, 137–138
of hemangioma, **131**
in hepatic cirrhosis, 135, **136**
Inversion recovery, 149t
  in NMR imaging, 150, 152, 153
Inversion time, in NMR imaging, 149t, 150
Iodiapamide acid, in hepatic scintigraphy, 51
Iodine, intravenous
  in computed angiotomography, 114, **115**
  for CT contrast, 111, **113, 114, 120**
  future developments in, 137–138
  and hemangioma, **131**
  and hepatic cirrhosis, 135, **136**
Ioglyamic acid, in hepatic scintigraphy, 51
Iron, hepatic deposits of, 132
  CT in, **133**
Isobutyl-2-cyanoacrylate, as embolic material, 278, 282
Ivalone, 299
  in arteriovenous portal fistulas, 294
  as embolic material, 277, 283, 290
  in metastatic hepatic malignancy, 303

K

Kupffer cell
  in cirrhosis, 70
  colloid uptake by, 70
  in focal nodular hyperplasia, 62

L

Lavage, peritoneal, 195
Left gastric artery injection, 258, 260
Left renal vein
  catheterization of, **255**
  collateral filling and, **256**
  evaluation of
    interpretation of, 253–254
    preoperative, **257**
  technique of, 253
Leukocyte, radiolabeled, for hepatic abscess, 65, **66**
Liver
  anatomy of
    with angiography, 216–218
    with CT, 116, **117–118,** 119
    with NMR imaging, 152–153, **155, 156**
    with plain films, 1–6, **2, 3, 4**
    with sonography, 84, **85,** 86
  calcification. *See* Hepatic calcification
  fatty infiltration of. *See* Fatty liver

metastases to. *See* Metastatic hepatic
  malignancy
parenchymal cells of, in scintigraphy, 51–52
reticuloendothelial cells of, in scintigraphy, 51
-spleen volumes, CT for, 137
Liver cell adenoma
  vs. focal nodular hyperplasia, 99–100
  sonography for, **100**
Liver function
  radiocolloid scanning evaluation of, 69
  scintigraphic evaluation of, 52
  tests of, 69
"Liver package," 250
  contraindications to, 260, 263
Lymph node, calcified granuloma of, 7
Lymphocytic interstitial pneumonia,
  precirrhotic, 39
Lymphoma
  CT in, 134
  hepatic, sonography for, 104, **105**

M

McArdle's disease, plain film diagnosis of,
  40, 40t
"Mercedes Benz" sign, gallstones and, **36**
Mesenteric artery injection
  left
    interpretation of, 255–257
    technique of, 254–255
    venous phase of, **259, 260, 261**
  superior
    following distal splenorenal shunt, 284–**288**
    in variceal embolization, 281
Mesocaval shunt, H-type graft, **268**
Metastatic hepatic malignancy
  angiography in, **236**, 237–238
  calcified, **88, 89**
  CT of, **110**, 121, **122**, 123–124, **158, 160, 161, 162**
    calcified, **123**
  hepatic calcification due to, 14–18
  hepatic embolization in, **302**–303
  incidence of, 55
  NMR imaging of, **158, 159, 160, 161**
  "poppyseed" pattern of, **17**
  scintigraphy for, 55–59
    differential diagnosis with, 55–56, **58**
    image patterns of, **56, 57**
    radiolabeled antibody for, 59–60
  sensitivity and specificity of, 57, 59
  special forms of, 59–60
  sonography for, 86–91
Methyl-2-cyanoacrylate, fibrosarcoma due
  to, 278
Morison's pouch, 33, **34**
Mucin, in hepatic calcification, 16
Mucopolysaccharide, in amyloidosis, 224
Multinodular hemangiomatosis, angiography
  for, 228

N

Needle, for hepatic biopsy, 197, 199
  in CT, 200
Neonatal hepatitis, vs. biliary atresia, 74, 77
Neoplasm, hepatic
  hepatic artery embolization in, 297, **298,**
    299, **300**–**302**
  hepatic calcification due to, 12–18
  survival rates for, 297
Norepinephrine, in angiography, 216
Nuclear magnetic resonance (NMR)
    imaging, hepatic
  of benign masses, **157**
  of cholangiocarcinoma, **157**
  vs. CT, 150, 152
  description of, 146–150, 152
  hepatic anatomy with, 152–153
  of hepatic cyst, **157**
  of hepatic metastases, **151**, 153–158, **159,
    160, 161**
  for infiltrative disease, 159
  of malignancies, **157**
  of normal liver, **155, 156**
  partial saturation in, 149t, 150
  spectroscopy, 159, 165

O

Omphalitis, hepatic calcification and, 22
Oral contraceptives
  adenomas and, 124, **125, 126**
  hepatoadenoma and, 62, **63**
  and peliosis hepatis, 219

P

Pain, embolization and, 303
Papaverine, in angiography, 216

315

Paragonimus westermani, hepatic
    calcification due to, 11
Parasites
  hepatic abscess due to, 30, **31**
  hepatic calcification due to, 8–12
  hepatic cysts due to, 96–97, 225, **226**, 227
Parenchymal cell, hepatic
  in scintigraphy, 51–52
  in sonography, 84, **85**, 86
Peliosis hepatis, angiography in, 219, **220**, 221
Peptic ulcer, internal biliary fistulae and, 27
Perfluorocytlbromide, 106
Peritoneal lavage, 195
Phagocytosis, of hepatic cells, in
    scintigraphy, 51
Pharmacoangiography, 216
  in hepatic metastases, 238
Plain film radiography, hepatic
  in anemia, 39
  for aneurysms, **222**
  in cholangitis, 42
  cirrhosisin, 34–39
  in cystic diseases, 42–43
  of echicoccal cyst, **226**
  of gallbladder gas, 24–28, **25, 26**
  in gallstone detection, 26–27
  in Gaucher's disease, 40, **41**
  in glycogen storage disease, 40
  hepatic radiolucencies on, 23–34
  in hepatic trauma
    advantages of, 172
    of flank-stripe sign, **170**
    of hepatic laceration, **171**
    of intraperitoneal blood, **172**
    limitations of, 173
    signs, 168–172
    of subcapsular hematoma, **169**
    technique of, 168
  in infectious liver calcifications, 7–12
  in liver calcifications, 6, 19–22
  manifestations
    of fat, 23–24, **24**
    of gas-air, 24–34
  in neoplastic calcification, 12–18
  normal hepatic anatomy and, 1–6
  in vascular calcifications, 18–19
  in Wilson's disease, 40–41
Pneumatosis, 24
  of gallbladder, 25
  intestinal, plain film diagnosis of, 30
Pneumoperitoneum, plain film diagnosis of, 33, **35**
Polyarteritis nodosa, angiography in, 221

Polycystic renal disease
  plain film diagnosis of, 42–43
  tomography of, **43**
Polyvinyl alcohol foam
  in arteriovenous portal fistula, 294
  as embolic material, 277, 283, 290
Pompe's disease, plain film diagnosis of, 40, 40t
Portal hypertension, *See also* Portal vein
  causes of, 246–249
  clinical considerations in, 245
  corrected sinusoidal pressure in, 252–253
  definition of, 243–244
  extrahepatic-postsinusoidal cause of, 248
  extrahepatic-presinusoidal cause of, 246–247
  hepatic wedge injection in, 250–252
  hyperkinetic, 246
  intrahepatic cause of, 248–249
  left renal vein and, 253–254
  liver package and, 250
  measurement of, 244
  risk of GI bleeding in, 245
  splenic artery injection and, 257–258
  superior mesenteric artery injection and, 254–257
Portal vein. *See also* Portal hypertension
  calcification in, 18–19, **20**
  cavernous transformation of, 246, **247**
  in hepatic sonography, 84, **85**, 86
  plain film manifestations of, 29–30, **29**
  thrombosis of, 246
    splenoportography for, 263–264
Portocaval shunt, **268**
Portography, 215
  transhepatic
    of coronary vein embolization, 279, **280**
    use of, 264–265
Priscoline (tolazoline hydrochloride), 250
  in angiography, 216
  and contrast injection, 260
Prostaglandins, in angiography, 216
Protein, hepatic-binding, in scintigraphy, 52
Pseudocyst, bile
  cholangiography for, 175–176
  sonography of, **178**
Pulse sequence, 149t
  in NMR imaging, 150, 152, 153
Pyridoxylidene glutamate, in hepatic
    scintigraphy, 51

R

Radiation, hepatic changes due to, CT of, 134
Radiocolloid. *See* Colloid(s)

Radiocolloid scanning, *See* Scintigraphy, hepatic
Radiography. *See specific type*
Radiolabeled antibody, for metastatic hepatic malignancy, 59–60
Radiolucencies
 fat, 23–24, **24**
 gas-air, 24–**28**
Radiopharmaceuticals
 experimental, 52
 in hepatic scintigraphy, 51–52
Radium, and angiosarcoma, 236–237
Real-time scanning, in hepatic sonography, 83–84
Red blood cell (RBC) scan, in hemangioma, 64–65, **66**
Renal vein, left
 catheterization of, **255**
 collateral filling, **256**
 evaluation of
  interpretation of, 253–254
  preoperative, **257**
  technique of, 253
Repetition time, in NMR imaging, 149t, 150
Reticuloendothelial cell, colloid uptake by, 70
Rheumatoid arthritis, colloid uptake in, 72
Riedel's lobe, 4, **4**
Rose bengal
 hepatic scintigraphy, 51
 in hepatobiliary scanning, 73, 77
Ru-97, in hepatobiliary imaging, 77

S

Sarcoid, hepatic calcification due to, 12
Schistosomiasis, cirrhosis due to, 249
Schistosomiasis japonica, hepatic calcification due to, 12
Scintigraphy, hepatic
 vs. CT, 82
 description of, 50
 in diffuse hepatic disease
  hepatobiliary, 72–77
  radiocolloid, 69–72
 focal increased uptake in, 66–69
 for focal liver disease, 52–55
  disadvantages of, 53
 for focal nodular hepatoadenoma, 62–64
 in focal nodular hyperplasia, 62–64, 100–101
 for hemangioma, 64–65
 for hepatic abscess, 65–66
 for hepatic cyst, 66
 for hepatic hematoma, **178**
 in hepatic trauma, 175
 for metastatic malignancy, 55–59
  sensitivity and specificity of, 57, 59
  special forms of, 59–60
 for primary hepatic malignancy, 60–62
 radiopharmaceuticals for, 51–52
Seldinger technique, 205–207
 and hepatic wedge technique, 250
Sengstaken-Blakemore tube, in variceal hemorrhage, 279
Septicemia, colloid uptake in, 72
Shunt procedures
 goals of, 267
 types of, **268, 269,** 271
Sickle cell disease, plain film diagnosis of, 39
Sonography, hepatic
 accuracy of, 105–106
 for aneurysms, **222**
 of benign cyst, **92**
 for bilomas, **178**
 in biopsy guidance, 199, 200
 vs. CT, 83–84, 106
 for cavernous hemangioma, 97–99
 in cirrhosis, 103–104, **239, 265**
 in diffuse liver disease, 101–103, **102**
 in fatty liver, 103
 in focal nodular hyperplasia, 99–101
 future developments in, 106
 in glycogen storage disease, 104–105
 of hematoma, **182, 183**
 for hepatic abscess, 101
 hepatic anatomy with, 84, **85,** 86
 for hepatic cysts, 91, **92, 94,** 95
 in hepatic hyatid disease, 96–97
 in hepatic lymphoma, 104
 in hepatic trauma
  advantages of, 179
  limitations of, 179–180
  signs, 177, 179
  technique of, 177
 in hepatitis, 103, **225**
 in hepatocellular carcinoma, 866
 for liver cell adenoma, 99–100
 in metastatic disease, 86–91, **96**
 patterns in, 86–87
 in peliosis hepatis, **220**
 technique of, 82
 transducers in, 83–84
Spectroscopy, NMR, hepatic, 159, **164**
Spider, in arteriovenous portal fistula, 294
"Spider web," in Budd-Chiari syndrome, 248, **249**

Spin echo, 149t
  in NMR imaging, 150, 152, 153
Spin-lattice relaxation time, in NMR
    imaging, 150, 152, 153
Spin-spin relaxation time, in NMR imaging,
    150, 152, 153
Spleen
  calcified granuloma of, 7, 8
  colloid uptake by, in cirrhosis, 71, **72**
Splenic artery injection
  interpretation of, 255–257, 258
  technique of, 257–258
  venous phase of, **259, 260, 261, 262**
Splenic vein
  calcified thrombus in, **19**
  splenoportography of, 263–264
Splenoportography, 215
  of collaterals, **244**
  technique of, 246
  in thrombosis, 19, 263–264
Splenorenal shunt, **268, 269, 270, 271**
  distal
    collateral pathways and, 289
    embolization following, 283, **284–288**
Static-B scanning technique, in hepatic
    sonography, 83–84
Steatosis. *See* Fatty liver
Stein-Leventhal syndrome, angiography in,
  233
Steroids, anabolic, and peliosis hepatis, 219
Storage disease, type I glycogen, sonography
    for, 104–105
Sulfur colloid. *See also* Colloid(s)
  for scintigraphy, in hepatic trauma, 175
Superior mesenteric artery, CT of, 116
Superior mesenteric artery arteriography
  following distal splenorenal shunt, **284–288**
  interpretation of, 255–257
  technique of, 254–255
  in variceal embolization, 281
  venous phase of, **259, 260, 261**
Syphilitic cirrhosis, hepatic calcification and,
    8

T

Taenia saginata, hepatic calcification due to,
    12
Taenia solium, hepatic calcification due to,
    12
Tapeworm, hepatic cysts due to, 96–97

Tc-99m
  for hemangiomas, 64–65
  in hepatic arterial perfusion scanning, 60
  in hepatic scintigraphy, 51, 52
    in hepatic trauma, 175
  hepatoadenoma and, 62, **63**
  in hepatobiliary scanning, 73, **75,** 77
  in hepatocellular carcinoma, **61**
Tc-99m neogalactoalbumin, in hepatic
    scintigraphy, 52
Thalassemia, plain film diagnosis of, 39
Thorium, 14
Thorotrast, 14
  and angiosarcoma, 236–237
Thrombosis
  calcification, 18–19
  extrahepatic portal, 246
  portal vein, splenoportography for, 263–264
  splenic vein, splenoportography for, 263–264
Time delay, in NMR imaging, 149t, 150
Tolazoline hydrochloride, 250
  in angiography, 216
  and contrast injection, 260
Tomography, computed. *See* Computed
    tomography (CT), hepatic
Transcatheter embolization
  in arteriovenous portal fistula, 294, **295–296**
  in hepatic neoplasms, 297
Transducers
  future development of, 106
  in hepatic sonography, 83–84
Transhepatic portography
  of coronary vein embolization, 279, **280**
  use of, 264–265
Trauma, hepatic
  angiography in, 173–175
  cholangiography in, 175–177
  conventional radiography in, 168–173
  CT in, 180–195
  hemobilia due to, 290–291
  hemorrhage following, hepatic artery
      embolization for, 290
  incidence of, 167
  mortality due to, 167
  radionuclide scintigraphy in, 175
  types of, 167–168
  ultrasonography in, 177–180
Triglycerides
  hepatic deposits of, 131–132
    CT of, **132, 133**

Trocar technique, 207, **208**
Tuberculosis
    and calcified liver granulomas, 7
    hepatic involvement in, 225
Tumor. *See also specific type*
    antibodies, in hepatic scintigraphy, 59–60
    differential diagnosis of, with NMR imaging, 153–154, 156
    hepatic calcification due to, 12–18
    intrahepatic, scintigraphy for, 52–55
    primary hepatic, radionuclide scanning for, 60–62, **60, 61**

U

Ulcer, peptic, internal biliary fistulae and, 27
Ultrasonography. *See* Sonography, hepatic

V

"Vacuum mechanism," definition of, 5–6
Variceal embolization, 279–280
    approaches to, 279–280
    following splenorenal shunt, 283, **284, 285, 286,** 289
    technique of, 280–283
Vasculitis, angiography in, 221
Vasoconstrictors, in angiography, 216
Vasodilators, in angiography, 216
Vasopressin, in angiography, 216

Vein. *See specific vessel*
Vena cava
    inferior
        calcification in, 18–19
        in hepatic sonography, 84, **85**
        obstruction of
            angiogram of, **68**
            radionuclide scan and, 66, 68–69, **69**
Venography, wedged hepatic, 215
Veno-occlusive disease, 248
Vinyl chloride
    and angiosarcoma, 236–237
    and peliosis hepatis, 219
Von Gierkes disease, plain film diagnosis of, 40, 40t

W

White blood cell (WBC) scan, for hepatic abscess, 65, **66**
Wilson's disease
    chondrocalcinosis in, 41, **42**
    CT in, 134
    plain film diagnosis of, 40, **41**
Window width, in CT, 111, **112**

Z

Zellweger's disease, plain film diagnosis of, 43